Melissa R. Marselle • Jutta Stadler • Horst Korn
Katherine N. Irvine • Aletta Bonn
Editors

Biodiversity and Health in the Face of Climate Change

Editors
Melissa R. Marselle
Department of Ecosystem Services
Helmholtz Centre for Environmental Research – UFZ
Leipzig, Germany

German Centre for Integrative Biodiversity Research (iDiv) Halle-Jena-Leipzig
Leipzig, Germany

Horst Korn
Federal Agency for Nature Conservation (BfN), Isle of Vilm
Putbus, Germany

Aletta Bonn
Department of Ecosystem Services
Helmholtz Centre for Environmental Research – UFZ
Leipzig, Germany

German Centre for Integrative Biodiversity Research (iDiv) Halle-Jena-Leipzig
Leipzig, Germany

Institute of Biodiversity
Friedrich Schiller University Jena
Jena, Germany

Jutta Stadler
Federal Agency for Nature Conservation (BfN), Isle of Vilm
Putbus, Germany

Katherine N. Irvine
Social, Economic and Geographical Sciences Research Group
The James Hutton Institute
Aberdeen, Scotland, UK

https://doi.org/10.1007/978-3-030-02318-8

Foreword I

The biosphere underlies the whole sustainable development concept, as the layer on which society and the economy rely. Nature and biodiversity fuel the natural cycles and life-support systems of the planet, on which humanity ultimately depends. Crucially, human health and well-being depend on functional ecosystems and the services they provide. That is why the Convention on Biological Diversity sets out the vision that biodiversity is to be valued, conserved, restored and wisely used, maintaining ecosystem services, sustaining a healthy planet, and delivering benefits essential for all people, including good health. Indeed, managing, restoring and protecting nature in both rural and urban areas provide multiple benefits to human societies. Ecosystem-based approaches to climate change, nature-based solutions for food production, and green infrastructure in cities and elsewhere all contribute to several societal objectives and have a great potential to positively affect human health.

However, it is well known that the world is facing a steady and dramatic rate of biodiversity loss from human causes, which may have severe consequences to human health and put in question a range of the Sustainable Development Goals. Further, we live in a context of climate change, which, on the one hand, impacts both health and biodiversity and, on the other, requires thriving ecosystems delivering for mitigation and adaptation. It is thus timely and important to stress the linkages and interdependencies of the climate-biodiversity-health nexus.

Recognizing our fundamental reliance on nature and the value of the services it provides to human health offers increased opportunities for the biodiversity agenda, be it in urban spaces, rural areas, or protected areas. In essence, we need innovative ways to tackle the biodiversity crisis and the societal challenges it contributes to, including exploring nature-based solutions that foster public health and biodiversity conservation. The alignment of the health and biodiversity agendas presents an opportunity to transcend institutional and sectoral siloes and to allow different communities to join forces. A coalition of partners from sectors such as public health, nature conservation, urban planning, tourism, climate adaptation and others would be a promising avenue to help pave the way for the transition to sustainability.

This volume brings together rich insights of how biological diversity matters to people and their physical, mental and spiritual health and well-being, particularly in the context of a changing climate. Notably, the volume takes a systemic approach to assembling evidence from the social, natural and health sciences, draws on practical expertise from applied case studies, and discusses findings in the frame of ongoing developments in policy and planning. By understanding the true value and potential of biodiversity for health, we can develop the policies, research and practice to safeguard and secure these crucial contributions from nature to society and to our future. This book helps understand what is at stake and what can be done. We should do it quickly, because we have no alternative – and Mother Nature is the timekeeper.

Humberto Delgado Rosa

Director for Natural Capital
Directorate-General Environment
European Commission
Brussels, Belgium

Foreword II

Effects of heat-waves, heavy precipitation, river floods, landslides, droughts, forest fires, avalanches and storm surges are all felt in Europe, and more and more frequently. These extreme weather- and climate-related events have large impacts on human health, the economy and ecosystems. They are exacerbated by ecosystem degradation. Climate projections show that the frequency and severity of most of these hazards will increase across Europe in the next decades. Thus, reducing their impacts on human health as well as the underlying ecosystem health, and in this way adapting to a changing climate have become top priorities for communities and public authorities.

Regarding impacts on human health, heat waves affect especially vulnerable groups such as elderly people by worsening respiratory and cardiovascular diseases, which are aggravated by air pollution. Flooding, landslides and forest fires also cause fatalities. Arguably, enhancing coherence among the many actors involved in the knowledge base, policy responses, and practices on these issues represents an urgent need. New models of governance need to be adopted between national and local levels and across sectors in Europe. Spatial planning and risk prevention policies as well as technical measures need to combine conventional engineering (e.g. raising dikes) with 'nature-based' solutions (e.g. making room for rivers). If carried out properly, such projects can be highly efficient and cost-effective and have multiple benefits – for example, building parks that cool cities in the summer – and thereby boost human well-being and also contribute to biodiversity conservation.

Updated European regulations and policies on water, agriculture and climate adaptation are driving the push for more sustainable investment solutions to address the challenges posed by climate to address human health and well-being as well as biodiversity. Financing transformational adaptation measures, i.e. measures that change the way a city is built and organized, can be easy or difficult to implement. Measures often fall under the responsibility of other sectors, including water management, transport, nature conservation/protection and health. Collaboration is needed.

Taking a comprehensive perspective of integrated and long-term urban development and considering the municipality as a whole can result in lower overall costs and many additional benefits. Demonstrating these multiple benefits will help to align sectors. The European Commission and the European Environment Agency are hosting the Climate-ADAPT portal to make better use of knowledge on adaptation in Europe. The portal provides information on, for example, adaptation policies and strategies, case studies and a database on adaptation resources, to enhance effective uptake by decision-makers and contribute to better coordination among sectors and governance levels.

This volume adds significantly to the knowledge base to show the interlinkages of biodiversity and health in a changing climate. The synthesis of knowledge across different disciplines is highly welcomed and will inform practical and actionable management options to climate adaptation to foster, ultimately and in a mutually dependent manner, human health and well-being and ecosystem resilience.

Head of Natural Systems and Sustainability Ronan Uhel
European Environment Agency
Copenhagen, Denmark

Acknowledgements

Synthesizing knowledge in this volume from different disciplines and sectors about biodiversity, health and climate change inter-relationships has been a productive and fruitful collaboration of all contributing authors. The transdisciplinary approach for this book brought together 64 experts from the natural and social sciences as well as from policy and planning representing 15 countries. Working on this volume has been an inspiring, enriching and rewarding journey for us as editors.

We are deeply grateful to all authors who contributed to the chapters within this volume. This book would not have been possible without the joint expertise and insights into the various interconnected issues on the topic of biodiversity and health in the face of climate change. We appreciate the stimulating discussion process and hope this dialogue will continue. We would also like to extend our gratitude to all practitioners and policy advisors who have contributed their expertise to the science and case studies in this volume, demonstrating the possibilities for bringing together the issues of biodiversity, health and climate change. Their efforts and active collaboration made this synthesis possible.

We are sincerely thankful to the following peer reviewers who provided valuable, constructive comments on earlier versions of the chapters in this book: Agnieszka Olszewska-Guizzo, Amber Pearson, Anja Byg, Aurora Torres, Benjamin Lee, Caroline Hägerhäll, Chantal van Ham, Christopher Coutts, Cynthia Skelhorn, Daniel Cox, David Eichenberg, Delphine Thizy, Elaine Fuertes, Emma Coombes, Emma White, Freddie Lymeus, Hans Keune, Jack Benton, Jana Verboom, Jenny Veitch, Jill Fisher, Kalevi Korpela, Karen Keenleyside, Kathryn Rossiter, Laura B. Cole, Manuel Wolff, Martin Dallimer, Martin Pfeffer, Mike Hardman, Nadja Kabisch, Nick Osborne, Paul Heintzman, Peter Cochrane, Pippin Anderson, Rachel McInnes, Robert Ryan, Ruth Hunter, Sjerp de Vries, Sonja Knapp, Sophus zu Ermgassen, Stephanie Thomas, Stephen Heiland, Suneetha Subramanian, Terry Hartig and Thomas Classen.

We are especially grateful to Margaret Deignan from the Springer publishing team and to our Springer project coordinator, Karthika Menon, for their helpful guidance.

This book developed out of the successful European conference "Biodiversity and Health in the Face of Climate Change" on 27–29 June 2017 in Bonn, Germany (for detailed conference documentation, see https://www.ecbcc2017jimdo.com/european-conference-on-biodiversity-and-climate-change-ecbcc/downloads-presentations/and https://doi.org/10.19217/skr509). The conference was organized by the German Federal Agency for Nature Conservation (BfN) and the climate change interest group of the Network of European Nature Conservation Agencies (ENCA) in collaboration with the Helmholtz Centre for Environmental Research – UFZ and the German Centre for Integrative Biodiversity Research (iDiv) Halle-Jena-Leipzig. The World Health Organization (WHO) Regional Office for Europe co-sponsored the conference. More than 220 experts from 31 countries convened to discuss the importance of the interlinkages between biodiversity, human health, and climate change at this conference. The large number of presented papers and posters illustrated the highly topical and relevant nature of this field in science, policy and practice, and fueled stimulating debate.

This work was supported by the BfN with funds of the German Federal Ministry for the Environment, Nature Conservation, and Nuclear Safety (BMU) through the research project "Conferences on Climate Change and Biodiversity" (BIOCLIM, project duration from 2014 to 2017, funding code: 3514 80 020A). Dr. Irvine's involvement was funded by the Rural and Environment Science and Analytical Services Division of the Scottish Government.

The editors have used their best endeavors to ensure URLs provided for external websites are correct and active at the time of going to press. However, the publisher has no responsibility for websites and cannot guarantee that contents will remain live or appropriate.

Leipzig, Germany	Melissa R. Marselle
Isle of Vilm, Germany	Jutta Stadler
Isle of Vilm, Germany	Horst Korn
Aberdeen, Scotland, UK	Katherine N. Irvine
Leipzig, Germany	Aletta Bonn

Contents

Abbreviations

ADHD	Attention deficit hyperactivity disorder
AR	Allergic rhinitis
ART	Attention Restoration Theory
BfN	German Federal Agency for Nature Conservation
BiodivERsA	European Research Network on Biodiversity and Ecosystem Services
BMI	Body mass index
CBD	United Nations Convention on Biological Diversity
COP	Conference of the Parties
COST	European Cooperation in Science and Technology
CVD	Cardiovascular disease
DOHaD	Developmental origins of health and diseases
EC	EcoHealth
ECDC	European Centre for Disease Prevention and Control
EcoHealth	The International Association for Ecology and Health
EEG	Electroencephalography
EFSA	European Food Safety Authority
EIA	Environmental Impact Assessment
EID	(Re-)Emerging infectious diseases
EKLIPSE	Knowledge and Learning Mechanism on Biodiversity and Ecosystem Services
ENCA	European Network of Heads of Nature Conservation Agencies
EROEI	Energy returned on energy invested
ESP	Ecosystem Service Partnership
ESS	Ecosystem services
EU	European Union
GI	Green infrastructure
GIS	Geographic information systems
GM	Genetic modifications
GP	General practitioner, a medical doctor
GPS	Global positioning system
GVCR	Global vector control response

HIA	Health Impact Assessment
HPHP	Healthy Parks Healthy People initiative
IPBES	Intergovernmental Science-Policy Platform on Biodiversity and Ecosystem Services
IPCC	Intergovernmental Panel on Climate Change
IUCN	International Union for Conservation of Nature
IVM	Integrated vector management
KAS	Knowledge-action systems
LCP	GIS-based least-cost path model
MAES	Mapping and Assessment of Ecosystems and their Services
MEA	Millennium Ecosystem Assessment
NBS	Nature-based solutions
NCD	Noncommunicable disease
NDVI	Normalized difference vegetation index
NEOH	Network for Evaluation of One Health
NESTA	UK National Endowment for Science, Technology and the Arts
NGOs	Nongovernmental organizations
NICA	US National Interfaith Coalition on Aging
NPPF	UK National Planning Policy Framework
OH	One Health
PES	Payment for ecosystem services
RCT	Randomized controlled trial
SBSTTA	CBD's Subsidiary Body on Scientific, Technical and Technological Advice
SDG	UN Sustainable Development Goal
SEA	Strategic Environmental Assessment
SES	Socio-economic status
SIT	Sterile insect technique
SRT	Stress Reduction Theory
TEEB	The Economics of Ecosystems and Biodiversity
TWG	Thematic Working Group
UGS	Urban green space
UHI	Urban heat island
UN	United Nations
UNEP	United Nations Environment Program
UNFCCC	United Nations Framework Convention on Climate Change
VBDs	Vector-borne diseases
WHO	World Health Organization

About the Editors and Contributors

Editors

Melissa R. Marselle Researcher in the Department of Ecosystem Services at the Helmholtz Centre for Environmental Research (UFZ) and the German Center for Integrative Biodiversity Research (iDiv). She is an environmental psychologist whose research focuses on the influence of biodiversity and contact with nature on mental health and well-being. She is a chartered psychologist with the British Psychological Society.

Jutta Stadler Senior scientific officer in the International Nature Conservation Division at the German Federal Agency for Nature Conservation. She has been organizing numerous conferences and workshops on nature conservation and climate change as well as on other biodiversity-related issues.

Horst Korn Head of the International Nature Conservation Division at the German Federal Agency for Nature Conservation. His special interest lies in the application of holistic approaches to the conservation and sustainable use of biodiversity and the further development and application of science-policy interfaces.

Katherine N. Irvine Senior researcher in conservation behavior and environmental psychology at the James Hutton Institute, UK. Her transdisciplinary research focuses on the people-nature relationship, evaluating effectiveness of interventions to facilitate use of nature to promote well-being and sustainable behavior, and the spiritual dimensions of well-being and biodiversity.

Aletta Bonn Professor of Ecosystem Services at Friedrich Schiller University Jena in Germany and head of the Department of Ecosystem Services at the Helmholtz Center for Environmental Research Germany (UFZ), and the German Center for Integrative Biodiversity Research (iDiv). With a working background at the science-policy interface in the UK and Germany, her research focuses on ecosystem services, biodiversity and human well-being, participatory conservation, and citizen science.

Contributors

Rebecca Bell-Williams Research fellow at the University of Nottingham, UK. Her research focuses on nature connection and spiritual well-being.

Matthias Braubach Technical officer of Urban Health Equity at the WHO European Centre for Environment and Health. He has a background in urban geography and public health. He assists the WHO European Region Member States in the development and implementation of urban policies and interventions that address environmental risks and associated environmental equity issues.

Anne Cleary PhD candidate in the School of Medicine at Griffith University, Australia. Her research focuses on the links between nature and health, with a specific focus on urban nature and mental well-being.

Penny A. Cook Professor of public health at the University of Salford, UK. Her research focuses on working with communities to improve health, using an asset-based community development approach. She is also interested in health behavior and carries out research into sedentary behavior, physical activity and the health benefits of green space.

Payam Dadvand Assistant Research Professor at the Barcelona Institute for Global Health (ISGlobal), Spain. He is a medical doctor by training and has a PhD in environmental epidemiology. His research focuses on the impacts of both environmental stressors (e.g. air pollution, climate change) and mitigation measures (e.g. green spaces) on human health, particularly on maternal and child health.

Martin Dallimer Associate Professor of Environmental Change at the University of Leeds, UK. His research applies and integrates research techniques from across different disciplines to better understand, and provide solutions for, the sustainable management of natural environments, biodiversity, and ecosystems in a human-dominated world.

Athanasios Damialis Aerobiologist at the University Centre for Health Sciences at the Augsburg Hospital, Germany (UNIKA-T), and the German Research Centre for Environmental Health. Since 1996, he has worked in plant and fungal ecology and biology, biometeorology and climate change, and environmental medicine. Two of his future goals are to protect environmental quality and to promote human health via real-time, personalized health information services.

Zoe G. Davies Professor of Biodiversity Conservation at the University of Kent, UK. She is a landscape ecologist who uses empirical data to address questions of importance to conservation management and policy. One of her key research interests is understanding biodiversity-human well-being relationships.

Sjerp de Vries Senior social scientist in environmental psychology at Wageningen Environmental Research (WENR), The Netherlands. His research focuses on cultural ecosystem services, especially on the effect of access to and contact with nature on human health and well-being.

Raymond De Young Associate Professor of Environmental Psychology and Planning at the University of Michigan, USA. His work explores behavioral responses to the urgent need to transition to a life lived within local resource limits. Despite dismal ecological forecasts, his work is decidedly optimistic but without illusions.

Matthew Dennis Lecturer in geographical information science in geography at the University of Manchester, UK. His research focuses on human-dominated systems employing a landscape approach to understanding patterns and processes that influence human health and social-ecological resilience.

Thomas Elmqvist Professor in Natural Resource Management at the Stockholm Resilience Centre, Stockholm University, Sweden. His research is focused on urbanization, urban ecosystem services and components of resilience including the role of social institutions. He has led the "Cities and Biodiversity project" (www.cbobook.org) and is currently leading a Future Earth project entitled "Urban Planet".

Kerstin Ensinger Environmental psychologist at the Black Forest National Park, Germany. She is the director of the social research program of the Black Forest National Park. Her research and teaching activities have focused on issues of the effects of wilderness and nature-based experiences on body and mind.

Jessica C. Fisher Conservation researcher at DICE, University of Kent, UK. While her background is in ecology, much of her current work crosses traditional disciplinary boundaries. She is particularly interested in understanding how human-wildlife interactions can help solve conservation challenges.

Kerstin Friesenbichler Policy officer and project manager at Umweltdachverband, an Austrian NGO environmental umbrella organisation. Her work mainly concerns biodiversity, nature conservation and protected areas, the interlinkages of biodiversity and human health, and awareness raising among decision-makers and the general public. She has a master's degree in nature conservation and biodiversity management.

Richard A. Fuller Professor of Conservation and Biodiversity at the University of Queensland, Australia. He studies how people have affected the natural world around them. Much of his work is interdisciplinary, focusing on the interactions between people and nature, how these can be enhanced, and how these relationships can be shaped to build solutions to the biodiversity crisis.

Mireia Gascon Environmental epidemiologist at the Barcelona Institute for Global Health (ISGlobal), Spain. During her PhD, she focused on estimating the impact of pre- and postnatal exposures to chemicals on child health. After obtaining her PhD, she focused her research on improving scientific understanding of the health impacts of the urban environment, particularly air pollution and green spaces and transport planning.

Franz Gatzweiler Professor at the Institute of Urban Environment, Chinese Academy of Sciences. He is executive director of the global science program on system science for urban health and well-being under the International Science Council. His research has focused on the value of ecosystems and biodiversity and institutional change in complex social and ecological systems.

Anna Gilchrist Lecturer in environmental planning at the University of Manchester, UK. Her research is focused on biodiversity and ecosystem responses to environmental change and the pressures that are created under changing sociopolitical conditions.

Alistair Griffiths Director of Science and Collections at the Royal Horticultural Society (RHS) in the UK and member of the RHS Executive Board. He leads a highly skilled team of scientists focused on research to provide evidence-based solutions to address environmental and horticultural challenges. Prior to the RHS, he was a key player in using horticulture science to create the award-winning Eden Project. His interest is in the science of gardening to benefit the health of biodiversity, the environment, and people.

Barbara Häsler Senior lecturer in Agrihealth at the Royal Veterinary College, University of London, UK. Her research focuses on the application of integrated health approaches to food systems, and how changes in those approaches affect food safety and food security. She also studies how to improve the well-being of people and animals through better resource allocation.

Stefan Heiland Professor of Landscape Planning and Development at the Technical University of Berlin, Germany. Currently his work focuses on adaptation to climate change by landscape planning, urban green infrastructure and its contributions to human well-being, and the transition of landscapes, for example, by renewable energies. He was head of the working group preparing the scientific basis of the German Federal Green Infrastructure Concept.

Astrid Hilgers Landscape ecologist and senior policy advisor at the Dutch Ministry of Agriculture, Nature and Food Quality. She is the national coordinator of the Convention of Biological Diversity (CBD) and of the Intergovernmental Panel on Biodiversity and Ecosystem Services (IPBES) for The Netherlands. She is an initiator of the international Coalition of the Willing on Pollinators.

Dusty Hoesly Lecturer in the departments of Religious Studies and Asian American Studies at the University of California, Santa Barbara, in the USA. His research focuses on contemporary American religions and the social scientific study of religion, specializing in how minority religions and spirtual movements shape modern American culture.

Jo Hopkins Chair of the IUCN WCPA Health and Well-being Specialist Group. In this role, she advocates for the vital role that parks and protected areas play in ensuring a healthy natural world. Jo is also the manager of National and International Engagement at Parks Victoria (Australia) and is responsible for the consolidation of partnerships that deliver on Government policy and facilitates initiatives with mutually beneficial outcomes between partners.

Michelle Howarth Senior lecturer in nursing at the University of Salford, UK. She is a specialist in the impact of nature-based interventions on health and well-being. Her current research explores the process, impact and mode of social prescribing as an emerging social movement and how this promotes a person-centred, salutogenic approach to well-being.

Ruth F. Hunter Researcher and lecturer in public health at Queen's University Belfast, UK. Her field of expertise is on green space interventions and health behavior change, with a focus on natural experiment methodology.

Jukka-Pekka Jäppinen Development manager and deputy director of the Biodiversity Centre at the Finnish Environment Institute (SYKE). He has a long career in working with the research and policy development on biodiversity and ecosystem services, Convention on Biological Diversity (e.g. ecosystem approach), nature management in forestry, nature-based solutions, business and biodiversity, and biodiversity and human health.

Beate Job-Hoben Scientific assistant in the Nature Conservation and Society Division at the German Federal Agency for Nature Conservation. Her fields of work include nature conservation and sustainable tourism, sports in nature, and health. She studied biology and chemistry in Bonn and ecology in Essen.

Nadja Kabisch Junior research group leader on GreenEquityHEALTH at the Humboldt University of Berlin, Germany. The project is funded for 5 years to study potential health outcomes of urban nature under global challenges of climate change and urbanization.

Vladimir Kendrovski Technical officer for climate change and health at the WHO European Centre for Environment and Health. A specialist in the field of health aspects of climate change, he provides and facilitates technical expertise to the WHO European Region Member States for the development and implementation of policies in relation to climate change, extreme events, and health issues.

Hans Keune Senior researcher at the Belgian Biodiversity Platform and the Research Institute for Nature and Forest (INBO). He works on critical complexity, inter- and transdisciplinary, action research, decision support, environment and health, ecosystem services, biodiversity and health, and One Health/Eco Health. He also coordinates the Chair in Care and the Natural Living Environment at the Faculty of Medicine and Health Sciences, University of Antwerp.

Elisabet Lindgren Physician and associate professor in sustainability science at the Stockholm Resilience Centre in Sweden. Her field of expertise is global environmental changes and human health, with focus on health and climate change and sustainable cities.

Sarah J. Lindley Professor of Geography at the University of Manchester and research director of the Department of Geography, University of Manchester, UK. She is a lead author for the IPBES Regional Assessment for Africa. She is an expert in climate change adaptation, particularly in relation to urban heat. Her main research interests are associated with urban air pollution, climate adaptation and urban ecosystem contributions to people, including regulating ecosystem functions for human health and well-being.

Jieling Liu PhD candidate in climate change and sustainable development policies at the University of Lisbon, Portugal. She has a background in political science and journalism. Her current research focuses on the institutional frameworks of urban ecological governance in China.

Barbara Livoreil Knowledge broker at the French Foundation for Research on Biodiversity (FRB). She works to promote the use of systematic reviews to support decision and negotiation. Her background is in animal behavior and she also spent 10 years in the field doing conservation biology. Her main interests currently are behavioural change, conservation psychology and mainstreaming biodiversity into society.

Kathy MacKinnon Chair of the IUCN World Commission on Protected Areas (WCPA). The IUCN WCPA is a global network of conservation protected areas professionals supporting well-managed and connected parks and other protected areas as natural solutions to biodiversity loss and other global challenges, including climate change and human health and well-being.

Iana Markevych Postdoctoral researcher in the Institute of Epidemiology at the German Research Center for Environmental Health. She is an environmental epidemiologist with a background in ecology. Among others, her interests lie in the field of green space benefits for childhood health.

Dörte Martens Researcher at the Eberswalde University for Sustainable Development, Germany. She completed her PhD in environmental psychology at the University of Zürich on the effects of different urban forests on psychological well-being. Her current research interests are psychological effects of nature experience areas for children in an urbanized environment.

Doreen Montag Lecturer in Global Public Health in the Barts and London School of Medicine at Queen Mary University of London, UK. Her interests lie in health-centred global environmental governance, political economy of planetary health, climate change, biodiversity, sustainable development and vector-borne diseases.

Ruth Müller Head of the Environmental Toxicology and Medical Entomology Department at Goethe University, Frankfurt in Germany and the head of the Ecology and Genetics Platform of Polo GGB, Italy. She is a vector biologist. Her basic and applied research focuses on mosquito-borne diseases and innovative, environmentally friendly control of aedine and anopheline vector species, in particular those altering their distribution with global climate changes.

Bram Oosterbroek PhD candidate at the International Centre for Integrated Assessment and Sustainable Development (ICIS), Maastricht University, The Netherlands. His research topic is on a healthy living environment, specialized in the method of spatial modeling. He is working on a GIS model to assess and map the human health impacts of urban green spaces.

Kate Reilly EU program officer for Nature-Based Solutions at the IUCN European Regional Office in Brussels, Belgium. She supports IUCN's work to promote nature-based solutions through a range of projects on urban nature and biodiversity, forest and aquatic ecosystem services, and ecosystem-based management.

Friederike Reuss PhD candidate at Goethe University Frankfurt in Germany and a research associate in the Department of Molecular Ecology, Senckenberg Biodiversity and Climate Research Centre, Germany. She has a scientific background in molecular biology. Her present research focuses on bioassays with culicid and drosophilid insects.

Cristina Romanelli Coordinator of the CBD and WHO joint work program on biodiversity and human health for the UN Secretariat of the Convention of Biological Diversity in Canada. She is an expert in global policy development, biodiversity and health mainstreaming, cross-sectoral partnerships, and capacity development. She was lead author of *Connecting Global Priorities: Biodiversity and Human Health.*

Robbert Snep Senior researcher in Regional Development and Spatial Use at Wageningen Environmental Research, The Netherlands. He is an ecologist. His research connects urban nature science with health and climate adaptation issues of cities. He collaborates with urban designers, developers, NGOs, and local governments in improving the quality of city life.

Hélène Soubelet Director of the French Foundation for Research on Biodiversity (FRB). She is a doctor of veterinary medicine and a master's degree in plant pathology. She has a background in public health as she worked for 10 years for the French Ministry of Agriculture and also spent 7 years in the field of biodiversity working for the French Ministry of Ecology.

Helena Ströher Scientific assistant in the Nature Conservation and Society division at the German Federal Agency for Nature Conservation. Helena deals with the implementation of the National Strategy on Biological Diversity and the United Nations Decade on Biodiversity.

Matti Tapaninen Senior advisor in Metsähallitus Parks and Wildlife Finland. Previously, he has worked in protected area management as a park director and regional manager. Matti also has a long international career in the field of protected area management.

Jessica Thompson Lead for Health and Well-being at City of Trees based in Manchester, UK. Her background is in community forestry and has worked to engage people in urban forestry initiatives since 2005. She has an MSc in Dementia focused on 'life-enabling' green environments. Jessica is a PhD candidate at the University of Salford, UK, exploring well-being impacts of neighborhood greening outreach work.

Claudia Traidl-Hoffmann Head of the Institute for Environmental Medicine at the University Centre for Health Sciences at Augsburg Hospital, Germany (UNIKA-T), and director the Institute of Environmental Medicine at the German Research Center for Environmental Health. She investigates human-environment interactions focusing on allergic diseases. Her research contributes to our understanding of how environmental factors act on the body's epithelial and immunological interface. In 2013 she was appointed to the board of directors of CK CARE Center for Allergy Research and Education.

Regina Treudler Senior physician and a professor in the Faculty of Medicine at the University of Leipzig as well as the head of the Leipzig Comprehensive Allergy Centre (LICA) at the University of Leipzig and consultant in the Department of Dermatology at the UMC Leipzig, Germany. She was educated at the Free University of Berlin and at the Université de Paris XII, France. Prof. Treudler received her board examination in dermatology and in allergology at the Charité Allergy center.

Chantal van Ham EU program manager for Nature-Based Solutions at the IUCN. She is responsible for IUCN's activities on urban biodiversity and the cooperation with cities and subnational governments in Europe. She develops and coordinates projects that help policy-makers, cities, and local and regional governments find nature-based solutions for sustainable development to improve quality of life and economic prosperity by mobilizing IUCN knowledge and best practices.

Eike von Lindern Co-founder of Dialog N, an independent research institute in Switzerland. He holds a PhD in social and environmental psychology. His work focuses on restorative environments research, health promotion, sustainable development, and the involvement of the (local) population with parks and protected areas.

Veikko Virkkunen Development manager in Metsähallitus Parks and Wildlife Finland. He works with projects that increase benefits from protected areas, such as health and well-being, recreation and tourism. His background is in visitor management and sustainability in protected areas.

Sara L. Warber Senior physician and emeritus professor of family medicine at the University of Michigan and the former director of the Integrative Medicine Program at the University of Michigan, USA. She is a clinician-scholar whose research focuses on the effects of nature-based programs and other complex psychosocial-spiritual interventions on human health and well-being. Examples include the health benefits of camps, retreats and national group walking programs in the USA and the UK.

Catharine Ward Thompson Professor of Landscape Architecture at the University of Edinburgh and director of OpenSpace, the research center for inclusive access to outdoor environments at the University of Edinburgh, UK. Her research focuses on salutogenic environments, with a particular focus on deprived populations, and quality of life in older age.

Julia Weidenweber Master's candidate in environmental planning at the Technical University of Berlin, Germany. Her master's thesis focuses on approaches to strengthen the integration of health issues into the German system of landscape planning.

C. Philip Wheater Professor of Environmental and Geographical Sciences at Manchester Metropolitan University, UK. As an ecologist and environmental scientist, he is interested in how people interact with their environment, especially in urban systems. He also works on conservation and biodiversity management and how it influences local communities, for example in health and education.

The original version of this book was revised: This book was inadvertently published with the incorrect copyright holder which has been corrected now. The correction to this book is available at https://doi.org/10.1007/978-3-030-02318-8_21

Chapter 1
Biodiversity and Health in the Face of Climate Change: Challenges, Opportunities and Evidence Gaps

Melissa R. Marselle, Jutta Stadler, Horst Korn, Katherine N. Irvine, and Aletta Bonn

Abstract Climate change presents significant challenges to human health and biodiversity. Increased numbers of extreme climate events, such as heat waves, droughts or flooding, threaten human health and well-being, both directly and indirectly, through impaired ecosystem functioning and reduced ecosystem services. In addition, the prevalence of non-communicable diseases is rising, causing ill health and accelerating costs to the health sector. Nature-based solutions, such as the provision and management of biodiversity, can facilitate human health and well-being, and mitigate the negative effects of climate change. The growing recognition of the importance of biodiversity's contribution to human health offers great potential for maximising synergies between public health, climate change adaptation and nature

M. R. Marselle (✉)
Department of Ecosystem Services, Helmholtz Centre for Environmental Research – UFZ, Leipzig, Germany

German Centre for Integrative Biodiversity Research (iDiv) Halle-Jena-Leipzig, Leipzig, Germany
e-mail: melissa.marselle@ufz.de

J. Stadler · H. Korn
Federal Agency for Nature Conservation (BfN), Isle of Vilm, Putbus, Germany
e-mail: jutta.stadler@bfn.de; horst.korn@bfn.de

K. N. Irvine
Social, Economic and Geographical Sciences Research Group, The James Hutton Institute, Aberdeen, Scotland, UK
e-mail: katherine.irvine@hutton.ac.uk

A. Bonn
Department of Ecosystem Services, Helmholtz Centre for Environmental Research – UFZ, Leipzig, Germany

German Centre for Integrative Biodiversity Research (iDiv) Halle-Jena-Leipzig, Leipzig, Germany

Institute of Biodiversity, Friedrich Schiller University Jena, Jena, Germany
e-mail: aletta.bonn@ufz.de

M. R. Marselle et al. (eds.), *Biodiversity and Health in the Face of Climate Change*, https://doi.org/10.1007/978-3-030-02318-8_1

conservation. This book identifies the contribution of biodiversity to physical, mental and spiritual health and well-being in the face of climate change, and considers implications across multiple sectors.

Keywords Climate change · Biodiversity · Health · Nature-based solutions · Nature conservation · Interdisciplinarity

Highlights

- Climate change poses significant challenges to both human health and biodiversity.
- Green spaces can improve human health and well-being, and mitigate biodiversity loss.
- The inter-relationships of biodiversity to human physical, mental and spiritual aspects of health and well-being are not yet well understood.
- There is great potential for synergies between public health, climate change adaptation and biodiversity conservation.

1.1 Background

Climate change poses significant challenges to human health and biodiversity. Increased numbers of heat waves, droughts and flooding events due to climate change have negative consequences for both human health and biodiversity (EEA 2016, Box 1.1). The 2003 summer heat wave in Europe gave rise to 70,000 deaths, both directly through temperature stress and indirectly by affecting air quality and respiratory systems (Wolf et al. 2015). The most vulnerable people in society – the elderly, those with chronic diseases and persons of lower socio-economic status – are often most affected. While susceptibility varies geographically and among groups, studies show that an increase of 1 °C in temperature above local comfort

Box 1.1: Definitions of Health, Climate Change and Biodiversity

Health is "a state of complete physical, mental and social well-being and not merely the absence of disease or infirmity" (WHO 1948).

Climate change is "any change in climate over time, resulting from natural variability or human activity" (IPCC 2007).

Biodiversity is "the variability among living organisms from all sources including, *inter alia*, terrestrial, marine and other aquatic ecosystems and the ecological complexes of which they are part; this includes diversity within species, between species and of ecosystems" (United Nations Convention on Biological Diversity 1992).

(For further definitions, see the Glossary, this volume).

thresholds can be associated with an increase in mortality of up to 12% (Gabriel and Endlicher 2011). The frequency and severity of heat waves and other weather-related events are expected to increase in Europe with a changing climate. This will have a significant impact on biodiversity and ecosystem functioning by worsening habitat conditions (EEA 2012).

Non-communicable diseases (NCDs), for example, diabetes, cardiovascular diseases, mental disorders, cancer and chronic respiratory diseases, are a significant risk to health and well-being (WHO 2017b). NCDs are a leading cause of death globally (WHO 2017a) and account for 85% of all deaths in Europe (WHO 2017b). These deaths are largely preventable and linked by common risk factors, such as physical inactivity, alcohol use and environmental factors (WHO 2017a). As such, population-level interventions are necessary to promote mental health and physical activity in order to prevent and control NCDs, and to reduce health-care costs. Supportive environments that facilitate healthier lifestyles and reduce exposure to stressors is one example of such an intervention. New approaches are needed to attenuate the negative effects of climate change and prevent NCDs in order to maximise opportunities for improving human health and preventing biodiversity loss.

Nature-based solutions (NBS) (Nesshöver et al. 2017), such as the management of green spaces to increase benefits for people and to mitigate stressors, might be one such approach. Work on NBS demonstrates the importance of green spaces for climate change adaptation and mitigation (Kabisch et al. 2017). Green spaces are also used as natural health clinics to promote human health and well-being (Mayer et al. 2009; Frumkin et al. 2017; Frumkin and Louv 2007), while at the same time providing habitats for a range of species (Niemela 1999; Goddard et al. 2010) and aiding conservation goals. A large body of research shows that contact with green space can improve human health and well-being, through for example reducing stress, depression and negative emotions, and improving positive emotions, mental well-being, cognitive abilities and increasing physical activity (Bowler et al. 2010b; Hartig et al. 2014; Markevych et al. 2017; Frumkin 2001; Irvine and Warber 2002), suggesting that nature can promote public health and prevent NCDs. Moreover, evidence suggests that positive experiences in nature contribute to feelings of connection to nature (Mayer et al. 2009), which could also result in greater acceptance of nature conservation activities (Prévot et al. 2018), and thereby protection of our foundation of life on earth (Geng et al. 2015; Zelenski et al. 2015; Capaldi et al. 2015).

In this context, there is growing recognition of the contribution of biodiversity to climate change adaptation and human health. Street trees and green space in cities can contribute to climate change adaptation by reducing the impact of high temperatures, poor air quality and high water flows (Bowler et al. 2010a, Gill et al. 2007). Biodiversity underpins ecosystem services that are essential for human health and well-being (Cardinale et al. 2012). Ecosystem services provided by biodiversity include the provision of food, timber and medicines as well as climate and water regulation, and cultural services such as the provision of opportunities for recreation (WHO & CBD 2015). Yet biodiversity loss can negatively influence physical health through loss of these vital services, diminished options for medicines and increased transmission of infectious diseases (WHO & CBD 2015; Sandifer et al. 2015; Hough 2014). Unsurprisingly then, biodiversity has been shown to be positively associated with good physical health (Hough 2014; Lovell et al. 2014). Less understood, however, are the impacts of biodiversity on other aspects of human health and well-being. Whilst a fast-growing field of research is investigating the influence of biodiversity on mental health and well-being (Aerts et al. 2018; Lovell et al. 2014; Dallimer et al. 2012; Fuller et al. 2007; Wheeler et al. 2015; Cox et al. 2017; Marselle et al. 2015, 2016; Carrus et al. 2015; Cracknell et al. 2016, 2017; Johansson et al. 2014), work is still progressing in this area, and evidence gaps remain. For example, the mechanistic pathways through which biodiversity influences mental health and well-being is undeveloped. Several models consider the pathways through which nature might influence various dimensions of health and well-being (Hartig et al. 2014; Markevych et al. 2017), yet it is unknown whether these same mechanistic pathways would hold for biodiversity and health and well-being relationships. In this book, we aim to synthesise existing studies and further develop the research agenda.

Increasingly, the importance of biodiversity for human health and well-being is being recognised by international governments and organizations (WHO & CBD 2015, CBD 2017a, ten Brick et al. 2016). The linkage between biodiversity and human health is at the heart of several high-level strategic decisions being taken at a national and international scale. The Convention of Biological Diversity (CBD) and the World Health Organization (WHO) are collaborating to promote the interlinkages between biodiversity and human health sectors as secured in the Conference of the Parties (COP) 12 Decision XII/21 and joint publications (WHO & CBD 2015, CBD 2017a, b, c). The Health 2020 policy framework of the WHO European Region identifies the importance of environmental conditions as health determinants, and has recently published a review of the evidence of urban green space for health (WHO 2017c). The United Nations 2030 Agenda on Sustainable Development has dedicated Sustainable Development Goals (SDGs) both for health and biodiversity, and current activities under the CBD aim to closely align health and biodiversity issues. The relevance of biodiversity to physical and mental health is also reflected in levels of EU research activity, the quantity of public and private expenditure, and the number of high-profile government initiatives on biodiversity and health (EKLIPSE 2017). High-profile international initiatives and research on biodiversity and health also highlight this burgeoning area (e.g. United Nations Environment Programme (UNEP), the International Association for Ecology and Health (Eco Health), and One Health).

Awareness of the significant potential for synergies between improvement of human health and adaptation to climate change with conservation of biodiversity is also increasing in applied resource management, urban planning, landscape architecture and protected areas management. In practice, there is growing interest in the use of green space in general, and biodiversity in particular, for physical, mental and/or spiritual health and well-being. For example, city urban planning projects encourage physical exercise through green infrastructure as a measure to improve human health (Marselle et al. 2013), while also contributing to climate change adaptation as well as to nature conservation. Use of green spaces for health has been advocated *inter alia* by the New Zealand Ministry of Health's 'Green Prescriptions' programme,[1] the USA National Park Service's 'Parks and Trails Prescription Partnerships' programme,[2] as well as by the German Government's 'Soziale Stadt'[3] and 'Grün in der Stadt'[4] initiatives, the German Federal Agency for Nature Conservation's 'Urban Biodiversity'[5] theme, the 'Outdoors for All' programme by Natural England[6] and Scottish Natural Heritage's 'Our Natural Health Service' initiative.[7] These co-benefits can only be achieved, however, through joined-up, collaborative, cross-sectoral and transdisciplinary working, and in this book we demonstrate with case studies good practice examples.

Awareness of the impacts of climate change and biodiversity on human health is growing. With this book, we hope to catalyse the discussion about the integral links between climate change, biodiversity and human health. Specifically, this book not only identifies the contribution of biodiversity to physical health, but also to mental and spiritual health and well-being in the face of climate change. The implications of the biodiversity–health relationship for public health, nature conservation, pro-environmental behaviour, protected areas and landscape architecture and design are detailed. The book compiles current policy and practice integrating biodiversity, human health and climate change adaptation at both national and international levels.

1.2 Scope of the Book

Integrating biodiversity, human health and climate change requires new approaches and transdisciplinary working. One of the challenges facing research, policy and practice on biodiversity and health is that the science has not fully joined together the different disciplines of biodiversity, ecology, public health, psychology, natural resource management, urban planning and landscape architecture to provide a

[1] http://www.health.govt.nz/our-work/preventative-health-wellness/physical-activity/green-prescriptions

[2] https://www.nps.gov/public_health/hp/hphp/partners_ptp.htm

[3] https://www.bmi.bund.de/DE/themen/bauen-wohnen/stadt-wohnen/staedtebau/soziale-stadt/soziale-stadt-node.html;jsessionid=9F4F2DB35101A11DD1530AE7BA605ABB.1_cid287

[4] https://www.gruen-in-der-stadt.de/

[5] https://www.bfn.de/themen/planung/siedlungsbereich.html

[6] http://www.gov.uk/government/publications/outdoors-for-all-fair-access-to-a-good-quality-natural-environment

[7] https://www.nature.scot/professional-advice/contributing-healthier-scotland/our-natural-health-service

cohesive evidence base for action. Whilst studies investigate the impacts of climate change on biodiversity and on human health, at present there is limited research detailing the inter-relationships of all three topics together. In applied resource management, nature conservation needs to better link to the health sector and vice versa (WHO & CBD 2015). The health sector, whilst it has begun to incorporate the health benefits of climate change adaptation (Watts et al. 2015), has yet to fully appreciate the influence of biodiversity. Likewise, the nature conservation community needs to harness synergies with public health and climate change adaptation. The scope of this book is to align these three areas of research and to link to application in policy and practice.

This book brings together experts from transdisciplinary fields in science, policy and practice to provide an overview of the current state of knowledge on biodiversity and health relationships in the face of climate change. As such, this book provides a synthesis of the current state of the knowledge drawing from ecology, geography, environmental psychology, public health, medical science and urban planning. Moreover, experts discuss the implications that the health benefits of biodiversity have for public health, nature conservation and environmental sustainability. The book also captures in-depth, practical expertise and experience from protected area managers and landscape architects. National and international policy and practice activities regarding biodiversity, health and climate change interrelationships from health and nature conservation agencies are also detailed.

The scope of this book is on biodiversity's contribution to physical, mental and spiritual health and well-being in the face of climate change. This makes it unique compared to other books that focus on the effect of biodiversity on human physical health (Morand and Lajaunie 2017, Chivian and Bernstein 2008, Grifo and Rosenthal 1997), the contribution of green spaces to physical and mental health (Nilsson et al. 2011, Pearlmutter et al. 2017) or social-environmental equity perspectives on nature-health relationships (Kopnina and Keune 2010). In addition, the recognition of climate change as an important factor influencing biodiversity as well as health takes up new aspects of the current debate, encouraging new thinking alongside joined-up collaboration and transdisciplinary working. Consequently, some topics of biodiversity and health, such as medicine, food and nutrition, are not covered in this book, as they have already been extensively covered elsewhere (see Morand and Lajaunie 2017, Chivian and Bernstein 2008, Grifo and Rosenthal 1997). As the book focuses on biodiversity in the natural environment, consideration of the human microbiome is also not included here.

Many of the topics discussed in this book were intensely discussed at the European conference 'Biodiversity and Health in the Face of Climate Change' that took place in Bonn, Germany, from 27–29 June 2017 (Marselle et al. 2018). The conference was organised by the German Federal Agency for Nature Conservation (BfN), the Helmholtz Centre for Environmental Research-UFZ, the German Centre for Integrative Biodiversity Research (iDiv) Halle-Jena-Leipzig, the Network of European Nature Conservation Agencies (ENCA), and co-sponsored by the WHO Regional Office for Europe. We hope this book contributes to an increased understanding of how green spaces and biodiversity can contribute to human health in a changing climate.

1.3 Structure and Contents of the Book

This book is structured in four main parts. The first two parts highlight the important contribution of green spaces and biodiversity to physical health on the one hand, and mental and spiritual health and well-being on the other hand, in a changing climate. Here we also touch on theoretical and methodological considerations. Part III discusses the implications of biodiversity on human health and well-being for specific sectors and describes the current policy and practice perspective. The final part addresses the co-benefits and the implementation challenges associated with the planning and management of urban green spaces for both biodiversity and human health.

1. Part I: Biodiversity and physical health
2. Part II: Biodiversity, mental health and spiritual well-being
3. Part III: Implications of the biodiversity and health relationship
4. Part IV: Planning and managing urban green spaces for biodiversity and health in a changing climate

The various chapters provide up-to-date scientific background information, address policy-related issues, lay out pressing urban planning and biological conservation management questions and identify knowledge gaps. Different chapters provide specific examples and applications of the use of urban green spaces for human health, nature conservation and climate change adaptation with case studies, mainly from Europe and North America. Here we provide a summative overview of each of the book's four parts.

1.3.1 Part I: Biodiversity and Physical Health

The first part considers the impacts that biodiversity has on physical health. The focus is on non-communicable diseases that can be caused or prevented by exposure to green space and biodiversity. The impacts of climate change on biodiversity-health relationships are additionally highlighted in the first three chapters.

In the first chapter, *Sarah Lindley and co-authors* provide a general overview of the interlinkages between biodiversity, health and climate change. They highlight the role that climate change has on human health and the adaptation role that NBS can play; this is illustrated with a case study from Manchester, England. *Athanasios Damialis and co-authors* discuss the impact of climate change on biodiversity and human health through the expanding geographical spread of allergies and allergenic pollen. Further negative effects of biodiversity on human health by vector-borne diseases, that may become more prevalent due to a changing climate, are reviewed by *Ruth Müller and co-authors*. The authors highlight how climate change shapes the distribution and abundance of disease vectors, and the role biodiversity can play in this relationship. The health effects of green space for different socio-economic and socio-demographic population groups is addressed by *Nadja Kabisch*. Conclusions are drawn about how to design green spaces that are beneficial for the health and well-being of all population groups to protect the most vulnerable in society. Complementing this chapter, *Payam Dadvand and co-authors* show how urban green spaces can affect the health and development of children living in urban environments. In their review, the authors identify how green spaces influence prenatal development and pregnancy outcomes, children's brain development as well as effects on respiratory conditions and physical activity.

1.3.2 Part II: Biodiversity, Mental Health and Spiritual Well-Being

Chapters in the second part of the book discuss the evidence of the impact of biodiversity on mental health and spiritual well-being. The first two chapters touch on theoretical and methodological issues for biodiversity and mental health and well-being relationships. The latter chapters review the evidence on the influence biodiversity has on mental health and spiritual well-being.

To set the scene, *Melissa Marselle* provides an overview of the theoretical frameworks that provide a perspective into the ways that biodiversity can influence mental well-being. Complementing this chapter, *Sjerp de Vries and Robbert Snep* highlight conceptual issues associated with the design of studies when investigating the effect of biodiversity on mental health, drawing out key methodological issues to be considered in future research on biodiversity-mental health relationships. The next chapter by *Melissa Marselle and co-authors* provides a comprehensive review of the scientific literature on how biodiversity can affect mental health and well-being based on a synthesis of 24 studies. *Katherine Irvine and colleagues* examine evidence of the inter-relationship between biodiversity and spiritual well-being.

1.3.3 Part III: Implications of the Biodiversity and Health Relationship

The third part of this book focuses on the policy and practice implications of biodiversity and health relationships. In particular, the implications of this relationship from the perspective of public health, nature conservation and efforts to promote pro-environmental behaviour are highlighted. The latter chapters review the national and international policy and practice support for biodiversity, climate change, and human health.

Penny Cook and co-authors provide a comprehensive overview of the scientific literature on the linkages between public health, climate change and biodiversity. The authors demonstrate how access to, and use of, urban green spaces can reduce social inequalities in health, a key goal of modern public health policies and programmes. Reflecting on the health and well-being benefits of nature, *Zoe Davies and colleagues* discuss the management options to ensure that both biodiversity conservation and people's health are considered. The authors argue that the evidence on biodiversity-health relationships suggests that green spaces should be managed for both people and biodiversity conservation. As the consequences of climate change and biodiversity loss will require humans to change their behaviour to consume far fewer resources in a resource finite world, *Raymond De Young* discusses how to initiate long-term behaviour change. The author argues for a "capacities-first approach" to support people to become "behavioural entrepreneurs" and self-initiate behaviour change. To assess how health agendas are embedded in biodiversity policies and vice versa, *Horst Korn and co-authors* review the international policy agendas with the potential to foster linkages between biodiversity conservation and human health, and identify alignments between sectors and avenues for implementation. Reflecting on institutional aspects and challenges of integrating nature and health, *Hans Keune and co-authors* highlight the need for increased and improved collaboration between the health and nature sectors, as well as science, policy and practice. The chapter presents several international/European examples of nature and health network initiatives as well as various national activities in Europe alongside summarising successes and challenges of each initiative.

1.3.4 Part IV: Planning and Managing Urban Green Spaces for Biodiversity and Health in a Changing Climate

The last part focuses on planning and managing green spaces in and around cities for nature conservation, health and climate change adaptation. In particular, this part discusses how managers of protected areas and urban green space can work with other sectors to maximise the benefits of these places, and how landscape planners can design urban environments that benefit both people and nature.

Kathy MacKinnon and colleagues provide a scene-setting chapter in which they highlight the benefits and services that NBS and protected areas provide for biodiversity, health and climate change adaptation, *inter alia* in the context of the SDGs. The authors discuss the need for increased and improved collaboration between sectors and stakeholders to foster the use of NBS and protected areas for these multiple benefits. Complementing this chapter, *Ruth Hunter and co-authors* review the effectiveness of urban green space interventions for improving health and biodiversity and provide recommendations for research, policy and practice regarding the design of these types of interventions. *Thomas Elmqvist and co-authors* propose applying systems thinking to foster sustainable urban development and resilience. They discuss Knowledge-Action-Systems for urban health, in which knowledge of complex urban system functions and interactions with climate change, and NBS for economic, environmental and social dimensions of urban development, are interlinked by constant feedback loops. The last chapter in this part by *Stefan Heiland and colleagues* refers to the opportunities for integrating human health into landscape planning projects in order to cope with climate change and societal change. The authors discuss planning policy opportunities for incorporating health issues in Germany and the UK, and provide examples of health-promoting landscape design.

The book is complemented with a conclusion chapter which summarises the main challenges for research, policy and practice described in the chapters, highlights opportunities for future developments, and presents recommendations for tackling the inter-related issues of biodiversity, health and climate change.

We hope this book provides important pointers to the flourishing debate on the importance of biodiversity to human health in this current time of climate change, and illustrates good practice with demonstration case studies. Ultimately, we hope this book can fuel further advances in science, policy and practice. Many of the themes have applications beyond urban systems as they focus on solutions for public health, biodiversity conservation and climate adaptation in a changing world.

Acknowledgements This work was supported by the German Federal Agency for Nature Conservation (BfN) with funds of the German Federal Ministry for the Environment, Nature Conservation, and Nuclear Safety (BMU) through the research project "Conferences on Climate Change and Biodiversity" (BIOCLIM, project duration from 2014 to 2017, funding code: 3514 80 020A). Dr. Irvine's involvement was funded by the Rural & Environment Science & Analytical Services Division of the Scottish Government.

References

Aerts R, Honnay O, Van Nieuwenhuyse A (2018) Biodiversity and human health: mechanisms and evidence of the positive health effects of diversity in nature and green spaces. Br Med Bull 127(1):5–22

Bowler DE, Buyung-Ali L, Knight TM, Pullin AS (2010a) Urban greening to cool towns and cities: a systematic review of the empirical evidence. Landsc Urban Plan 97:147–155. https://doi.org/10.1016/j.landurbplan.2010.05.006

Bowler DE, Buyung-Ali L, Knight T, Pullin AS (2010b) A systematic review of evidence for the added benefits to health of exposure to natural environments. BMC Public Health 10:456. https://doi.org/10.1186/1471-2458-10-456

Capaldi CA, Passmore H, Nisbet EK, Zelenski JM, Dopko RL (2015) Flourishing in nature: a review of the benefits of connecting with nature and its application as a wellbeing intervention. Int J Wellbeing 5(4):1–16. https://doi.org/10.5502/ijw.v5i4.449

Cardinale BJ, Duffy JE, Gonzalez A et al (2012) Biodiversity loss and its impact on humanity. Nature 486:59–67. https://doi.org/10.1038/nature11148

Carrus G, Scopelliti M, Lafortezza R et al (2015) Go greener, feel better? The positive effects of biodiversity on the well-being of individuals visiting urban and peri-urban green areas. Landsc Urban Plann 134:221–228

CBD (2017a) Biodiversity and human health. Secretariat of the Convention on Biological Diversity, Montreal, Canada. https://www.cbd.int/doc/c/72d6/b5bb/9244e977048688ec45735d2c/sbstta-21-04-en.pdf. Accessed 30 Jan 2018

CBD (2017b) Recommendation adopted by the subsidiary body on scientific, technical and technological advice. XXI/3. Health and biodiversity. Secretariat of the Convention on Biological Diversity, Montreal, Canada. https://www.cbd.int/doc/recommendations/sbstta-21/sbstta-21-rec-03-en.pdf. Accessed 12 Jan 2018

CBD (2017c) Workshop on biodiversity and health for the European Region. Secretariat of the Convention on Biological Diversity, Montreal, Canada. https://www.cbd.int/health/european/default.shtml. Accessed 12 Jan 2018

Chivian E, Bernstein A (eds) (2008) Sustaining life: how our health depends on biodiversity. Oxford University Press, Oxford

Cox DTC, Shanahan DF, Hudson HL et al (2017) Doses of neighborhood nature: the benefits for mental health of living with nature. Bioscience 67:147–155. https://doi.org/10.1093/biosci/biw173

Cracknell D, White MP, Pahl S, Nichols WJ, Depledge MH (2016) Marine biota and psychological well-being: a preliminary examination of dose–response effects in an aquarium setting. Environ Behav 48(10):1242–1269. https://doi.org/10.1177/0013916515597512

Cracknell D, White MP, Pahl S, Depledge MH (2017) A preliminary investigation into the restorative potential of public aquaria exhibits: a UK student-based study. Landsc Res 42(1):18–32. https://doi.org/10.1080/01426397.2016.1243236

Dallimer M, Irvine KN, Skinner AMJ et al (2012) Biodiversity and the feel-good factor: understand associations between self-reports human well-being and species richness. Bioscience 62(1):47–55

EEA (2012) Climate change, impacts and vulnerability in Europe 2012. An indicator-based report. European Environment Agency, Copenhagen, Denmark. https://www.eea.europa.eu/publications/climate-impacts-and-vulnerability-2012

EEA (2016) Extreme temperatures and health. European Environment Agency, Copenhagen, Denmark. https://www.eea.europa.eu/data-and-maps/indicators/heat-and-health-2/assessment

EKLIPSE (2017) Types and components of natural or man-made urban and suburban green and blue spaces affecting human mental health *and mental well-being*. Available: http://www.eklipse-mechanism.eu/documents/32503/0/Final_DoW_Health_08092017.pdf/d5e269a2-da6b-4809-9458-fd9747ca383c. Accessed 15 Jan 2018

Frumkin H (2001) Beyond toxicity: human health and the natural environment. Am J Prev Med 20(3):234–240

Frumkin H, Louv R (2007) The powerful link between conserving land and preserving health. Land Trust Alliance, Washington, DC

Frumkin H, Bratman GN, Breslow SJ et al (2017) Nature contact and human health: a research agenda. Environ Health Perspect 125(7):075001. https://doi.org/10.1289/EHP1663

Fuller RA, Irvine KN, Devine-Wright P, Warren PH, Gaston KJ (2007) Psychological benefits of greenspace increase with biodiversity. Biol Lett 3:390–394

Gabriel KM, Endlicher WR (2011) Urban and rural mortality rates during heat waves in Berlin and Brandenburg, Germany. Environ Pollut 159:2044–2050

Geng L, Xu J, Ye L, Zhou W, Zhou K (2015) Connection with nature and environmental behaviors. PLoS One 10(5):e0127247. https://doi.org/10.1371/journal.pone.0127247

Gill SE, Handley JF, Ennos AR, Pauleit S (2007) Adapting cities for climate change: the role of the green infrastructure. Built Environ 33:155–133

Goddard M, Dougill AJ, Benton TG (2010) Scaling up from gardens: biodiversity conservation in urban environments. Trends Ecol Evol 25:90–98. https://doi.org/10.1016/j.tree.2009.07.016

Grifo F, Rosenthal J (eds) (1997) Biodiversity and human health. Island Press, Washington, DC

Hartig T, Mitchell R, de Vries S, Frumkin H (2014) Nature and health. Annu Rev Public Health 35:207–228. https://doi.org/10.1146/annurev-publhealth-032013-182443

Hough R (2014) Biodiversity and human health: evidence for causality? Biodivers Conserv 23:267–288

IPCC (2007) Climate change 2007: the physical science basis. In: Solomon S, Qin D, Manning M, Chen Z, Marquis M, Averyt KB, Tignor M, Miller HL (eds) Contribution of working group I to the fourth assessment report of the intergovernmental panel on climate change. Cambridge University Press, Cambridge. http://www.ipcc.ch/publications_and_data/ar4/wg1/en/contents.html

Irvine KN, Warber SL (2002) Greening healthcare: practicing as if the natural environment really mattered. Altern Ther Health Med 8(5):76–83

Johansson M, Gyllin M, Witzell J, Küller M (2014) Does biological quality matter? Direct and reflected appraisal of biodiversity in temperate deciduous broad-leaf forest. Urban For Urban Green 13:28–37

Kabisch N, Stadler J, Korn H, Bonn A (eds) (2017) Nature-based solutions to climate change in urban areas – Linkages between science, policy and practice, Theory and Practice of Urban Sustainability Transitions. Springer International Publishing, Cham

Kopnina H, Keune H (2010) Health and environment: social science perspectives. Nova Science Publishers, New York

Lovell R, Wheeler BW, Higgins SL, Irvine KN, Depledge MH (2014) A systematic review of the health and wellbeing benefits of biodiverse environments. J Toxicol Environ Health B Crit Rev 17(1):1–20. https://doi.org/10.1080/10937404.2013.856361

Markevych I, Schoierer J, Hartig T et al (2017) Exploring pathways linking greenspace to health: theoretical and methodological guidance. Environ Res 158:301–317. https://doi.org/10.1016/j.envres.2017.06.028

Marselle MR, Irvine KN, Warber SL (2013) Walking for well-being: are group walks in certain types of natural environments better for well-being than group walks in urban environments? Int J Environ Res Public Health 10:5603–5628

Marselle MR, Irvine KN, Lorenzo-Arribas A, Warber SL (2015) Moving beyond green: exploring the relationship of environment type and indicators of perceived environmental quality on emotional well-being following group walks. Int J Environ Res Public Health 12(1):106. https://doi.org/10.3390/ijerph120100106

Marselle MR, Irvine KN, Lorenzo-Arribas A, Warber SL (2016) Does perceived restorativeness mediate the effects of perceived biodiversity and perceived naturalness on emotional well-being following group walks in nature? J Environ Psychol 46:217–232

Marselle MR, Stadler J, Korn H, Bonn A (eds) (2018) Proceedings of the European Conference "Biodiversity and Health in the Face of Climate Change – Challenges, Opportunities and Evidence Gaps". BfN-Skripten 509. Federal Agency for Nature Conservation, Bonn, Germany. https://www.bfn.de/fileadmin/BfN/service/Dokumente/skripten/Skript509.pdf

Mayer FS, Frantz CM, Bruehlman-Senecal E, Dolliver K (2009) Why is nature beneficial? The role of connectedness to Nature. Environ Behav 41(5):607

Morand S, Lajaunie C (eds) (2017) Biodiversity and health: linking life, ecosystems and societies. Elsevier, Oxford

Nesshöver C, Assmuth T, Irvine KN et al (2017) The science, policy and practice of nature-based solutions: an interdisciplinary perspective. Sci Total Environ 579:1215–1227

Niemela J (1999) Ecology and urban planning. Biodivers Conserv 8:119–131

Nilsson K, Sangster M, Gallis C et al (eds) (2011) Forest, trees and human health. Springer, Dordrecht

Pearlmutter D, Calfapietra C, Samson R et al (eds) (2017) The urban forest: cultivating green infrastructure for people and the environment. Springer, Cham

Prévot A-C, Cheval H, Raymond R, Cosquer A (2018) Routine experiences of nature in cities can increase personal commitment toward biodiversity conservation. Biol Conserv 226:1–8. https://doi.org/10.1016/j.biocon.2018.07.008

Sandifer PA, Sutton-Grier AE, Ward BP (2015) Exploring connections among nature, biodiversity, ecosystem services, and human health and well-being: opportunities to enhance health and biodiversity conservation. Ecosyst Serv 12:1–15. https://doi.org/10.1016/j.ecoser.2014.12.007

ten Brick P, Mutafogla K, Schweitzer J et al. (2016) The health and social benefits of nature and biodiversity protection. Institute for European Environmental Policy (IEEP), London/Brussels. https://ieep.eu/publications/new-study-on-the-health-and-social-benefits-of-biodiversity-and-nature-protection. Accessed 30 July 2018

United Nations Convention on Biological Diversity (1992) Convention on Biological Diversity. https://www.cbd.int/doc/legal/cbd-en.pdf. Accessed 12 July 2018

Watts N, Adger WN, Agnolucci P et al (2015) Health and climate change: policy responses to protect public health. Lancet 386:1861–1914

Wheeler BW, Lovell R, Higgins SL et al (2015) Beyond greenspace: an ecological study of population general health and indicators of natural environment type and quality. Int J Health Geogr 14(1):17. https://doi.org/10.1186/s12942-015-0009-5

WHO (2017a) Fact sheets on sustainable development goals: health targets for noncommunicable diseases. World Health Organization Regional Office for Europe, Copenhagen, Denmark. http://www.euro.who.int/__data/assets/pdf_file/0007/350278/Fact-sheet-SDG-NCD-FINAL-25-10-17.pdf?ua=1. Accessed 30 July 2018

WHO (2017b) Noncommunicable diseases. World Health Organization regional Office for Europe, Copenhagen, Denmark. http://www.euro.who.int/en/health-topics/noncommunicable-diseases. Accessed 13 July 2018

WHO (2017c) Urban green space interventions and health: a review of impacts and effectiveness. World Health Organization regional Office for Europe, Copenhagen, Denmark. http://www.euro.who.int/__data/assets/pdf_file/0010/337690/FULL-REPORT-for-LLP.pdf?ua=1. Accessed 30 July 2018

WHO & CBD (2015) Connecting global priorities: biodiversity and human health. A state of the knowledge review. World Health Organization & Secretariat of the Convention on Biological Diversity. http://www.who.int/globalchange/publications/biodiversity-human-health/en/. Accessed 30 July 2018

Wolf T, Lyne K, Martinez GS, Kendrovski V (2015) The health effects of climate change in the WHO European region. Climate 3:901–936

World Health Organization (1948) Constitution of WHO: principles. http://www.who.int/about/mission/en/

Zelenski JM, Dopko RL, Capaldi CA (2015) Cooperation is in our nature: nature exposure may promote cooperative and environmentally sustainable behavior. J Environ Psychol 42:24–31

Part I
Biodiversity and Physical Health

Chapter 2
Biodiversity, Physical Health and Climate Change: A Synthesis of Recent Evidence

Sarah J. Lindley, Penny A. Cook, Matthew Dennis, and Anna Gilchrist

Abstract We are at a point in history marked by unprecedented changes in the environmental foundations of human health and well-being. At the same time, the demands from human populations have never been greater, with profound differences in how we engage with the natural environment. By the middle of this century, when climate change impacts are further increasing, the United Nations expects the global population to be approaching 10 billion. In this chapter, we provide a synthesis of published evidence of the complex and important relationships between elements of biodiversity, health and climate change. We draw primarily on reviews conducted in the past five years supplemented with evidence on additional themes. We also develop a detailed case study example focused on urban climate, climate change and biodiversity, taken from the perspective of a large and representative conurbation. The case study uses a body of existing published evidence together with new data and insights to demonstrate important pathways, impacts and outcomes. We end by identifying a set of research questions and stress the need for even more extensive multi-disciplinary and multi-sector approaches. Nevertheless, despite the need for more knowledge, it is already clear that more effective action could, and should, be taken.

Keywords Biodiversity · Health · Climate · Review · Mechanisms · Urban

---

S. J. Lindley (✉) · M. Dennis
Department of Geography, School of Environment, Education and Development, University of Manchester, Manchester, UK
e-mail: sarah.lindley@manchester.ac.uk

P. A. Cook
School of Health and Society, The University of Salford, Salford, UK
e-mail: p.a.cook@salford.ac.uk

A. Gilchrist
Department of Planning and Environmental Management, School of Environment, Education and Development, University of Manchester, Manchester, UK
e-mail: anna.gilchrist@manchester.ac.uk

M. R. Marselle et al. (eds.), *Biodiversity and Health in the Face of Climate Change*, https://doi.org/10.1007/978-3-030-02318-8_2

Highlights

- Biodiversity, health and climate change have multi-scale and interdependent links.
- Few studies explicitly connect climate change with biodiversity and physical health.
- The full extent of human health impacts from biodiversity losses is unclear.
- Action is needed due to climate projections, biodiversity losses and health demands.
- New research agendas demand ambitious, multi-disciplinary and cross-sector approaches.

2.1 Introduction

Few would now dispute that important links exist between the natural environment and human physical health. Nevertheless, despite considerable progress in conceptualising and understanding relationships, there is still much to learn about particular connections, their underlying mechanisms, causality and inter-relationships (Sandifer et al. 2015; Ziter 2016; Cameron and Blanusa 2016).

Biodiversity is considered one of the underlying requirements for beneficial functioning of ecosystems for human health and well-being and is enshrined as such within policy-focused arenas (Lovell et al. 2014; Sandifer et al. 2015). However, the many interpretations of the term biodiversity, the ways in which it is measured and its inter-relationships with other factors, including climate, present considerable challenges for building and testing hypotheses (Schmeller et al. 2018). Where hypotheses relate to impacts on human health, there are still more elements to consider, including an appreciation of direct and indirect pathways, relevant controls and the interdependencies between psychological and physiological processes.

Climate change is known to be modifying the natural environment and how it functions in relation to human health (Bonebrake et al. 2018). For example, climate affects ecological states and processes. As climate changes, it affects the functioning of ecosystems in terms of the quantity and quality of functions with a beneficial role for human physical health. Climate change is also affecting the relative balance of benefits and disbenefits. Furthermore, it has been implicated as one of the mechanisms driving global biodiversity loss, though in fact it is just one of a suite of factors that remove and degrade associated ecosystems. Data from 63 protected areas in Germany collected over 29 years has shown a three-quarters reduction in the biomass of flying insects, a much higher loss than previously supposed (Hallmann et al. 2017). However, analysis of climate variables suggested no strong climate signal to explain the decline. While not all climate-related factors could be discounted, other large-scale factors were also thought to be contributing, in this case agricultural intensification. Similarly, although climate change leads to health impacts, such as through climate extremes like high temperatures and climate-related events like flooding, health trends are also influenced by social, political and wider environmental factors.

Climate and biodiversity act as important 'boundary conditions' for human health and well-being. These boundary conditions exert an influence on many of the other elements that affect the health and well-being of individuals through natural environments and associated ecosystem functions (Barton and Grant 2006; Dahlgren and Whitehead 2007). The health status of any one person can be seen as a composite of: individual characteristics (e.g. hereditary genetics), the living environment and life experiences, both physical and social (Fig. 2.1 (left)). Health is determined not only through external ecosystem-related processes and factors, but also internal ones, for example, recognising that the human body itself hosts complex and biodiverse ecosystems that have differing impacts on physical health (Garrett 2015; Ruokolainen et al. 2017) (Fig. 2.1 (right)). External factors include the abundance, type and quality of the natural environment underpinned by 'external' biodiversity. Other external factors include social connections (e.g. family and community), access to health infrastructure and income (e.g. through diet). Inevitably, all are related to some extent to wider socio-economic and political contexts.

The overarching aim of this chapter is to summarise the current evidence of the links between nature, biodiversity, health and climate change, with a particular emphasis on physical health and well-being, defined as "*the quality and performance of bodily functioning. This includes having the energy to live well, the capacity to sense the external environment and our experiences of pain and comfort*"

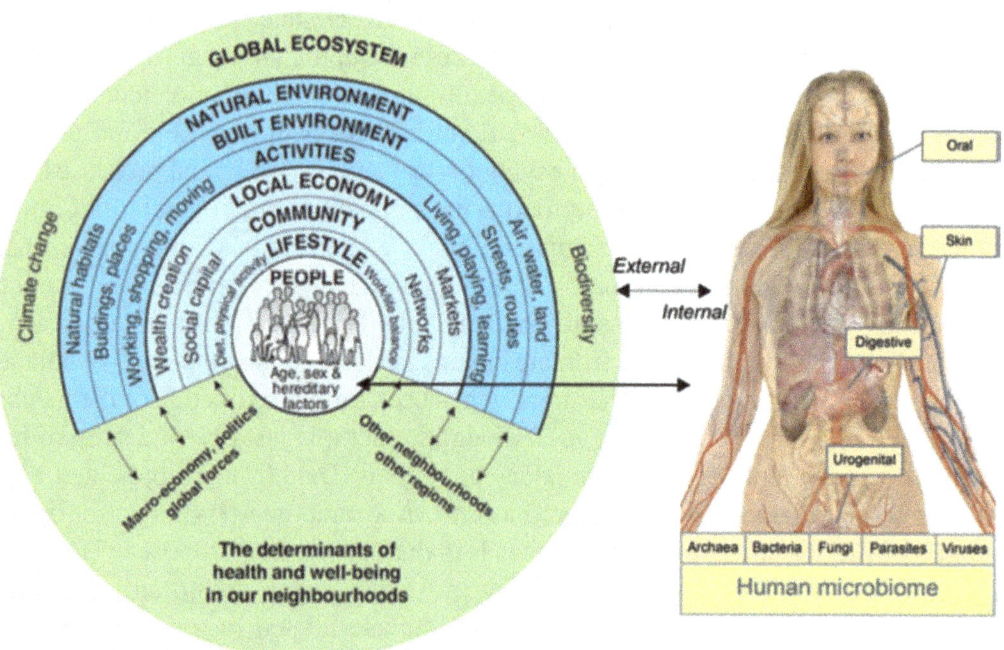

Fig. 2.1 Determinants of human health and well-being (Barton and Grant 2006, based on Dahlgren and Whitehead 1991), including biodiversity at the human scale (after Garrett 2015, Ruokolainen et al. 2017)

(Linton et al. 2016). In the summary, we primarily draw on existing reviews conducted in the past five years supplemented with review evidence on additional themes such as diet. The chapter also covers three sub-aims. First, we consider the evidence for nature's contributions to physical health from the broad perspective of the natural environment (see Sect. 2.2). We look at direct and indirect ways that natural systems influence human health and well-being with reference to the 11 body systems. Given that the body's systems are highly interconnected, the discussion inevitably connects with material presented in other chapters in this volume (e.g. Cook et al. Chap. 11, this volume). Within the scope of this review and synthesis, it is also inevitable that not all of the evidence can be covered. Nevertheless, the section shows some of the key mechanisms through which human physical health is influenced, according to the most recent literature. Second, we aim to take a closer look at the importance of different forms of 'nature', but with a particular focus on biodiversity (see Sect. 2.3). In cities, nature is often thought of as essential urban green infrastructure – the means through which vital ecological and biodiversity-related functions (e.g. habitat provision and landscape connectivity) and most nature-derived human benefits are delivered (Benedict and McMahon 2002). However, cities and their populations cannot be considered in isolation. Therefore, the chapter touches on how the protective role of biodiversity operates through diverse pathways, how it functions at different human and geographical scales and when it is most significant during the life course. The protective role includes, but is not limited to, the regulation of disease emergence, micro-nutrient availability for human sustenance and the promotion of contact with symbiotic bacteria necessary for building up tolerances to environmental allergens (Ruokolainen et al. 2017; Rogalski et al. 2017). Thirdly, we provide an overview of some of the important ways that climate change impacts physical health and the natural environment, including through biodiversity (see Sect. 2.4). A particular emphasis is given to how climate change increases potential poor health burdens (including for example in terms of high temperatures and air pollution in urban areas) and also how extreme climate-related events and long-term climatic trends can erode the beneficial physical health effects of nature, green spaces and biodiversity (LWEC 2015; European Environment Agency 2017). Before concluding on emerging research agendas, the chapter ends with a detailed case study example, focused on urban climate, climate change and biodiversity, primarily from the perspective of how the regulating functions of different plant species vary (see Sect. 2.5).

Much of the focus of this chapter is on urban areas. Urban areas are where the majority of the population now resides – nearly three quarters in Europe, with 41% in the most densely populated centres (European Environment Agency 2018) – where stressors on human health and well-being tend to be most extreme. Evidence is drawn primarily from a European context, supplemented with evidence from elsewhere, where possible. It is recognized that this focus gives a particular perspective on connections and the challenges faced that may not be echoed in all contexts.

2.2 Nature's Contributions to Physical Health

In this section, we consider how ecosystems influence human physical health. We discuss direct and indirect pathways which connect the natural environment to human physical health with a particular emphasis on ecosystem regulatory functions (e.g. modification of environmental stressors) and provisioning functions (such as the use of ecosystems by people for food, fresh water and fuel). For example, direct pathways include the health benefits from the consumption of nutritious food and indirect pathways include health benefits due to increased physical activity rates associated with the natural environment. In making this distinction, it is important to note that beyond the more obvious examples given above, the type and form of pathways are not always fully clear. Whether a process is considered direct or indirect may differ depending on the primary consideration in hand, be it human biological systems, physical environmental systems or some specific form of exposure. We consider the evidence from the perspective of the commonly recognised body organ systems, each of which provides a particular function for physical health. The identified body systems are then referenced in subsequent sections of the chapter.

The body has 11 interlinked systems: reproductive, integumentary (skin/hair), skeletal, muscular, nervous (brain/brain activity), circulatory/cardiovascular (blood/transport of nutrients), endocrine (glands/hormones), lymphatic (associated with immune functions), digestive (food), respiratory (breathing) and urinary/renal (waste). Numerous physiological parameters associated with these systems can be measured to determine physical health. In turn, each parameter can be assessed in order to establish underlying mechanisms for the influence of nature, whether through evidenced processes or through ones that are currently only hypothetical. Psychological parameters have been the focus of much of the existing body of research on exposure to nature and the connection between nature and human health. Associated study outcomes have tended to identify positive links between nature and health (Keniger et al. 2013). However, the range of health benefits is much wider, including in terms of cognitive function, social interaction and improved resilience (Sandifer et al. 2015).

Sandifer et al. (2015) identify no fewer than 27 published examples of the physiological health benefits of interaction with nature (broadly defined as living things and associated landscapes in a wide variety of settings). While some are very broad indicators, others refer to specific physiological metrics, including reduced sympathetic/parasympathetic nerve activity, faster healing after illness, surgery or trauma and positive influences on diabetes. Nevertheless, some reviews point to a more inconsistent picture for specific physiological outcomes. For example, positive outcomes are shown for circulatory/cardiovascular, endocrine and immune systems but with a good deal of mixed evidence (Haluza et al. 2014). Figure 2.2 considers evidence from the perspective of different pathways, but also highlights inconsistencies in the evidence base.

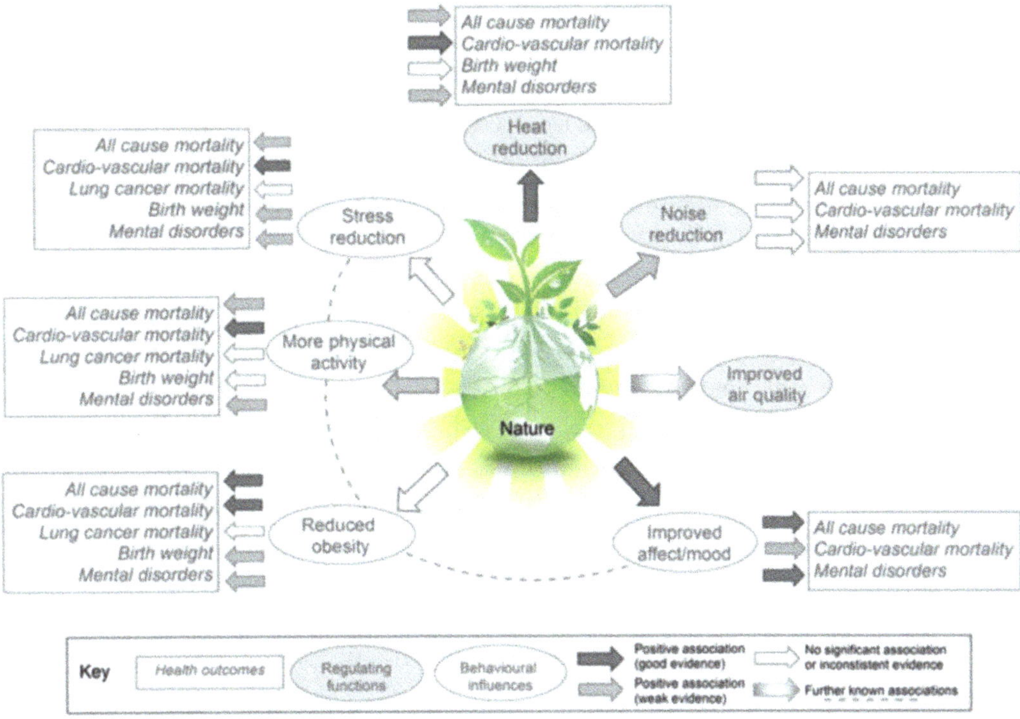

Fig. 2.2 Pathways for physiological outcomes associated with 'exposure to natural environments' (after van den Bosch and Sang 2017)

Interestingly, much of the evidence cited in Haluza et al. (2014) is related to Japan's 'Shinrin-Yoku' (forest-bathing) with most consistency shown for evidence of short-term restorative effects in physiological parameters associated with the cardiovascular, endocrine and immune systems. Studies covered a range of activity types, time periods and populations, but bias is a potential issue due to underreporting of negative or inconclusive findings and a tendency towards short-term studies (Hartig et al. 2014; Haluza et al. 2014). There is less evidence for cumulative effects and therefore how they may translate into measurable mortality and morbidity outcomes (ibid.).

Some of the published evidence relates to effects that are seen as a result of simply being in 'natural' spaces (Haluza et al. 2014). In this context, at least some of the associated mechanisms may be direct, for example physiological responses linked to feelings of well-being inspired by direct engagement with green and blue space (see also Marselle Chap. 7, this volume). Feelings of well-being may come about through impacts on the nervous system and are thus difficult to separate from aspects of psychology and mental health. Nevertheless, the identification of possible direct impacts is important since it suggests that not all of the physical health benefits are associated with physical activity-related physiological responses (given that exercise results in some of the same physiological benefits wherever it is undertaken). That green and blue spaces tend to help to encourage physical exercise is of course also important. More than three quarters of 50 reviewed studies reported positive associations between how green an environment is and physical activity rates (Kaczynski and Henderson 2007 in Coutts and Hahn 2015). Similar positive associations are also found between 'blue' spaces and physical activity rates (Grellier et al. 2017; White et al. 2014) (see also Hunter et al. Chap. 17, this volume). Encouragement of physical activity is particularly important in the context of increases in non-communicable diseases (NCDs) related to inactivity, such as Type 2 diabetes (Cook et al. Chap. 11, this volume).

The other important, and increasingly well recognised, pathway explaining why physiological responses might be seen at rest in 'natural' spaces is due to the regulating functions of green and blue spaces through moderating noise, air quality and temperatures. In other words, some health benefits are due to the influence that green and blue spaces have on removing or reducing environmental stressors, especially in busy, densely populated urban centres (Hartig et al. 2014; Coutts and Hahn 2015; Markevych et al. 2017). Indeed, this also makes physical activity undertaken in urban green spaces potentially more healthy since it could otherwise lead to increased exposure to harmful levels of air pollutants with acute or chronic effects on the respiratory and cardiovascular systems (Mölter and Lindley 2015). However, the 'absence of stressors' argument does not explain all associations, such as have been found in studies where physiological responses are seen in response to visual cues with no direct contact, something that points to psychological and socio-cultural factors (Clark et al. 2014). Due to the interwoven biophysical, psychological and socio-cultural elements underpinning connections between nature and health some conceptualisations are based on grouped biopsychosocial pathways, specifically pathways that positively influence health through reducing the potential for harm (reducing environmental stresses), restoring capacities (improving recovery functions) and building capacities (reducing individual susceptibility to harm) (Hartig et al. 2014; Markevych et al. 2017) (see also Marselle et al. Chap. 9, this volume).

The role of reduced exposure to environmental noise is one particularly interesting example given that reductions in noise exposure have been given relatively little emphasis in earlier models, e.g. Hartig et al. (2014), compared to those developed more recently, e.g. Markevych et al. (2017) and van den Bosch and Sang (2017). Explanatory mechanisms have also been proposed to link noise stress with impacts on cardiovascular, respiratory, immune response and metabolic health through stress-response models (Recio et al. 2016). Similar processes may apply to some of the other common environmental stressors, in addition to the better known, but still imperfectly understood connections. For example, new research is finding a wider range of connections between air pollution and human health than ever before, not just through morbidity and mortality from cardiovascular and respiratory diseases but also through neurodevelopmental disorders and birth defects (Landrigan et al. 2018). It should be remembered that environmental stresses also affect other animals and have been linked to biodiversity loss. Although an issue that is particularly acute in urban areas, anthropogenic sources have been found to elevate noise levels in more than a fifth of protected areas in the USA, reaching levels known to have negative effects on wildlife (Buxton et al. 2017).

Direct physical health outcomes from ecosystem functions may be difficult to evidence for some pathways, but one more obvious direct way that nature influences physical health is through human sustenance and micro-nutrient availability. Primary production from plant materials is the initial source of food energy for all living beings, and humans directly consume 25–50% of the energy embodied in plant-life even before considering the consumption of animals that plants also sustain (Coutts and Hahn 2015). However, human health is not just a matter of the quantity of energy consumed but also its diversity. Diversity in diet and the micro-nutrient supply this provides is something that can be linked to wider ecological biodiversity too (see Sect. 2.3).

Plants and other natural sources are also responsible for a large proportion of the medicines currently in use today, contributing to almost a third of all marketed drug products sold (Coutts and Hahn 2015). Bioactive compounds, and their role in disease prevention and ageing, are still the subject of much important research. For example, evidence for the anti-microbial properties of phenolics in berries is important in the context of growing antibiotic resistance (Paredes-Lopez et al. 2010). Polyphenols from berries also have a range of other positive functional properties, including anti-inflammatory, neuro-protective, anti-oxidant, anti-cancer and anti-mutagenic roles (Nile and Park 2014). Polyphenols are just one of the bioactive compound groups found in berries, which are also rich sources of vitamins and minerals (ibid.). Brassica vegetables are associated with anti-cancer properties as well as a range of other health benefits (Moreno et al. 2006). Other food groups have similar beneficial properties, such as seaweed and fungi.

These provisioning functions of ecosystems (such as the use of ecosystems by people for food, fresh water, fuel and animal forage) are a critical component of human health with a huge literature and evidence base. Fuel from ecosystem sources (e.g. wood) impacts health too, including cooking, facilitating water purification and also via the improved ability for people to moderate living conditions. The connections between provisioning functions and health can be indirect, for example through the role of pollinators in agricultural systems (IPBES 2016). Relationships can be complex with both beneficial and detrimental roles for human health, varying between and within species and also in response to local environmental factors. For example, a recent study of crops across five continents found that some 39% of crop flower visits are from insects other than bee species (such as flies and wasps) and the relative importance varies considerably by crop type and location (Rader et al. 2016). In other contexts, some of these species are regarded as pests and can be associated with negative health effects, such as via food contamination.

2.3 Biodiversity and Physical Health

In this section, we consider the range of connections and pathways between biodiversity and human physical health, beginning with the scale of the human body before looking at processes operating at wider spatial scales. Given that much of the evidence in the previous section considered the natural environment in a broad sense, here we examine how biodiversity metrics are linked to ecosystem functions affecting physical health.

In considering the role of biodiversity on human health it is useful to start by recognising the human body as an ecosystem, with both internal and external microbiota, something that has been termed the human core microbiome (Karkman et al. 2017). The human gut alone contains some 1,014 bacterial strains and species as well as other micro-organisms and viruses, the mix of which is unique to each individual and which changes during the life course (Odamaki et al. 2016; Seksik and Landman 2015). The concept of the exposome has been developed to recognize the role of factors shown in Fig. 2.1 in determining human health and well-being, the significance of environment and how human health is affected by cumulative influences over time, and therefore the life course (Renz et al. 2017). Renz et al. (2017) further propose the meta-exposome as a means of connecting human exposures with those of the wider biosphere and linking ecosystem health at all scales to human health (Fig. 2.3), a notion that is echoed elsewhere (e.g. Sandifer et al. 2015).

Major microbiota colonisation events are associated with particular parts of the human life cycle, such as birth, but continue throughout the life course dependent on lifestyle, environment and exposure (Ruokolainen et al. 2017). The so-called 'old friends' hypothesis also relates to this process of gaining health benefits from beneficial symbiotic microbes. Benefits are associated with many of the body organ systems and are multi-functional. For example, as well as helping with the healthy development of the immune system, beneficial microbes can also perform protective roles when human hosts encounter allergens (Rook 2013; Ruokolainen et al. 2017). Both environmental and behavioural factors are involved in the development of dysbiosis, where alterations in microbiota may result in a negative cycle of ill-heath (Fig. 2.3). Dysbiosis is also implicated in problems associated with the integumentary, digestive and urinary/renal systems as well as disorders in the respiratory and cardiovascular systems (Carding et al. 2015; Renz et al. 2017). Lack of contact with sources of symbiotic microbiota is one of the outcomes of people's growing 'extinction of experience' of natural environments, and lack of contact even of itself tends to promote greater disassociation (Cox and Gaston 2018).

Of course, biodiversity does not just affect human health through the body's own ecosystem. As well as affecting humans directly, such microbiota relationships also underpin the healthy functioning of wider ecosystems on which humans depend (Flandroy et al. 2018). Biodiversity is also important at community, neighbourhood and regional scales. For example, in Australia, where 31% of the population are estimated to be affected by long-term respiratory conditions, after socio-economic factors, the second and third most important determinants of

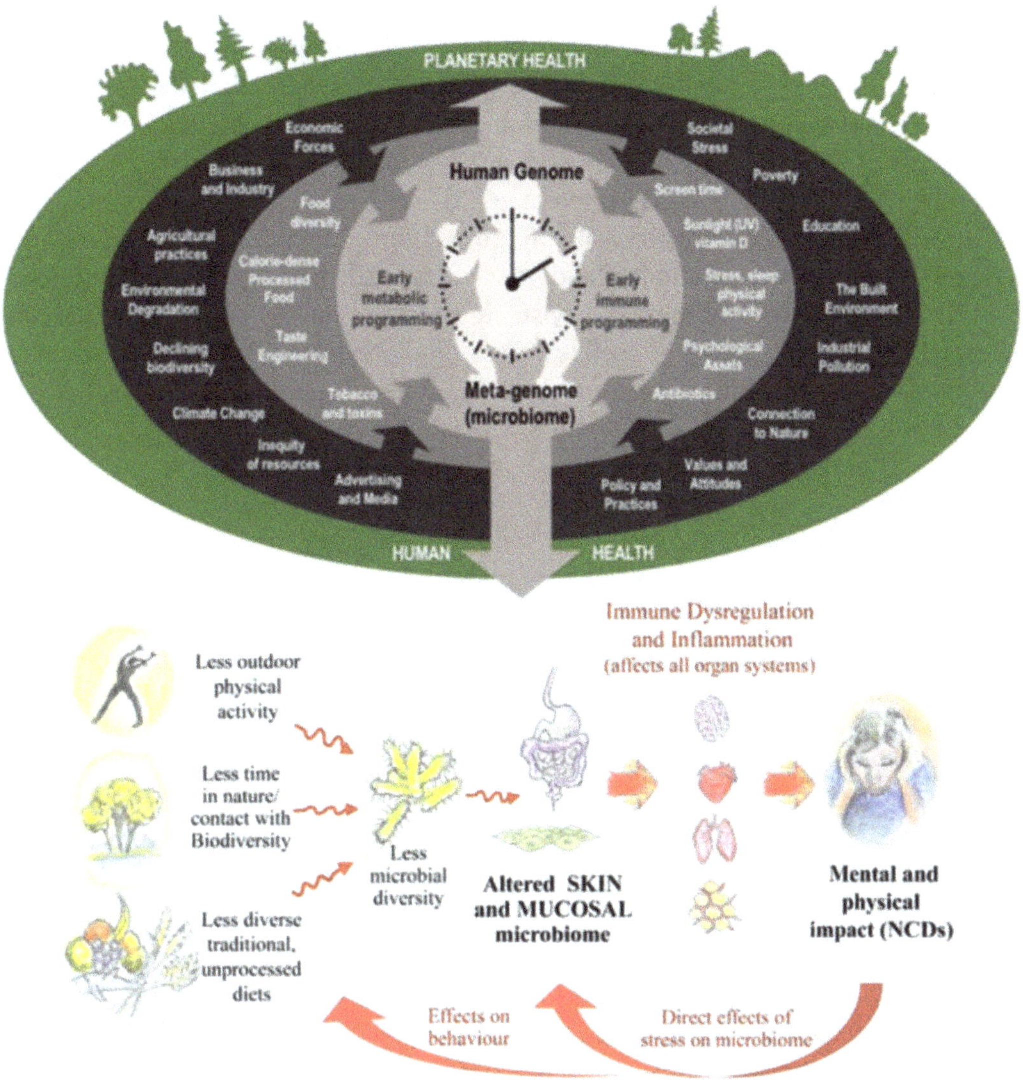

Fig. 2.3 The inter-relationships between human and ecological health as expressed through the exposome concept (top) and the pathways to reductions in physical health through dysbiosis (bottom) (Renz et al. 2017)

positive respiratory health are associated with landscape biodiversity (vegetation diversity and species richness) (Liddicoat et al. 2018). Many critical ecosystem processes operate on much larger spatial scales and ultimately impact global processes through the effect that ecosystems exert on wider natural systems, such as climate, water and air quality, and the impact that they have on food nutritional quality and diversity (Harrison et al. 2014; Ziter 2016; Schwarz et al. 2017). Nutritional diversity is important for ensuring good physical health (Lovell et al. 2014), but biodiversity in agricultural systems is important for a range of other reasons, such as supporting ecosystem health (and therefore functions such as pollination and soil regulation) and protecting against potential problems from pests and diseases in large areas of monoculture crops (Dobson et al. 2006). In turn, biodiversity ultimately affects human health by making agricultural systems more inherently resilient and less liable to large scale losses (Dobson et al. 2006). Evidence also suggests a link between biodiversity and the productivity of systems for human use, for example more biodiverse woodlands and fisheries are more productive for fuel and food (Harrison et al. 2014).

In order to understand mechanisms in more detail, it is necessary to unpack the concept of biodiversity and understand how, where and when its different elements are important. Otherwise, there is considerable potential for uncertainty and the potential to equate 'ecosystem services' and 'biodiversity' so that they are seen as essentially the same thing (Mace et al. 2012). Indeed, there is still considerable disagreement about which ecosystem and biodiversity metrics should be considered (ibid.), with most reviews considering metrics beyond those implied by the definition used to frame this volume. Figure 2.4 shows two examples of diagrammatic representations of biodiversity metrics and the functions of ecosystems known to influence human health, a number of which relate to the pathways that have already been identified in Sect. 2.2.

Figure 2.4 (top) identifies a range of biodiversity metrics of different levels of complexity and summarises the available evidence on how they relate to ecosystem functions that have a useful role for people in urban areas. Some of the connections are identified as being positive (red – beneficial for functions) while others are negative (blue – detrimental for functions). For example, Schwarz et al. (2017) (Fig. 2.4 (top)) reviewed 82 studies that examined taxonomic diversity and its links to useful ecosystem functions in urban areas. The studies identified positive connections through pollination, soil protection and fertility, pest control, fresh water and environmental regulation. However, the studies also identified some negative connections, even for these same pathways. Therefore, even taking the one example of urban ecosystems, the extent to which there are positive compared to negative effects depends on context and perspective (Díaz et al. 2018). Some of the biodiversity metrics, such as functional identity (associated with 22 studies) were found to have only positive effects on urban ecosystem functions. While it may be assumed that these effects are then positive for human health, this claim cannot be made on the basis of the review findings alone. Figure 2.4 (bottom) identifies ecological elements acting as 'Ecosystem Service Providers', i.e. the conduits through which the various biotic attributes listed act to benefit or harm human beings. For example, a wide range of function providers exist for pest regulation, from single species to functional groups and whole habitats. In this case, most studies have connected pest regulation to species within single functional groups. There are fewer studies considering multiple functional groups which makes cross-connections more difficult to determine. Ultimately considering the impacts of environmental stressors, including climate change, will require the systematic investigation of cross connections and whole ecosystem responses.

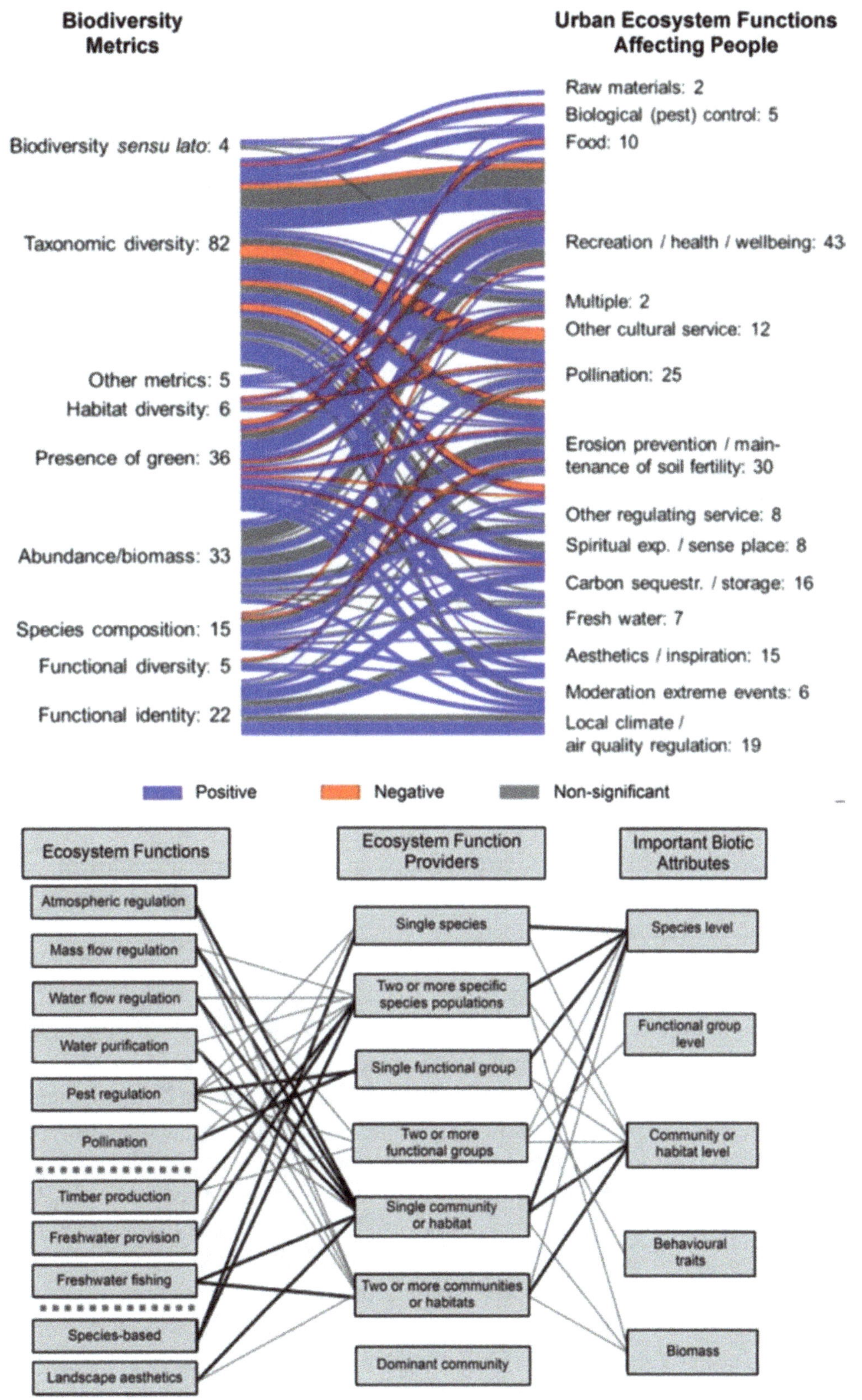

Fig. 2.4 Biodiversity metrics and some of the ecosystem functions underpinning physical human health (top – Schwarz et al. 2017; bottom – Harrison et al. 2014). Linear connections denote the metrics that have been explored, line-width shows the relative proportion of studies and line-colours (top only) indicate the type of associations found

2.4 Climate Change and Physical Health

Climate is an inherent part of the natural systems that are associated with both biodiversity and physical health. Therefore, climate change is similarly interconnected with the processes discussed in the previous two sections, particularly in the context of rapid changes that go beyond the pace of autonomous adaptive capacity and in the context of other drivers of change, such as urbanisation (Fisher et al. 2017). Climate change has direct and indirect influences on the underlying mechanisms of processes discussed in the previous sections. Direct impacts on human health include, for example, the influence of higher temperatures on heat stress in urban dwellers. Indirect impacts include how climate change affects evaporative cooling in urban areas through which people's exposure to high temperature events may be reduced. In this section, we consider the ways in which climate change affects physical health and the role of the natural environment, both generally and through biodiversity. Since biodiversity is also affected by climate change, the section ends with an assessment of climate impacts on the biosphere, particularly in terms of the functions and processes identified in the previous sections as being important for human health.

There are numerous reviews of the deleterious effects of accelerated anthropogenic climate change on natural systems and on human health, as well as those that point to some of the possible benefits. Reviews include the following direct/indirect and primary/secondary pathways (LWEC 2015; European Environment Agency 2017; Fig. 2.5).

- *Health effects of heat and heat waves*

Heat-waves are estimated to have resulted in cumulative death rates of 129.0 people per million in Europe between 1991 and 2015, 24 times higher than the next highest most severe extreme weather-related hazards in terms of death rates (which are cold- and flood-related events at 5.3 and 6.4 people per million respectively; European Environment Agency 2017). Heat-waves are well known to be associated with excess deaths particularly in older people, people with pre-existing health problems and people living in urban areas, for example based on analyses of the 2003 European heat-wave (Johnson et al. 2004; Grize et al. 2005; Poumadere et al. 2005). Excess death rates have also been recorded in cities across the world, e.g. in Chicago, Melbourne and Moscow, including cities with populations already adapted to relatively high temperatures (Norton et al. 2015; Burkart et al. 2014). Evidence from the UK suggests that cardiovascular causes result in the larger number of deaths, though tending to be more associated with atrial fibrillation or pulmonary heart disease compared to other heart diseases. Furthermore, excessive heat seems to be most strongly associated with causes of deaths related to the endocrine, nervous and urinary/renal systems (Arbuthnott and Hajat 2017). People with dementia and on some prescribed medications may also be susceptible to heat-related hospitalisation and mortality, possibly due to higher potential for dehydration and/or reduced ability to sweat (Stollberger et al. 2009). The frequency and severity

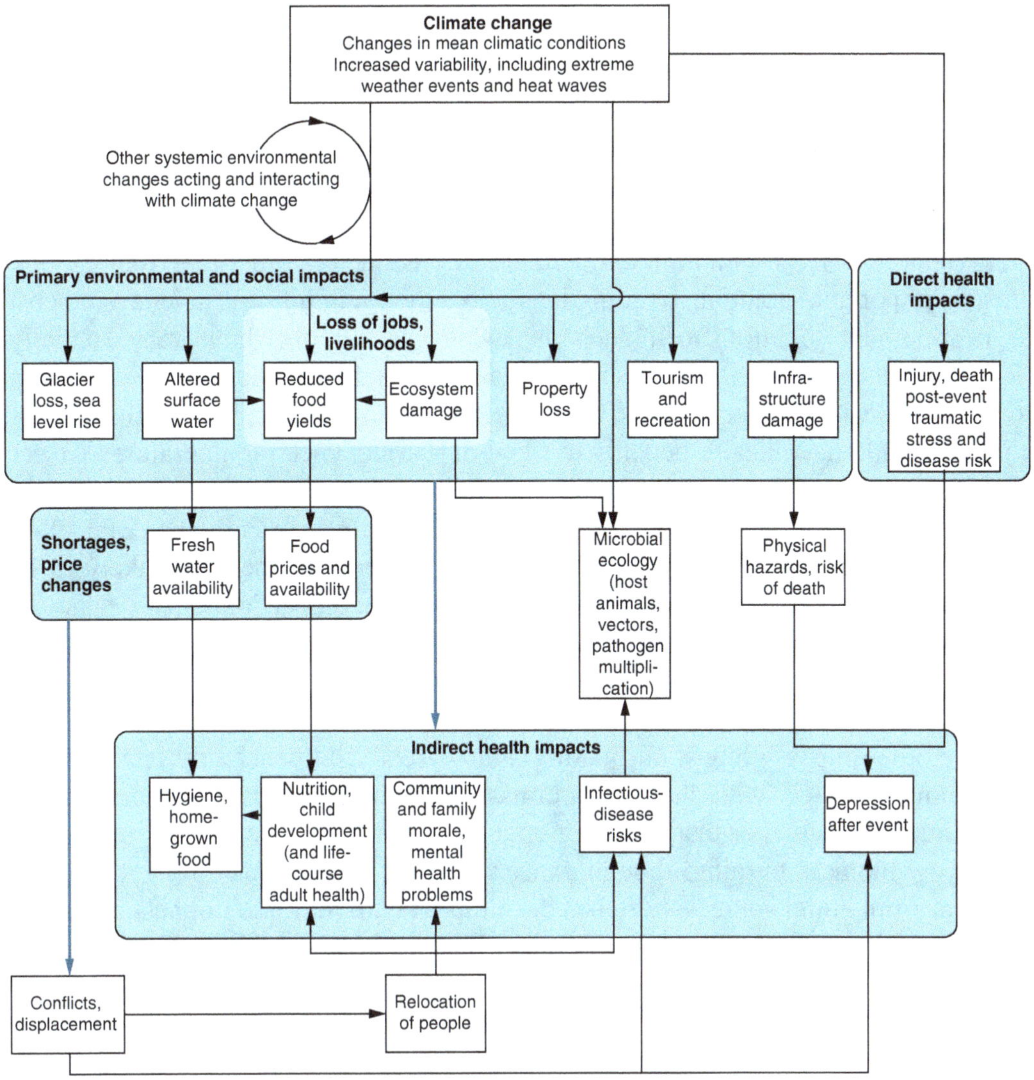

Fig. 2.5 Pathways through which climate change can influence human health and well-being, including though ecosystem-related effects. (McMichael 2013 in European Environment Agency 2017)

(duration and intensity) of events are expected to increase in the future and to be compounded further by other influencing trends, such as an ageing population with higher sensitivity to impacts, the potential for maladaptation in some health and social care systems and the potential for combined impacts from other climate-related hazards, such as drought, fire and poor air quality (European Environment Agency 2017; Curtis et al. 2017). However, there are also moderating factors, for example, analyses over recent decades in the south of England found no evidence of a substantial worsening of heat-related mortality trends, something that analysts have attributed to successes in national scale adaptation actions and improvements in health and health systems more generally (Arbuthnott and Hajat 2017).

- *Health effects of milder winters*

Cold weather events are well known to be associated with excess mortality and morbidity (European Environment Agency 2017). For example, all of the UK's devolved nations report increases in all-cause mortality with reducing temperatures below health-related baselines, though mortality tends to be due to secondary impacts on the cardiovascular and respiratory systems rather than due to hyperthermia (Hajat 2017). As with high temperature events, factors other than temperature are also important, including building insulation, the availability, efficiency and cost of heating and social factors, such as awareness, all of which vary spatially (Robinson et al. 2018). By extension, milder winters do not necessarily result in a reduction in cold weather impacts. Nevertheless, all other things being equal milder winters should have health benefits in view of warmer mean temperatures (fewer Heating Degree Days) and fewer extreme cold-weather events (European Environment Agency 2017). Incidence rates and timings of influenza and other infectious diseases are linked to climatic drivers, therefore there are likely to be secondary effects. Although changes have been observed in influenza peaks and seasons, climatic and other determinants are currently uncertain (Caini et al. 2018).

- *Outdoor air quality*

Like other impact groups, air quality is also greatly influenced by factors other than climate change, with changes in emissions being particularly important over short time horizons. For example, regional haze in South East Asia is ultimately caused by biomass burning, though exacerbated by other climate-related factors. Even far from initial sources, haze has been linked with multiple impacts on physical health, including through the respiratory and cardiovascular systems due to the predominance of fine particulate matter (<2.5 μm) as well as impacts on agriculture and tourism (Latif et al. 2018). Despite the influence of other factors, studies suggest that over the longer term there are likely to be climate penalties associated with a number of air pollutants known to impact both human and ecosystem health e.g. ozone and particulate matter (though with considerable uncertainty). Dust storms are more directly associated with climatic factors and changes in wind and precipitation are likely to affect the distribution and extent of associated health burdens, including respiratory, cardiovascular and infectious diseases (Schweitzer et al. 2018). Alongside more gradual changes to baseline air quality affecting annual average concentrations and chronic human health effects, climate change therefore also has a role in determining the frequency and severity of meteorological conditions that give rise to episodes of poor air quality. Air quality episodes with elevated concentrations of air pollutants can lead to a range of chronic and acute diseases, evidenced by health outcomes that include increased hospital admissions and excess morbidity and mortality rates. The stagnation events associated with air quality episodes can also be associated with summer heat waves and therefore have cumulative outcomes for human health (Doherty et al. 2017).

- *Flooding and health*

Flood events are frequently associated with storms and landslips, which themselves have high numbers of people directly affected, but there are also long-term and indirect impacts from events, such as increased exposure to disease (European Environment Agency 2017). There are numerous pathways through which health impacts are felt and they operate both during flood events and after them, frequently affecting people who have heightened sensitivity due to age or existing health status. Drowning, electrocution and other physical injury may lead to mortality during these events, as well as morbidity associated with injuries, illness from water-borne disease, carbon monoxide poisoning due to the use of generators and cardiovascular effects due the stress of being affected (Lowe et al. 2013). Many of these morbidity factors are also associated with the period following flood events, which is sometimes long and exacerbated by displacement. Lack of power and water supply disproportionately affects people with pre-existing illness and poor mobility and inhibits access to health and social care services, something that can be particularly important when essential medicines have been lost or contaminated (Fernandez et al. 2002; Klinger et al. 2014).

- *Emerging infections*

Infectious disease is inevitably influenced by human factors and mobility. However, redistributions of species through climatic change and climatic triggers are also recognised as having a key role in major events in history, such as the bubonic plague in Europe (Bonebrake et al. 2018). Novel species assemblages are expected to be associated with new emergences in the future. See Müller et al. (Chap. 4, this volume) for more on vector-borne diseases and climate change.

- *Impacts of extreme events on health services and social care*

In addition to differences in levels of demand for services, the services themselves can be impacted, indirectly affecting physical health. Social, institutional and physical infrastructure systems are interconnected and impacts on one will affect how others are able to operate during heat waves, cold weather events and other climate-related hazards, for example affecting mobility/transport, storage/distribution of medicines, the operation, reliability and efficiency of energy systems, availability of fresh water and access to record systems (Curtis et al. 2017).

- *Food- and water-borne disease and contamination*

There are known linkages between climate and the prevalence of food and water borne diseases. They include: campylobacter (seasonal, related to rainfall amounts/timing and higher temperatures), salmonella (warmer temperatures and flooding, due to potential for contamination), listeria (humidity), vibrio (summer, brackish water), cryptosporidium (drinking/recreational water affected by heavy rain/flooding) and norovirus (winter, flooding/high rainfall) (European Environment Agency 2017). However, the likelihood of higher incidence rates depends on many other factors. For example, strong positive associations between elevated temperatures and cases of food poisoning from salmonella could lead to increases in future cases, but future estimates need to be considered in the light of successes in interventions that have led to a low incidence rate in recent years. While the picture for salmonella is one of relative control and decline, this is not true for all intestinal infectious diseases and sometimes knowledge of climatic responses is insufficient to make full assessments (Lake 2017).

- *Pollens and other allergens*

Changing human behaviour is also a factor in terms of the extent to which exposures are changed due to a changing climate, something that is likely to affect a range of other stressors. These issues are discussed in more detail in Damialis et al. (Chap. 3, this volume).

- *Drought and water scarcity*

The availability of, and access to, water resources is a basic human need and one that is inextricably linked with physical health. Climate change is known to be modifying the cryosphere and affecting fresh water resources (European Environment Agency 2017). Although not the only determinant of water scarcity – where much is driven by socio-political factors and other issues such as water quality and distribution – no account of climate change and physical health would be complete without recognising the essential associations between water and other aspects of health.

- *Wildfires and health*

Climate change influences the likelihood and severity of wildfires as a result of extending the ‘fire season’, the higher susceptibility of vegetation to burn when coming in contact with ignition sources (e.g. due to being water stressed) and the greater likelihood of spread due to the potential for increased growth rates (European Environment Agency 2017; Carporn and Emmett 2009). In the United States it has been estimated that annual respiratory hospital admissions ranged from 5200 to 8500 and cardiovascular hospital admissions from 1500 to 2500 between 2008 and 2012 due to $PM_{2.5}$ associated with wildland fires (Fann et al. 2018).

Although not an exhaustive list, a considerable number of the themes above are clearly related to ecosystems. Climate change is recognised as one of the main pressures on ecosystems, alongside habitat change and fragmentation, invasive species, land management changes and pollution (European Environment Agency 2017). Climate induced changes have been observed in all land (e.g. changes in species ranges and phenological responses), freshwater (e.g. changes in flow, also related to changes in human extraction rates which are partly climate-related) and marine ecosystems (e.g. changes in species ranges, acidification and sea level rise) (ibid.). Agricultural systems can see both benefits and stresses, the former in terms of increased opportunities through extension of the growing season and the potential for enhanced photosynthesis, but also tempered with the potential for climate extremes, irrigation demand and availability, increased incidence and new emergence of pests and diseases, and unintended consequences resulting from changes to farming practices (European Environment Agency 2017; Bonebrake et al. 2018).

The balance between positive and negative influences is likely to vary geographically and over time and issues of the transmission of risk must also be considered (Challinor et al. 2018).

Human factors are a key component of the systems through which health effects occur. For example, climate affects transportation networks with higher temperatures making the distribution of perishable goods more challenging and higher rainfall potentially increasing the probability of contamination. Given the increasing concentration of people in urban areas, remote from areas of production, these challenges become more acute. Climate can also affect the nutritional value of some produce. Picking up the example of berries from Sect. 2.2, it is known that climate factors have an influence on the concentrations of phenolics. Phenolic concentrations can also be affected by storage conditions and ripeness as well as species, variety, location and associated environmental interactions (Teixeira et al. 2013; Kellogg et al. 2010; Paredes-Lopez et al. 2010). Thus, the potential for changes in nutritional values of crops as well as their yields under climate change is also a consideration. Diseases and changing distributions of pests and weeds may also affect livestock and fisheries both directly and indirectly (e.g. through the availability of foodstocks) with secondary impacts on human health (European Environment Agency 2017). We have much still to learn of the impact of climate change on ecosystems and biodiversity, including how the interconnections are being felt through mechanisms like the human biome.

2.5 Exploring a Subset of Interactions Through an Urban Case Study

The previous sections have shown the complexities of interconnections between biodiversity, climate change and physical health. To explore the complexities further we present a case study which synthesizes evidence from some of the identified links for Manchester, UK. The conurbation of Greater Manchester in the north of England has a population of around 2.6 million people and covers an area of around 1,280 km^2. Despite being one of England's largest city-regions, Greater Manchester has been used as a representative urban case in previous studies (Lindley et al. 2006). The case for Greater Manchester being representative has been made due to its varied population and urban character. It is also exposed to a range of different hazards and although some parts of the city are affected by flooding – some of them severely – there is no single hazard which dominates the conurbation as a whole in terms of population risk, physical health or associated decision-making. Accordingly, the representativeness and body of existing research for Greater Manchester make it a good basis for a more focused examination compared with cities that are more distinctive in environmental or political terms. The case study starts from the perspective of high temperatures and heat-waves and through that considers wider impacts and links with other environmental characteristics and processes, including some of the biodiversity metrics underpinning how ecosystems influence health outcomes examined in the previous sections.

The Urban Heat Island (UHI) effect is the well-recognised phenomenon whereby cities and towns are often much warmer than surrounding rural areas, particularly at night after calm, sunny days (Oke 1982). The effect can exacerbate the potential for human exposures during periods of high temperature (Wilby 2003). The UHI effect is primarily generated as a result of the physical properties of urban materials, their structure and – to a lesser extent – their use, e.g. through anthropogenic heat emissions (Smith et al. 2009). Built materials have different radiative and thermal storage properties compared to natural surfaces, with the former tending to absorb direct and diffuse short-wave radiation during the day and later re-radiate stored energy back to the atmosphere as long-wave radiation. Where there is higher sky-view factor (the amount of sky which is visible from a point on the ground) stored energy can be re-radiated quickly. However, geometries in cities are complex and low sky-view factor tends to inhibit the loss of long-wave radiation leading to a heating of overlying air during periods of low wind speeds and/or due to inhibited wind flows (Lindberg 2007). In urban areas there is also a relative lack of vegetation and water, which provide cooling functions through evapotranspiration and surface shading in the case of large vegetation stands (Sproken-Smith and Oke 1999). Due to their cooling properties, large areas of vegetation and water within cities play an important role in offsetting urban temperatures, with even modest amounts having an effect (Bowler et al. 2010).

An analysis of temperature records for Manchester has shown that UHI intensities have been increasing over time (Levermore et al. 2017). If trends continue to the end of the century, increases will be similar to those expected with climate change (medium emissions scenario). Increased UHI intensities are likely to be associated with more severe heat-wave events in the future. In the north west of England, a heat-wave is defined as a period of time where the maximum temperature exceeds 30 °C for 2 days with a minimum temperature of ≥ 15 °C in the intervening night. Using this definition, the number of heat waves is not expected to increase dramatically by the 2050s (according to the central estimate of the UKCIP09 projections (high emissions scenario)) (Cavan 2010). However, estimates based on climate projections do not explicitly consider the additional UHI effect on temperatures (Jenkins et al. 2009). Even without the UHI effect being considered, the number of days exceeding 30 °C is expected to be around three per annum by the 2050s (Cavan 2010). Monitoring of the UHI carried out between May and August 2010 demonstrated that the UHI effect can add up to 6 °C (day) and 8 °C (night) in some locations in Greater Manchester (Cheung 2011). The conurbation could also see up to a 3.4 °C (2.4 °C) increase in the temperature of the warmest summer day (night), according to the central estimate of the UKCIP09 projections (high emissions scenario) with these highest increases expected for the upland Pennine fringe (Cavan 2010).

Archival studies show that high temperatures in Manchester, even those that could be considered relatively modest elsewhere, are associated with increased hospital admissions rates and excess mortality. In July 2006, an estimated 140 excess deaths in the region were associated with elevated temperatures which reached a peak of 31.3 °C measured at the airport on the southern periphery of the Greater Manchester urban area (Smith and Lawson 2012). Some of the excess deaths from past high temperature events in Greater Manchester are not only directly heat-related but also due to drownings from swimming in open waters and waterways as well as respiratory problems due to elevated air pollution concentrations and extremely high pollen counts (ibid.). Other impacts include from infrastructure damage and delay (road and rail), water restrictions and fires, both within the city and in the upland hinterlands (see Box 2.1).

Box 2.1 Heat-Related Events and Their Impacts: Evidence from Summer 2018 in the Case Study Area

Late June/early July 2018 saw a particularly long warm, dry period in Greater Manchester. Between 22 June and 6 July 2018 there were more than five consecutive dry days with ten of those dry days seeing peak temperatures >25 °C. This is compared with a longer-term June/July average of 64.5/67.3 mm rainfall, 9.7/11.7 rain days (>1 mm rain) and peak temperatures of 18.4/20.2 °C (1982–2010 averages) (Met Office 2018). At the time of writing the event was ongoing, with a Level 3 Heatwave action issued and with the national meteorological office reporting a probable lack of rainfall lasting a month (Manchester Evening News 2018). Peak temperatures exceeded 30 °C (Fig. 2.6 (top)) and were certainly considerably higher in the city centre where there is no official meteorological station.

The warm, dry conditions contributed to the development of a moorland fire on Saddleworth moor (near Oldham, Greater Manchester), which was so extreme that the army was called to assist fire fighters, schools were closed and local residents evacuated (BBC 2018). The resultant smoke was extensive and severe enough to trigger smoke alarms in buildings in Manchester city centre more than 15 km away (University of Manchester, *pers. com.*). At least two other large moorland fires on Bolton's Winter Hill to the north of the city also affected an area greater than 10 km^2 (BBC 2018). At least one industrial fire occurred in Rochdale to the north east of the conurbation. The combined effects of the fires, high temperatures and wind flows led to elevated air pollutant concentrations in terms of ozone, fine particulate matter and nitrogen dioxide (Fig. 2.6 (bottom)).

All of these pollutants are regulated for public health. Although no evidence of health effects has yet emerged, it is highly likely that they occurred. Fig. 2.7 provides a rich picture of the expected links between ecosystems, human health and key climate-related indicators.

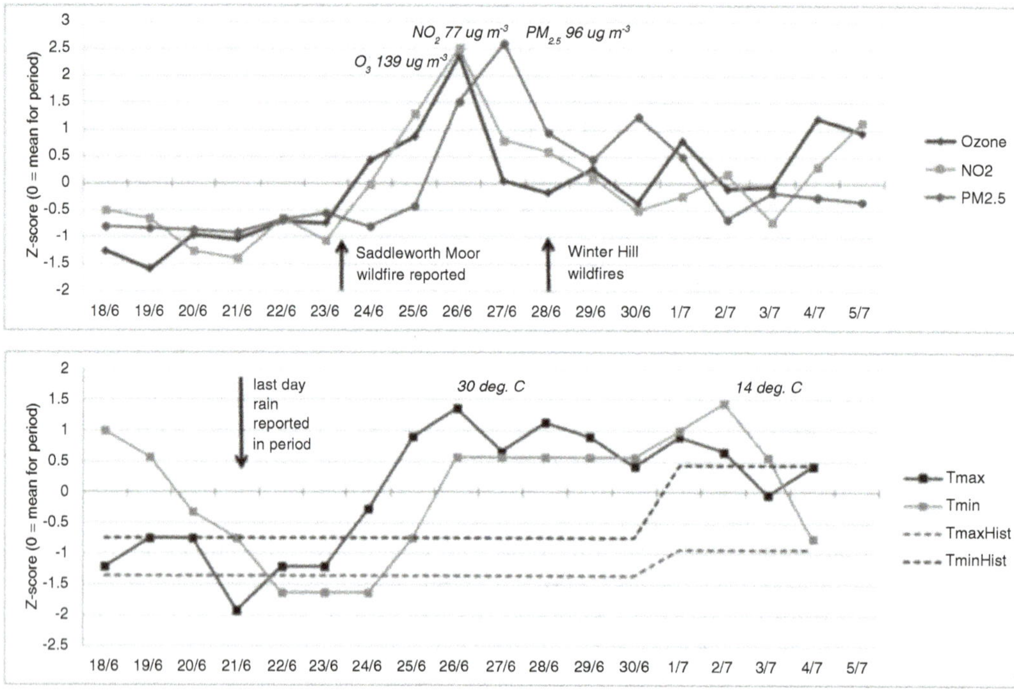

Fig. 2.6 Peak daily concentrations of air pollutants monitored for human health (top) and maxima and minima air temperatures (bottom). The x-axis represents the mean for the period with the y-axis showing the extent of deviation around that mean (as standard deviations). Actual values are shown for the peak days/hours (developed from data sourced from: Defra, Rainchester.com, Accuweather, Met Office, Manchester Evening News and the BBC)

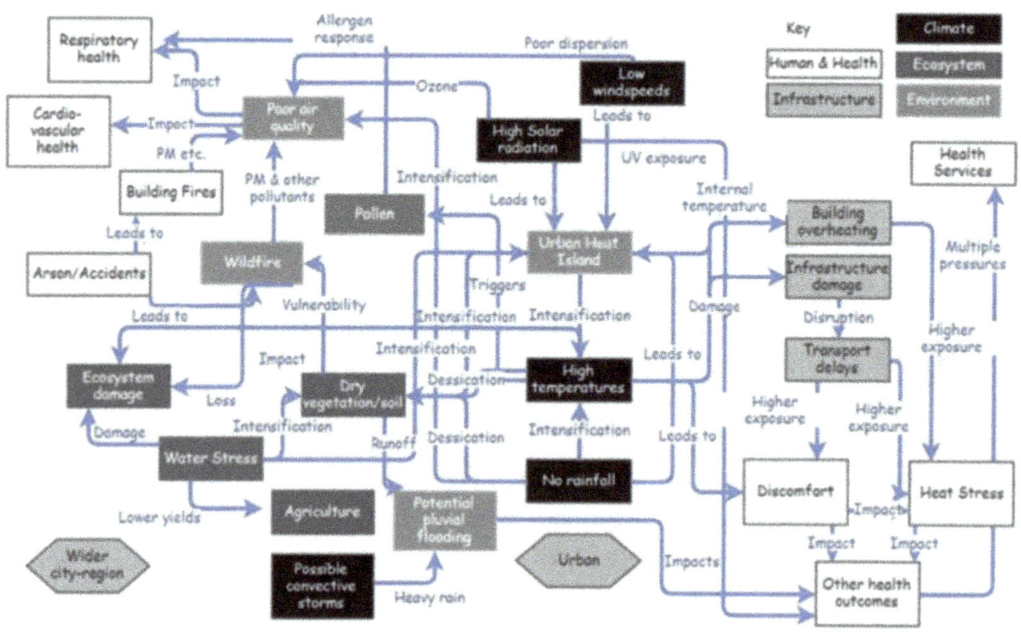

Fig. 2.7 Complex interactions of high temperature events with environmental stressors and health effects. Synthesis of evidence from Box 2.1 and Sect. 2.5

The trend towards an increasing frequency and severity of heat-related events is significant not only due to impacts on human health, but also due to the implications for energy demand for space cooling as people start to autonomously adapt. Even in relatively cool Manchester, modelling studies suggest that the summer UHI increases air conditioning loads by ~7–8% (Skelhorn et al. 2017). The UHI effect is then an additional factor to consider on top of the estimated mean of 13 cooling degree days per year (days where the mean temperature exceeds 22 °C) under the high emissions scenario central estimate for the 2050s (Cavan 2010). More chiller energy is likely to be required to maintain comfortable temperatures, particularly for people who have higher sensitivities to ill-effects, e.g. due to age or pre-existing health conditions (Lindley et al. 2011). It is also highly likely that autonomous adaptation will lead to increases in air conditioning, but only for those who can afford it.

One of the drivers of increasing UHI is urban densification and associated losses of green cover. For example, green cover around Manchester's urban weather station has reduced by ~11% (2000–2009). Impacts are corroborated by modelling, showing that replacing all vegetation with asphalt would lead to air temperature increases of up to 3.2 °C in parts of the city (Skelhorn et al. 2014). Presence and abundance of biomass are two of the biodiversity metrics that are positively connected with moderation of extreme events and local climate/air quality regulation (Fig. 2.4) along with taxonomic diversity, species composition, functional diversity and functional identity.

In addition to green space losses a range of other ecosystem and biodiversity metrics are influential in affecting spatial and temporal patterns in the urban microclimate, such as species type and functional traits. There is also the issue of green space degradation and/or modification due to urban factors, including through impacts on biodiversity. Urban ecosystems have distinct abiotic characteristics: higher temperatures, modified/drier soils, higher surface sealing, higher light levels due to artificial lighting and more fragmentation (Schwarz et al. 2017). Urban ecosystems also differ in their composition, functional traits and structures as a result of abiotic factors and management practices (Ziter 2016; Schwarz et al. 2017). The effect can be to modify regulating functions, sometimes reversing beneficial functions for health and well-being. For example, inappropriate management of a large, 30-year-old green roof in Manchester was found to increase both air and surface temperatures. Peak air temperatures above a damaged green roof exceeded those above an adjacent bare roof during some of the hottest periods of an experimental study (Speak et al. 2013a, b). In the damaged roof case, impacts were exacerbated by the removal of vegetation (largely grasses) during an extended drought period. Natural re-colonization to a 'meadow' form took two growing seasons during which time temperature regulating functions continued to be compromised, as well as the other functions that the green roof had been providing, including air pollution removal and regulation of water runoff and water quality (Speak et al. 2012, 2013a, b, 2014).

Clearly, for green spaces to be able to retain their beneficial functions, it will be necessary to adapt associated management practices and consider what sorts of metrics are used to assess change. Fortunately, in terms of temperature, a relatively modest 5% increase in mature tree cover in suburban areas (e.g. *Acer campestre* (Field Maple), *Acer platanoides Globosum* (Norway Maple), *Acer pseudoplatanus* (Sycamore) and *Quercus robur* (English Oak)) can reduce surface temperatures by ~1 °C. In turn, there are positive impacts for climate mitigation through reductions in energy demand (Skelhorn et al. 2016, 2017). Evidence from studies like these can help fill the void between knowledge and practice by beginning to link specific plant assemblages and species to benefits (Cameron and Blanusa 2016). However, potential trade-offs must also be considered. For example, how effective is evapotranspiration from urban trees under drought conditions and what implications are there for water management for other types of green spaces? Cameron and Blanusa (2016) pose the question of what is the right 'plant palette' for multi-functional green infrastructure, such as aesthetically pleasing road-side amenity green space, which can provide noise and air pollution removal, encourage physical activity, offer pedestrian shading and contain food for pollinators while also being able to tolerate the harsh environment of urban areas in terms of water, nutrients and temperatures. Decisions also need to consider whether some species, despite delivering positive functions, may have drawbacks, e.g. in terms of becoming invasive, generating large amounts of pollen or perhaps being associated with 'nuisance' issues that impact public acceptability, such as damage to pavements with secondary consequences for accessibility, or honeydew release, which itself is an indicator of ecosystem health due to the increased likelihood of tree disease.

There is also the issue that wider urban planning systems are not yet set up to recognise and protect functional traits that link types of green infrastructure to human health benefits (see Heiland et al. Chap. 19, this volume). In the UK, the most common method for evaluating tree loss caused by development is to calculate the change in the number of trees for individual planning applications. However, the number of trees lost or gained in a development reveals little about the associated impacts on human health. Indeed, simple loss/gain metrics can be a serious misrepresentation of the more important biodiversity metrics which underpin benefits. For example, an unpublished study of tree removal on the University of Manchester campus demonstrated that when calculated by number, the proportion of trees lost to development was lower than if calculated by loss of total leaf area and much less if calculated by loss of canopy area (Fig. 2.8). Yet canopy extent (surface shading) is important for temperature regulation. There was also a loss of species richness, albeit one that was lower proportionally compared to the loss of tree numbers. According to estimates generated by the i-Tree Eco tool (produced by the US Forestry Service), the proportion of air pollutants (carbon monoxide, nitrogen dioxide, ozone, sulphur dioxide and $PM_{2.5}$) being captured by campus trees had declined by 23.4%. Of the trees that were felled between 2013 and 2017, the top 10% ($n = 28$) most effective absorbers of air pollution captured 26% of the total air pollution removed by campus trees. The results point to a disproportional loss of beneficial functions for human health even if replacement – usually less mature – trees are planted to compensate for losses.

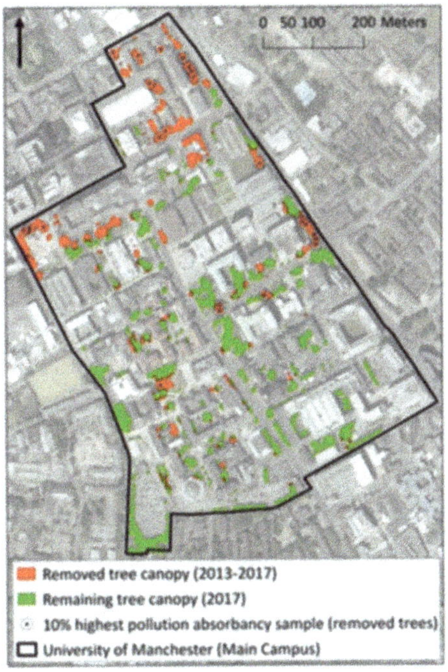

Indicator	2013	2017	Change (n)	Change (%)
Number of Trees	1149	874	-275	-23.9
Canopy Area (ha)	5.4	3.7	-1.7	-32
Leaf Area (ha)	21.3	16.1	-5.2	-24.4
Species Richness	112	92	-20	-17.9

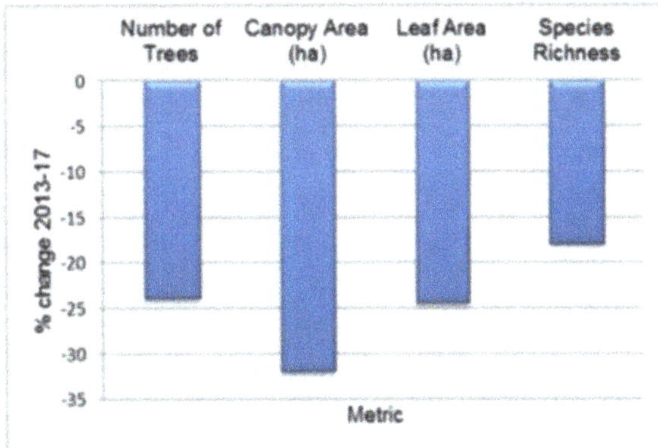

Fig. 2.8 Comparison of metrics associated with tree felling from 2013 to 2017 in an urban district of Manchester (© Getmapping Plc)

2.6 Conclusion

In this chapter, we have presented a summary and synthesis of the current evidence for the links between nature, biodiversity, physical health and climate change with a particular focus on urban areas. We have mainly drawn on recent review papers from the peer reviewed academic literature, supplemented by additional materials from a range of disciplinary fields. Much of the literature is still discipline-based, but increasingly informed by multi-disciplinary research projects and related endeavours. We feel that this is a necessary and positive development, and the greater availability of papers with large and diverse authorships is a positive sign that research is increasingly attempting to draw disciplines together to provide insights into the bigger and most critically important questions for human health and well-being. Nevertheless, we have found little evidence from investigations that explicitly sought to connect climate change with biodiversity and human physical health.

The evidence that does exist suggests that links between biodiversity, physical health and climate change are multiple, interconnected, multi-scale and interdependent. Their interdependence puts into sharp focus the importance of a holistic approach to the major global challenges of health, biodiversity and climate change. Indeed, a holistic approach in policy and practice is as important as it is in scientific research (see Korn et al. Chap. 14; Keune et al. Chap. 15, both this volume). Some of the existing, and newly emerging, challenges for health can be tackled through technological development and research into new interventions, such as new medicines and treatments. However, the extent to which the trends in losses of biodiversity will curtail the potential for future responses is unclear. Protecting ecosystems and associated biodiversity through a 'maintenance of options' insurance function is important for this reason alone (Díaz et al. 2018). It is also important for helping to address inequalities and for promoting social and environmental justice (Kabisch Chap. 5, this volume), given that in developing countries there is an even stronger reliance on ecosystems for health and well-being than in the developed world (Roy et al. 2018). Ironically, despite developing countries containing most of the world's untapped genetic diversity, developing countries are also where pressures such as urbanisation, demographics and population need, are greatest.

Uncertainties remain about some of the evidence for the links between biodiversity, human physical health and climate change. However, we know enough about the human health-biodiversity-climate change relationship to argue strongly to protect biodiversity and mitigate against climate change. Conceptual and theoretical work, empirical evidence and process modelling are all contributing to an improving evidence base, with increasing emphasis on integrative methods (Calvin and Bond-Lamberty 2018). Nevertheless, the complexities of environmental, social and governance factors mean that there is some way to go for a more complete understanding. Underpinning evidence will need to consider a range of settings and scales, including spatio-temporal dynamics in different climate zones and biomes as well as in the distinct urban habitat that now defines the majority of people's lives. We will also need to further develop our understanding of links between mental and physical health, connections between different body organ systems and the environmental determinants of health/ill-health from the perspective of biodiversity and the natural environment (see de Vries and Snep Chap. 8; Marselle et al. Chap. 9; Cook et al. Chap. 11, all this volume). Studies of the life course also have something to offer here, including environment-focused population cohort studies (see Dadvand et al. Chap. 6, this volume).

Our review reveals that there is still a need for extensive further research into relationships between biodiversity, climate change and human physical health. We still know little about trade-offs and the balance between benefits and harms. Such research is multi-layered and inherently multi-disciplinary. Complexities are compounded due to differing perspectives on issues, for example with some researchers using health as a primary starting point and other researchers starting from the perspective of environmental or ecological processes. The different perspectives are important for developing fuller understandings, but still make the challenges of integrated research all the more demanding, especially at the science-practice interface.

Ultimately, the most pressing questions also include some recognition of the need for action in the light of climate change projections, biodiversity losses and public health demands (De Young Chap. 13, this volume). It will be important to understand and resolve the web of connecting pathways between biological and functional diversity, and human health and well-being (Box 2.1) to identify the main protective roles and ensure that they are retained and enhanced in a range of ecosystems. Given urban growth and economic imperatives, it will be necessary to explore what sort of configurations can be promoted for multiple beneficial ecosystem functioning in different geographical, temporal and social settings. It will also be important to understand how climate change and related stresses will modify functions and functional groups, including the development of measurable and robust indicators that can be monitored over time. Other questions then emerge, how can wider landscapes be productive, diverse and climate resilient? How far are climate and other stressors likely to modify the beneficial functioning of the human biome in terms of physical health outcomes? What habitat types and elements of biodiversity in green and blue spaces in urban areas help promote physical health through the normal functioning of the human biome at different stages of the life course? How can these types and elements be considered within the planning process and within health and social care systems? Making progress on these questions is not easy. However, given the finite nature of the planetary boundary and the mounting pressures from a wide range of human drivers they remain some of the most important and urgent for researchers and practitioners alike.

References

Arbuthnott KG, Hajat S (2017) The health effects of hotter summers and heat-waves in the population of the United Kingdom: a review of the evidence. Environ Health 16(Suppl 1):119

Barton H, Grant M (2006) A health map for the local human habitat. J R Soc Promot Health 126(6):252–253

BBC (2018) England Moor fires. https://www.bbc.co.uk/news/topics/cq5p6wx822pt/england-moor-fires. Accessed 6 July 2018

Benedict M A, McMahon E T (2002) Green infrastructure: smart conservation for the 21st century. [Online] Available at: wwwsactreeorg/assets/files/greenprint/toolkit/b/greenInfrastructurepdf. Accessed 16 June 2014

Bonebrake TC, Brown CJ, Bell JD, Blanchard JL, Chauvenet A, Champion C, Chen IC, Clark TD, Colwell RK, Danielsen F (2018) Managing consequences of climate-driven species redistribution requires integration of ecology, conservation and social science. Biol Rev 93:284–305

Bowler DE, Buyung-Ali L, Knight TM, Pullin AS (2010) Urban greening to cool towns and cities: a systematic review of the empirical evidence. Landsc Urban Plan 97(3):147–155

Burkart K, Breitner S, Schneider A, Khan MMH, Krämer A, Endlicher W (2014) An analysis of heat effects in different subpopulations of Bangladesh. Int J Biometeorol 58(2):227–237

Buxton RT, McKenna MF, Mennitt D, Fristrup K, Crooks K, Angeloni L, Wittemyer G (2017) Noise pollution is pervasive in U.S. protected areas. Science 356(6337):531–533. https://doi.org/10.1126/science.aah4783c

Caini S, Schellevis F, El-Guerche Séblain C, Paget J (2018) Important changes in the timing of influenza epidemics in the WHO European region over the past 20 years: virological surveillance 1996 to 2016. Eur Secur 23(1):17-00302

Calvin K, Bond-Lamberty B (2018) Integrated human-earth system modeling–state of the science and future directions. Environ Res Lett 13(6):063006

Cameron RW, Blanusa T (2016) Green infrastructure and ecosystem services – is the devil in the detail? Ann Bot 118:377–339

Carding S, Verbeke K, Vipond DT, Corfe BM, Owen LJ (2015) Dysbiosis of the gut microbiota in disease. Microb Ecol Health Dis 26(26191). https://doi.org/10.3402/mehd.v26.26191

Carporn SJM, Emmett BA (2009) Threats from air pollution and climate change to upland systems: past, present and future. In: Bonn A, Allott T, Hubacek K, Stewart J (eds) Drivers of environmental change in uplands. Routledge, Oxon, pp 34–58

Cavan G (2010) Climate change projections for Greater Manchester. Manchester: EcoCities project, University of Manchester. Available at: http://media.adaptingmanchester.co.uk.ccc.cdn.faelix.net/sites/default/files/Climate_change_projections_GM_final.pdf. Accessed 6 July 2018

Challinor AJ et al (2018) Transmission of climate risks across sectors and borders. Phil Trans R Soc A 376:20170301

Cheung HKW (2011) An urban heat island study for building and urban design. Manchester: PhD thesis, University of Manchester

Clark NE, Lovell R, Wheeler BW, Higgins SL, Depledge MH, Norris K (2014) Biodiversity, cultural pathways, and human health: a framework. Trends Ecol Evol 29(4):198–204

Coutts C, Hahn M (2015) Green infrastructure, ecosystem services, and human health. Int J Environ Res Public Health 12:9768–9798

Cox DTC, Gaston KJ (2018) Human–nature interactions and the consequences and drivers of provisioning wildlife. Phil Trans R Soc 373:20170092

Curtis S, Fair A, Wistow J, Val DV & Oven K (2017) Impact of extreme weather events and climate change for health and social care systems. Environ Health 16(Suppl 1):128

Dahlgren G, Whitehead M (1991) Policies and strategies to promote social equity in health. Institute for Futures Studies, Stockholm

Dahlgren G, Whitehead M (2007) European strategies for tackling social inequities in health: levelling up, part 2. WHO Regional Office for Europe, Copenhagen

Díaz S, Pascual U, Stenseke M, Martín-López B, Watson RT, Molnár Z, Hill R, Chan KMA, Baste IA, Brauman KA, Polasky S, Church A, Lonsdale M, Larigauderie A, Leadley PW, van Oudenhoven APE, van der Plaat F, Schröter M, Lavorel S, Aumeeruddy-Thomas Y, Bukvareva E, Davies K, Demissew S, Erpul G, Failler P, Guerra CA, Hewitt CL, Keune H, Lindley S, Shirayama Y (2018) Assessing nature's contributions to people. Science 359(6373):270–272

Dobson A, Cattadori I, Holt RD, Ostfeld RS, Keesing F, Krichbaum K, Rohr JR, Perkins SE, Hudson PJ (2006) Sacred cows and sympathetic squirrels: the importance of biological diversity to human health. PLoS Med 3(6):714–718

Doherty RM, Heal MR, O'Connor FM (2017) Climate change impacts on human health over Europe through its effect on air quality. Environ Health 16(Suppl 1):1–18

European Environment Agency (2017) Climate change, impacts and vulnerability in Europe: an indicator based report. European Environment Agency, Copenhagen

European Environment Agency (2018) About urban environment. [Online] Available at: https://www.eea.europa.eu/themes/sustainability-transitions/urban-environment/about-urban-environment. Accessed 10 Jan 2018

Fann N, Alman B, Broome RA, Morgan GG, Johnston FH, Pouliot G, Rappold AG (2018) The health impacts and economic value of wildland fire episodes in the US: 2008–2012. Sci Total Environ 610–611:802–809

Fernandez LS, Byard D, Lin C-C, Benson S (2002) Frail elderly as disaster victims: emergency management strategies. Prehosp Disaster Med 17(2):67–74

Fisher JE, Andersen ZJ, Loft S, Pedersen M (2017) Opportunities and challenges within urban health and sustainable development. Curr Opin Environ Sustain 25:77–83

Flandroy L, Poutahidis T, Berg G, Clarke G, Dao M-C, Decaestecker E, Furman E, Haahtela T, Massart S, Plovier H (2018) The impact of human activities and lifestyles on the interlinked microbiota and health of humans and of ecosystems. Sci Total Environ 627:1018–1038

Garrett WS (2015) From cell biology to the microbiome: an intentional infinite loop. J Cell Biol 210(1):7–8

Grellier J, White MP, Albin M, Bell S, Elliott LR, Gascón M, Gualdi S, Mancini L, Nieuwenhuijsen MJ, Sarigiannis DA (2017) BlueHealth: a study programme protocol for mapping and quantifying the potential benefits to public health and well-being from Europe's blue spaces. BMJ Open 7:e016188

Grize L, Huss A, Thommen O, Schindler C, Braun-Fahrländer C (2005) Heatwave 2003 and mortality in Switzerland. Swiss Med Wkly 135:200–205

Hajat S (2017) Health effects of milder winters: a review of evidence from the United Kingdom. Environ Health 16(Suppl 1):109

Hallmann CA, Sorg M, Jongejans E, Siepel H, Hofland N, Schwan H, Stenmans W, Müller A, Sumser H, Hörren T (2017) More than 75 percent decline over 27 years in total flying insect biomass in protected areas. PLoS One 12(10):1–21

Haluza D, Schönbauer R, Cervinka R (2014) Green perspectives for public health: a narrative review on the physiological effects of experiencing outdoor nature. Int J Environ Res Public Health 11:5445–5461

Harrison PA, Berry PM, Simpson G, Haslett JR, Blicharska M, Bucur M, Dunford R, Egoh B, Garcia-Llorente M, Geamănă N, Geertsema W, Lommelen E, Meiresonne L, Turkelboom F (2014) Linkages between biodiversity attributes and ecosystem services: a systematic review. Ecosyst Serv 9:191–203

Hartig T, Mitchell R, de Vries S, Frumkin H (2014) Nature and health. Annu Rev Public Health 35:207–228

IPBES (2016) Pollinators, pollination and food production. Secretariat of the Intergovernmental Science-Policy Platform on Biodiversity and Ecosystem Services, Bonn

Jenkins G, Murphy J, Sexton S, Lowe J, Jones P, Kilsby C (2009) UK climate projections: briefing report. Met Office Hadley Centre, Exeter

Johnson H, Kovats S, McGregor G, Stedman J, Gibbs M, Walton H, Cook L (2004) The impact of the 2003 heat-wave on mortality and hospital admissions in England. Epidemiology 15(4):6–11

Kaczynski A, Henderson K (2007) Environmental correlates of physical activity: a review of evidence about parks and recreation. Leis Sci 29:315–354

Karkman A, Lehtimäki J, Ruokolainen L (2017) The ecology of human microbiota: dynamics and diversity in health and disease. Ann N Y Acad Sci 1399(1):78–92

Kellogg J, Wang J, Flint C, Ribnicky D, Kuhn P, De Mejia EGl, Raskin I, Lila MA (2010) Alaskan wild berry resources and human health under the cloud of climate change. J Agric Food Chem 58(7):3884–3900

Keniger LE, Gaston KJ, Irvine KN, Fuller RA (2013) What are the benefits of interacting with nature? Int J Environ Res Public Health 10:913–935

Klinger C, Landeg O, Murray V (2014) Power outages, extreme events and health: a systematic review of the literature from 2011–2012. PLOS Curr Disasters, Issue Edition 1

Lake IR (2017) Food-borne disease and climate change in the United Kingdom. Environ Health 16:117

Landrigan PJ, Fuller R, Acosta NJ, Adeyi O, Arnold R, Baldé AB, Bertollini R, Bose-O'Reilly S, Boufford JI, Breysse PN (2018) The lancet commission on pollution and health. Lancet 391:462–512

Latif MT, Othman M, Idris N, Juneng L, Abdullah AM, Hamzah WP, Khan MF, Sulaiman NMN, Jewaratnam J, Aghamohammadi N (2018) Impact of regional haze towards air quality in Malaysia: a review. Atmos Environ 177:28–44

Levermore G, Parkinson J, Lee K, Lindley S (2017) The increasing trend of the urban heat island intensity. Urban Climate 24:360–368

Liddicoat C, Bi P, Waycott M, Glover J, Lowe AJ, Weinstein P (2018) Landscape biodiversity correlates with respiratory health in Australia. J Environ Manag 206:113–122

Lindberg F (2007) Modelling the urban climate using a local governmental geo-database. Meteorol Appl 14:263–273

Lindley SJ, Handley JF, Theuray N, Peet E, McEvoy D (2006) Adaptation strategies for climate change in the adaptation strategies for climate change in the related risk in UK urban areas. J Risk Res 9(5):543–568

Lindley S, O'Neill J, Kandeh J, Lawson N, Christian R, O'Neill M (2011) Climate change, justice and vulnerability. Joseph Rowntree Foundation, York

Linton M-J, Dieppe P, Medina-Lara A (2016) Review of 99 self-report measures for assessing well-being in adults: exploring dimensions of well-being and developments over time. BMJ Open 6:e010641

Lovell R, Wheeler BW, Higgins SL, Irvine KN, Depledge MH (2014) A systematic review of the health and Well-being. J Toxicol Environ Health B 17:1–20

Lowe D, Ebi KL, Forsberg B (2013) Factors increasing vulnerability to health effects before, during and after floods. Int J Environ Res Public Health 10(12):7015–7067

LWEC (2015) Living with environmental change: health report card. [Online] Available at: http://www.nerc.ac.uk/research/partnerships/ride/lwec/report-cards/health/. Accessed 23 Feb 2018

Mace GM, Norris K, Fitter AH (2012) Biodiversity and ecosystem services: a multilayered relationship. Trends Ecol Evol 27(1):19–26

Manchester Evening News (2018) Firefighters continue to tackle Winter Hill blaze which has caused 'pure devastation' – live updates. https://www.manchestereveningnews.co.uk/news/greater-manchester-news/winter-hill-fire-updates-manchester-14842549. Accessed 6 July 2018

Markevych I, Schoierer J, Hartig T, Chudnovsky A, Hystad P, Dzhambov AM, de Vries S, Triguero-Mas M, Brauer M, Nieuwenhuijsen MJ, Lupp G, Richardson EA, Astell-Burt T, Dimitrova D, Feng X, Sadeh M, Standl M, Heinrich J, Fuertes E (2017) Exploring pathways linking greenspace to health: theoretical and methodological guidance. Environ Res 158:301–317

McMichael AJ (2013) Globalization, climate change, and human health. N Engl J Med 368:1335–1343

Met Office (2018) Woodford climate 1981–2010. https://www.metoffice.gov.uk/public/weather/climate/gcqrqyr80. Accessed 6 July 2018

Mölter A, Lindley S (2015) Influence of walking route choice on primary school children's exposure to air pollution–a proof of concept study using simulation. Sci Total Environ 530:257–262

Moreno DA, Carvajal M, López-Berenguer C, García-Viguera C (2006) Chemical and biological characterisation of nutraceutical compounds of broccoli. J Pharm Biomed Anal 41(5):1508–1522

Nile SH, Park SW (2014) Edible berries: bioactive components and their effect on human health. Nutrition 30:134–144

Norton BA, Coutts AM, Livesley SJ, Harris RJ, Hunter AM, Williams NSG (2015) Planning for cooler cities: a framework to prioritise green infrastructure to mitigate high temperatures in urban landscapes. Landsc Urban Plan 134:127–138

Odamaki T, Kato K, Sugahara H, Hashikura N, Takahashi S, Xiao J-z, Abe F, Osawa R (2016) Age-related changes in gut microbiota composition from newborn to centenarian: a cross-sectional study. BMC Microbiol 16(90):12

Oke T (1982) The energetic basis of the urban heat island. Q J R Meteorol Soc 108(445):1–24

Paredes-Lopez O, Cervantes-Ceja ML, Vigna-Pérez M, Hernández-Pérez T (2010) Berries: improving human health and healthy aging, and promoting quality life–a review. Plant Foods Hum Nutr 65(3):299–308

Poumadere M, Mays C, Le Mer S, Blong R (2005) The 2003 heat wave in France: dangerous climate change here and now. Risk Anal 25(6):1483–1494

Rader R, Bartomeus I, Garibaldi LA, Garratt MP, Howlett BG, Winfree R, Cunningham SA, Mayfield MM, Arthur AD, Andersson GK (2016) Non-bee insects are important contributors to global crop pollination. PNAS 113 (1):146–151

Recio A, Linares C, Ramón Banegas J, Díaz J (2016) Road traffic noise effects on cardiovascular, respiratory, and metabolic health: an integrative model of biological mechanisms. Environ Res 146:359–370

Renz H, Holt PG, Inouye M, Logan AC, Prescott SL, Sly PD (2017) An exposome perspective: early-life events and immune development in a changing world. J Allergy Clin Immunol 140(1):24–40

Robinson C, Bouzarovski S, Lindley S (2018) Underrepresenting neighbourhood vulnerabilities? The measurement of fuel poverty in England. Energy Res Soc Sci 36:79–93

Rogalski MA, Gowler CD, Shaw CL, Hufbauer RA, Duffy MA (2017) Human drivers of ecological and evolutionary dynamics in emerging and disappearing infectious disease systems. Philos Trans B 372 (1712):20160043

Rook G (2013) Regulation of the immune system by biodiversity from the natural environment: an ecosystem service essential to health. Proc Natl Acad Sci 110(46):18360–18367

Roy M, Shemdoe R, Hulme D, Mwageni N, Gough A (2018) Climate change and declining levels of green structures: life in informal settlements of Dar es Salaam, Tanzania. Landsc Urban Plan 180:282–293

Ruokolainen L, Lehtimäki J, Karkman A, Haahtela T, von Hertzen L, Fyhrquist N (2017) Holistic view on health: two protective layers of biodiversity. Ann Zool Fenn 54:39–49

Sandifer PA, Sutton-Grier AE, Ward BP (2015) Exploring connections among nature, biodiversity, ecosystem services and human health and well-being: opportunities to enhance health and biodiversity conservation. Ecosyst Serv 12:1–15

Schmeller DS, Weatherdon LV, Loyau A, Bondeau A, Brotons L, Brummitt N, Geijzendorffer IR, Haase P, Kuemmerlen M, Martin CS (2018) A suite of essential biodiversity variables for detecting critical biodiversity change. Biol Rev 93(1):L55–L71

Schwarz N, Moretti M, Bugalho MN, Davies ZG, Haase D, Hack J, Hof A, Melero Y, Pett TJ, Knapp S (2017) Understanding biodiversity-ecosystem service relationships in urban areas: a comprehensive literature review. Ecosyst Serv 27:161–171

Schweitzer MD, Calzadilla AS, Salamo O, Sharifi A, Kumar N, Holt G, Campos M, Mirsaeidi M (2018) Lung health in era of climate change and dust storms. Environ Res 163:36–42. https://doi.org/10.1016/j.envres.2018.02.001

Seksik P, Landman C (2015) Understanding microbiome data: a primer for clinicians. Dig Dis 33(suppl 1):11–16. https://doi.org/10.1159/000437034

Skelhorn CP, Lindley SJ, Levermore G (2014) The impact of vegetation types on air and surface temperatures in a temperate city: a fine scale assessment in Manchester, UK. Landsc Urban Plan 121:129–140

Skelhorn CP, Levermore G, Lindley SJ (2016) Impacts on cooling energy consumption due to the UHI and vegetation changes in Manchester, UK. Energ Build 122:150–159

Skelhorn CP, Lindley SJ, Levermore G (2017) Urban greening and the UHI: seasonal trade-offs in heating and cooling energy consumption in Manchester, UK. Urban Clim 23:173–187

Smith C, Lawson N (2012) Exceeding climate thresholds: extreme weather impacts on the environment and population of greater Manchester. North West Geography, Issue 1

Smith C, Lindley S, Levermore G (2009) Estimating spatial and temporal patterns of urban anthropogenic heat fluxes for UK cities: the case of Manchester. Theor Appl Climatol 98:19–35

Speak AF, Rothwell JJ, Lindley SJ, Smith CL (2012) Urban particulate pollution reduction by four species of green roof vegetation in a UK city. Atmos Environ 61:283–293

Speak AF, Rothwell JJ, Lindley SJ, Smith CL (2013a) Rainwater runoff retention on an aged intensive green roof. Sci Total Environ 461:28–38

Speak A, Rothwell JJ, Lindley S, Smith C (2013b) Reduction of the urban cooling effects of an intensive green roof due to vegetation damage. Urban Clim 3:40–55

Speak AF, Rothwell JJ, Lindley SJ, Smith CL (2014) Metal and nutrient dynamics on an aged intensive green roof. Environ Pollut 184:33–43

Sproken-Smith RA, Oke TR (1999) Scale modelling of nocturnal cooling of urban parks. Bound-Layer Meteorol 93:287–312

Stollberger C, Lutz W, Finsterer J (2009) Heat-related side-effects of neurological and non-neurological medication may increase heat wave fatalities. Eur J Neurol 16(7):879–882

Teixeira A, Eiras-Dias J, Castellarin SD, Gerós H (2013) Berry Phenolics of grapevine under challenging environments. Int J Mol Sci 14(9):18711–18739

van den Bosch M, Sang AO (2017) Urban natural environments as nature-based solutions for improved public health – a systematic review of reviews. Environ Res 158:373–384

White MP, Wheeler BW, Herbert S, Alcock I, Depledge MH (2014) Coastal proximity and physical activity: is the coast an under-appreciated public health resource? Prev Med 69:135–140

Wilby RL (2003) Past and projected trends in London's urban heat island. Weather 58(7):251–259

Ziter C (2016) The biodiversity–ecosystem service relationship in urban areas: a quantitative review. Oikos 125:761–768

Chapter 3
Climate Change and Pollen Allergies

Athanasios Damialis, Claudia Traidl-Hoffmann, and Regina Treudler

Abstract This chapter reviews the emerging importance of pollen allergies in relation to ongoing climate change. Allergic diseases have been increasing in prevalence over the last decades, partly as the result of the impact of climate change. Increased sensitisation rates and more severe symptoms have been the partial outcome of: increased pollen production of wind-pollinated plants resulting in long-term increased abundance of pollen in the air we breathe; earlier shifts of airborne pollen seasons making occurrence of allergic symptoms harder to predict and deal with efficiently; increased allergenicity of pollen causing more severe health effects in allergic individuals; introduction of new, invasive allergenic plant species causing new sensitisations; environment-environment interactions, such as plants and hosted microorganisms, i.e. fungi and bacteria, which comprise a complex and dynamic system, with additive, presently unforeseeable influences on human health;

A. Damialis (✉)
Chair of Environmental Medicine (UNIKA-T), Technical University of Munich, Augsburg, Germany

Institute of Environmental Medicine, Helmholtz Zentrum München – German Research Center for Environmental Health, Augsburg, Germany
e-mail: thanos.damialis@tum.de

C. Traidl-Hoffmann
Chair of Environmental Medicine (UNIKA-T), Technical University of Munich, Augsburg, Germany

Institute of Environmental Medicine, Helmholtz Zentrum München – German Research Center for Environmental Health, Augsburg, Germany

CK-CARE – Christine Kühne Center for Allergy Research and Education, Davos, Switzerland
e-mail: c.traidl-hoffmann@tum.de

R. Treudler
Department of Dermatology, Venerology and Allergology, University of Leipzig Medical Centre, Leipzig, Germany

Leipzig Interdisiplinary Centre for Allergology (LICA), University of Leipzig Medical Centre, Leipzig, Germany
e-mail: allergie-hautklinik@medizin.uni-leipzig.de

M. R. Marselle et al. (eds.), *Biodiversity and Health in the Face of Climate Change*, https://doi.org/10.1007/978-3-030-02318-8_3

environment-human interactions, as the consequence of a combination of environmental factors, like air pollution, global warming, urbanisation and microclimatic variability, which create a multi-resolution spatiotemporal system that requires new processing technologies and huge data inflow in order to be thoroughly investigated. We suggest that novel, real-time, personalised pollen information services, like mobile-app risk alerts, must be developed to provide the optimum first line of allergy management.

Keywords Climate change · Environmental medicine · Pollen allergy

Highlights
- Climate change contributes significantly to increasing allergy prevalence worldwide.
- This chapter overviews the emerging challenges with regard to allergic diseases.
- More abundant and more allergenic pollen over time will affect allergic patients.
- New allergenic pollen and spatial shifts in pollen occurrence will increase sensitisation.
- Real-time pollen risk alerts are needed as the first line of allergy management.

3.1 Introduction

International reports have documented a progressive global increase in the burden of allergic diseases across the industrialised world over the past half century. Clinical evidence reveals a general increase in both the incidence and the prevalence of respiratory diseases, including allergic rhinitis and asthma (Bieber et al. 2016; Bunne et al. 2017; Burney et al. 1994; Ninan and Russell 1992; Strachan and Ross Anderson 1992; Wüthrich et al. 1995). Such phenomena may be related not only to air pollution and changes in lifestyle, but also to an actual increase in the amount and allergenicity of airborne allergenic pollen (Ziello et al. 2012; Beck et al. 2013). However, the exact relationship between these factors is not yet clear. The amount of allergenic pollen has increased in specific bioclimatic regions or for specific pollen types (Ziello et al. 2012), and allergenicity has been documented for only some pollutants and plant species (e.g. the ozone impact on birch; Beck et al. 2013). A large gap in our knowledge still exists regarding global trends across different biogeographical regions and for a wider diversity of pollen taxa. In addition, because of ongoing climate change, emerging challenges must be dealt with, such as newly introduced allergenic pollen, changing environmental parameters leading to unpredictable changing health effects, an urgent need for allergy risk alerts, and personalised environmental medicine services. In this chapter, we provide an overview of the state of the art of this topic and discuss multi-disciplinary and timely interaction between humans and the environment.

3.2 Clinical Implications of Pollen-induced Respiratory Allergy

Allergies represent a major public health problem, one that has increased rapidly in recent decades in both developed and developing countries and one that is recognised as an important global epidemic carrying a considerable economic burden (Bieber et al. 2016; Linneberg 2016; Traidl-Hoffmann 2017).

For the clinical manifestation of allergic symptoms, there is a need for allergic sensitisation to pollen allergens resulting in IgE antibody production. IgE antibodies bind to an IgE-specific receptor on the surface of immune cells (mast cells and basophils), and if later exposure to the same allergen occurs, the allergen can bind to the IgE molecules on the surface of these cells, thereby activating them. Activated mast cells and basophils undergo degranulation, during which they release histamine and other inflammatory chemical mediators into the surrounding tissue, causing vasodilation, mucous secretion, nerve stimulation and smooth muscle contraction (Averbeck et al. 2007).

In pollen allergies, the most common symptoms induced by allergens are sneezing, itchy nose, rhinorrhea and nasal congestion (Averbeck et al. 2007). Inhaled allergens can also result in exacerbation of bronchial allergic asthma, with coughing, wheezing, shortness of breath, chest tightness, pain or pressure.

In industrialised countries, allergic rhinitis (AR) can affect more than 20% of the population, as has been reviewed by Linneberg (2011). This percentage varies among cities, countries and continents because of environmental and other factors, and can exceed 40% (e.g. Brożek et al. 2017; Morais-Almeida et al. 2013; Sibbald and Strachen 1995). For example, the lifetime prevalence of allergic diseases in adults in Germany is 8.6% (95% CI) for asthma and 14.8% (95% CI) for rhinitis, as measured by self-reported doctor-diagnosed allergies within the Study on Adult Health in Germany of the Robert Koch Institute for rhinitis (Bergmann et al. 2016; Langen et al. 2013; Haftenberger et al. 2013). Regarding allergic sensitisation, in tests on 50 common single allergens and two mixtures comprising either inhalant allergens or grass pollen allergens, 48.6% of participants exhibited at least one allergic sensitisation (specific IgE antibody detection). Overall, 33.6% of participants were sensitised to inhalant allergens (Haftenberger et al. 2013). Table 3.1 shows sensitisation rates to 17 different pollens in atopic patients across the globe: the various pollen types refer to the most widespread and allergenic ones worldwide, and the spatial variability and relative occurrence can be concluded based on the different cohorts studied all over the world.

A comparison of data on adults from 1998 (Federal Health Survey/Bundes-Gesundheitssurvey 1998, [BGS98] of the Robert Koch Institute) and 2008–2011 (DEGS1) documented an increase in the rate of sensitisation to inhalant allergens, from 29.8% to 33.6% (Haftenberger et al. 2013). The Germany-wide lifetime prevalence of allergic diseases in children and adolescents (Study on the Health of Children and Adolescents in Germany/Studie zur Gesundheit von Kindern und

Table 3.1 Epidemiological studies on the allergenic properties of airborne pollen from different plant taxa

Pollen taxon	Studied species or genus (according to the authors)	Country	Number of atopic patients	Positive skin prick tests (%)	Citation
Alnus	*A. glutinosa*	Spain	210	20.9	Cosmes Martín et al. (2005)
Alnus	*A. glutinosa*	Turkey	130	32.3	Erkara et al. (2009)
Ambrosia	*A. artemisiifolia*	Australia	1000	13.4	Mueller et al. (2000)
Ambrosia	*A. elatior*	Croatia	750	20.3	Peternel et al. (2008)
Ambrosia		Czech Republic	300	19.0–25.0	Rybníček et al. (2000)
Ambrosia		France	59	56.0	Boralevi et al. (2008)
Ambrosia		Hungary	1139	82.7–84.8	Kadocsa and Juhasz (2002)
Ambrosia		Switzerland	1274	16.7	Frei et al. (1995)
Artemisia		Hungary	1139	48.8–54.8	Kadocsa and Juhasz (2002)
Artemisia	*A. vulgaris*	Poland	676	12.0	Stach et al. (2007)
Artemisia	*A. vulgaris*	Portugal	371	17.6	Loureiro et al. (2005)
Artemisia	*A. vulgaris*	Spain	891	13.0	Barber et al. (2008)
Artemisia		Switzerland	1274	22.6–28.0	Frei et al. (1995)
Betula		Finland	357	28.0	Varjonen et al. (1992)
Betula		Hungary	1139	8.7–17.0	Kadocsa and Juhasz (2002)
Betula		Italy	6750	18.0	Marogna et al. (2006)
Betula		Switzerland	1274	46.1–54.0	Frei et al. (1995)
Betula	*B. verrucosa*	Turkey	130	33.8	Erkara et al. (2009)
Betula	*B. verrucosa*	USA	371	32.9	Lin et al. (2002)
Chenopodiaceae/ Amaranthaceae	*Amaranthus retroflexus*	Australia	1000	16.6	Mueller et al. (2000)
Chenopodiaceae/ Amaranthaceae		Greece	1311	18.3	Gioulekas et al. (2004)

(continued)

Table 3.1 (continued)

Pollen taxon	Studied species or genus (according to the authors)	Country	Number of atopic patients	Positive skin prick tests (%)	Citation
Chenopodiaceae/ Amaranthaceae		Hungary	1139	10.6–15.8	Kadocsa and Juhasz (2002)
Chenopodiaceae/ Amaranthaceae	*Chenopodium*	India	2568	16.3	Mandal et al. (2008)
Chenopodiaceae/ Amaranthaceae		Spain	338	49.3	Alfaya Arias and Marqués Amat (2003)
Corylus		Hungary	1139	6.3–16.7	Kadocsa and Juhasz (2002)
Corylus		Switzerland	1274	46.7–47.2	Frei et al. (1995)
Corylus	*C. avellana*	Turkey	130	30.8	Erkara et al. (2009)
Cupressaceae		Greece	1311	12.7	Gioulekas et al. (2004)
Cupressaceae		Italy	547	13.3	Copula et al. (2006)
Cupressaceae	*C. sempervirens*	Spain	891	14.9	Barber et al. (2008)
Cupressaceae	*C. sempervirens*	Turkey	455	14.3	Sin et al. (2008)
Fraxinus	*F. excelsior*	Austria	5416	17.6	Hemmer et al. (2006)
Fraxinus		Switzerland	1274	30.4–35.9	Frei et al. (1995)
Fraxinus	*F. americana*	USA	371	26.0	Lin et al. (2002)
Olea	*O. europaea*	Greece	1311	31.8	Gioulekas et al. (2004)
Olea	*O. europaea*	Portugal	371	27.5	Loureiro et al. (2005)
Olea	*O. europaea*	Spain	210	71.9	Cosmes Martín et al. (2005)
Olea	*O. europaea*	Turkey	127	15.0	Kirmaz et al. (2005)
Pinaceae		Greece	1311	9.3	Gioulekas et al. (2004)
Pinaceae	*Pinus radiata*	Portugal	371	7.5	Loureiro et al. (2005)
Plantago	*P. lanceolata*	Australia	1000	15.3	Mueller et al. (2000)
Plantago		Greece	1311	14.8	Gioulekas et al. (2004)

(continued)

Table 3.1 (continued)

Pollen taxon	Studied species or genus (according to the authors)	Country	Number of atopic patients	Positive skin prick tests (%)	Citation
Plantago		Hungary	1139	14.2–27.7	Kadocsa and Juhasz (2002)
Plantago	*P. lanceolata*	Japan	160	12.8	Nakamaru et al. (2005)
Plantago	*P. lanceolata*	Portugal	371	10.6	Loureiro et al. (2005)
Platanus	*P. orientalis*	Turkey	130	27.7	Erkara et al. (2009)
Poaceae	*Phleum pratense*	Finland	357	35.5	Varjonen et al. (1992)
Poaceae		Greece	1311	40.4	Gioulekas et al. (2004)
Poaceae		Hungary	1139	56.7–56.8	Kadocsa and Juhasz (2002)
Poaceae		Italy	726	46.6	Asero (2004)
Poaceae	*Dactylis glomerata*	Kyrgyzstan	633	70.5	Kobzar (1999)
Poaceae	*Phleum pratense*	Kyrgyzstan	633	57.8	Kobzar (1999)
Poaceae		Portugal	371	44.9	Loureiro et al. (2005)
Poaceae		Spain	459	83.7	Belver et al. (2007)
Poaceae	*Dactylis glomerata*	Spain	614	87.0	Subiza et al. (1995)
Poaceae	*Phleum pratense*	Spain	891	27.2–80.0	Barber et al. (2008)
Poaceae		Switzerland	1274	71.6–81.0	Frei et al. (1995)
Poaceae	*Festuca pratensis*	Turkey	130	60.8	Erkara et al. (2009)
Poaceae	*Phleum pratense*	Turkey	130	37.7	Erkara et al. (2009)
Poaceae		USA	189	71.0	Wu et al. (1999)
Populus	*P. alba*	Spain	614	29.0	Subiza et al. (1995)
Populus	*P. nigra*	Spain	210	32.3	Cosmes Martín et al. (2005)
Populus	*P. deltoides*	USA	371	20.6	Lin et al. (2002)
Quercus	*Q. alba*	USA	371	34.3	Lin et al. (2002)

(continued)

Table 3.1 (continued)

Pollen taxon	Studied species or genus (according to the authors)	Country	Number of atopic patients	Positive skin prick tests (%)	Citation
Rumex	*R. crispus*	Australia	1000	26.5	Mueller et al. (2000)
Ulmaceae	*Ulmus pumila*	Australia	1000	11.6	Mueller et al. (2000)
Ulmaceae	*Ulmus*	Hungary	1139	6.0–17.9	Kadocsa and Juhasz (2002)
Ulmaceae	*Trema orientalis*	India	2568	13.8	Mandal et al. (2008)
Ulmaceae	*Ulmus americana*	USA	371	24.6	Lin et al. (2002)
Urticaceae	*Parietaria*	Greece	150	27.5–28.0	Kaleyias et al. (2001)
Urticaceae	*Parietaria*	Italy	507	23.0	Verini et al. (2001)
Urticaceae	*Parietaria*	Portugal	371	23.4	Loureiro et al. (2005)

For each study, the taxon whose properties were studied, the country where the research was conducted, the sample size of atopic patients examined and the percentage of positive reactions to skin prick tests are given. Taxa are presented in alphabetical order. Empty cells signify lack of information

Sources: Scopus and Web of Science; references without an abstract in English are not included

Jugendlichen in Deutschland, (KiGGS initial survey, 2003–2006 of the Robert Koch Institute)) was shown to be 4.7% (95% CI) for allergic bronchial asthma and 10.7% (95% CI) for allergic rhinitis (Bergmann et al. 2016). Allergic rhinitis was shown to have a negative impact on quality of life, by using validated questionnaires like the five-dimension EuroQol QOL survey (EQ-5D, the Sino-Nasal Outcome Test (SNOT-22) or the Nasal Obstruction Severity Evaluation (NOSE) scale (e.g. Höhle et al. 2017).

In addition to respiratory symptoms, a number of pollen-allergic patients, especially those with birch allergy, suffer from concomitant pollen-related food allergies, which means that they develop allergy symptoms after ingestion of certain foods. Symptoms may manifest as oral itching, swelling of the lips, itchy exanthema, shortness of breath, diarrhoea or even circulation problems (Treudler et al. 2017). Overall, the majority of IgE-mediated food allergies in adults are based on sensitisation to aeroallergens (in particular pollen), followed by (cross-) reactions to structurally related, often unstable, allergens, especially in (plant) foods such as fruit, vegetables and spices (Treudler et al. 2017). This type of food allergy has been referred to as a secondary food allergy, as distinct from the primary form, which is presumed to involve sensitisation via the gastrointestinal tract. The types of fruit most commonly involved in pollen-related food allergy belong to the Rosaceae plant family (e.g. apples) and to the Corylaceae family (e.g. hazel) (Treudler and Simon 2017). Recently, birch-related soy allergy has gained much attention as soy products (i.e. soy drinks) have been promoted as healthy foods and are being consumed in increasing amounts in many European countries (Treudler et al. 2017).

Different allergen families, which are also present in plant tissues, can become airborne, as well as be found in foods, and they are associated with different types of clinical reactions (i.e. sensitisation to pathogenesis-related (PR) protein-10, like Bet v 1 homologues). These reactions are mostly seen in Northern Europe and they are associated with oral itching and swelling. In contrast, sensitisation to lipid transfer proteins (LTPs) occurs more frequently in Southern Europe and is associated with anaphylaxis (severe immediate-type reactions involving several organ systems).

3.3 Allergenic Pollen and Epidemiology

There are differences within pollen-producing plants with regard to their ability to induce allergic sensitisation. There have been numerous studies worldwide over the past several decades that have documented such sensitisation rates. Nonetheless, a huge variability may exist, because of (but not limited to) climatic, air quality, environmental, social and genetic differences. A short overview is provided in Table 3.1, which gives the sensitisation rates of the most important allergenic pollen types.

The international literature documents grass pollen as the leading aeroallergen worldwide (e.g. Lewis et al. 1983; Weeke and Spieksma 1991; Wu et al. 1999; García-Mozo 2017). The reason for this is the wide distribution of grass species, along with their pollen's high allergenicity. The grass (Poaceae) family comprises one of the largest and most common plant families worldwide and, noticeably, consists mostly of wind-pollinated species (e.g. Wodehouse 1971; Lewis et al. 1983). It includes both annual and perennial herbaceous species, many of which are highly cosmopolitan and, hence, they are found in a wide variety of latitudes and biogeographical zones, in both urban or natural habitats (e.g. Pignatti 1982; Lewis et al. 1983). The grass species most implicated in respiratory allergies are orchard grass (*Dactylis glomerata*), fescue grass (*Festuca* spp.), ryegrass (*Lolium perenne*), timothy grass (*Phleum pratense*) and bluegrass (*Poa* spp.) (e.g. Lewis et al. 1983). Sensitisation rates to grass pollen can exceed 80% of the atopic population according to many epidemiological and clinical studies carried out across the globe (Table 3.1).

Other allergologically important plants are birch (*Betula* spp.), alder (*Alnus* spp.), hazel (*Corylus* spp.) and – recently of growing interest – the invasive ragweed (*Ambrosia* spp.). Sensitisation rates for the above pollen types can exceed 50% for the Corylaceae and Betulaceae families, whereas sensitisation to ragweed pollen can reach up to 80% (Table 3.1).

However, if investigating the exact relationship of the actual pollen exposure to the respiratory allergic symptoms of sensitised individuals, there are specific prerequisites. The exact pollen season occurrence and intensity need to be defined on a spatial and a temporal scale. Pollen allergy symptoms are mostly observed during the main pollen season. Even though the exact relationship between symptoms (pulmonary, nasal or ocular) and pollen occurrence and abundance is not yet clear, there are some recent reports clarifying this interaction (e.g. Berger et al. 2013; Bastl et al. 2014; Karatzas et al. 2014; Osborne et al. 2017; Voukantsis et al. 2015; Damialis et al. 2019). Overall, there are indications that there is a positive correlation between allergic symptoms and pollen abundance. However, this relationship can differ significantly among different bioclimatic regions, among different atopic patients, and for each different pollen type, and of course the relationship itself is not linear and there is usually a variable time lag between the actual pollen exposure and the occurrence of the allergic symptoms. The above do make pollen season forecasting (and consequent symptom forecasting) rather complex, thus highlighting the need for additional research in order to achieve accurate and operational predictive models.

Knowing the exact pollen season (in terms of occurrence, magnitude and shape) increases the capacity to accurately and in a timely way forecast the potential pollen exposure significantly and constitutes the first-line tool for allergy prevention. As an example, in Germany (Fig. 3.1), the main pollen season is confined to only a few months, usually commencing in March with the highly allergenic and cross-reactive pollen of hazel, alder and birch, and extending to the end of summer with the also very allergenic pollen from grasses and ragweed. A big allergy risk may exist even with shorter pollen seasons; even though a shorter duration of relevant allergic symptoms could then be hypothesised, such seasons tend to be highly peaked, thus potentially causing extreme exacerbations of symptoms even during these short intervals. Overall, in order to define the exposure to pollen beyond which respiratory

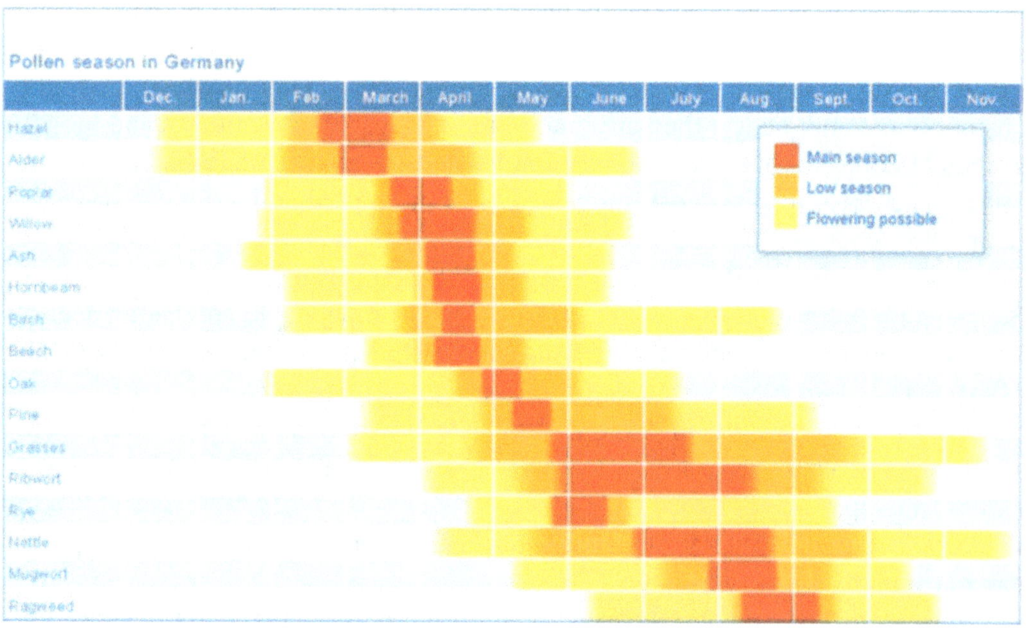

Fig. 3.1 Typical pollen seasons in Germany according to the Polleninformationsdienst (averages from pollen data from 2007–2011; www.pollenstiftung.de). Ragweed pollen has been added to this diagram only recently

symptoms are manifested, it is crucial to define the threshold of airborne concentrations of pollen that provoke these symptoms. However, it is well known that defining such thresholds involves highly demanding and complicated investigations, with values varying between sites, countries, geoclimatic regions, different years and per pollen type (de Weger et al. 2013).

3.4 Adjuvant Factors from Pollen and Impact of Environmental Factors

When we are exposed to pollen, it is not only the allergenic proteins that we inhale that affect us, but also our mucosa and/or skin are exposed to biochemically complex particles. Indeed, the allergenicity of pollen is not only the result of the allergen but also of adjuvant factors from pollen, such as lipids and pollen-derived adenosine (Dittlein et al. 2016; Gilles-Stein et al. 2016). Thus, exposure to allergens is necessary but not sufficient for the development of allergy (Gilles et al. 2009). By analysing the pollen's metabolome, Gilles et al. (2011) found that pollens release a wide array of different bioactive substances such as sugars, lipids, secondary metabolites and hormones. Notably, these bioactive mediators bind to receptors on human immune cells, which could promote allergic sensitisation to pollen-derived proteins or boost already manifested allergic immune responses. These substances, apart from the allergen itself, could be responsible for the potency of the allergenicity of pollen. Furthermore, these adjuvant mediators are influenced by environmental factors such as ozone (Beck et al. 2013). Only recently has part of the pollen microbiome been discovered (Obersteiner et al. 2016). This microbiome of pollen is not only species-specific, but also influenced by environmental factors (Obersteiner et al. 2016).

3.5 New Pollen Allergies: The Case of Ragweed

The European and Mediterranean Plant Protection Organization has reported the species *Ambrosia artemisiifolia* L. (common ragweed; Fig. 3.2) as an invasive and alien plant (Brunel et al. 2010). Apart from being a harmful weed, its pollen is highly allergenic. As ragweed has become naturalised in Europe, it is now quite common in regional flora in many areas across the continent (Smith et al. 2013). This expansion in European flora is expected to be reflected in human health by increasing sensitisation rates in allergic individuals (Burbach et al. 2009). These rates have already been reported as extremely high, often reaching 80% (Table 3.1). The most commonly implicated allergen is Amb a 1. There is already evidence of increasing long-term trends in *Ambrosia*-specific IgE antibodies from 20% in the

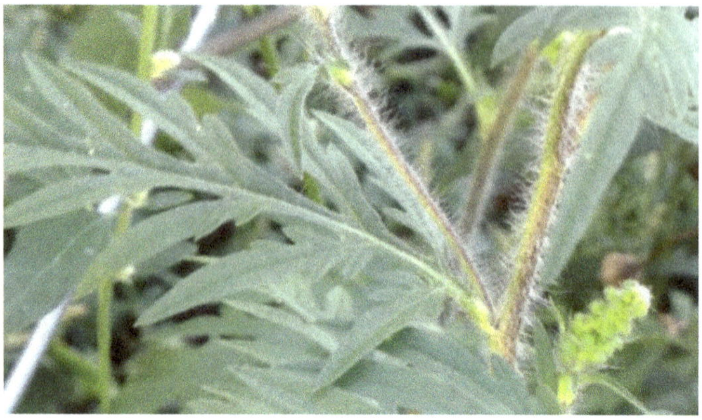

Fig. 3.2 Ragweed (*Ambrosia artemisiifolia*) plant, stems, leaves and flowers

late 1980s to about 30% at the end of the 1990s among patients with inhalation allergic diseases in Vienna, Austria (Buters et al. 2008).

Because of these factors, there is already awareness of the threats posed through the establishment and expansion of ragweed populations in Europe and, consequently, a European Commission Cooperation in Science and Technology (COST) Action FA1203 'SMARTER' (http://ragweed.eu) was approved in order to deal with this international problem. Among other goals, it aimed to describe the existing status of the threat, assess the European pollen abundance levels of ragweed, and attempt to make recommendations for the sustainable management of *Ambrosia* plants across Europe. Sikoparija et al. (2017), within this COST Action, have recently implied that only a few significant trends in the magnitude and frequency of atmospheric *Ambrosia* pollen exist at present (8% for the mean sum of daily average *Ambrosia* pollen concentrations and 14% for the mean number of days that *Ambrosia* pollen were recorded in the air). The direction of any trends (increasing or decreasing) varied locally.

Nonetheless, even in regions where ragweed has not yet been established, the probability of this occurring in the near future is quite high. For example, in Germany, which is located near the main source of ragweed pollen, the Pannonian Plain, ragweed does not seem to be as abundant, and therefore as noxious, yet as for neighbouring countries. As reported by Haftenberger in 2013, from the population-based German Health Study DEGS, IgE sensitisation rates to *A. artimisiifolia* were 8.2% of German adults, and this prevalence is quickly rising, with even very low concentrations (5–10 pollen grains per m^3 of air) being sufficient to trigger allergic reactions in sensitive patients. Thus, ragweed pollen may represent a new allergen, potentially responsible for new asthma incidents, and expected to occur much more frequently than other pollen types (Sikoparija et al. 2017).

3.6 Climate Change Effects

Airborne pollen measurements are among the longest term datasets of biological origin, therefore representing a valuable proxy of ongoing climate change. Extensive research over the last decade has shown that airborne pollen has increased in abundance but pollen seasons have also shifted to an earlier timeframe and may last longer (Ziello et al. 2012). It is still not clear, though, if this is the result of increased pollen production per floral unit or per individual plant, or the consequence of land use changes, ongoing climate change, eutrophication, global warming or a combination of these and many other factors. To date, some of the main causative factors for these changes have been considered air pollutants and higher air temperatures associated with global warming, or urbanisation rates and land use changes (e.g. Voltolini et al. 2000; Sofiev et al. 2009).

In parallel with this, allergic reactions to pollen in sensitised individuals have increased in both frequency and severity over the last decades, which is in accordance with the above-mentioned increase in airborne pollen concentrations (Linneberg et al. 1999). Although the reason for this synchronicity is not thoroughly understood and the cause-effect relationship not completely determined, a correlation between pollen abundance and pollen sensitisation has been considered to be real (e.g. Troise et al. 1992; Ault 2004).

Overall, a very large number of factors are expected (but not limited) to be influenced by climate change (anthropogenic or not) and together to contribute to the exacerbated provocation of allergic symptoms in sensitised individuals. There was an extensive review by Sofiev et al. in 2009 where the authors discuss plant-induced human allergy, from plant pollination and pollen dispersion to modelling and forecasting of airborne pollen concentrations. The following are some of the factors thought to be most important, although the list cannot be exhaustive:

- Plant growth, as influenced by the combination of air pollutants (i.e. carbon dioxide) and elevated air temperature, because of increased plant biomass.
- Pollen production, as expressed by increased pollen or flower production per inflorescence, or by a higher number of inflorescences per plant.
- Onset and duration of the pollen season, as influenced by meteorological and climatic factors, per site, among sites and among years and for each pollen type.
- Pollen allergenicity, as influenced by air pollutants (e.g. ozone and nitrogen dioxide) and air temperature, but, notably, in inverse correlation to pollen production per plant, after taking into account available resources as a limiting factor.
- Plant microbiome (plant, leaf, inflorescence and pollen microbiome), as determined by a wide variety of environmental factors, including biodiversity per se and its temporal variability.

- Pollution, including air, water, soil and other forms of pollution, on various spatial and temporal scales.
- Weather events, including drought or extreme rainfall, wind gusts, thunderstorms and any kind of extreme micro- and macro-meteorological effects.
- Land use changes, land management, habitat fracturing and moving to the north because of global warming.

Plant phenological traits (like flowering, leaf and bud formation, fruit and pollen production) are well known to be very sensitive to environmental stress and especially to temperature variability. This is particularly true for flowering and pollen production (e.g. Damialis et al. 2011; Menzel et al. 2006; Parmesan and Yohe 2003). There have been strong indications that plants produce more pollen, and earlier, when temperatures are higher, that is, at urban locations, lower elevations or southern exposure slopes, or during warmer years (e.g. Damialis et al. 2011; Fotiou et al. 2011). Higher rainfall prior to the inflorescence production and pollen formation and liberation also favour increased pollen and flower production (Damialis et al. 2011). However, the implicated processes are excessively complex and influence of many other factors is involved, for example microclimatic conditions in the examined site. Likewise, temperature seems to have a direct effect on allergen release, as revealed by the inter-annual variability in a study on birch pollen in Germany (Buters et al. 2008).

Air pollutants are also responsible for higher biomass production (including flower and pollen production). Wan et al. (2002) and Wayne et al. (2002) experimentally found that, especially in combination with elevated air temperature, increased carbon dioxide (CO_2) did not alter pollen production per se, but increased plant biomass in *Ambrosia artemisiifolia* and, consequently, individual plants produced more pollen. Ziska et al. (2003) studied the same species but in real-life conditions in a gradient simulating different climatic scenarios and, likewise, found that plants exhibited higher biomass, pollen production and earlier flowering dates. Ziska et al. (2003) additionally concluded that plant expansion rates and regional abundance may also increase with increasing CO_2, thus increasing allergenic pollen exposure rates on a wider spatial scale.

Air pollution and climate change do not only affect plant growth, pollen and flower production, and duration of the whole pollen season, but can also display more direct health effects by increasing the amount of allergenic proteins of the pollen (Zhao et al. 2016, 2017). According to Zhao et al. (2016), elevated levels of certain pollutants, like nitrogen dioxide (NO_2), which is traffic-related and hence more prevalent in urban locations, increase overall pollen allergenicity, thus also increasing the relevant allergy risk for sensitised individuals. El Kelish et al. (2014), as well as Zhao et al. (2017), showed that elevated pollutants change the transcriptome of ragweed pollen; therefore, under global change scenarios, the allergenic potential of pollen is also expected to change. Vehicular-exhaust pollution has been reported to influence the allergenicity of ragweed pollen: pollen along high-traffic roads showed an overall higher allergenicity than pollen from low-traffic roads and vegetated areas (Ghiani et al. 2012). Beck et al. (2013) documented a positive relationship between atmospheric ozone (O_3) levels and the amount of Bet v 1 in pollen samples collected from birch trees in outdoor stands in Bavaria, Germany. However, further clarification is needed regarding what the combined effect of ozone, nitrogen dioxide, carbon dioxide and air temperature on pollen allergenicity is on a plant population or ecosystem level. Epidemiological studies have demonstrated that urbanisation, high levels of vehicle emissions and a Westernised lifestyle are correlated with an increase in the frequency of pollen-induced respiratory allergy, which is more prominent in people who live in urban areas compared to those who live in rural areas (Haftenberger et al. 2013).

3.7 Pollen Information Services

Airborne pollen is routinely monitored worldwide, mainly for providing information on pollen season occurrence with a view to allergy prevention. Hirst-type devices are the most widely used pollen samplers worldwide (e.g. Galán et al. 2014). The device is volumetric and samples with a stable suction of airflow (10 l min^{-1}). Captured pollen grains are processed in the laboratory and then analysed under an optical microscope (manually identified and counted by expert scientists). The identification level is usually per genus for woody taxa and per family for herbaceous taxa. All measurements are expressed as numbers of pollen per cubic metre of air (e.g. British Aerobiology Federation 1995; Galán et al. 2014).

Pollen data from Hirst-type traps do not allow for real-time pollen measurements and timely dissemination of airborne pollen concentrations, even though their main purpose is to provide information on airborne particle abundance to allergic individuals. Hence, predictions with a minimum of a weekly forecasting horizon had to be developed. Additionally, a lot of effort and time are required because of the laborious nature of the microscopical identification technique. It is evident that there is an overall need for faster, near real-time reporting of airborne pollen concentrations. To date, high-risk pollen exposure alerts have been provided only via mid-term pollen season forecasting models, which are often not of good accuracy for operational and everyday medical practice. The future aim is to disseminate airborne pollen measurements using a novel automatic, real-time pollen sampler, in order to provide timely and accurate warning alerts to allergic patients throughout the duration of the pollen season, with the ultimate aim of more efficiently managing allergic diseases.

A new generation of automated, near real-time pollen measurements is currently being developed, and has already been able, in some cases, to work on an operational basis (Oteros et al. 2015; Häring et al. 2017). The most well-developed, promising or already operating automated pollen measuring devices are located in

(1) Japan (KH-3000) (Kawashima et al. 2017), which until now has been able to provide information only on one pollen type (*Cryptomeria japonica*, Cupressaceae family) and not on the complete pollen diversity, (2) the USA (Pollen Sense) (http://pollensense.com/), where it is still under calibration and not in fully operational mode, (3) Switzerland (PA-300 Rapid E) (Crouzy et al. 2016), where it is under calibration, and (4) Germany (BAA500), which has been in fully operational mode for the last half decade (e.g. Oteros et al. 2015; Häring et al. 2017).

The aforementioned automated pollen measuring device in Germany, the BAA500 Pollen Monitor, is an automated pollen monitoring system that is able to successfully recognise more than 10 pollen taxa, among which the allergenic *Alnus*, *Artemisia*, *Betula*, *Corylus*, *Fraxinus*, Poaceae and *Taxus* (Oteros et al. 2015). This system uses an image recognition algorithm on batch-collected pollen. The obtained pollen data exhibit a delay of only 3 h (Oteros et al. 2015). Oteros et al. (2015) have reported that the BAA500 manages to correctly identify all different pollen types in >70% of all cases (except for *Salix* pollen), with false-positive reports only occurring rarely.

3.8 Conclusions and Future Challenges

Climate change has been responsible for changes in biodiversity and species richness. Air quality, vegetation and land use changes, plant diversity and distribution have been altering pollen seasons, pollen abundance and allergenicity. In a changing world working towards optimum health management, it is crucial to take quick counter-measures, as suggested below.

First, a reliable, fully operational, real-time aeroallergen monitoring programme across the globe, needs to be urgently implemented, and must include all allergy-implicated pollen types, mainly birch, grasses and ragweed. This also includes setting up an automated system of free dissemination of the obtained results. Automated monitoring ought to be extended to other allergenic bioaerosols as well, such as the notorious fungal spore types of *Alternaria* and *Cladosporium*: if we consider that we spend more than two-thirds of our life indoors, at home or at work, it is critical that we evaluate the exposure risk and consequent symptoms due to indoor aeroallergens as well.

Secondly, special attention must be paid to changing aeroallergen seasons and spatial variability as this could increase sensitisation rates. Invasive plant species like ragweed and relevant eradication programmes have to be focused on. Likewise, *Alternaria* growth and production of spores have to be extensively investigated in the frame of future climate change, as it has been reported that this will dramatically change in 2100 climatic scenarios, growing faster but likely producing fewer spores, thus indicating an alteration in life strategy (Damialis et al. 2015).

It is crucial that all research approaches reflect real-life conditions as much as possible; it is important to focus mainly on the interaction effects between plant biological, physiological and ecological processes under varying environmental stress conditions, so as to be able to foresee the consequent health impacts.

Above all, more emphasis needs to be placed on environmental research, transforming the current status quo from anthropocentric research to the harmonic interaction of human-environment. The development of modern, automatic, real-time environmental health services is urgently needed, with the aim of providing, in the future, efficient guidelines for allergy prevention and management. Exposure risk alerts, e-health infrastructure and personalised forecasts on allergy management are seen as the (near) future of allergy research.

References

Alfaya Arias T, Marqués Amat L (2003) Pollinosis in the Lleida (former Lérida) province. Alergol Inmunol Clin 18:84–88

Asero R (2004) Analysis of new respiratory allergies in patients monosensitized to airborne allergens in the area north of Milan. J Investig Allergol Clin Immunol 14:208–213

Ault A (2004) Report blames global warming for rising asthma. Lancet 363:1532

Averbeck M, Gebhardt C, Emmrich F et al (2007) Immunologic principles of allergic disease. J Dtsch Dermatol Ges 5:1015–1028

Barber D, de la Torre F, Feo F et al (2008) Understanding patient sensitization profiles in complex pollen areas: a molecular epidemiological study. Allergy 63:1550–1558

Bastl K, Kmenta M, Jäger S et al (2014) Development of a symptom load index: enabling temporal and regional pollen season comparisons and pointing out the need for personalized pollen information. Aerobiologia 30:269–280

Beck I, Jochner S, Gilles S et al (2013) High environmental ozone levels lead to enhanced allergenicity of birch pollen. PLoS One 8:e80147

Belver MT, Caballero MT, Contreras J et al (2007) Associations among pollen sensitizations from different botanical species in patients living in the northern area of Madrid. J Investig Allergol Clin Immunol 17:157–159

Berger U, Karatzas K, Jaeger S et al (2013) Personalized pollen-related symptom-forecast information services for allergic rhinitis patients in Europe. Allergy 68:963–965

Bergmann KC, Heinrich J, Niemann H (2016) Current status of allergy prevalence in Germany: position paper of the environmental medicine commission of the Robert Koch institute. Allergo J Int 25:6–10

Bieber T, Akdis C, Lauener R et al (2016) Global allergy forum and 3rd Davos declaration 2015: atopic DERMATITIS/eczema: challenges and opportunities toward precision medicine. Allergy 71:588–592

Boralevi F, Hubiche T, Léauté-Labrèze C et al (2008) Epicutaneous aeroallergen sensitization in atopic dermatitis infants – determining the role of epidermal barrier impairment. Allergy 63:205–210

British Aerobiology Federation (1995) Airborne pollens and spores. A guide to trapping and counting. National Pollen and Hayfever Bureau, Rotherham

Brożek JL, Bousquet J, Agache I et al (2017) Allergic rhinitis and its impact on asthma (ARIA) guidelines-2016 revision. J Allergy Clin Immunol 140:950–958

Brunel S, Branquart E, Fried G et al (2010) The EPPO prioritization process for invasive alien plants. Bull OEPP/EPPO 40:407–422

Bunne J, Moberg H, Hedman L et al (2017) Increase in allergic sensitization in schoolchildren: two cohorts compared 10 years apart. J Allergy Clin Immunol 5:457–463

Burbach GJ, Heinzerling LM, Röhnelt C et al (2009) Ragweed sensitization in Europe – GA(2) LEN study suggests increasing prevalence. Allergy 64:664–665

Burney PG, Luczynska C, Chinn S et al (1994) The European community respiratory health survey. Eur Respir J 7:954–960

Buters JTM, Kasche A, Weichenmeier I et al (2008) Year-to-year variation in release of bet v 1 allergen from birch pollen: evidence for geographical differences between west and South Germany. Int Arch Allergy Immunol 145:122–130

Copula M, Carta G, Sessini F et al (2006) Epidemiologic investigation of the pollen allergy to Cupressaceae in a population at risk for atopy. Ped Med Chir Med Surg Ped 28:91–94

Cosmes Martín PM, Moreno Ancillo A, Domínguez Noche C et al (2005) Sensitization to Castanea sativa pollen and pollinosis in northern Extremadura (Spain). Allergol Immunopathol 33:145–150

Crouzy B, Stella M, Konzelmann T et al (2016) All-optical automatic pollen identification: towards an operational system. Atmos Environ 140:202–212

Damialis A, Fotiou C, Halley JM et al (2011) Effects of environmental factors on pollen production in anemophilous woody species. Trees 25:253–264

Damialis A, Mohammad AB, Halley JM et al (2015) Fungi in a changing world: growth rates may be elevated, but spore production will decrease in future climates. Int J Biometeorol 59:1157–1167

Damialis A, Häring F, Gökkaya M, Rauer D, Reiger M, Bezold S, Bounas-Pyrros N, Eyerich K, Todorova A, Hammel G, Gilles S, Traidl-Hoffmann C (2019) Human exposure to airborne pollen and relationships with symptoms and immune responses: indoors versus outdoors, circadian patterns and meteorological effects in alpine and urban environments. Sci Total Environ 653:190–199

de Weger L, Bergmann KC, Rantio-Lehtimäki A et al (2013) Impact of pollen. In: Sofiev M, Bergmann K-C (eds) Allergenic pollen. A review of the production, release, distribution and health impacts. Springer, Dordrecht/Heidelberg/New York/London, pp 161–215

Dittlein DC, Gilles-Stein S, Hiller J et al (2016) Pollen and UV-B radiation strongly affect the inflammasome response in human primary keratinocytes. Exp Dermatol 25:991–993

El Kelish A, Zhao F, Heller W et al (2014) Ragweed (*Ambrosia artemisiifolia*) pollen allergenicity: superSAGE transcriptomic analysis upon elevated CO_2 and drought stress. BMC Plant Biol 14:176

Erkara IP, Cingi C, Ayranci U et al (2009) Skin prick test reactivity in allergic rhinitis patients to airborne pollens. Environ Monit Assess 151:401–412

Fotiou C, Damialis A, Krigas N et al (2011) Parietaria judaica flowering phenology, pollen production, viability and atmospheric circulation, and expansive ability in the urban environment: impacts of environmental factors. Int J Biometeorol 55:35–50

Frei T, Torricelli R, Peeters AG et al (1995) The relationship between airborne pollen distribution and the frequency of specific pollen sensitization at two climatically different locations in Switzerland. Aerobiologia 11:269–273

Galán C, Smith M, Thibaudon M et al (2014) Pollen monitoring: minimum requirements and reproducibility of analysis. Aerobiologia 30:385–395

García-Mozo H (2017) Poaceae pollen as the leading aeroallergen worldwide: a review. Allergy 72:1849–1858

Ghiani A, Aina R, Asero R et al (2012) Ragweed pollen collected along high-traffic roads shows a higher allergenicity than pollen sampled in vegetated areas. Allergy 67:887–894

Gilles S, Mariani V, Bryce M et al (2009) Pollen allergens do not come alone: pollen associated lipid mediators (PALMS) shift the human immune systems towards a TH2-dominated response. Allergy Asthma Clin Immunol 5:3

Gilles S, Fekete A, Zhang X et al (2011) Pollen metabolome analysis reveals adenosine as a major regulator of dendritic cell-primed T(H) cell responses. J Allergy Clin Immunol 127:454–461

Gilles-Stein S, Beck I, Chaker A et al (2016) Pollen derived low molecular compounds enhance the human allergen specific immune response in vivo. Clin Exp Allergy 46:1355–1365

Gioulekas D, Papakosta D, Damialis A et al (2004) Allergenic pollen records (15 years) and sensitization in patients with respiratory allergy in Thessaloniki, Greece. Allergy 59:174–184

Haftenberger M, Laußmann D, Ellert U et al (2013) Prevalence of sensitisation to aeraoallergens and food allergens: results of the German health interview and examination survey for adults (DEGS1). Bundesgesundheitsblatt Gesundheitsforschung Gesundheitsschutz 56:687–697

Häring F, Glaser M, Buters J et al (2017) Towards automatic, real-time pollen monitoring for allergic patients: need for health information services. Allergy 72(S103):80–81

Hemmer W, Focke M, Wantke F et al (2006) Ash (*Fraxinus excelsior*)-pollen allergy in Central Europe: specific role of pollen panallergens and the major allergen of ash pollen, Fra e 1. Allergy 55:923–930

Höhle LP, Speth MM, Phillips KM et al (2017) Association between symptoms of allergic rhinitis with decreased general health-related quality of life. Am J Rhinol Allergy 31:235–239

Kadocsa E, Juhasz M (2002) Study of airborne pollen composition and allergen spectrum of hay fever patients in South Hungary (1990-1999). Aerobiologia 18:203–209

Kaleyias J, Papaioannou D, Manoussakis M et al (2001) Skin-prick test findings in atopic asthmatic children: a follow-up study from childhood to puberty. Ped Allergy Immunol 13:368–374

Karatzas K, Voukantsis D, Jaeger S, Berger U, Smith M, Brandt O, Zuberbier T, Bergmann KCh (2014) The patient's hay-fever diary: three years of results from Germany. Aerobiologia 30(1):1–11

Kawashima S, Thibaudon M, Matsuda S et al (2017) Automated pollen monitoring system using laser optics for observing seasonal changes in the concentration of total airborne pollen. Aerobiologia 33:351–362

Kirmaz C, Yuksel H, Bayrak P et al (2005) Symptoms of the olive pollen allergy: do they really occur only in the pollination season? J Investig Allergol Clin Immunol 15:140–145

Kobzar VN (1999) Aeropalynological monitoring in Bishkek, Kyrgyzstan. Aerobiologia 15:149–153

Langen U, Schmitz R, Steppuhn H (2013) Prevalence of allergic diseases in Germany: results of the German health interview and examination survey for adults (DEGS1). Bundesgesundheitsblatt Gesundheitsforschung Gesundheitsschutz 56:698–706

Lewis WH, Vinay P, Zenger VE (1983) Airborne and allergenic pollen of North America. The Johns Hopkins University Press, Baltimore, pp 105–121

Lin RY, Clauss AE, Bennett ES (2002) Hypersensitivity to common tree pollens in New York city patients. Allergy Asthma Proc 23:253–258

Linneberg A (2011) The increase in allergy and extended challenges. Allergy 66:1–3

Linneberg A (2016) Burden of allergic respiratory disease: a systematic review. Clin Mol Allergy 28:14

Linneberg A, Nielsen NH, Madsen F et al (1999) Increasing prevalence of allergic rhinitis symptoms in an adult Danish population. Allergy 54:1194–1198

Loureiro G, Rabaca MA, Blanco B et al (2005) Aeroallergens' sensitization in an allergic paediatric population of Cova da Beira, Portugal. Allergol Immunopathol 33:192–198

Mandal J, Chakraborty P, Roy I et al (2008) Prevalence of allergenic pollen grains in the aerosol of the city of Calcutta, India: a two year study. Aerobiologia 24:151–164

Marogna M, Massolo A, Berra D et al (2006) The type of sensitizing allergen can affect the evolution of respiratory allergy. Allergy 61:1209–1215

Menzel A, Sparks TH, Estrella N et al (2006) European phenological response to climate change matches the warming pattern. Glob Chang Biol 12:1969–1976

Morais-Almeida M, Santos N, Pereira AM et al (2013) Prevalence and classification of rhinitis in preschool children in Portugal: a nationwide study. Allergy 68:1278–1288

Mueller RS, Bettenay SV, Tideman L (2000) Aero-allergens in canine atopic dermatitis in South-Eastern Australia based on 1000 intradermal skin tests. Austr Vet J 78:392–399

Nakamaru Y, Maguchi S, Oridate N et al (2005) Plantago lanceolata (English plantain) pollinosis in Japan. Auris Nasus Larynx 32:251–256

Ninan TK, Russell G (1992) Respiratory symptoms and atopy in Aberdeen schoolchildren: evidence from two surveys 25 years apart. Brit Med J 304:873–875

Obersteiner A, Gilles S, Frank U et al (2016) Pollen-associated microbiome correlates with pollution parameters and the allergenicity of pollen. PLoS One 11:e0149545

Osborne NJ, Alcock I, Wheeler BW et al (2017) Pollen exposure and hospitalization due to asthma exacerbations: daily time series in a European city. Int J Biometeorol 61:1837–1848

Oteros J, Pusch G, Weichenmeier I et al (2015) Automatic and online pollen monitoring. Int Arch Allergy Immunol 167:158–166

Parmesan C, Yohe G (2003) A globally coherent fingerprint of climate change impacts across natural systems. Nature 421:37–42

Peternel R, Milanović SM, Srnec L (2008) Airborne ragweed (*Ambrosia artemisiifolia* L.) pollen content in the city of Zagreb and implications on pollen allergy. Ann Agr Environ Med 15:125–130

Pignatti S (1982) Flora d' Italia, vol 1-3. Edagricole, Bologna

Rybníček O, Novotná B, Rybníčkova E et al (2000) Ragweed in the Czech Republic. Aerobiologia 16:287–290

Sibbald B, Strachen D (1995) Epidemiology of rhinitis. In: Busse W, Holgate S (eds) Asthma and rhinitis. Blackwell Scientific Publications, Boston, pp 32–34

Sikoparija B, Skjøth CA, Celenk S et al (2017) Spatial and temporal variations in airborne *Ambrosia* pollen in Europe. Aerobiologia 33:181–189

Sin AZ, Ersoy R, Gulbahar O et al (2008) Prevalence of cypress pollen sensitization and its clinical importance in Izmir, Turkey, with cypress allergy assessed by nasal provocation. J Investig Allergol Clin Immunol 18:46–51

Smith M, Cecchi L, Skjoth CA et al (2013) Common ragweed: a threat to environmental health in Europe. Environ Int 61:115–126

Sofiev M, Bousquet J, Linkosalo T et al (2009) Pollen, allergies and adaptation. In: Ebi KL, Burton I, McGregor GR (eds) Biometeorology for adaptation to climate variability and change. Springer, London, pp 75–106

Stach A, García-Mozo H, Prieto-Baena JC et al (2007) Prevalence of *Artemisia* species pollinosis in western Poland: impact of climate change on aerobiological trends, 1995–2004. J Investig Allergol Clin Immunol 17:39–47

Strachan DP, Ross Anderson H (1992) Trends in hospital admission rates for asthma in children. Brit Med J 304:819–820

Subiza J, Jerez M, Jiménez JA et al (1995) Clinical aspects of allergic disease. Allergenic pollen and pollinosis in Madrid. J Allergy Clin Immunol 96:15–23

Traidl-Hoffmann C (2017) Allergy – an environmental disease. Bundesgesundheitsbl Gesundheitsforsch Gesundheitsschutz 60:584–591

Treudler R, Simon J-C (2017) Pollen-related food allergy: an update. Allergo J Int 26:273–282

Treudler R, Franke A, Schmiedeknecht A et al (2017) BASALIT trial: double-blind placebo-controlled allergen immunotherapy with rBet v 1-FV in birch-related soya allergy. Allergy 72:1243–1253

Troise C, Voltolini S, Delbono G et al (1992) Allergy to pollens from Betulaceae and Corylaceae in a Mediterranean area (Genoa, Italy). A 10-year retrospective study. J Inv Allergol Clin Immunol 2:313–317

Varjonen E, Kalimo K, Lammintausta K et al (1992) Prevalence of atopic disorders among adolescents in Turku, Finland. Allergy 47:243–248

Verini M, Rossi N, Verroti A et al (2001) Sensitization to environmental antigens in asthmatic children from a central Italian area. Sci Total Environ 270:63–69

Voltolini S, Minale P, Troise C et al (2000) Trend of herbaceous pollen diffusion and allergic sensitisation in Genoa, Italy. Aerobiologia 16:245–249

Voukantsis D, Berger U, Tsima F et al (2015) Personalized symptoms forecasting for pollen-induced allergic rhinitis sufferers. Int J Biometeorol 59:889–897

Wan S, Yuan T, Bowdish S et al (2002) Response of an allergenic species, *Ambrosia psilostachya* (Asteraceae), to experimental warming and clipping: implications for public health. Am J Bot 89:1843–1846

Wayne P, Foster S, Connolly J et al (2002) Production of allergenic pollen by ragweed (*Ambrosia artemisiifolia* L.) is increased in CO_2-enriched atmospheres. Ann Allergy Asthma Immunol 88:279–282

Weeke ER, Spieksma FTM (1991) Allergenic significance of Gramineae (Poaceae). In: D'Amato G, Spieksma FTHM, Bonini S (eds) Allergenic pollen and pollinosis in Europe. Blackwell Scientific Publications, Oxford/London/Edinburgh/Boston/Melbourne/Paris/Berlin/Vienna, pp 109–112

Wodehouse RP (1971) Hayfever plants, 2nd edn. Hafner, New York, p 280

Wu LYF, Steidle GM, Meador MA et al (1999) Effect of tree and grass pollens and fungal spores on spring allergic rhinitis: a comparative study. Ann Allergy Asthma Immunol 83:137–143

Wüthrich B, Schindler C, Leuenberger P et al (1995) Prevalence of atopy and pollinosis in the adult population of Switzerland (SAPALDIA study). Int Arch Allergy Immunol 106:149–156

Zhao F, Elkelish A, Durner J et al (2016) Common ragweed (*Ambrosia artemisiifolia* L.): allergenicity and molecular characterization of pollen after plant exposure to elevated NO_2. Plant Cell Environ 39:147–164

Zhao F, Durner J, Winkler JB et al (2017) Pollen of common ragweed (*Ambrosia artemisiifolia* L.): illumina-based de novo sequencing and differential transcript expression upon elevated NO_2/O_3. Environ Pollut 224:503–514

Ziello C, Sparks TH, Estrella N et al (2012) Changes to airborne pollen counts across Europe. PLoS One 7:e34076

Ziska LH, Gebhard DE, Frenz DA et al (2003) Cities as harbingers of climate change: common ragweed, urbanization, and public health. J Allergy Clin Immunol 111:290–295

Chapter 4
Vector-Borne Diseases

Ruth Müller, Friederike Reuss, Vladimir Kendrovski, and Doreen Montag

Abstract Vector-borne diseases (VBDs) are illnesses caused by parasites, viruses or bacteria that are transmitted by a vector such as mosquitoes, ticks, sandflies, triatomine bugs, tsetse flies, fleas, black flies, aquatic snails and lice. In this chapter, we aim to show how climate change impacts VBDs and what role biodiversity (and its loss) plays for VBDs. (1) We show how climatic changes shape the distribution and abundance of disease vectors. To point out current triple vulnerabilities regarding climate change, biodiversity and VBDs, we selected ticks and mosquitoes as examples. (2) We point out important knowledge gaps on VBDs and biodiversity, which make prognoses for VBDs under climate change challenging. (3) We review vector control tools as well as policy options and related infrastructural responses to manage VBDs under climate and biodiversity changes.

R. Müller (✉)
Institute of Occupational, Social and Environmental Medicine, Goethe University, Frankfurt am Main, Germany

Polo d'Innovazione di Genomica, Genetica e Biologia (PoloGGB), Terni, Italy
e-mail: ruth.mueller@med.uni-frankfurt.de

F. Reuss
Institute of Occupational, Social and Environmental Medicine, Goethe University, Frankfurt am Main, Germany

Senckenberg Biodiversity and Climate Research Centre, Frankfurt am Main, Germany

Institute for Ecology, Diversity and Evolution, Goethe University, Frankfurt am Main, Germany
e-mail: friederike.reuss@senckenberg.de

V. Kendrovski
European Centre for Environment and Health, WHO Regional Office for Europe, Bonn, Germany
e-mail: kendrovskiv@who.int

D. Montag
Barts and the London School of Medicine, Centre for Primary Care and Public Health, Queen Mary University of London, London, UK
e-mail: d.montag@qmul.ac.uk

M. R. Marselle et al. (eds.), *Biodiversity and Health in the Face of Climate Change*, https://doi.org/10.1007/978-3-030-02318-8_4

Keywords Mosquito-borne · Tick-borne · One Health · Planetary health · Vector diversity · Vector control

Highlights

- Climatic change shapes the regional distribution and abundance of disease vectors.
- There are important knowledge gaps with relation to VBDs and biodiversity.
- A variety of new biological and genetic vector control tools are under development.
- VBD control needs a trans-sectoral One Health approach, not just the health sector.
- VBD control and elimination should be based on a wider understanding of planetary health.

4.1 Triple Vulnerability: Climate Change, Biodiversity and Vector-Borne Diseases

Both climate change and biodiversity loss are current challenges to humankind. Climate and biodiversity change have health impacts that range widely from direct effects such as progressive temperature increases from global warming, flooding or heat waves due to increased climate variability and extreme weather events, to indirect effects such as changes in ecosystem services, food productivity or species distributions (Montag et al. 2017). Indirect effects also include the redistribution of vector species or extended seasonal transmission periods and spatial extension, as well as the disappearance of vector-borne diseases (VBDs).

VBDs are illnesses caused by parasites, viruses or bacteria that are transmitted by a vector, such as mosquitoes, ticks, sandflies, triatomine bugs, tsetse flies, fleas, black flies, aquatic snails and lice (Table 4.1, WHO 2017a). The current spatial distributions of ten important vector-borne diseases are shown in Fig. 4.1.

Currently, on average, 77,000 people living in Europe fall sick from VBDs every year, but numbers are predicted to increase as vector species emerge (e.g. the Asian tiger mosquito, *Aedes albopictus*) or re-emerge (e.g. the yellow fever mosquito, *Aedes aegypti*) (http://www.euro.who.int/en/media-centre/sections/press-releases/2014/77-000-europeans-fall-sick-every-year-with-vector-borne-diseases). Globally, every year there are more than 700,000 deaths from zoonotic vector-borne diseases such as malaria, dengue, schistosomiasis, human African trypanosomiasis, leishmaniasis, Chagas disease, yellow fever, Japanese encephalitis and onchocerciasis (WHO 2017a). These zoonotic diseases account for around 17% of the estimated global burden of communicable diseases and disproportionately affect poorer populations that live in environmentally degraded environments and housing conditions that are favourable to VBDs (WHO 2017a). They impede economic

Table 4.1 Main vectors and diseases they transmit

Mosquitoes			Ticks	Sandflies	Triatomine bugs	Tsetse flies	Fleas	Black flies	Aquatic snails	Lice
Aedes	*Anopheles*	*Culex*	*Ixodes, Dermacentor, Hyalomma*	*Phlebotomia*	*Triatominae*	*Glossina*		*Simuliidae*	*Biomphalaria, Bulinus*	
Chikungunya, Dengue fever, Lymphatic filariasis, Rift Valley fever, yellow fever, Zika	Malaria, Lymphatic filariasis	Japanese encephalitis, lymphatic filariasis, West Nile fever	Crimean-Congo haemorrhagic fever, Lyme disease, relapsing fever (borreliosis), Rickettsial diseases (spotted fever and Q fever), Tick-borne encephalitis, Tularaemia	Leishmaniasis, sandfly fever (phelebotomus fever)	Chagas disease (American trypanosomiasis)	Sleeping sickness (African trypanosomiasis)	Plague (transmitted by fleas from rats to humans), Rickettsiosis	Onchocerciasis (river blindness)	Schistosomiasis (bilharziasis)	Typhus and louse-borne relapsing fever

Adapted from the WHO fact sheet *Vector-borne diseases* (WHO 2017a)

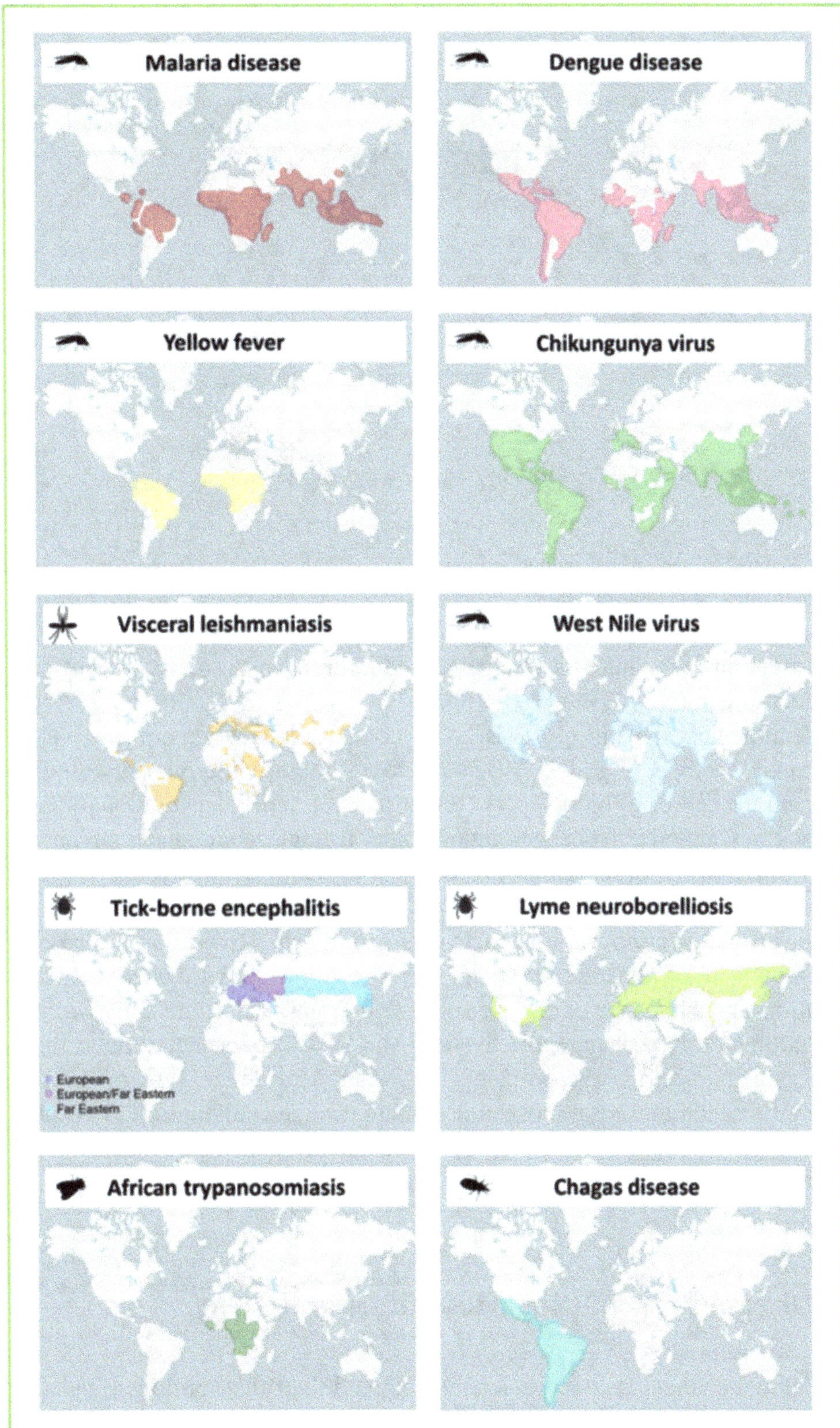

Fig. 4.1 Overview of countries/territories where ten important vector-borne diseases/related pathogens have been reported: malaria disease[1], dengue disease[2], yellow fever[3], chikungunya virus[4], visceral leishmaniasis[5], West Nile virus[6], tick-borne encephalitis[7], Lyme neuroborreliosis[8], African trypanosomiasis, and Chagas disease[10]. (Data sources: [1]Centers for Disease Control and Prevention (CDC), 2017; [2]World Health Organization (WHO), 2013, [3,4]CDC, 2018, [5]WHO, 2010, [6]CDC, 2012, [7]Holbrook (2017) *Viruses* 9(5):97, based on CDC and WHO data, [8]Pachner & Steiner (2007) *Lancet Neurology* 6(6):544–52, [9]WHO, 2016, [10]WHO, 2004)

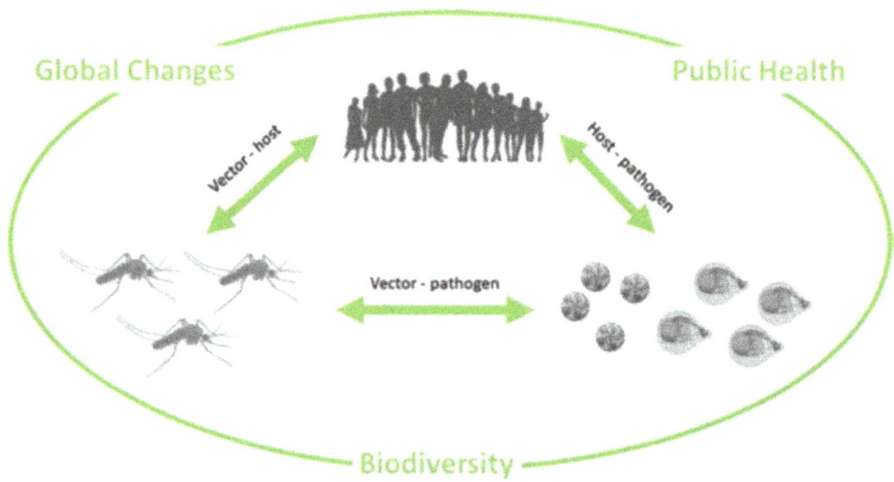

Fig. 4.2 Scheme of vector-host-pathogen interactions indicating the complex interplay of public health, biodiversity and global changes

development through direct medical costs and indirect costs such as loss of productivity and tourism (Narrod et al. 2012).

Epidemiological dynamics of VBDs are complex interactions of the vector, the pathogen and the host (Fig. 4.2). VBDs are clearly highly intertwined with climatic change and the degree of biodiversity (Engering et al. 2013). In addition to temperature alterations and rainfall changes, among other factors, heterogeneity of landscapes (Chaves et al. 2011), urbanisation (Wood et al. 2017) and local forest degradation (Brownstein et al. 2005) are extrinsic factors determining VBD risk or burden.

In this chapter, we show how climate change impacts VBDs and what role biodiversity (and its loss) plays for VBDs. (1) We show how climatic changes shape the distribution and abundance of disease vectors. To point out current triple vulnerabilities regarding climate change, biodiversity and VBDs, we selected ticks and mosquitoes as examples. (2) We point out important knowledge gaps on VBDs and biodiversity, which make prognoses for climate change challenging. (3) We review policy options to manage VBDs under climate and biodiversity changes and related infrastructural responses.

4.2 Disease-Transmitting Mosquitoes and Ticks

Due to global change, vector species may expand their distributions (Ogden et al. 2006; Gould and Higgs 2009) and shift their seasonal and spatial occurrences (Lafferty 2009), the latter particularly to higher latitudes and altitudes (Siraj et al. 2014; Dhimal et al. 2014a, b, 2015). This leads to increased species richness, e.g. a higher biodiversity of the vector species and pathogens at time of arrival in newly invaded regions. However, invasive species show a tendency to successfully establish in a new environment and outcompete native species sharing the same ecological niche. Thus, biodiversity can even decrease rather than increase under certain ecological conditions.

4.2.1 Influence of Temperature on Vector Mosquitoes and Associated Pathogens

In holometabolous vector mosquitoes, larval rearing temperature influences development times (Delatte et al. 2009; Reiskind and Janairo 2015; Couret et al. 2014; Müller et al. 2018), larval survival (Chang et al. 2007; Delatte et al. 2009; Couret et al. 2014; Müller et al. 2018), adult longevity (Aytekin et al. 2009; Delatte et al. 2009), length of female gonotrophic cycle (Delatte et al. 2009), and adult body size (Briegel and Timmermann 2001; Mohammed and Chadee 2011; Muturi et al. 2011). In arboviruses, temperature effects plaque growth (Jia et al. 2007) and replication speed (Kilpatrick et al. 2008). In addition, mosquito-arbovirus interactions such as virus susceptibility (Turell 1993; Kilpatrick et al. 2008; Westbrook et al. 2010), prevalence of dissemination (Turell 1993, Kilpatrick et al. 2008, Westbrook et al. 2010), transmission rate (Kilpatrick et al. 2008) and extrinsic incubation period (Chan and Johansson 2012) are influenced by temperature (reviewed in Samuel et al. 2016).

Altogether, temperature plays a key role in determining the viral transmission areas (Bayoh and Lindsay 2003; Lambrechts et al. 2010; Kilpatrick et al. 2008). Studies have shown that the ambient rearing temperature at immature stages influences the virus susceptibility and dissemination rate at adult stages for chikungunya virus in *Aedes albopictus* (Westbrook et al. 2010), Rift Valley fever virus and Venezuelan equine encephalitis virus in *Ae. taeniorhynchus* (Turell 1993) and Sindbis virus in *Ae. aegypti* (Muturi et al. 2011). Adult females of *Ae. albopictus* produced from larvae reared at 18 °C were more likely infected and disseminated with chikungunya virus than females from larvae reared at 32 °C (Westbrook et al. 2010) and *Ae. taeniorhynchus* females reared at 19 °C as larvae had a higher susceptibility and dissemination-prevalence for Rift Valley fever virus and Venezuelan equine encephalitis virus than larval cohorts reared at 26 °C (Turell 1993). *Ae. aegypti* females showed significantly higher infection and insemination rates with Sindbis virus when reared at their optimal larval temperature (25 °C) than when reared under temperature stress at 32 °C (Muturi et al. 2011). Therefore, knowledge on temperature effects triggering vector mosquitoes' mortality and development is important to explain disease outbreaks (Bangs et al. 2006).

4.2.2 Distributional Changes of Mosquito Vector Species

Climate change will not uniformly increase the burden of VBDs, but changes will differ between regions. In Ecuador, a modelling study examining the distributional changes of 14 vector species under climate change demonstrated that some arthropod vector species will become extinct in certain regions, while other regions, and in particular the Andean highlands, will experience a novel VBD burden (Escobar et al. 2016) (see Box 4.1). In accordance, the expansion of other VBDs such as

Box 4.1 VBD Risk Modelling for Climate Change Conditions and Suitable Policy Interventions in Ecuador

In their article, Escobar et al. (2016) analyse the current and potential future impact of climate change on vector diversity and geographical distribution in Ecuador through ecological niche modelling. The authors applied broader scale climate modelling concerning the current distribution of vectors, using remote sensing data. They defined suitable vector environments as potential high-risk areas, which were used to do future risk VBD modelling under climate change. Overall, they analysed current, medium-term and long-term predictions for vector distribution that can transmit dengue, malaria, Chagas and leishmaniasis. The model for the dengue transmitting vectors *Aedes aegypti* and *Ae. albopictus*, the latter not being officially reported in Ecuador but in neighboring countries, indicates a currently reduced, but future increased, risk for dengue transmission in highland regions, and long-term high risk in the coastal and Northeastern Amazonian areas. Importantly, climate change models predicted a change in vector-suitability environments, proposing an increased risk in western Andean valleys, which will pose additional public health and intervention challenges.

Escobar et al. (2016) present overall a higher risk for vector-borne diseases under future climate regimes, particularly in part of the Ecuadorian coast, valleys of the Northeastern Amazonian and western Andean region. Mitchell-Foster et al. (2015) have presented an integrated policy intervention that could propose a lasting option to vector-borne disease prevention and control, empowering communities and building future community health leaders. In their randomised controlled study in Machala, on the southwestern coast of Ecuador, they employed an integrated eco-bio-social approach among school children, aged 8–12 years, to significantly reduce the pupa per person index. Mitchell-Foster et al. (2015) used 20 clusters of 100 households, selected based on a two-stage-sampling design. Ten clusters were used for the integrated eco-bio-social approach and ten as control clusters. In addition, different forms of geographical mapping and pupa per person index (PPI) were used as an outcome measurement. The overall result showed a decreased PPI, and in those households where there were not any changes noted through monthly control visits, particular engagement activities were deployed (Mitchell-Foster et al. 2015, p.128). The integrative eco-bio-social approach among school children allowed for social empowerment, capacity building of future leaders and vector control. Given the projections for future dengue risk by Escobar et al. (2016), the findings of Mitchell-Foster's et al. (2015) randomised controlled study would present a suitable policy intervention, which could easily be scaled up on a national level.

Japanese encephalitis, dengue, chikungunya, lymphatic filariasis and visceral leishmaniasis towards a cooler mountainous region has been reported from Nepal (Dhimal et al. 2014a, 2015; Ostyn et al. 2015). Altitude is often used as a proxy for temperature changes, so one may speculate that this trend might also be true for more northern/temperate regions.

In Europe, four exotic *Aedes* types of mosquitoes are currently found (partly reviewed in Medlock et al. 2012): the Asian tiger mosquito (*Ae. albopictus*; Adhami and Reiter 1998), the yellow-fever mosquito (*Ae. aegypti*; Goncalves et al. 2008), the Asian bush mosquito (*Ae. japonicus japonicus*; Schaffner et al. 2009) and *Ae. koreicus* (Versteirt et al. 2012). Particularly, the Asian tiger mosquito *Ae. albopictus* with widespread European distribution is a competent vector for several VBDs and therefore poses human public health risks. It is suspected that the Asian tiger mosquito was the main vector for dengue viruses in France in 2015 (Succo et al. 2016) and for chikungunya virus in Italy in 2007 and 2017 (Rezza 2018) (autochthonous cases in Europe 2007–2012 reviewed in Tomasello and Schlagenhauf 2013). These cases show how human transport activities and temperature change facilitate the establishment of vector species and highlight the importance of actively preventing such establishments (Eritja et al. 2017; Ducheyne et al. 2018, Reuss et al. 2018, Dhimal et al. 2018).

Despite temperature, climate change will lead to hydrological changes. For *Ae. albopictus* in Europe, it is projected that Mediterranean locations will become more unsuitable habitats due to climatic variables and changed water regimes, while suitability is increased in middle and northern Europe up to 55°N (Fischer et al. 2014). Climate and photoperiod also alter the host-seeking and feeding activity in ticks as well as the seasonal occurrence of vector stages (Altizer et al. 2013; Kurtenbach et al. 2006).

4.2.3 Distributional Changes of Ticks in Europe

There are objective grounds that climate change influences the distribution and seasonal activity of disease-transmitting ticks (Ogden et al. 2014). The tick *Ixodes ricinus* is medically highly relevant as a vector for spirochaete bacteria *Borrelia burgdorferi*, with Lyme disease extending its distribution northwards in Europe, in a warmer climate (Lindgren et al. 2000). The taiga tick (*Ixodes persulcatus*), transmitting the 'early summer' meningo-enzephalitis virus, is currently spread from Russia west-northwards to Scandinavia (Jaenson et al. 2016). Ticks of the genera *Dermacentor* with a previously Mediterranean distribution, for instance the *Coxiella burnetti*-transmitting sheep tick *Dermacentor marginatus* (Q fever,) are now established in cold-temperate Germany (Földvári et al. 2016). The Mediterranean tick *Hyalomma marginatum* is the main vector for the emerging pathogen Crimean-Congo Hemorrhagic Fever in Europe. International livestock trading guarantees the tick's mobility, as ticks live on domestic animals, while the degradation of agricultural land favours the mass development of *Hyalomma marginatum* (Estrada-Pena et al. 2012). This tick species has established populations in southern and eastern Europe but may extend its distribution to some areas of Italy, the Balkans and southern Russia when climatic conditions are improved, especially in autumn (Estrada-Pena et al. 2012).

4.3 Biodiversity and VBDs: The Large Unknowns

4.3.1 Pathogen Diversity

The diversity of potential human pathogens, the species diversity and phenotypic plasticity of vectors and the biodiversity of their reservoir hosts is largely unexplored. On our planet, an immense but largely unknown diversity of viral species is hosted by mammals and birds (estimate over 1.3 million, http://www.globalviromeproject.org/overview/). Approximately 38% of these viral species could result in VBDs in humans. The Global Virome Project will explore this biodiversity of viruses over the next 10 years, which may result in many surprises for the VBD research community.

4.3.2 Vector Diversity

The understanding of spatio-temporal phenotypic diversity and genetic architectures of vector populations under current and climate change conditions is crucial for vector control management. Local knowledge on phenotypic diversity to insecticide resistance can foster success in chemical vector control. The worldwide insecticide resistance network WIN is currently tracking insecticide resistance in mosquito disease vectors on a global scale and consults with the WHO and member states on how to improve insecticide resistance surveillance and implement alternative vector control tools (https://win-network.ird.fr/). Likewise, the understanding of vector ecology and in particular the understanding of age-structure of field populations, the adaptive behaviour of vectors, and context-dependence of vector capacities fundamentally affect the success rate of biotechnological interventions. The efficiency of biological and genetic vector control is in some cases defined by the available number of targeted life stages. In others, the ratio of released *Wolbachia* contaminated insects and genetically modified or radiation-sterilised males and the virgin wildtype counterparts in a field population determines the suppression rate of vector populations and hence the degree of disease control (Iturbe-Ormaetxe et al. 2011; Ross et al. 2017). Our lack of basic ecological knowledge even with a prominent vector such as *Anopheles gambiae* for malaria disease could blunt our new biotechnological weapons for vector control (Alphey and Alphey 2014; Ferguson et al. 2010).

4.3.3 *Host Diversity*

Mosquitoes and ticks feed on a wide range of hosts, and their pathogens circulate in diverse animal species. Lyme disease is caused by *Borrelia burgdorferi*, which is transmitted to humans through the bite of *Ixodes* ticks. For *Borrelia burgdorferi* sensu *lato*, a broad range of reservoir hosts have been identified, for instance nine small mammals, seven medium-sized mammals and 16 bird species in Europe (Gern et al. 1998), and eight small mammals in the USA (summarised in Salkeld et al. 2008). As another example, the Zika virus is known to circulate in monkey and wild mammal populations in Africa, and has been detected in domestic sheep, goats, horses, cows, ducks, rodents, bats, orangutans and carabaos in Indonesia and Pakistan (Vorou 2016). However, large knowledge gaps on the diversity of reservoir hosts for mosquito- and tick-borne pathogens in old and new areas of distribution still exist (Baráková et al. 2018; Hashiguchi et al. 2018). Certainly, these gaps will never be closed given the complex dynamics of adaptations between pathogens, vectors and hosts.

The conceptual model of the dilution effect in Lyme disease (Ostfeld and Keesing 2012) is the textbook example about how biodiversity on the level of the host species can directly influence the transmission of an arthropod-transmitted disease. Humans are aberrant hosts for the pathogen, because the pathogens cannot replicate in humans. In a natural cycle of *Borrelia burgdorferi*, the bacteria are maintained by small mammals and birds (reservoir hosts). The dilution effect model in the Lyme-disease system states that the relative abundance of host individuals should be evenly distributed across host species to decrease the potential for an encounter of the tick with the most competent reservoir host. This model also applies to other vector-host systems in which a generalist vector uses many host species of which only a few are competent reservoir hosts (Swaddle and Calos 2008; Civitello et al. 2015). The smaller the risk for a host to become infected and thereby maintain and release pathogens, the more species-diverse and abundant is the host community (Civitello et al. 2013; Levi et al. 2016). However, this dilution effect is still under academic debate (e.g. Civitello et al. 2015 and Salkeld et al. 2015), and there is an urgent need for further research.

4.4 How to Manage VBDs?

Different public health measures exist, ranging from epidemic control through vector control (of mosquitoes, bugs, flies, fleas) and eradication of diseases through vaccination, case treatment and breeding site elimination (WHO 2017b). Vector control tools target specific life stages of arthropod vectors and are of a chemical (e.g. pyrethroid insecticides), biological (e.g. *Wolbachia* bacteria) or transgenic nature (e.g. genetically modified mosquitoes). Chemical insecticides are additionally used for preventive measures such as insecticide-treated bed nets, insecticide-treated livestock or indoor residual spraying in highly VBD endemic areas, which complements other preventive actions such as source reduction and information campaigns. All pest control measures can influence biodiversity in manifold ways, whereas prospective evaluations of positive and negative effects of pest control under global changes is rarely available in the VBD context.

4.4.1 Chemical Insecticides

Arthropod pest control in epidemic regions is based on chemical insecticides, which work efficiently against vectors, but are mostly associated with undesirable side effects for biodiversity. The past use of dichloro-diphenyl-trichloroethane (DDT), for example, successfully eliminated malaria in North America and Europe and significantly decreased the number of deaths in other regions of the world (WHO 2008; Keiser et al. 2005). However, DDT is highly persistent in the environment, accumulates in fatty tissues of organisms, and biomagnifies from low trophic levels to predators such as ice bears and eagles (e.g. reviewed in Van den Berg 2009). The high ecotoxicological risk of DDT for wildlife and ecosystem functioning was first discovered by Rachel Carlson in 1962 (Carson 2002). Consequently, the Stockholm Convention on Persistent Organic Pollutants (2001) banned DDT and a number of other chemicals that were used as insecticides in the past (NO 2005). The use of DDT is, however, allowed under the Stockholm Convention for disease vector control, within the recommendations and guidelines of the WHO until locally effective and affordable substitutes and methods are available. Concerted large-scale efforts are now underway to reduce both the burden of VBDs and the use of DDT (Van den Berg 2009).

The generations of insecticides following DDT were organophosphates (e.g. parathion), carbamates, pyrethroids (e.g. deltamethrin) and neonicotinoids (e.g. imidacloprid), all designed to increase the efficiency to kill pest insects, overcome problems with insecticide resistance in pest species, and lower the environmental burden by increasing specificity (and thereby decreasing applied amounts for the same efficiency). In every insecticide class, however, negative health effects on human and/or wildlife occurred. For example, pyrethroids are recommended for indoor spraying and bed net treatment by the WHO. However, pyrethroid resistance evolved in several insect species and hence vector control cannot rely exclusively on this insecticide class in the long term (Hemingway and Ranson 2000). As another example, neonicotinoids, the most recent insecticide class (developed in the 1990s) are discussed as a good candidate (clothianidin) for indoor residual spraying in areas with pyrethroid-resistant mosquito populations (Agossa et al. 2018). Neonicotinoids are currently under restricted use in the European market due to increasing evidence of toxic effects on honey bees (honey-bee colony-collapse disorder), wild pollinators and indirectly on insectivorous birds, which are already challenged by climate change (e.g., Le Conte and Navajas 2008; Hladik et al. 2018).

On 17 May 2018, the European Commission banned the neonicotinoids imidacloprid, clothianidin and thiamethoxam for field applications in EU member states.

With climatic changes, the efficiency of chemical insecticides can change (thermal-dependent toxicity of specific chemicals; Kreß et al. 2014) and the distribution of chemical insecticides in the environment will alter (Op de Beeck et al. 2017). Probably enhanced by a warmer climate, insecticide resistance of arthropod vectors to chemical insecticides will evolve further (Maino et al. 2018). In contrast, non-target organisms in aquatic environments are threatened by manifold stressors, while the combined effects of pesticides and warming may accelerate the ongoing biodiversity loss (Liess et al. 2016). Thus, even if the use of chemical insecticides currently appears to be an easy-to-use tool, in the long term, we need new, eco-friendly and sustainable vector control tools.

4.4.2 Biological Insecticides

There is a consensus between researchers, that biodiversity is a valuable resource for discovering novel insecticides (Silva-Filha 2017; Huang et al. 2017). The ongoing dramatic loss of biodiversity under climate and other global changes may empty this treasure chest faster than new biological insecticides can be discovered.

For a few decades, control measures have made use of natural insect toxins from *Bacillus israelensis thuringiensis* (B.t.i.) and the bacterial endoparasite *Wolbachia* spp. (mostly *W. pipientis*) (Baldacchino et al. 2015). The application of B.t.i. in wetlands against floodwater mosquitoes, which are primarily annoying insects but are also known as vectors for Usutu and West Nile viruses, is assumed to be environmentally safe, although discussions on this topic are highly controversially discussed (Niemi et al. 2015; Jakob and Poulin 2016). Unfortunately, first resistance against B.t.i. has been observed, for instance in the dengue vector *Aedes aegypti*, and is expected to be supported by a warming climate (Paris et al. 2011).

A great success story is the contamination of *Aedes* mosquitoes with natural *Wolbachia* bacteria (Iturbe-Ormaetxe et al. 2011). The presence of the bacteria inhibits the dengue and West Nile virus replication and hence reduces the pathogen load of mosquitoes (Ant et al. 2018). This biological technique can also be used to suppress mosquito populations since wild females become sterilised when mating with a *Wolbachia*-contaminated male mosquito. The World Mosquito Program developed a *Wolbachia* method that enables the transmission of *Wolbachia* to offspring and spreads through the whole population (http://www.eliminatedengue.com/our-research/wolbachia). This theoretically self-sustaining *Wolbachia* method is now in the large-scale trial phase (reviewed in Mishra et al. 2018).

Many other biological approaches have been discussed (Huang et al. 2017). As one example, copepods have been used for a long time to control *Aedes* species (e.g. Vu et al. 1998) and are now also proposed as biological agents against *Culex* mosquitoes. Copepods feed on mosquito larvae (and other prey) and hence suppress populations. Since the growth rates of both prey and predator strongly depend on temperature, the *Relative Control Potential* metric has been developed to allow the right selection of a living biological control agent for specific temperature conditions (Cuthbert et al. 2018).

4.4.3 New Genetic Tools in Vector Control

Recent advances to modernise and develop new vector control and surveillance tools mean that there has never been a better time to reinvigorate vector control. The genetic control of vectors will add to the existing vector control toolbox. Certain genetic vector control strategies have a greater advantage as they will perform even better when climatic conditions favour vector population growth and development. Furthermore, genetic vector control targets only one species and thereby could avoid direct negative effects on non-target species.

The sterile insect technique (SIT) is based on the release of sterile mosquito males, produced by irradiation or sterilising chemicals, mating with wild females and thereby suppressing the mosquito population growth. However, the successful implementation of SIT requires a repeated release of a high number of mosquitoes with ideally no fitness costs if compared to wild counterparts. Therefore mass-rearing facilities have been set up and several sex-sorting techniques for pupae have been developed. SIT successfully eliminates or suppresses populations, as shown for *Cx. quinquefasciatus* on an island in Florida and *Anopheles albimanus* in El Salvador or *Ae. albopictus* in Italy (reviewed in Baldacchino et al. 2015). Alternatively, insects can be sterilised or immunised by genetic modifications (GMs), which is a more precise procedure and goes along with less fitness costs for male mosquitoes. The release of transgenic sterile male mosquitoes carrying a dominant lethal genetic system (RIDL technique) has been successfully applied for dengue-carrying mosquitoes in the Caribbean (Harris et al. 2011), Malaysia (Lacroix et al. 2012) and Brazil (Carvalho et al. 2015). However, as with SIT, repeated releases with large numbers of males are necessary to efficiently control insect vectors and agricultural pest insects.

The release of gene-drive insects for population suppression or vector immunisation might be an even more promising technique. Preliminary studies have confirmed the feasibility of using gene drive-based modifications for vector control (Hammond et al. 2016; Burt et al. 2018). Gene-drives rely on an endonuclease cassette (e.g. CRISPR-Cas9) targeting genes important for fitness of the vector or inhibit parasite development. This endonuclease cassette spreads through the target population by modifying/cutting the DNA of target genes in the germline of every offspring. When the DNA in wild-type insects is repaired, the DNA of genetically modified insects serves as the DNA template. As a result, the endonuclease cassette copies to the wild-type DNA. This way, the gene-drive construct passes via germline modification to almost every offspring and from generation to generation. This hypothetical self-sustaining behaviour of gene-drives might be a clear advantage, because the reduction of release efforts is necessary to save costs, lower infrastructural needs and may also work in large and remote areas. However, the technique lacks post-release control and the required data for environmental risk assessment are not yet available. Further research is needed before allowing the release of gene-drive insects to the wild.

4.4.4 Sustainable Control Programs

The ecological risk assessment of chemical, biological and genetic vector control measures on non-target biodiversity will remain difficult because our basic knowledge on non-VBD biodiversity as well as on cryptic viral, microbiological, genetic, phenotypic and reservoir host biodiversity under global changes is so fragmentary. One may also hope for the future, that biodiverse nature endows us with new biological insecticides and medically active compounds to help us to treat VBDs. Such ecosystem services could deliver a very good reason to preserve existing biodiversity and respect traditional lifestyles and related knowledge of local communities.

Traditionally, single-intervention approaches such as insecticide treatment dominated the toolbox of vector control managers in the past. The Integrated Vector Control Management (IVM) makes use of vector surveillance, risk mapping and a variety of vector prevention and control tools, and adjusts the set of applied tools to local conditions in a time- and dose-dependent manner. However, it must be kept in mind that just a reduction of mosquito breeding sites (prevention), use of insecticides (control), IVM or SIT have brought only few benefits in the attempt to control the vector populations (Baldacchino et al. 2015). Building sustainable control programs that are resilient in the face of technical, operational and financial challenges will in addition require the engagement and collaboration of local communities.

Efforts to limit the breeding of disease vectors are often hampered by lack of community awareness of the interconnections between disease, vectors and viruses/parasites. On the other hand, community mobilisation and the implementation of an integrated community-based approach can probably render dengue fever control effective (Andersson et al. 2015; Mitchell-Foster et al. 2015). Lessons learned from previous studies should be used to inform previously VBD-unaffected populations. For example, a study from Nepal shows that only 12% of the sample population had good knowledge of dengue fever and those living in the lowlands with regular outbreaks of mosquito-borne diseases were five times more likely to possess good knowledge than highlanders experiencing rare or zero outbreaks of mosquito-borne diseases (Dhimal et al. 2014b). Thus, VBD-naïve populations such as in remote mountainous regions may be at special risk under the impact of climate change fostering the spread of disease vectors to cooler ecoregions (Dhimal et al. 2014a, b, c, 2015; Escobar et al. 2016). The same might be true for northern/temperate regions if considering altitude as a proxy for temperature conditions.

4.5 Responses to VBDs Along with Biodiversity Loss and Climate Change

4.5.1 *Target the Complexity*

Though the world is complex, our understanding of VBDs comes mainly from individual research disciplines. Who is at a high risk of VBDs is determined by biological, ecological, climatic, social, cultural, historical, political and economic factors (Lacey 2012; Marmot and Wilkinson 2005). Ecological factors refer, for example, to micro-climate, the natural landscape and anthropogenic settings. Biological factors relate to population dynamics of vectors and the transmission dynamics of pathogens. Socio-cultural, political and economic factors comprise a number of variables relating to conservation of biodiversity, mitigation and adaption strategies of climate change impacts and health systems, including vector control, health services, the political context, public and private services (such as water supply), 'macro-social' events (such as urbanisation), and community and household-based practices, and how these are shaped by large-scale forces (such as gender, ethnicity, education, social and economic status) (Chu-Agor et al. 2012; Huffaker 2015). All those factors need to be understood in a systemic context, rather than as individual factors, if we want to understand altered geographical and temporal distributions of VBDs. To give an example, dengue and chikungunya viruses are transmitted by the mosquitoes *Aedes albopictus* and *Aedes aegypti.* Their local transmission of dengue and chikungunya viruses is coupled with meteorological and climatological conditions, and ecological, socio-economic, demographic and cultural factors (Morrison 2014; Teurlai et al. 2015; Harapan et al. 2017, 2018).

4.5.2 *Interconnecting People and Knowledge*

There are several promising developments to interconnect people and knowledge in Europe and beyond.

At the G7 summit on 7 and 8 June 2015, G7 member states committed themselves to research and development in the field *Neglected Tropical Diseases*, which includes many VBDs such as Zika, dengue, chikungunya and leishmaniasis. As a result, for example, the four German ministries Federal Ministry of Education and Research, Federal Ministry of Food and Agriculture, Federal Ministry of Health and Federal Ministry of Defence signed a research agreement on One Health that supports interdisciplinary research on zoonotic diseases for the health of animals and humans. In accordance, the national network on zoonoses (https://www.gesundheitsforschung-bmbf.de/de/nationales-forschungsnetz-zoonotische-infektionskrankheiten-6820.php) was founded in 2017, which interacts strongly with the German Research platform for zoonoses (http://www.zoonosen.net/EnglishSite/Home.aspx). Both German initiatives aim to improve our understanding of zoonotic diseases and to improve the knowledge transfer from science to practice and *vice versa*.

At the European level, the European Food Safety Authority (EFSA) and the European Centre for Disease Prevention and Control (ECDC) support the European VectorNet initiative. The VectorNet network assembles data on vector distributions and cases of animal and human VBDs. The information on biogeography of vectors and latest VBD outbreaks can be freely accessed at https://ecdc.europa.eu/en/about-us/partnerships-and-networks/disease-and-laboratory-networks/vector-net. Moreover, the European Union funds the InfraVec2 project, which offers free access to European infrastructures for research on insect vectors and their pathogens and thereby interconnects the VBD research community (https://infravec2.eu/). The InfraVec2 project aims to set up common quality standards and operating frameworks in the field of arthropod VBDs (standardise test procedures, develop accepted, traceable reference standards for biological material, etc.) and thus improve inter-laboratory reproducibility and finally the quality of research outcomes.

4.5.3 Policy Options

The recent unprecedented global spread of dengue and chikungunya viruses and the outbreaks of Zika virus and yellow fever in 2015–2016 have highlighted the challenges faced by countries. The need has never been greater for a comprehensive approach to vector control. Most VBDs can be prevented through vector control, but only if it is implemented effectively. This is, however, hampered by numerous challenges that include: lack of capacity and capability (human, infrastructural and institutional) in country programmes; lack of a comprehensive national strategy for vector control and the necessary legal framework; a limited toolbox of interventions; lack of community involvement; and ongoing environmental and social changes that result in the proliferation and geographic expansion of vectors. The global vector control response 2017–2030 (GVCR) approved by the World Health Assembly provides strategic guidance to countries and development partners for urgent strengthening of vector control, preventing disease and responding to outbreaks (WHO 2017a, b). In addition, WHO provides fact sheets on *VBDs* and *Climate change and Health* in different languages for lay people and public health workers. To achieve the re-alignment of vector control programs and increased technical capacity, improved infrastructures, strengthened monitoring and surveillance systems, and greater community mobilisation are required. One of the priority activities outlined in the GVCR is for countries to conduct or update their vector control needs assessment. This information can then be utilised to develop or update countries' vector control strategies and to plan necessary activities. This Framework for a National Vector Control Needs Assessment sets the standards for baseline assessment and progress tracking in line with the goals, targets, milestones and priorities of the GVCR. Ultimately, all these activities will support implementation of a comprehensive approach to vector control, disease surveillance and VBD research that will enable the achievement of disease-specific national and global goals and contribute to achievement of the Sustainable Development Goals and Universal Health Coverage (WHO 2017a, b).

One important policy area is with climate change mitigation policies under the Paris Agreement. Keeping global warming under 2 °C in relation to global temperatures before the Industrial Revolution will have an impact on VBD's spread to zones that have previously been uninhabitable for vectors. However, with current global warming we are already seeing an impact (Dhimal et al. 2014a, 2015; Ostyn et al. 2015); therefore, climate change adaptation policies are also directly linked to VBD control and elimination, particularly in those areas that have previously not shown any risk to VBD's or evidence of prevalence.

VBD control and elimination need to be addressed from an interdisciplinary and trans-sectoral approach, not just in the health sector. It is highly important to situate VBD control and elimination within a wider understanding of planetary health (Whitmee et al. 2015). Global policy approaches need to address a One Health approach, which interlinks human and animal health within planetary ecosystem processes that are determined by human action and therefore global change (Steffen et al. 2015; Whitmee et al. 2015).

Another policy area is influenced by Sustainable Development Goals that guide regional, national and local policies and practices and are directly interlinked with VBD control (Table 4.2).

We argue that Sustainable Development Goals will only be lasting if ensuring good health and well-being, which will rely on effective vector control as well as on initiatives for clean water and sanitation (Goal 6), sustainable cities and communities (Goal 11), climate action (Goal 13), life on land and biodiversity (Goal 15), among others. Multiple approaches that are implemented by different sectors will be required for control and elimination of VBDs, such as those promoting healthy environments (Pruss-Ustun et al. 2016).

Recognition that climate change mitigation and adaptation strategies can have substantial benefits for both health and biodiversity conservation presents policy options that are potentially both more cost-effective and socially attractive than are those that address these priorities independently. Any policy, for example the move and expansion of vectors, through transportation and livestock trade and movement on a local, national and sub-national level, needs to be coordinated in a regional context addressing global change challenges.

Acknowledgements We are grateful to our funders: Ruth Müller is funded by the Federal Ministry of Education and Research of Germany (BMBF) under the project AECO (number 01KI1717), part of the National Research Network on Zoonotic Infectious Diseases. Friederike Reuss is funded by the Hessian Centre on Climate Change of the Hessian Agency for Conservation, Environment and Geology.

Table 4.2 Relationship between Sustainable Development Goals and control of VBDs

SDG	Relationship to VBDs	Example
Goal 3. *Ensure healthy lives and promote well-being for all at all ages*	VBDs are a major contributor to global morbidity and mortality	VBDs account for > 17% of the global burden of infectious diseases; > 80% of the global population is at risk from one VBD, with > 50% at risk of two or more VBDs.
Goal 6. *Ensure access to water and sanitation for all*	Investment in clean water and sanitation can reduce the risk from VBDs	Open stored water containers are a major habitat for immature dengue, chikungunya and Zika virus vectors worldwide; provision of piped water and/or mosquito-proof water storage containers can reduce the transmission of these diseases.
Goal 11. *Make cities inclusive, safe, resilient and sustainable*	Ending VBDs makes cities (and slums) safer	Resilience against VBDs needs to be included in strategic planning for urban development.
Goal 13. *Take urgent action to combat climate change and its impacts*	Mitigating the impacts of climate change has the potential to reduce VBDs	VBDs are highly sensitive to climatic conditions, especially temperature, rainfall and relative humidity; patterns of epidemiology change more rapidly than health policy can respond; climate change can impact all VBDs.
Goal 15. *Sustainably manage forests, combat desertification, halt and reverse land degradation, halt biodiversity loss*	Maintaining terrestrial ecosystems and halting biodiversity loss will help reduce VBDs in some places, but increase it in others	Bio-reserves can harbour vector populations in protected areas. Biodiversity loss (such as that associated with deforestation) may enhance the risk of some diseases such as malaria, while biodiversity gains (such as that associated with reforestation) could sometimes increase the risk for other diseases
	Significantly reduce the impact of invasive alien species on land and water ecosystems	Invasive vector species (e.g. *Aedes albopictus*)
	Promote fair and equitable sharing of the benefits arising from the utilisation of genetic resources and promote appropriate access to such resources	Biological vector control

Adapted from: WHO (2017a, b). The Global vector control response (GVCR) 2017–2030

References

Adhami J, Reiter P (1998) Introduction and establishment of *Aedes (Stegomyia) albopictus* Skuse (Diptera: Culicidae) in Albania. J Am Mosq Control Assoc 14(3):340–343

Agossa FR, Padonou GG, Koukpo CZ, Zola-Sahossi J, Azondekon R, Akuoko OK, Ahoga J, N'dombidje B, Akinro B, Fassinou AJYH, Sezonlin M, Sezonlin M (2018) Efficacy of a novel mode of action of an indoor residual spraying product, SumiShield® 50WG against susceptible and resistant populations of *Anopheles gambiae* (sl) in Benin, West Africa. Parasit Vectors 11(1):293

Alphey L, Alphey N (2014) Five things to know about genetically modified (GM) insects for vector control. PLoS Pathog 10(3):e1003909

Altizer S, Ostfeld RS, Johnson PTJ, Kutz S, Harvell CD (2013) Climate change and infectious diseases: from evidence to a predictive framework. Science 341:514

Andersson N, Nava-Aguilera E, Arosteguí J, Morales-Perez A, Suazo-Laguna H, Legorreta-Soberanis J, Hernandez-Alvarez C, Fernandez-Salas I, Paredes-Solís S, Balmaseda A (2015) Evidence based community mobilization for dengue prevention in Nicaragua and Mexico (Camino Verde, the green way): cluster randomized controlled trial. Br Med J 351:h3267

Ant TH, Herd CS, Geoghegan V, Hoffmann AA, Sinkins SP (2018) The *Wolbachia* strain wAu provides highly efficient virus transmission blocking in *Aedes aegypti*. PLoS Pathog 14(1):e1006815

Aytekin S, Aytekin AM, Alten B (2009) Effect of different larval rearing temperatures on the productivity (R0) and morphology of the malaria vector *Anopheles superpictus* Grassi (Diptera: Culicidae) using geometric morphometrics. J Vector Ecol 34(1):32–42

Baldacchino F, Caputo B, Chandre F, Drago A, della Torre A, Montarsi F, Rizzoli A (2015) Control methods against invasive *Aedes* mosquitoes in Europe: a review. Pest Manag Sci 71(11):1471–1485

Bangs MJ, Larasati RP, Corwin AL, Wuryadi S (2006) Climatic factors associated with epidemic dengue in Palembang, Indonesia: implications of short-term meteorological events on virus transmission. Southeast Asian J Trop Med Public Health 37(6):1103–1116

Baráková I, Derdáková M, Selyemová D, Chvostáč M, Špitalská E, Rosso F, Collini M, Rosà R, Tagliapietra V, Girardi M, Ramponi C (2018) Tick-borne pathogens and their reservoir hosts in northern Italy. Ticks Tick-borne Dis 9(2):164–170

Bayoh MN, Lindsay SW (2003) Effect of temperature on the development of the aquatic stages of *Anopheles gambiae* sensu stricto (Diptera: Culicidae). Bull Entomol Res 93:375–381

Briegel H, Timmermann SE (2001) *Aedes albopictus* (Diptera: Culicidae): physiological aspects of development and reproduction. J Med Entomol 38(4):566–571

Brownstein JS, Skelly DK, Holford TR, Fish D (2005) Forest fragmentation predicts local scale heterogeneity of Lyme disease risk. Oecologia 146(3):469–475

Burt A, Coulibaly M, Crisanti A, Diabate A, Kayondo JK (2018) Gene drive to reduce malaria transmission in sub-Saharan Africa. J Respon Innov 5(suppl 1):66–80

Carson R (2002) Silent spring. Houghton Mifflin Harcourt, Boston

Carvalho DO, McKemey AR, Garziera L, Lacroix R, Donnelly CA, Alphey L, Malavasi A, Capurro ML (2015) Suppression of a field population of *Aedes aegypti* in Brazil by austained release of transgenic male mosquitoes. PLoS Negl Trop Dis 9:e0003864

Chan M, Johansson MA (2012) The incubation periods of dengue viruses. PLoS One 7(11):e50972

Chang LH, Hsu EL, Teng HJ, Ho CM (2007) Differential survival of *Aedes aegypti* and Aedes albopictus (Diptera: Culicidae) larvae exposed to low temperatures in Taiwan. J Med Entomol 44(2):205–210

Chaves LF, Hamer GL, Walker ED, Brown WM, Ruiz MO, Kitron UD (2011) Climatic variability and landscape heterogeneity impact urban mosquito diversity and vector abundance and infection. Ecosphere 2(6):art70

Chu-Agor ML, Munoz-Carpena R, Kiker GA, Aiello-Lammens ME, Akcakaya HR, Convertino M, Linkov I (2012) Simulating the fate of Florida snowy plovers with sea-level rise: exploring research and management priorities with a global uncertainty and sensitivity analysis perspective. Ecol Model 224(1):33–47

Civitello DJ, Cohen J, Fatima H, Halstead NT, Liriano J, McMahon TA, Ortega N, Sauer EL, Sehgal T, Young S, Rohr JR (2015) Biodiversity inhibits parasites: broad evidence for the dilution effect. Proc Natl Acad Sci 112(28):8667–8671

Civitello DJ, Pearsall S, Duffy MA, Hall SR (2013) Parasite consumption and host interference can inhibit disease spread in dense populations. Ecol Lett 16(5):626–634

Couret J, Dotson E, Benedict MQ (2014) Temperature, larval diet, and density effects on development rate and survival of *Aedes aegypti* (Diptera: Culicidae). PLoS One 9(2):e87468

Cuthbert RN, Dick JT, Callaghan A, Dickey JW (2018) Biological control agent selection under environmental change using functional responses, abundances and fecundities; the relative control potential (RCP) metric. Biol Control 121:50–57

Delatte H, Gimonneau G, Triboire A, Fontenille D (2009) Influence of temperature on immature development, survival, longevity, fecundity, and gonotrophic cycles of Aedes albopictus, vector of chikungunya and dengue in the Indian Ocean. J Med Entomol 46(1):33–41

Dhimal M, Ahrens B, Kuch U (2014a) Altitudinal shift of malaria vectors and malaria elimination in Nepal. Malar J 13(S1):P26

Dhimal M, Gautam I, Kreß A, Müller R, Kuch U (2014b) Spatio-temporal distribution of dengue and lymphatic filariasis vectors along an altitudinal transect in Central Nepal. PLoS Negl Trop Dis 8(7):e3035

Dhimal M, Aryal KK, Dhimal ML, Gautam I, Singh SP, Bhusal CL, Kuch U (2014c) Knowledge, attitude and practice regarding dengue fever among the healthy population of highland and lowland communities in Central Nepal. PLoS One 9(7):e102028

Dhimal M, Ahrens B, Kuch U (2015) Climate change and spatiotemporal distributions of vector-borne diseases in Nepal–a systematic synthesis of literature. PLoS One 10(6):e0129869

Dhimal M, Dahal S, Dhimal ML, Mishra SR, Karki KB, Aryal KK, Haque U, Kabir I, Guin P, Butt AM, Harapan H, Liu Q, Chu C, Montag D, Groneberg DA, Pandey BD, Kuch U, Müller R (2018) Threats of Zika virus transmission for Asia and its Hindu-Kush Himalayan region. Infect Dis Pov 7:40

Ducheyne E, Minh NNT, Haddad N, Bryssinck W, Buliva E, Simard F, Malik MR, Charlier J, De Waele V, Mahmoud O, Mukhtar M, Bouattour A, Hussain A, Hendrick G, Roiz D (2018) Current and future distribution of *Aedes aegypti* and *Aedes albopictus* (Diptera: Culicidae) in WHO eastern mediterranean region. Int J Health Geogr 17(1):4

Engering A, Hogerwerf L, Slingenbergh J (2013) Pathogen–host–environment interplay and disease emergence. Emerg Microb Infect 2(2):e5

Eritja R, Palmer JRB, Roiz D, Sanpera-Calbet I, Bartumeus F (2017) Direct evidence of adult *Aedes albopictus* dispersal by car. Sci Rep 7:14399. https://doi.org/10.1038/s41598-017-12652-5

Escobar LE, Romero-Alvarez D, Leon R, Lepe-Lopez MA, Craft ME, Borbor-Cordova MJ, Svenning JC (2016) Declining prevalence of disease vectors under climate change. Sci Rep 6:39150

Estrada-Pena A, Sanchez N, Estrada-Sanchez A (2012) An assessment of the distribution and spread of the tick *Hyalomma marginatum* in the western Palearctic under different climate scenarios. Vector Borne Zoonotic Dis 12(9):758–768

Ferguson HM, Dornhaus A, Beeche A, Borgemeister C, Gottlieb M, Mulla MS, Gimnig JE, Fish D, Killeen GF (2010) Ecology: a prerequisite for malaria elimination and eradication. PLoS Med 7(8):e1000303

Fischer D, Thomas SM, Neteler M, Tjaden N, Beierkuhnlein C (2014) Climatic suitability of Aedes albopictus in Europe referring to climate change projections: comparison of mechanistic and correlative niche modeling approaches. Eur Secur 19:34–46

Földvári G, Široký P, Szekeres S, Majoros G, Sprong H (2016) *Dermacentor reticulatus*: a vector on the rise. Parasit Vectors 9(1):314

Gern L, Estrada-Pena A, Frandsen F, Gray JS, Jaenson TG, Jongejan F, Kahl O, Korenberg E, Mehl R, Nuttall PA (1998) European reservoir hosts of *Borrelia burgdorferi sensu lato*. Zentralblatt für Bakteriol 287(3):196–204

Goncalves Y, Silva J, Biscoito M (2008) On the presence of *Aedes (Stegomyia) aegypti* Linnaeus, 1762 (Insecta, Diptera, Culicidae) in the island of Madeira (Portugal). Boletim do Museu Municipal do Funchal (Funchal, Portugal) 58(322):53–59

Gould EA, Higgs S (2009) Impact of climate change and other factors on emerging arbovirus diseases. Trans R Soc Trop Med Hyg 103(2):109–121

Hammond A, Galizi R, Kyrou K, Simoni A, Siniscalchi C, Katsanos D, Gribble M, Baker D, Marois E, Russell S, Burt A, Windbichler N, Crisanti A, Nolan T (2016) A CRISPR-Cas9 gene drive system targeting female reproduction in the malaria mosquito vector *Anopheles gambiae*. Nat Biotechnol 34(1):78

Harapan H, Bustamam A, Radiansyah A, Angraini P, Fasli R, Salwiyadi S, Bastian RA, Oktiviyari A, Akmal I, Iqbalamin M, Adil J, Henrizal F, Groneberg DA, Kuch U, Müller R (2017) Dengue prevention: confirmatory factor analysis of relationships between economic status, knowledge, attitudes and practice, vaccine acceptance and willingness to participate in a study. Southeast Asian J Trop Med Public Health 48(2):297–305

Harapan H, Rajamoorthy Y, Anwar S, Bustaman A, Radiansyah A, Angraini P, Fasli R, Salwiyadi S, Bastian RA, Oktiviyari A, Akmal I, Iqbalamin M, Adil J, Henrizal F, Darmayanti D, Pratama R, Setiawan AM, Mudatsir M, Hadisoemarto PF, Dhimal ML, Kuch U, Groneberg DA, Imrie A, Dhimal M, Müller R (2018) Knowledge, attitude, and practice regarding dengue virus infection among inhabitants of Aceh, Indonesia: a cross-sectional study. BMC Infect Dis 18:96

Harris AF, Nimmo D, McKemey AR, Kelly N, Scaife S, Donnelly CA, Beech C, Petrie WD, Alphey L (2011) Field performance of engineered male mosquitoes. Nat Biotechnol 29:1034–1037

Hashiguchi Y, Cáceres AG, Velez LN, Villegas NV, Hashiguchi K, Mimori T, Uezato H, Kato H (2018) Andean cutaneous leishmaniasis (Andean-CL, uta) in Peru and Ecuador: the vector *Lutzomyia* sand flies and reservoir mammals. Acta Trop 178:264–275

Hemingway J, Ranson H (2000) Insecticide resistance in insect vectors of human disease. Annu Rev Entomol 45(1):371–391

Hladik ML, Main A, Goulson D (2018) Environmental risks and challenges associated with neonicotinoid insecticides. Environ Sci Technol. https://doi.org/10.1021/acs.est.7b06388

http://www.eliminatedengue.com/our-research/wolbachia. Accessed 30 May 2018

http://www.euro.who.int/en/media-centre/sections/press-releases/2014/77-000-europeans-fall-sick-every-year-with-vector-borne-diseases. Accessed 30 May 2018

http://www.globalviromeproject.org/overview/. Accessed 30 May 2018

http://www.zoonosen.net/EnglishSite/Home.aspx. Accessed 30 May 2018

https://ecdc.europa.eu/en/about-us/partnerships-and-networks/disease-and-laboratory-networks/vector-net. Accessed 30 May 2018

https://ecdc.europa.eu/en/publications-data/rhipicephalus-sanguineus-current-known-distribution-april-2017. Accessed 30 May 2018

https://infravec2.eu/. Accessed 30 May 2018

https://win-network.ird.fr/. Accessed 30 May 2018

https://www.gesundheitsforschung-bmbf.de/de/nationales-forschungsnetz-zoonotische-infektionskrankheiten-6820.php. Accessed 30 May 2018

Huang YJS, Higgs S, Vanlandingham DL (2017) Biological control strategies for mosquito vectors of arboviruses. Insects 8(1):21

Huffaker R (2015) Building economic models corresponding to the real world. Appl Econ Perspect Policy 37(4):ppv021

Iturbe-Ormaetxe I, Walker T, Neill SLO (2011) *Wolbachia* and the biological control of mosquito-borne disease. EMBO Rep 12:508–518

Jaenson TG, Värv K, Fröjdman I, Jääskeläinen A, Rundgren K, Versteirt V, Estrada-Peña A, Medlock JM, Golovljova I (2016) First evidence of established populations of the taiga tick *Ixodes persulcatus* (Acari: Ixodidae) in Sweden. Parasit Vectors 9(1):377

Jakob C, Poulin B (2016) Indirect effects of mosquito control using Bti on dragonflies and damselflies (Odonata) in the Camargue. Insect Conserv Divers 9(2):161–169

Jia Y, Moudy RM, Dupuis AP II, Ngo KA, Maffei JG, Jerzak GV, Franke MA, Kauffman EB, Kramer LD (2007) Characterization of a small plaque variant of West Nile virus isolated in New York in 2000. Virology 367(2):339–347

Keiser J, Singer BH, Utzinger J (2005) Reducing the burden of malaria in different eco-epidemiological settings with environmental management: a systematic review. Lancet Infect Dis 5(11):695–708

Kilpatrick AM, Meola MA, Moudy RM, Kramer LD (2008) Temperature, viral genetics, and the transmission of West Nile virus by *Culex pipiens* mosquitoes. PLoS Pathog 4(6):e1000092

Kreß A, Kuch U, Oehlmann J, Müller R (2014) Impact of temperature and nutrition on the toxicity of the insecticide λ-cyhalothrin in full-lifecycle tests with the target mosquito species *Aedes albopictus* and *Culex pipiens*. J Pest Sci 87(4):739–750

Kurtenbach K, Hanincova K, Tsao JI, Margos G, Fish D, Ogden NH (2006) Fundamental processes in the evolutionary ecology of Lyme borreliosis. Nat Rev Microbiol. https://doi.org/10.1038/nrmicro1475

Lacey J (2012) Climate change and Norman Daniel's theory of just health: an essay on basic needs. Med Health Care Philos 5:3–14

Lacroix R, McKemey AR, Raduan N, Kwee Wee L, Hong Ming W, Guat Ney T, Rahidah AAS, Salman S, Subramaniam S, Nordin O, Hanum ATN, Angamuthu C, Marlina Mansor S, Lees RS, Naish N, Scaife S, Gray P, Labbé G, Beech C, Nimmo D, Alphey L, Vasan SS, Han Lim L, Wasi AN, Murad S (2012) Open field release of genetically engineered sterile male *Aedes aegypti* in Malaysia. PLoS One 7:e42771

Lafferty KD (2009) The ecology of climate change and infectious diseases. Ecology 90(4):888–900

Lambrechts L, Scott TW, Gubler DJ (2010) Consequences of the expanding global distribution of *Aedes albopictus* for dengue virus transmission. PLoS Negl Trop Dis 4(5):e646

Le Conte Y, Navajas M (2008) Climate change: impact on honey bee populations and diseases. Revue Scientifique et Technique-Office International des Epizooties 27(2):499–510

Levi T, Keesing F, Holt RD, Barfield M, Ostfeld RS (2016) Quantifying dilution and amplification in a community of hosts for tick-borne pathogens. Ecol Appl 26(2):484–498

Liess M, Foit K, Knillmann S, Schäfer RB, Liess HD (2016) Predicting the synergy of multiple stress effects. Sci Rep 6:32965

Lindgren E, Tälleklint L, Polfeldt T (2000) Impact of climatic change on the northern latitude limit and population density of the disease-transmitting European tick *Ixodes ricinus*. Environ Health Perspect 108(2):119

Maino JL, Umina PA, Hoffmann AA (2018) Climate contributes to the evolution of pesticide resistance. Glob Ecol Biogeogr 27(2):223–232

Marmot M, Wilkinson RG (2005) Social determinants of health. Oxford University Press, Oxford

Medlock JM, Hansford KM, Schaffner F, Versteirt V, Hendrick G, Zeller H, Bortel WV (2012) A review of the invasive mosquitoes in Europe: ecology, public health risks, and control options. Vector-Borne Zoonotic Dis 12(6):435–447

Mishra N, Shrivastava NK, Nayak A, Singh H (2018) Wolbachia: a prospective solution to mosquito borne diseases. Int J Mosq Res 5(2):01–08

Mitchell-Foster K, Ayala EB, Breilh J, Spiegel J, Wilches AA, Leon TO, Delgado JA (2015) Integrating participatory community mobilization processes to improve dengue prevention: an eco-bio-social scaling up of local success in Machala, Ecuador. Trans R Soc Trop Med Hyg 109(2):126–133

Mohammed A, Chadee DD (2011) Effects of different temperature regimens on the development of *Aedes aegypti* (L.) (Diptera: Culicidae) mosquitoes. Acta Trop 119:38–43

Montag D, Kuch U, Rodriguez L, Müller R (2017) Overview of the panel on biodiversity and health under climate change. In: Rodríguez L, Anderson I (eds) Secretariat of the convention on biological diversity. The Lima declaration on biodiversity and climate change: contributions from science to policy for sustainable development, Technical series no.89. Secretariat of the Convention on Biological Diversity, Montreal, pp 91–108. 156 pages

Morrison TE (2014) Reemergence of chikungunya virus. J Virol 88(20):11644–11647

Müller R, Knautz T, Vollroth S, Berger R, Kreß A, Reuss F, Groneberg DA, Kuch U (2018) Larval superiority of *Culex pipiens* to *Aedes albopictus* in a replacement series experiment: prospects for coexistence in Germany. Parasit Vectors 11:80

Muturi EJ, Kim CH, Alto BW, Berenbaum MR, Schuler MA (2011) Larval environmental stress alters *Aedes aegypti* competence for Sindbis virus. Tropical Med Int Health 16(8):955–964

Narrod C, Zinsstag J, Tiongco M (2012) A one health framework for estimating the economic costs of zoonotic diseases on society. EcoHealth 9(2):150–162

Niemi GJ, Axler RP, Hanowski JM, Hershey AE, Lima AR, Regal RR, Shannon LJ (2015) Evaluation of the potential effects of methoprene and BTI (*Bacillus thurinqiensis israelensis*)

on wetland birds and invertebrates in Wright County, MN, 1988 to 1993. Retrieved from the University of Minnesota Digital Conservancy, http://hdl.handle.net/11299/187246

NO, Treaty Series (2005) Stockholm convention on persistent organic pollutants

Ogden NH, Maarouf A, Barker IK, Bigras-Poulin M, Lindsay LR, Morshed MG, O'Callaghan CJ, Ramay F, Waltner-Toews D, Charron DF (2006) Climate change and the potential for range expansion of the Lyme disease vector *Ixodes scapularis* in Canada. Int J Parasitol 36(1):63–70

Ogden NH, Radojevic M, Wu X, Duvvuri VR, Leighton PA, Wu J (2014) Estimated effects of projected climate change on the basic reproductive number of the Lyme disease vector *Ixodes scapularis*. Environ Health Perspect 122(6):631

Op de Beeck L, Verheyen J, Olsen K, Stoks R (2017) Negative effects of pesticides under global warming can be counteracted by a higher degradation rate and thermal adaptation. J Appl Ecol 54(6):1847–1855

Ostfeld RS, Keesing F (2012) Effects of host diversity on infectious disease. Annu Rev Ecol Evol Syst 43:157

Ostyn B, Uranw S, Bhattarai NR, Das ML, Rai K, Tersago K, Pokhrel Y, Durnez L, Marasini B, Van der Auwera G, Dujardin J-C, Coosemans M, Argaw D, Boelaert M, Rijal S, Dujardin JC (2015) Transmission of *Leishmania donovani* in the hills of eastern Nepal, an outbreak investigation in Okhaldhunga and Bhojpur districts. PLoS Negl Trop Dis 9(8):e0003966

Paris M, David JP, Despres L (2011) Fitness costs of resistance to Bti toxins in the dengue vector *Aedes aegypti*. Ecotoxicology 20(6):1184–1194

Pruss-Ustun A, Wolf J, Corvalan C, Bos R, Neira M (2016) Preventing disease through health environments: a global assessment of the burden of disease from environmental risks. World Health Organization, Geneva

Reiskind MH, Janairo MS (2015) Late-instar behaviour of *Aedes aegypti* (Diptera: Culicidae) larvae in different thermal and nutritive environments. J Med Entomol 52(5):789–796

Reuss F, Wiesner A, Niamir A, Bálint M, Kuch U, Pfenninger M, Müller R (2018) Thermal experiments with the Asian bush mosquito (*Aedes japonicus japonicus*) (Diptera: Culicidae) and implications for its distribution in Germany. Parasit Vectors 11(1):81

Rezza G (2018) Chikungunya is back in Italy: 2007–2017. J Travel Med 25(1):tay004

Ross PA, Axford JK, Richardson KM, Endersby-Harshman NM, Hoffmann AA (2017) Maintaining *Aedes aegypti* mosquitoes infected with Wolbachia. J Vis Exp 126:e56124

Salkeld DJ, Leonhard S, Girard YA, Hahn N, Mun J, Padgett KA, Lane RS (2008) Identifying the reservoir hosts of the Lyme disease spirochete *Borrelia burgdorferi* in California: the role of the western gray squirrel (*Sciurus griseus*). Am J Trop Med Hyg 79(4):535–540

Salkeld DJ, Padgett KA, Jones JH, Antolin MF (2015) Public health perspective on patterns of biodiversity and zoonotic disease. Proc Natl Acad Sci U S A 112(46):E6261–E6261

Samuel GH, Adelman ZN, Myles KM (2016) Temperature-dependent effects on the replication and transmission of arthropod-borne viruses in their insect hosts. Curr Opin Insect Sci 16:108–113

Schaffner F, Kaufmann C, Hegglin D, Mathis A (2009) The invasive mosquito *Aedes japonicus* in Central Europe. Med Vet Entomol 23:448–451

Silva-Filha MHNL (2017) Resistance of mosquitoes to entomopathogenic bacterial-based larvicides: current status and strategies for management. In: Bacillus thuringiensis and Lysinibacillus sphaericus. Springer, Cham, pp 239–257

Siraj AS, Santos-Vega M, Bouma MJ, Yadeta D, Carrascal DR, Pascual M (2014) Altitudinal changes in malaria incidence in highlands of Ethiopia and Colombia. Science 343(6175):1154–1158

Steffen W, Richardson K, Rockström J, Cornell SE, Fetzer I, Bennett EM, Biggs R, Carpenter SR, de Vries W, de Wit CA, Folke C, Gerten D, Heinke J, Mace GM, Persson LM, Ramanathan V, Reyers B, Sörlin S (2015) Planetary boundaries: guiding human development on a changing planet. Science 347(6223):1259855

Stockholm Convention on Persistent Organic Pollutants (2001) Stockholm convention on persistent organic pollutants. United Nations Environment Programme, Geneva

Succo T, Leparc-Goffart I, Ferré JB, Roiz D, Broche B, Maquart M, Noel H, Catelinois O, Entezam F, Caire D, Jourdain F, Esteve-Moussion I, Cochet A, Paupy C, Rousseau C, Paty

M-C, Golliot F, Jourdain F (2016) Autochthonous dengue outbreak in Nîmes, South of France, July to September 2015. Eur Secur 21(21):30240

Swaddle JP, Calos SE (2008) Increased avian diversity its associated with lower incidence of human West Nile infection: observation of the dilution effect. PLoS One 3(6):e2488

Teurlai M, Menkès CE, Cavarero V, Degallier N, Descloux E, Grangeon J-P (2015) Socio-economic and climate factors associated with dengue fever spatial heterogeneity: a worked example in New Caledonia. PLoS Negl Trop Dis 9(12):e0004211

Tomasello D, Schlagenhauf P (2013) Chikungunya and dengue autochthonous cases in Europe, 2007–2012. Travel Med Infect Dis 11(5):274–284

Turell MJ (1993) Effect of environmental temperature on the vector competence of *Aedes taeniochynchus* for rift valley fever and Venezuelan equine encephalitis virus. Am J Trop Med Hyg 49(6):672–676

Van den Berg H (2009) Global status of DDT and its alternatives for use in vector control to prevent disease. Environ Health Perspect 117(11):1656

Versteirt V, De Clercq EM, Fonseca DM, Pecor J, Schaffner F, Coosemans M, Van Bortel W (2012) Bionomics of the established exotic mosquito species *Aedes koreicus* in Belgium, Europe. J Med Entomol 49(6):1226–1232

Vorou R (2016) Zika virus, vectors, reservoirs, amplifying hosts, and their potential to spread worldwide: what we know and what we should investigate urgently. Int J Infect Dis 48:85–90

Vu SN, Nguyen TY, Kay BH, Marten GG, Reid JW (1998) Eradication of *Aedes aegypti* from a village in Vietnam, using copepods and community participation. The American Journal of Tropical Medicine and Hygiene 59(4):657–660

Westbrook CJ, Reiskind MH, Pesko KN, Greene KE, Lounibos LP (2010) Larval environmental temperature and the susceptibility of *Aedes albopictus* Skuse (Diptera: Culicidae) to Chikungunya virus. Vector-Borne Zoonotic Dis 10(3):241–247

Whitmee S, Haines A, Beyrer C, Boltz F, Capon AG, de Souza Dias BF, Ezeh A, Frumkin H, Gong P, Head P, Horton R (2015) Safeguarding human health in the Anthropocene epoch: report of the Rockefeller Foundation–lancet commission on planetary health. Lancet 386(10007):1973–2028

WHO (2008) Global malaria control and elimination: report of a technical review. World Health Organization, Geneva

WHO (2017a) Fact sheet: vector-borne diseases. Available at: http://www.who.int/mediacentre/factsheets/fs387/en/

WHO (2017b) The global vector control response (GVCR) 2017–2030. World Health Organization, Geneva

Wood CL, McInturff A, Young HS, Kim DH, Lafferty KD (2017) Human infectious disease burdens decrease with urbanization but not with biodiversity. Philos Trans R Soc B 372:20160122

Chapter 5
The Influence of Socio-economic and Socio-demographic Factors in the Association Between Urban Green Space and Health

Nadja Kabisch

Abstract Green spaces can help preventing potential negative health outcomes from climate change and urbanisation. Urban green spaces may reduce cardiovascular diseases exaggerated by heat stress or noise because of their climate regulation and noise-buffering potential. Urban green space may also promote physical activity and social interactions, and thus improve the physical and mental health of residents who tend to be more stressed in urban environments. Research findings on associations between urban green space and health outcomes are, however, not consistent, and potential relationships are often affected by confounding factors. In this chapter, a systematic review of the association between urban green space and health is presented, with a particular focus on socio-economic and socio-demographic confounders that may over-ride potential associations. Results show that there is some positive effect of urban green space on mental health and cardiovascular diseases. However, evidence is weak as many other studies show that socio-economic confounders, such as household income or neighbourhood deprivation, have the highest impact. The mediating effect of urban green space to decrease health inequality among different socio-economic groups may be more important. Based on the results of the review, conclusions are drawn on how to design green space that is beneficial for the health and well-being of all population groups including the vulnerable groups of children, the elderly and deprived people. This field of research is growing, and important prospects for future research on urban green and health are highlighted.

Keywords Green space · Urban · Health · Well-being · Confounder

---

N. Kabisch (✉)
Department of Geography, Humboldt-Universität zu Berlin, Berlin, Germany
e-mail: nadja.kabisch@geo.hu-berlin.de

M. R. Marselle et al. (eds.), *Biodiversity and Health in the Face of Climate Change*, https://doi.org/10.1007/978-3-030-02318-8_5

Highlights

- A systematic review of the association between urban green space and health is presented.
- The focus has been on socio-economic and socio-demographic confounders.
- Results show some positive association between urban green space, mental health and cardiovascular diseases.
- Evidence is rather weak, and socio-economic confounders have the highest impact on health outcome effects.
- The mediating effect of urban green space to decrease health inequality among different socio-economic groups may be more important.

5.1 Introduction

The value of urban nature has been considered within a range of societal challenge areas in cities, such as water management, air quality, urban biodiversity, and human health and well-being (Raymond et al. 2017). Assessments of these values – mostly using the ecosystem services (ESS) concept – are now informing urban policy and planning across the world. For example, at the international level, the Intergovernmental Panel on Biodiversity and Ecosystem Services discusses the benefits of nature for people as one way to promote nature's values in environmental decision-making, for example, through the ESS concept and other human-nature inter-relations (Díaz et al. 2018). The integrated view to sustainable urban development is also highlighted in the 2030 Agenda for Sustainable Development and its sustainable development goals (SDGs), the New Urban Agenda adopted at the United Nations' HABITAT III conference and promoted by the European Commission's research and innovation policy on nature-based solutions. In particular, Goal 11 of the SDGs underlines that "Making cities safe and sustainable [...] involves [...] creating green public spaces, and improving urban planning and management in a way that is both participatory and inclusive" (The United Nations Development Programme (UNDP) 2015). Urban green spaces such as parks, allotment gardens, street trees, urban gardens, cemeteries, green roofs and green facades were shown to increase sustainability in urban areas. Urban green spaces ameliorate high temperatures in cities (Bowler et al. 2010), reduce noise, help filter pollutants from the air, and improve water inflow in times of extreme precipitation events (Haase et al. 2014). When developing new green spaces to make cities (more) sustainable, a key component for urban planning is to consider the spatial location of urban green spaces within the urban area, in order to understand their potential role in mediating improved health outcomes for groups of people.

Interest in research has recently increased regarding the role that urban green spaces may play in improving the health of urban residents (Hartig et al. 2014). One aspect that has been discussed is whether urban green can act as a health promoter by encouraging more active lifestyles, or as a disease preventer through reducing the impact of negative environmental conditions such as extreme weather events, air pollution, noise or heat (Kabisch et al. 2017; van den Bosch and Ode Sang 2017).

The reduction of the impact of negative environmental conditions is hypothesised to occur through providing ecosystem services, as presented above. In particular, van den Bosch and Ode Sang (2017) showed that urban green space contributes to the health of city residents by decreasing all-cause and cardiovascular disease–related mortality, adverse birth outcomes and mental disorders, particularly through providing regulating and provisioning ESS and through cultural ESS linked to socio-behavioural pathways. The authors, however, did not find significant results for sufficient evidence for stress reduction and physical activity as the mediating pathway.

They conclude that the impact of improving environmental conditions through urban green spaces is often spatially explicit, with an unequal distribution of environmental burdens and goods. In particular, disadvantaged and minority groups often bear higher environmental burdens such as noise or air pollution (Wolch et al. 2014), while they have less access to urban green spaces and the benefits they provide (Cook et al. Chap. 11, this volume). Clark et al. (2014) showed that low-income people are disproportionately exposed to air pollution in the USA, whereas Richardson et al. (2013) demonstrated a similar relationship for particular areas in Europe. Wolch et al. (2005) found that park availability is reduced in deprived neighbourhoods. Street trees, as a particular part of the green infrastructure network, have also been found to be differently distributed according to neighbourhood socio-economic status (Landry and Chakraborty 2009). Interestingly, Timperio et al. (2007) could not find any statistically significant relationship that urban green spaces are more scarce in low-income or minority neighbourhoods in Australia (Timperio et al. 2007). A recent review of park access by Rigolon (2016) also showed inconclusive findings for distance to parks but striking differences for size and quality of parks, with smaller park sizes and lower quality of parks for neighbourhoods of low socio-economic and minority groups. This suggests a more complex link between urban green space availability and accessibility and socio-economic differences, which depends on the indicators used for measuring greenness, availability and quality features of urban green spaces.

The relationships between environmental burdens, green space accessibility, socio-economic factors and potential health outcomes are still not clearly understood, and vary between studies. A structured systematic review is presented in this chapter to help close this gap in the research. In particular, effects of urban green spaces on urban health depending on accessibility and socio-economic status/trends are investigated. The term 'socio-economic confounder' is used in this chapter to describe factors that have a potential effect on health and that may even over-ride a potential association between urban green space and health outcomes.

5.2 Methods

A systematic, structured and quantitative literature review of peer-reviewed articles that were published in international scientific journals was conducted in November 2017. This review identified 140 papers of which the highest proportion were

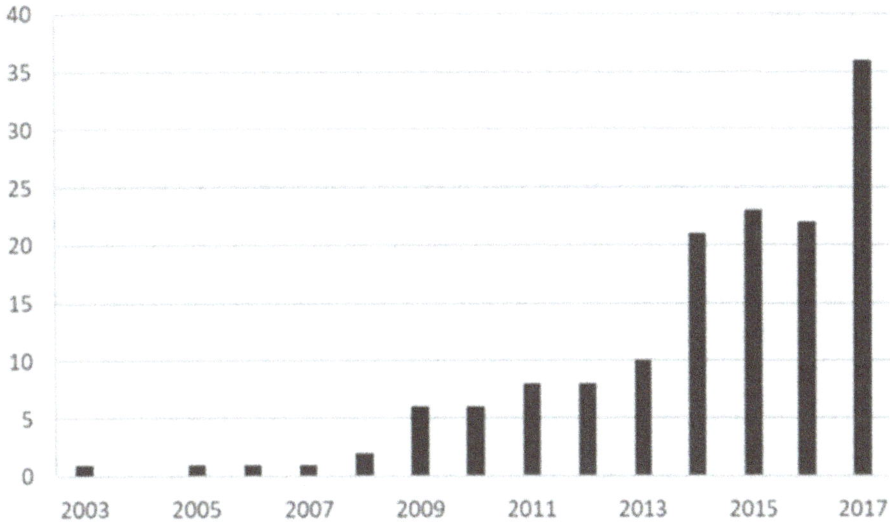

Fig. 5.1 Number of papers published in Web of Science on the relationship between urban green spaces and potential health effects

published within the last 5 years (2013–2017, Fig. 5.1). The analysis was therefore restricted to papers published in English from 2013 onward to highlight recent advances in the subject. Web of Knowledge© was used as the scientific search engine to find appropriate articles. The search profile was based on a number of primary search terms related to particular categories related to the topic. The first main term related to the topic 'urban green', the second to 'availability' and 'access', the third to socio-economic and socio-demographic profile of neighbourhoods or affected populations, and included key search terms such as 'income', 'age' or 'class', and the fourth to health including terms such as 'health', 'disease' and 'well-being'. The respective terms were chosen based on the author's own experiences with the topic and other reviews, existing theories and initial literature studies that revealed some inconsistent relationships on the green space associability link. The operators AND between and OR within categories were used. It was decided to restrict the search to scientific peer-reviewed papers. Excluded from the literature search were research reports and other non-scientific publications or bibliographies. However, these were used in searches for additional literature as was done with other existing reviews that touched on the topic (Kabisch et al. 2017; van den Bosch and Ode Sang 2017). Articles found through the search strategy were screened and included in the final sample if the content matched the main research objectives. An article was evaluated as not relevant if no direct link to health outcomes related to urban green could be found, or when the article presented a method only as main content. This strategy resulted in a total of 25 papers. All final articles were analysed using a standardised data extraction sheet based on pre-defined questions for review. This included general information such as publication date, case-study location, respective scale of interest, particular assessment method or data used.

5.3 Results

The relationship between urban green spaces and potential health effects is a growing research field, with an increasing number of publications, particularly since 2013 (Fig. 5.1). The research discussed here focusses on those studies that considered differences in the socio-economic and socio-demographic context of the population groups studied. In addition, the particular green space metrics, buffers and data used in the study are considered as it was assumed that there might be a difference in health outcome results when different measures are used. Only 25 papers were directly related to a health outcome linked to urban green space use or availability. The remaining papers indirectly address a health outcome by mentioning a potential health benefit of green space exposure for different population groups in the abstract but not analysing health outcome as a main aim. Papers that address health directly mostly deal with mental health outcomes followed by studies on physical activity, birth outcome, overweight, general health and cardiovascular diseases. Results are presented in Table 5.1 and summarised with main associations indicated in Fig. 5.4.

5.3.1 *Mental Health and General Health*

Cohen-Cline et al. (2015) studied potential associations between access to green space and self-reported depression, stress and anxiety. When adjusted for confounding factors such as income, the association between urban green space and less depression remained significant. Mukherjee et al. (2017) found a similar association between the nearest park size and depression even when controlling for confounders such as household wealth and education. They showed that a smaller size of the nearest park was associated with higher odds of depression. Controlling for socio-economic status, Triguero-Mas et al. (2015) identified that surrounding green spaces were associated with better mental health. Mitchell et al. (2015) found improved mental health in lower income groups when access to green space and recreational areas improved. A similar relationship was found by Feda et al. (2015), who showed an inverse association between accessibility of urban parks and perceived stress among adolescents when controlled for socio-economic status. Thompson et al. (2016) identified that higher quantity and better access to green spaces including gardens and allotments were significantly related to decreased stress levels in deprived communities.

For 3- to 5-year-old children, Flouri et al. (2014) found that in lower income groups, children with a higher percentage of green space in their neighbourhood had fewer emotional problems. For a study of 4- to 6-year-old children, those with comparatively more park and natural area space around their homes had better mental health outcomes. Interestingly, Astell-Burt et al. (2014) showed that the green space-mental health association varies across the life course and between

Table 5.1 The main characteristics and results of studies on greenness and health by confounding factors

References	Country, city	Aim	HEALTH	Study design	Green space metrics and buffer	Confounder	Main results
Abelt and McLafferty (2017)	U.S., New York	Assessment of relationship between mothers' exposure to green and blue spaces and adverse birth outcomes.	Birth outcome	Mixed-effects linear and logistic regression models; GIS analysis	NDVI in buffers of 100 m, 250 m and 500 m, NYC Street Tree Census	Neighborhood deprivation, education, race, marital status, population density, birth place	No consistent significant relationship between adverse birth outcomes and residential greenness in fully adjusted models. Deprived tracts were less "green" and closer to major roads and industrial land use. Significant association between street trees surrounding the home and reduced odds of preterm birth were identified
Allan et al. (2017)	UK, England	Investigation of health variations by residential contexts, its causes and sensitivity to rural–urban classifications	General health (Limiting long-term illness)	Logistic regression models applied to UK census data (2001)	Rural-urban classification, no buffer used	Employment status, education, age, sex, marital status, ethnicity	A positive urban–rural health gradient was identified, with the exception of a protective "capital city" effect.
Astell-Burt et al. (2014)	UK, country scale	Analysis of variation in minor psychiatric morbidity	Mental health	Longitudinal study with data from nine annual waves of the British Household Panel Survey (1996–2004) using multi-level linear regression	Green space, no buffer used	Employment status, income, education, tenure status, age, gender, marital status	Psychiatric morbidity appeared less prevalent among residents living in greener neighbourhoods. In those areas, residents had higher household income. The link between urban green space and health varied across the lifecourse

Calogiuri et al. (2016)	Norway, country scale	Examination of green exercise as a physical activity across social groups.	Physical activity	Questionnaire survey (2168), reported weekly green exercise and other forms of physical activity, specific forms of GE, and perceived factors that promote GE	Green exercise (=physical activity taking place in natural environments), no buffer used	Income, education, sex, age	Green exercise was represented among the elderly. No associations were identified to sex, centrality, education level or household income
Cohen-Cline et al. (2015)	U.S., Washington	Assessment of the association between green space access and self-reported depression, stress and anxiety in between twin pairs.	Mental health (self-reported depression, stress and anxiety)	Multi-level random intercept model of same-sex twin pairs (4338 individuals) from the community-based University of Washington Twin Registry	NDVI based, no buffer used	Income, neighborhood deprivation, sex, age, ethnicity, population density, physical activity	Only the association between green space and depression was significant in fully adjusted models. Association between green space and stress became non-significant when adjusted for confounders
Cusack et al. (2017)	U.S., Portland and Austin	Identification of a relationship between multiple urban green space metrics and associations with term birth weight.	Birth outcome (term birth weight)	Vital Statistics data for a birth cohort (2005–2009). Correlation between green space metrics and mixed models	NDVI, % tree cover, % green space, % street tree buffering and access to parks (using US EPA EnviroAtlas Data), multiple buffer distances: 50 m, 250 m, 300 m, 500 m, 1000 m	Education, income, age, sex, ethnicity, population density	In fully adjusted significant associations disappeared. Maternal race, ethnicity and education as confounders were mostly reducing green space and birth weight associations

(continued)

Table 5.1 (continued)

References	Country, city	Aim	HEALTH	Study design	Green space metrics and buffer	Confounder	Main results
Feda et al. (2015)	U.S., Buffalo	Assessment of the association between neighbourhood park area and perceived stress among adolescents, while controlling for physical activity.	Mental health (perceived stress)	10-week Neighbourhood Environment study, GIS analysis, multivariate regression model	Parks, classification of high/low park access using a park access index, 800 m buffer distance	Socio-economic status (SES), race/ ethnicity, housing density, physical activity	Park area was significantly associated to perceived stress also when controlling for socio-economic status. Physical activity and gender were not significant as confounder in fully adjusted models
Flouri et al. (2014)	UK, England	Analysis of the effect of urban neighbourhoodgreen space on young children's emotional and behavioural adjustment and resilience.	Mental health (emotional and behavioural problems from early to middle childhood)	2000–2007 Millenium Cohort Study data on families in England whose children had emotional and behavioural problems living in urban neighbourhoods	Neighbourhood green space was measured using the 2001 Generalised Land Use Database, excluding domestic gardens, no buffer used	Tenure status, income support, poverty, education, sex, ethnicity, age, household composition	Green space appeared unrelated to child adjustment on the whole, but it predicted emotional resilience. Poor children with more green space in their neighbourhood had fewer emotional problems from age 3 to 5, relative to those living in less green neighbourhoods
Kihal-Talantikite et al. (2013)	France, Lyon	Exploration of a risk cluster of infant mortality according to neighbourhood characteristics	Infant mortality	Cluster analysis assessing spatial aggregation. 715 cases of infant deaths (2000–2009) obtained by city halls in Lyon	Green space index, calculated by using land cover datasets, no buffer used	Neighbourhood deprivation	Spatial distribution of infant mortality resulted to be not random but the high-risk cluster disappeared after controlling for greenness level and socio-economic deprivation. Both deprivation and greenness levels seem to have an independent effect

Jenkin et al. (2015)	New Zealand, country scale	Identification of neighbourhood characteristics associated with children's unhealthy behaviour.	Obesity (BMI), and weight-related behaviours (physical activity, diet, etc.)	Logistic regression models with individual-level data for children from 2006/7 New Zealand Health Survey	Green space (measured in distance and proportion in neighbourhood), no buffer used	Neighbourhood deprivation, income, education, employment status, tenure status, age, sex, ethnicity, household composition	Greater access to green space was significantly associated with lower sugar-sweetened beverage consumption next to neighbourhood deprivation, which was also significantly positively associated with other negative health behaviours
McMorris et al. (2015)	Canada, country scale	Analysis of associations between residential greenness and physical activity.	Physical activity	2001 Canadian Community Health Survey data, logistic regression	NDVI around home, buffer distances: 30 m, 500 m	Income, sex, age, marital status	Association was most significant for those in the higher income groups but positive associations were observed between greenness and physical activity in all income groupings
							Higher income households lived in areas with higher greenness
Michael et al. (2014)	U.S., Portland	Examination of the effect of a neighborhood-changing intervention on changes in obesity in older women	Obesity (BMI)	Retrospective cohort design, change in BMI and neighborhood built environment over 18-year period (1986–2004) among older women; structured interviews and clinical examinations	Green space proximity using Euclidian distance from participant's residence to closest edge of the nearest public park or green space. no buffer used	Occupational manual labor = employment status?, socio-economic status (SES), age, education	No significant association between changes in neighborhood walkability or parks and green spaces and variation in BMI over time was identified in fully adjusted models. SES, education, age among others appeared to be significant in adjusted models

(continued)

Table 5.1 (continued)

References	Country, city	Aim	HEALTH	Study design	Green space metrics and buffer	Confounder	Main results
Mitchell et al. (2015)	Europe, urban areas	Identification of potential neighbourhood characteristics associated with narrower socio-economic inequalities in mental well-being.	Mental health	Multi-level regression models using data of the 2012 European Quality of Life Survey	recreational/green areas non-specific, no threshold, participants were asked about accessibility (with great difficulty, with some difficulty, etc.)	Education, employment status, sex	Socio-economic inequality in mental well-being was significantly narrower among respondents reporting good access to green/recreational areas, compared with those with poorer access
Mukherjee et al. (2017)	India, Delhi	Analysis of the association between park availability and major depression.	Mental health (depression)	Questionnaire survey data from the baseline cross-sectional survey of the Centre for Cardio-Metabolic Risk Reduction in South Asia (CARRS); mixed-effects logistic regression models; development of park availability index with GIS	Park availability index with a buffer of 1-km distance	Education, employment status, income, age, gender, marital status, household composition	In adjusted models a significant association between area of nearest park and major depression remained and smaller park areas were associated with higher odds of depression

Nichani et al. (2017)	New Zealand, country scale	Analysis of association between green space exposure during pregnancy and depression	Mental health (antenatal depression)	Adjusted logistic mixed effect models; data from the Growing Up in New Zealand study, a longitudinal pre-birth cohort study; GIS analysis	Proportion of green space within Census Area Unit including parks, beaches, urban parklands/ open spaces, forests, grasslands, and croplands, but excluded private gardens, no buffer used	Education, employment status, neighbourhood deprivation, age, ethnicity, marital status, socio-economic status	No associations between green space and antenatal depression could be found. Even when adjusted for relevant factors such as deprivation
Padilla et al. (2016)	France, Nice	Assessment of diverse socio-economic, health, accessibility, and exposure factors to explain how they are linked to environmental health inequalities related to infant and neonatal mortality	Infant and neonatal mortality	Creation of environmental indicators with GIS. Multiple Component Analysis, Hierarchical Clustering and standard Poisson regression models using official statistics collected from death certificates in the city halls of Nice municipalities	Green space provided by Corine Land Cover data including natural area but not agricultural areas. Proportion of green area in census block with 10 m^2 of green space per habitant	Neighbourhood deprivation	Identified a significant relationship between infant and neonatal mortality risk and level of deprivation, but the link to urban green space and other exposure variables was not entirely clear. Deprivation was significantly positively correlated to proximity to high-traffic roads and negatively correlated to the proportion of green space as well as to the distance to respective health-care facilities

(continued)

Table 5.1 (continued)

References	Country, city	Aim	HEALTH	Study design	Green space metrics and buffer	Confounder	Main results
Paquet et al. (2013)	Australia, Adelaide	Assessment of associations between accessibility, greenness, size, and type of public open spaces and clinical risk markers for cardiometabolic diseases and mediating factors.	Cardiometabolic risk	Data from the 2000–2003 North West Adelaide Health Study, a longitudinal cohort; Poisson regression models; GIS analysis	NDVI, accessibility of public open spaces within 1000 m road-distance from participant's residence buffer	Education, income, socio-economic status (SES), gender, age	The number and proportion of public open spaces were not statistically significantly related to cardiometabolic health but greenness, size, and type were inversely related to cardiometabolic health
Pearson et al. (2014)	New Zealand, country scale	Assessment of environmental factors in reducing obesity and promoting physical activity.	Weight (overweight, obesity, both), weight-related behaviours (physical activity, vegetable and fruit consumption)	Logistic regression models using data from the 2006/2007 New Zealand Health Survey based on face-to-face interviews	environmental characteristics (e.g. food outlets and green space [...], Accessibility of useable green space, Proportion of meshblock consisting of useable green space), no buffer used	Neighbourhood deprivation, age, gender, ethnicity	Increased neighbourhood deprivation and decreased access to neighbourhood green space were significantly associated with risk of overweight and/or obesity. Increased access to green space was associated with high levels of walking. Significant trend for low levels of walking was additionally positively associated with neighbourhood deprivation

Richardson et al. (2017a)	U.S., Pittsburgh	Examination of influence of neighbourhood green space, walkability and crime on physical activity in low-income African American adults.	Physical activity	Self-reported data on demographics, functional limitations, objective measures of physical activity using accelerometry, neighbourhood green space using GIS, and walkability via street audits in 791 predominantly African-American neighbourhoods	Calculation of green space area surrounding each participant's household within 1-km network buffer	Income, education, number of crimes reported, age, marital status	No significant association was found between neighbourhood green space, walkability, incidents of crime and physical activity
Richardson et al. (2017b)	UK, Scotland	Assessment of a potential relationship between neighbourhood natural space and private garden access and children's developmental change over time	Mental health (emotional and behavioural difficulties)	Longitudinal data of 4- to 6-year-old urban children from the Growing Up in Scotland (GUS) survey; random-intercept repeated-measures linear models	Area (%) of total natural space and parks within 500 m of child's home using Scotland's Greenspace Map, buffer of 500 m	Education, income, neighbourhood deprivation, age, sex	Groups with more park or total natural space close to their homes had slightly better social, emotional and behavioural health outcomes. Having access to a garden was related to sizeable mental health benefits (children from degree-educated households over those from households with no educational qualifications)

(continued)

Table 5.1 (continued)

References	Country, city	Aim	HEALTH	Study design	Green space metrics and buffer	Confounder	Main results
Roe et al. (2016)	UK, London, West Midlands, Greater Manchester	Exploration of relationship between general health and individual, social and physical environmental predictors in deprived white British and black and minority ethnic groups.	Self-reported general health, physical activity	Household questionnaires (face-to-face interviews); Chi-Squared Automatic Interaction Detection (CHAID) segmentation analyses, Correlated Component Regression analyses	Wards identified via land use classifications, perception and use of local green space asked in interviews, no buffer used	Income, employment status, age, ethnicity, gender	General health in the "worst" health group (i.e. ethnicities within the Mixed group) was significantly more likely to be predicted by urban green space usage and perception variables than in any other ethnic group
Roe et al. (2017)	UK, two areas in Central Scotland	Analysis of the effect of urban nature on stress reduction in different segments of deprived urban communities.	Mental health (stress reduction)	A cross-sectional household questionnaire administered by a survey company, using a face-to-face, computer-assisted interviews; Latent Class Analysis	Green space includes parks, woodlands, scrub and other natural environments. Perception of green space access, quantity and quality and motivation for visiting green space was asked in survey, quantity of green space through a datazone green space measure, no buffer used	Education, neighbourhood deprivation, age, gender	Our study found that the opportunities in the immediate neighbourhood for stress reduction vary by age. Stress coping in youth is likely supported by being social and keeping physically active outdoors, including local green space visits. By contrast, local green space appears not to support stress regulation in young–middle-aged and older adults, who choose to stay at home

Thompson et al. (2016)	Scotland, Edinburgh and Dundee	Assessment if the use of local green space is associated with stress in deprived urban communities.	Mental health (stress)	Cross-sectional survey of 406 adults in four communities of high urban deprivation in Scotland, UK; Correlated Component Regression	Self-reported access to green space asked in survey. Green space based on reclassifications of the Ordnance Survey MasterMap and a city-wide audit of green space for Edinburgh and cross-referencing, no buffer used	Education, neighbourhood deprivation, employment status, age, sex, marital status	Quantity of green space in the neighbourhood, and access to garden or allotment, were significantly predicting of stress in deprived communities
Triguero-Mas et al. (2015)	Spain, Catalonia	Assessment of the association between natural outdoor environments and general and mental health.	Self-reported general and mental health	Cross-sectional data from adults interviewed in Catalonia (Spain) between 2010 and 2012 as part of the Catalonia Health Survey; logistic regression and negative binominal models	NDVI, access to green spaces, access to blue spaces, exposure to natural outdoor environments within 300 m from residence; sensitivity analyses used 100-m, 500-m, and 1- km buffers	Education, socio-economic status (SES), gender, age, marital status, population density	Green spaces were significantly associated with better self-perceived general health and better mental health, particularly. Results remained significant for different buffers, and when stratifying for socio-economic status. No association between green spaces and social contacts and physical activity. The results for blue spaces were not conclusive

(continued)

Table 5.1 (continued)

References	Country, city	Aim	HEALTH	Study design	Green space metrics and buffer	Confounder	Main results
Xu et al. (2017)	China, Hong Kong	Analysis of the relationship between green space and mortality.	Mortality (cardiovascular, diabetes, chronic respiratory, lung cancer mortality)	Mortality data for every registered death during the period of 2006–2011 from the Hong Kong Census and Statistics Department; Negative binomial regression models; Generalised Estimating Equations; GIS analysis	NDVI, no buffer used	Income, education, employment status, population density, sex	Higher NDVI values were significantly associated with lower cardiovascular and diabetes mortality, and non-significantly associated with lower chronic respiratory mortality. Associations were stronger for males and low-income area residents

gender. For males, the benefit of green space emerged in early adulthood, while no association was identified for women until later in life. Finally, Nichani et al. (2017) did not identify any associations between green space and depression in pregnant women.

Relatively consistent results show that urban green space has some positive effect on mental health in most age groups, in particular for children, but also for different deprived groups. The effect mostly remained even after controlling for socio-economic confounders such as SES, area deprivation, household income or educational status.

5.3.2 *Birth Outcome*

Abelt and McLafferty (2017) found no consistent significant relationship between birth outcomes and residential greenness. They did, however, identify an inverse relationship between street-level vegetation (street trees) and odds of preterm birth, which remained after controlling for the mother's socio-economic status. Adverse birth outcomes, such as preterm birth or low birth weight, were generally higher among women residing in deprived areas. These deprived areas were less green and had lower numbers of street trees. Similar inconsistencies in results were identified by Cusack et al. (2017). They could not show significant associations between green space and birth weight in full models that take confounders such as ethnicity into account. They did, however, find some consistent associations for the high density urban areas and green space measured at small buffer distances. Adjusted models showed that parents' race/ethnicity had the strongest influence on model predictions, whereas the inclusion of environmental confounders such as NO_2 and air pollution had no effect on the NDVI and birth-weight association (see also Dadvand et al. Chap. 6, this volume). Kihal-Talantikite et al. (2013) also included deprivation as a confounding variable to greenness, and showed that there was no difference in the results for infant mortality. Nevertheless, infant mortality rates were not randomly distributed over the study area, showing that both greenness and deprivation may have an impact. Padilla et al. (2016) could not identify a significant association between neonatal mortality and urban green-space exposure. Kihal-Talantikite et al. (2013) and Padilla et al. (2016) found a significant association between neonatal mortality risk and level of deprivation.

Clearly, there is a major link between socio-economic status or deprivation and birth outcomes. Only some studies could show a relationship with urban green space.

5.3.3 Overweight

Three of the reviewed studies have researched the link between green space availability and overweight or obesity in urban areas. Pearson et al. (2014) showed that deprivation and decreased access to green space in the neighbourhood were both significantly linked with higher odds of being overweight or obese. However, for a sample of older women, Michael et al. (2014) could not identify any association with overweight or body mass index (BMI) and changes in the urban environment through, for example, green-space improvements. They did, however, as shown above, again identify a link between being overweight and socio-economic status. A higher socio-economic status of the neighbourhood was associated with a healthier BMI value. Jenkin et al. (2015) found unexpected results, in that more green space in the neighbourhood was associated with lower sugar consumption values. As shown, they also found neighbourhood deprivation to be significantly linked to obesity-related behaviours such as fast-food consumption.

The link between lower socio-economic status and risk of being overweight was identified in the presented studies, whereas the association with urban green space was only identified in one study.

5.3.4 Physical Activity, Cardiovascular Disease and Mortality

Recent research suggests that urban green space is associated with participation in physical activity and has, through this, a positive effect on health (see also Dadvand et al. Chap. 6 and Cook et al. Chap. 11, both this volume). McMorris et al. (2015) showed that residents living in areas with the highest share of green space were significantly more likely to be physically active during leisure-time. This relationship appeared in all income groups. Likewise, Pearson et al. (2014) showed that increased access to urban green space was directly associated with higher levels of walking. Low levels of walking were significantly positively associated with neighbourhood deprivation. By contrast, Richardson et al. (2017a) found no significant relationship between physical activity and neighbourhood green space in low-income African-American adults in a US city.

Paquet et al. (2013) showed that larger, greener and more locally available green spaces in particular were associated with better cardiometabolic health, which is particularly mediated through physical activity. Xu et al. (2017) showed that greater greenness was significantly associated with lower cardiovascular and diabetes mortality, and non-significantly associated with lower chronic respiratory mortality. Relationships were identified to be stronger for residents living in low-income areas.

Although one study could not find any significant association between physical activity and green space, all other review studies showed that urban residents are more physically active in greener neighbourhoods, although one study highlighted a lower degree of activity in deprived areas.

5.3.5 Green Space Metrics, Buffers and Data Used

A number of studies estimated green space or urban greenness with the average Normalised Difference Vegetation Index (NDVI; Abelt and McLafferty 2017; Cohen-Cline et al. 2015; McMorris et al. 2015; Paquet et al. 2013; Triguero-Mas et al. 2015; Xu et al. 2017). The NDVI is a measure of urban greenness based on remote sensing data.

Others use green space classifications based on land use or land cover data in official statistics (Feda et al. 2015; McMorris et al. 2015; Abelt and McLafferty 2017; Cusack et al. 2017; Mukherjee et al. 2017). Several studies use a distinct distance or buffer size from the residential place ranging from 30 m to 1000 m (Cusack et al. 2017; McMorris et al. 2015; Abelt and McLafferty 2017; Mukherjee et al. 2017; Feda et al. 2015). Remaining studies apply land-use and land cover data from official national or local statistics. Here urban green is classified as urban parks, urban woodlands or forest areas. Nearly half of the studies use buffer sizes of 500 m around a residential place or neighbourhood followed by a 250-m and 300-m distance. Those areas should reflect a walking distance of around 10 min to the next available green space of a certain size.

In general, it cannot be concluded that the results differ depending on the green space measurement, data or buffer size used (for further discussion, see de Vries and Snep Chap. 8, this volume).

5.3.6 Confounding Factors

Many studies researched the relationship between health outcome and urban green space exposure or availability while controlling for confounding factors in their statistical models. The articles selected for our review used a number of different socio-economic and socio-demographic variables (Figs. 5.2 and 5.3). Socio-economic

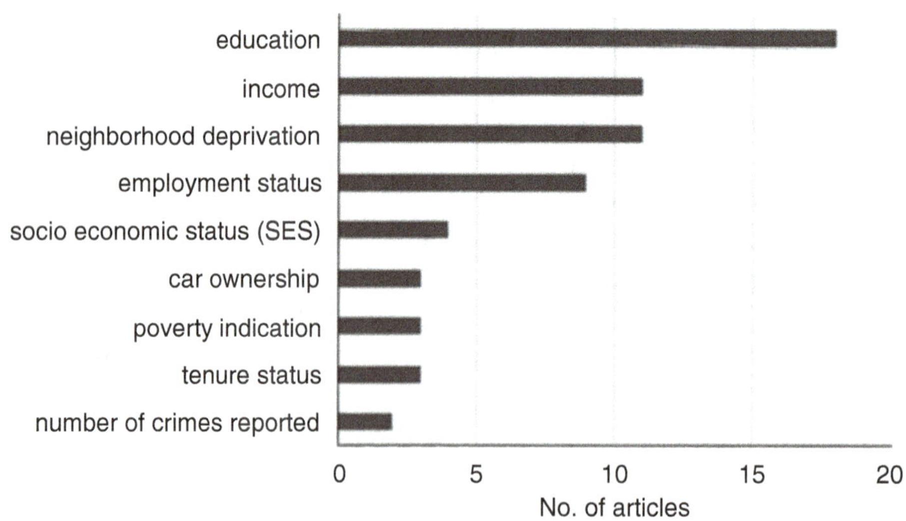

Fig. 5.2 Socio-economic confounders

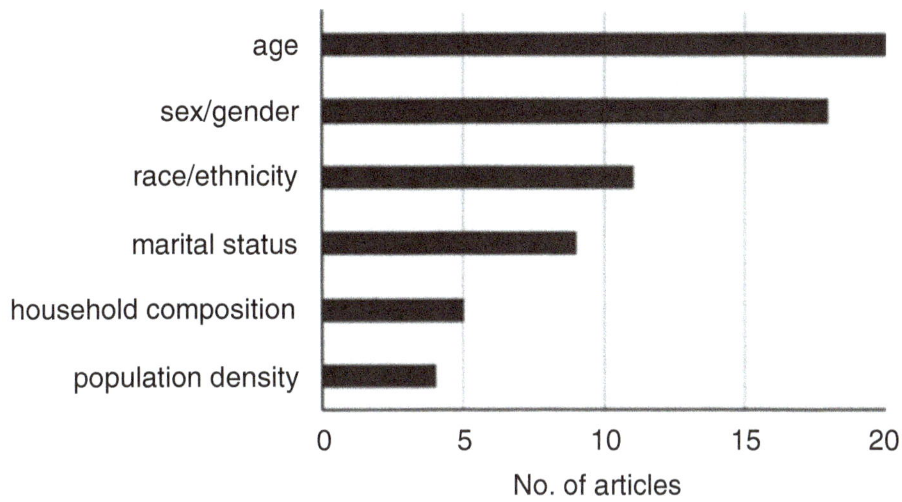

Fig. 5.3 Socio-demographic confounders

confounders mostly address variables of social status that include education of survey participants or households, followed by income or employment status.

For income, it was shown that a higher household income was found to be less likely for residents with psychiatric morbidity, and that this was less prevalent in greener neighbourhoods (Astell-Burt et al. 2014). Significant associations between greenness and physical activity were identified in all income groups (McMorris et al. 2015). Mukherjee et al. (2017) showed that park size was significantly negatively associated with depression even when models were adjusted for confounders such as income, education or employment status, but also for age, gender, marital status and household composition. Similarly, Calogiuri et al. (2016) and Nichani et al. (2017) found that socio-economic inequality in mental well-being was significantly lower among respondents reporting good access to a green space compared with those who had less access. Other studies, however, could not find any relationship between health outcome and socio-economic or socio-demographic confounders (Calogiuri et al. 2016; Nichani et al. 2017) or showed that significant associations between green space and health outcome became non-significant after models were adjusted for confounders (Cusack et al. 2017; Richardson et al. 2017a). For example, Padilla et al. (2016) showed that the significant association between green space and stress disappeared when models were adjusted for socio-economic confounders. A case study city in France showed a significant relationship between infant and neonatal mortality risk and level of deprivation, but could not clearly explain the link to urban green space (Kihal-Talantikite et al. 2013) (Fig. 5.4).

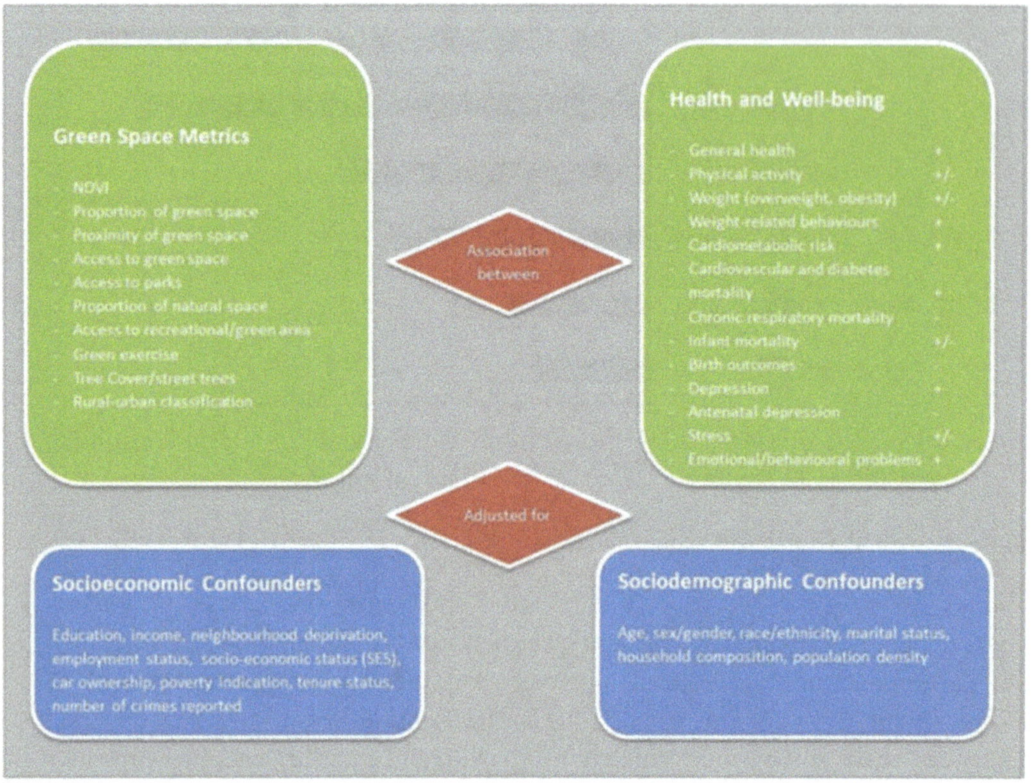

Fig. 5.4 The relationships between urban green space, and health outcomes and confounders, as treated in existing reviews. The strength of the evidence is indicated behind each health outcome: + significant association with evidence, – no signification association found; +/– weak evidence and no consistent results

5.4 Discussion

5.4.1 Urban Green Space and Health Outcomes in Relation to Socio-demographic and Socio-economic Confounders

This study presents the results of a systematic quantitative review that focuses on the association between green spaces and health outcomes with a particular focus on potential socio-economic and socio-demographic confounding factors. Based on the results of this review, it can be concluded that there is a positive association between urban green space and health outcome variables related to, for example, mental health, birth outcome, general health, overweight and other factors. The most consistent results were identified for the association between urban green space and mental health, in particular for children and adolescents. In a detailed review on the benefits of nature contact for children, Chawla (2015) impressively showed the protective effect of nature for psychological well-being irrespective of the method of measurement.

In a number of studies, the positive association between urban green space and health outcome remained even after controlling for socio-economic confounders such as SES, area deprivation, household income or educational status. However, associations are not significant in all studies and partly disappeared when statistical models were adjusted for socio-economic and socio-demographic confounding variables. The strongest remaining significance was shown here for mental health and physical activity. A similar conclusion was presented by Kabisch et al. (2017) for an association between urban greenness and health outcome for particular vulnerable groups of children and elderly. Consistent results were also shown for physical activity but not for overweight or obesity. We can conclude that results demonstrate a multi-factor association between socio-economic, socio-demographic and environmental/green factors and potential health outcomes.

Socio-economic and socio-demographic factors are particularly relevant, and often explain health outcomes to a greater extent than green space availability only. Variables that relate to a lower socio-economic status of participants explain more negative health outcomes. However, for mental well-being, inequalities were smaller among urban residents who reported good access to green spaces, compared with those reporting less access. Similar results were also found for health outcome variables other than mental health. Mitchell and Popham (2008) found that, in general, populations that are exposed to the greenest environments were also identified to have the lowest levels of health inequality linked to income deprivation (for further discussion, see Cook et al. Chap. 11, this volume). Further, the mediating effect of urban green space was highlighted for lower income or deprived groups (Flouri et al. 2014; Mitchell et al. 2015; Roe et al. 2017). Some green space and health relationships appeared to be stronger for those living in low-income areas (Xu et al. 2017). The mediating effect of urban green space may be particularly important for lower status groups. Chawla (2014) reported the importance of nature as a green refuge, with particular importance for children in the context of poverty and displacement.

Reasons for some inconsistencies in the results of the potential association between urban green space health outcomes depend on the particular inclusion variables. Some authors suggested that their results are different from other studies because of the non-inclusion of particular confounding factors such as environmental and neighbourhood characteristics of deprivation, crime, air pollution, etc. (Pearson et al. 2014). Furthermore, inconsistencies might be explained by the difference in green space provision in urban areas in different case studies (Richardson et al. 2017a).

5.4.2 *Implications for Urban Policy and Planning*

What can urban planning and policy-making learn from the studies discussed in this review? Goal 11 from the SDGs clearly states that creating green public spaces will be integratively linked to sustainable and safe urban development. But how is a green space that is most beneficial for all population groups including the vulnerable groups of children, the elderly and deprived people designed?

In the review, green space assessments were conducted that focus on different types of green space, such as parks, street trees or house gardens. Small-scale urban green space such as tree canopies in cities have been shown to improve health effects such as birth outcome, mortality and restoration (Abelt and McLafferty 2017) (see also Lindley et al. Chap. 2, this volume). Small green spaces such as street trees, paths, greenways or gardens provide effective opportunities for restoration and stress reduction as types of micro-restorative settings (Mitchell et al. 2015; Triguero-Mas et al. 2015). The increase in the number of street trees in an urban neighbourhood and the maintenance of existing trees might be of particular importance in disadvantaged neighbourhoods as this could go hand-in-hand with potential positive effects for environmental justice (Landry and Chakraborty 2009; Abelt and McLafferty 2017). In the study by Cusack et al. (2017), it was shown that an increase in urban green space on smaller scales is particularly important in high density urban areas to improve birth outcomes. Further, a stronger association between green space and lower mortality rates was highlighted for those living in areas with higher population densities (Xu et al. 2017). The authors argue that the beneficial effects of green space, including physical exercise opportunities, pollution and urban heat island reduction, and stress relief, may be more needed among people living in more urbanised settings. To conclude, the implementation and maintenance of small-scale green spaces in the form of trees, but also green space within a 50-m distance, is particularly beneficial in high-density urban areas (Markevych et al. 2014; Casey et al. 2016).

In many articles, the authors pointed to the fact that the availability, accessibility and quality of urban green spaces is important for health benefits (Paquet et al. 2013). The size of the park might be one quality criteria that particularly relates to physical activity and mental health outcomes. It has been argued that larger parks in particular are related to a lower risk of cardiometabolic diseases and greater levels of physical activity, whereas studies that only focus on accessibility distance measures without considering any quality aspect could often not find any significant relationship between health outcomes and urban green space (Michael et al. 2014; Nichani et al. 2017). Mukherjee et al. (2017) found an inverse association between park size and depression. They suggested that large parks in particular may provide more benefits of green space exposure, because in their case study of Delhi, they are better maintained, have more natural spaces and diverse landscapes, and are more frequently visited, which translates into more opportunities to socialise. It can be concluded that the quality and a certain size but also the availability within a certain distance of an urban green space all play a role in motivating individuals to use outdoor spaces for physical activity (Jenkin et al. 2015; Mukherjee et al. 2017). Furthermore, the review results showed how green spaces equipped with playgrounds, sport areas, benches, toilets, lights, trees to provide shade, and good sidewalk quality and connectivity can play a more important role in green space use for health and well-being and should be considered in urban planning and decision-making (Michael et al. 2014). Particularly for children, green spaces provide places to explore, play, discover and engage with nature, all important resources for mental well-being (Chawla 2015). This calls for green spaces that are not perfectly manicured but include diverse components of green such as adventure areas, wilderness areas, playgrounds, amongst others. This has been achieved in the development of the park 'Gleisdreieck' in the inner city area of Berlin, where local residents also took an active role in shaping and planning their local green space (Kabisch 2015; Rall et al. 2015).

With regard to the social and socio-economic context criteria, Richardson et al. (2017a, b) showed that children from low-education households had significantly less natural space in their neighbourhoods, and McMorris et al. (2015) found significant relationships between greenness and physical activity for all income groups. Increasing levels of greenness do therefore benefit all population groups, which should be taken into consideration in urban planning for future green space development and maintenance (Cook et al. Chap. 11, Davies et al. Chap. 12, and Heiland et al. Chap. 19, all this volume). Roe et al. (2016) highlighted the fact that particular patterns of use of urban green spaces differ significantly according to different ethnic and gender groups and needs to be considered by planners and policy-makers in a way to steer green space provision appropriately. This suggests that developing new green spaces needs to consider the local context carefully and sensitively.

Safety plays a major role in green space use. Urban green space might be available in significant quantity but is not used by the residential population because of safety concerns (Cohen et al. 2010). Perceived safety concerns and poor environmental quality of local green spaces may discourage residents from using these spaces (Dadvand et al. Chap. 6, this volume). Policy-makers and urban planners should act in these instances to make areas safer and decrease environmental pollution.

5.4.3 Directions for Future Research

Several studies have discussed that exposure and use of urban green space differs according to social and demographic background. Astell-Burt et al. (2014) discussed that exposure to green space varies in different stages in life and that these differences manifest in health disparities. People of different age groups may have different needs with regard to urban green spaces, which in turn translates into diverse health outcome effects (Roe et al. 2017). McMorris et al. (2015) identified an age-specific relationship to green space use for physical activity with significant results for associations between younger adults and women and lower associations with increasing age. In addition, Roe et al. (2017) showed that the use of green space and perception of green space quality does not only vary by age group but also by deprivation: Whilst younger people (youth) are using nearby green space regularly and are satisfied with its quality, the same (or similar) outdoor space is not supporting the needs of young to middle-aged adults. The authors showed that judgements about the quality aspects of urban green space vary across age groups, but place more importance on utilising green space than either on the size of green space or on proximity. Understanding how all these attributes interact and translate into health outcomes is one direction for future research.

Interestingly, results of only two studies were based on objective health measurements (Michael et al. 2014 through clinical examination for detecting obesity; Richardson et al. 2017a using accelerometry for detecting physical activity). All other studies under review used secondary data from official statistics or data from health questionnaires where respondents reported their health status themselves, mostly through well-developed Likert scale measurements for perceived health. In the two studies using objective measures, no consistent association between health and urban green space was identified. One could argue that objectively measured health is the most reliable because it might be less biased by indirect indicators or perceptions. There are, however, other studies that use objective measures to assess potential links between stress levels and urban green space, e.g. through cortisol levels or electroencephalography (Ward Thompson et al. 2012; Aspinall et al. 2013). In these studies, stress levels were found to decrease in greener environments. Stress levels, however, always depend on many different aspects that may lead to an increase or decrease in stress levels. A combination of both subjective and objective measurements is an important field for future research.

Focus on the method of measurement is worth discussing here. All studies used and produced quantitative data and conducted statistical analyses. The review showed that important results were produced from this approach. No study in this review used qualitative research methods, such as an ethnographic approach that includes assessments of observing free behaviour. For children of a particular age group, Chawla (2015) pointed out that ethnographic approaches show how green space can contribute to the development of children's capabilities and to their "complete physical, mental and social well-being". Echoing Chawla (2015), future research should combine qualitative and quantitative approaches that include ethnographic assessment (see Kabisch and Haase 2014; Low 2013 for further details), but also experimental and correlational methods that, when used together, may increase the understanding of health and the environment.

The selection of particular search terms for the review has, of course, produced somewhat narrow results. Using other search terms may have contributed to a larger evidence base on the urban green space-health outcome association, e.g. through increasing the scope to other types of nature, such as trees. However, the focus of this review was to look at potential confounding factors that may explain health-outcome results, and to urban green spaces as a broad group of urban nature. Further, by limiting the review to recent studies, older studies are omitted, although they certainly are as important to review and discuss, especially as they relate to confounding variables.

5.5 Conclusion

Research studies on the association between urban green space and health shows that availability, proximity and use of urban green space such as parks or even allotment gardens, helps to improve the mental health of urban residents even when controlling for socio-economic or socio-demographic confounders. Studies that focus on other health outcomes, such as overweight or birth outcomes, show that significant relationships partly disappear when statistical models are adjusted for socio-economic variables. Income, deprivation or education are amongst the most important variables that confound the green space–health-outcome relationship. Nevertheless, a mediating role of urban green space for socio-economic inequality in health outcome was identified. The results have led to important planning recommendations and directions for future research, which have been presented and discussed here.

This area of research is gaining widespread attention through the promotion of the Sustainable Development Goals and related larger project financing, considering recent calls under the European Commission Research and Innovation Programme. A number of important studies are expected to be conducted in the near future.

Acknowledgments This work was supported by the project "Environmental-health Interactions in Cities (GreenEquityHEALTH) – Challenges for Human Well-being under Global Changes" (2017–2022) funded by the German Federal Ministry of Education and Research (BMBF) (funding code: 01LN1705A).

References

Abelt K, McLafferty S (2017) Green streets: urban green and birth outcomes. Int J Environ Res Public Health 14(7). https://doi.org/10.3390/ijerph14070771

Allan R, Williamson P, Kulu H (2017) Unravelling urban-rural health disparities in England. Popul Space Place 23(8):e2073. https://doi.org/10.1002/psp.2073

Aspinall P et al (2013) The urban brain: analysing outdoor physical activity with mobile EEG. Br J Sports Med 1. https://doi.org/10.1136/bjsports-2012-091877

Astell-Burt T, Mitchell R, Hartig T (2014) The association between green space and mental health varies across the lifecourse. A longitudinal study. J Epidemiol Community Health 68(6):578–583. https://doi.org/10.1136/jech-2013-203767

Bowler DE et al (2010) Urban greening to cool towns and cities: a systematic review of the empirical evidence. Landsc Urban Plann Elsevier B.V. 97(3):147–155. https://doi.org/10.1016/j.landurbplan.2010.05.006

Calogiuri G, Patil GG, Aamodt G (2016) Is green exercise for all? A descriptive study of green exercise habits and promoting factors in adult Norwegians. Int J Environ Res Public Health 13(11). https://doi.org/10.3390/ijerph13111165

Casey JA et al (2016) Greenness and birth outcomes in a range of Pennsylvania communities. Int J Environ Res Public Health 13(3). https://doi.org/10.3390/ijerph13030311

Chawla L (2014) Children's engagement with the natural world as a ground for healing. In: Krasny ME, Tidball GG (eds) Greening in the red zone: disaster, resilience and community greening. Springer, Heidelberg, pp 111–124

Chawla L (2015) Benefits of nature contact for children. J Plan Lit 30(4):433–452. https://doi.org/10.1177/0885412215595441

Clark LP, Millet DB, Marshall JD (2014) National patterns in environmental injustice and inequality: outdoor NO2 air pollution in the United States. PLoS One 9(4):e94431. https://doi.org/10.1371/journal.pone.0094431

Cohen DA et al (2010) Parks and physical activity: why are some parks used more than others? Prevent Med Elsevier Inc 50(SUPPL):S9–S12. https://doi.org/10.1016/j.ypmed.2009.08.020

Cohen-Cline H, Turkheimer E, Duncan GE (2015) Access to green space, physical activity and mental health: a twin study. J Epidemiol Commun Health. Department of Epidemiology, School of Public Health, University of Washington, Seattle, Washington, USA: BMJ Publishing Group. https://doi.org/10.1136/jech-2014-204667

Cusack L et al (2017) Associations between multiple green space measures and birth weight across two US cities. Health Place 47:36–43. https://doi.org/10.1016/j.healthplace.2017.07.002

Díaz S et al (2018) Assessing nature's contributions to people. Science 359(6373):270–272. https://doi.org/10.1126/science.aap8826

Feda DM et al (2015) Neighbourhood parks and reduction in stress among adolescents: results from Buffalo, New York. Indoor Built Environ 24(5):631–639. https://doi.org/10.1177/1420326X14535791

Flouri E, Midouhas E, Joshi H (2014) The role of urban neighbourhood green space in children's emotional and behavioural resilience. J Environ Psychol 40:179–186. https://doi.org/10.1016/j.jenvp.2014.06.007

Haase D et al (2014) A quantitative review of urban ecosystem service assessments: concepts, models, and implementation. AMBIO 43(4):413–433. https://doi.org/10.1007/s13280-014-0504-0

Hartig T et al (2014) Nature and health. Annu Rev Public Health 35:207–228. https://doi.org/10.1146/annurev-publhealth-032013-182443

Jenkin GL et al (2015) Neighbourhood influences on children's weight-related behaviours and body mass index. AIMS Public Health 2(3):501–515. https://doi.org/10.3934/publichealth.2015.3.501

Kabisch N (2015) Ecosystem service implementation and governance challenges in urban green space planning–the case of Berlin, Germany. Land Use Policy Elsevier Ltd 42:557–567. https://doi.org/10.1016/j.landusepol.2014.09.005

Kabisch N, Haase D (2014) Green justice or just green? Provision of urban green spaces in Berlin, Germany. Landscape and Urban Planning. Institute of Geography, Humboldt Universität zu Berlin, Unter den Linden 6, 10099 Berlin, Germany 122:129–139. https://doi.org/10.1016/j.landurbplan.2013.11.016

Kabisch N, van den Bosch M, Lafortezza R (2017) The health benefits of nature-based solutions to urbanization challenges for children and the elderly – a systematic review. Environ Res 159(January):362–373. https://doi.org/10.1016/j.envres.2017.08.004

Kihal-Talantikite W, Padilla CM, Lalloué B et al (2013) Green space, social inequalities and neonatal mortality in France. BMC Preg Childbirth 13:191. https://doi.org/10.1186/1471-2393-13-191

Landry SM, Chakraborty J (2009) Street trees and equity: evaluating the spatial distribution of an urban amenity. Environ Plan A 41:2651–2670

Low S (2013) Public space and diversity: distributive, procedural and interactional justice for parks. In: Young G, Stevenson D (eds) The Ashgate research companion to planning and culture. Ashgate Publishing, Surrey, pp 295–310

Markevych I et al (2014) A cross-sectional analysis of the effects of residential greenness on blood pressure in 10-year old children: results from the GINIplus and LISAplus studies. BMC Public Health. Institute of Epidemiology i, Helmholtz Zentrum München, German Research Centre for Environmental Health, Ingolstädter Landstr, 1, 85764 Neuherberg, Germany: BioMed Central Ltd. 14(1). https://doi.org/10.1186/1471-2458-14-477

McMorris O et al (2015) Urban greenness and physical activity in a national survey of Canadians. Environ Res 137:94–100. https://doi.org/10.1016/j.envres.2014.11.010

Michael YL et al (2014) Does change in the neighborhood environment prevent obesity in older women? Soc Sci Med 102:129–137. https://doi.org/10.1016/j.socscimed.2013.11.047

Mitchell R, Popham F (2008) Effect of exposure to natural environment on health inequalities: an observational population study. Lancet 372(9650):1655–1660. https://doi.org/10.1016/S0140-6736(08)61689-X

Mitchell RJ et al (2015) Neighborhood environments and socioeconomic inequalities in mental Well-being. Am J Prev Med 49(1):80–84. https://doi.org/10.1016/j.amepre.2015.01.017

Mukherjee D et al (2017) Park availability and major depression in individuals with chronic conditions: is there an association in urban India? Health Place 47:54–62. https://doi.org/10.1016/j.healthplace.2017.07.004

Nichani V et al (2017) Green space and depression during pregnancy: results from the growing up in New Zealand study. Int J Environ Res Public Health 14(9). https://doi.org/10.3390/ijerph14091083

Padilla CM et al (2016) Use of geographic indicators of healthcare, environment and socioeconomic factors to characterize environmental health disparities. Environ Health 15(1):79. https://doi.org/10.1186/s12940-016-0163-7

Paquet C et al (2013) Are accessibility and characteristics of public open spaces associated with a better cardiometabolic health? Landsc Urban Plan 118:70–78. https://doi.org/10.1016/j.landurbplan.2012.11.011

Pearson AL et al (2014) Associations between neighbourhood environmental characteristics and obesity and related behaviours among adult New Zealanders. BMC Public Health 14. https://doi.org/10.1186/1471-2458-14-553

Rall EL, Kabisch N, Hansen R (2015) A comparative exploration of uptake and potential application of ecosystem services in urban planning. Ecosys Ser Elsevier:1–13. https://doi.org/10.1016/j.ecoser.2015.10.005

Raymond CM, Berry P, Breil M, Nita MR, Kabisch N, de Bel M, Enzi V, Frantzeskaki N, Geneletti D, Cardinaletti M, Lovinger L, Basnou C, Monteiro A, Robrecht H, Sgrigna G, Munari L, Calfapietra C (2017) An impact evaluation framework to support planning and evaluation of nature-based solutions projects. Report prepared by the EKLIPSE expert working group on nature-based solutions to promote climate resilience in urban areas. Centre for Ecology & Hydrology, Wallingford, United Kingdom

Richardson EA et al (2013) Particulate air pollution and health inequalities: a Europe-wide ecological analysis. Int J Health Geogr 12(1):34. https://doi.org/10.1186/1476-072X-12-34

Richardson AS et al (2017a) One size doesn't fit all: cross-sectional associations between neighborhood walkability, crime and physical activity depends on age and sex of residents. BMC Public Health 17. https://doi.org/10.1186/s12889-016-3959-z

Richardson EA et al (2017b) The role of public and private natural space in children's social, emotional and behavioural development in Scotland: a longitudinal study. Environ Res 158:729–736. https://doi.org/10.1016/j.envres.2017.07.038

Rigolon A (2016) A complex landscape of inequity in access to urban parks: a literature review. Landsc Urban Plan 153:160–169. https://doi.org/10.1016/j.landurbplan.2016.05.017

Roe J, Aspinall PA, Thompson CW (2016) Understanding relationships between health, ethnicity, place and the role of urban green space in deprived urban communities. Int J Environ Res Public Health 13(7). https://doi.org/10.3390/ijerph13070681

Roe JJ, Aspinall PA, Thompson CW (2017) Coping with stress in deprived urban neighborhoods: what is the role of green space according to life stage? Front Psychol 8. https://doi.org/10.3389/fpsyg.2017.01760

The United Nations Development Programme (UNDP) (2015) Sustainable development goals: introducing the 2030 agenda for sustainable development. Available at: file:///C:/iDiv/orga/Anträge/ESCALATE/SDGs_Booklet_Web_En.pdf

Thompson CW et al (2016) Mitigating stress and supporting health in deprived urban communities: the importance of green space and the social environment. Int J Environ Res Public Health 13(4). https://doi.org/10.3390/ijerph13040440

Timperio A et al (2007) Is availability of public open space equitable across areas? Health Place 13(2):335–340. https://doi.org/10.1016/j.healthplace.2006.02.003

Triguero-Mas M et al (2015) Natural outdoor environments and mental and physical health: relationships and mechanisms. Environ Int 77:35–41. https://doi.org/10.1016/j.envint.2015.01.012

van den Bosch M, Ode Sang Å (2017) Urban natural environments as nature-based solutions for improved public health – a systematic review of reviews. Environ Res 158:373–384. https://doi.org/10.1016/j.envres.2017.05.040

Ward Thompson C et al (2012) More green space is linked to less stress in deprived communities: evidence from salivary cortisol patterns. Landsc Urban Plann Elsevier BV 105(3):221–229. https://doi.org/10.1016/j.landurbplan.2011.12.015

Wolch J, Wilson J, Fehrenbach J (2005) Parks and park funding in Los Angeles: an equity-mapping analysis. Urban Geogr 26(1):4–35. https://doi.org/10.2747/0272-3638.26.1.4

Wolch JR, Byrne J, Newell JP (2014) Urban green space, public health, and environmental justice: the challenge of making cities "just green enough". Landsc Urban Plann Elsevier BV 125:234–244. https://doi.org/10.1016/j.landurbplan.2014.01.017

Xu L et al (2017) An ecological study of the association between area-level green space and adult mortality in Hong Kong. Climate 5(3). https://doi.org/10.3390/cli5030055

Chapter 6
Green Spaces and Child Health and Development

Payam Dadvand, Mireia Gascon, and Iana Markevych

Abstract The ongoing urbanisation worldwide has led to an increasing number of children living in urban areas. Urban children, compared to children from rural areas, are generally exposed to higher levels of a number of environmental hazards such as air pollution, noise and heat, and have limited access to natural environments, including green spaces. At the same time, urban lifestyle is predominantly associated with lower levels of physical activity and higher exposure to crime and psychological stress. Contact with green spaces, on the other hand, is thought to have a defining role in human brain development. An accumulating body of evidence has also associated such contact with improved mental and physical health in children. This chapter aims to present a synopsis of the current state-of-the-art of research linking green space and child health and development. Towards this aim, we (1) elaborate on potential mechanisms underlying health effects of green spaces, (2) highlight the importance of prenatal and postnatal periods as windows of vulnerability, and (3) provide an overview of the available evidence on effects of green spaces on (a) pregnancy outcomes, (b) brain development including structural brain development, as well as behavioural and cognitive development, (c) respiratory and allergic conditions, and (d) cardiometabolic risk factors.

P. Dadvand (✉)
Barcelona Institute for Global Health (ISGlobal), Barcelona, Spain
e-mail: payam.dadvand@isglobal.org

M. Gascon
Barcelona Institute for Global Health (ISGlobal), Barcelona, Spain

Universitat Pompeu Fabra (UPF), Barcelona, Spain

CIBER Epidemiología y Salud Pública (CIBERESP), Barcelona, Spain
e-mail: mireia.gascon@isglobal.org

I. Markevych
Institute and Clinic for Occupational, Social and Environmental Medicine, University Hospital, LMU Munich, Munich, Germany

Institute of Epidemiology, Helmholtz Zentrum München – German Research Centre for Environmental Health, Neuherberg, Germany
e-mail: Iana.Markevych@med.uni-muenchen.de

M. R. Marselle et al. (eds.), *Biodiversity and Health in the Face of Climate Change*, https://doi.org/10.1007/978-3-030-02318-8_6

Keywords Green space · Built environment · Biodiversity · Child health · Child development · Biophilia

Highlights

- Pre- and postnatal periods are important windows of vulnerability.
- Contact with green spaces is associated with improved pregnancy outcomes.
- Green spaces are beneficial for child brain (cognitive and behavioural) development.
- There is inconsistent evidence on the association with respiratory and allergic conditions.
- There is inconsistent evidence on the association with obesity and physical activity.

6.1 Potential Mechanisms

Mechanisms through which green spaces could exert their health benefits for foetuses and children are yet to be established. However, stress reduction; increase in social contacts and cohesion; enhanced physical activity; mitigation of urban-related environmental hazards such as air pollution, noise and heat; and enrichment of environmental microbiota have been suggested to play a role. The available evidence is still limited. Of the aforementioned mechanisms, mitigation of air pollution has been investigated the most. A study of 52 pregnant women in Barcelona, Spain, reported that higher residential surrounding greenness was associated with lower personal exposure to particulate air pollution, as measured by personal monitors (Dadvand et al. 2012). Another study reported that higher greenness within and surrounding 39 schools in Barcelona, Spain, was associated with lower indoor (e.g. classroom) and outdoor (e.g. yard) levels of traffic-related air pollution in these schools (Dadvand et al. 2015b). A second study of schoolchildren from these schools showed that 20–65% of the associations between school greenness and cognitive development could be explained by lower air pollution levels (Dadvand et al. 2015a). However, other studies did not support a mediatory role of air pollution in the associations between green spaces and foetal growth and blood pressure in children (Dadvand et al. 2012b; Hystad et al. 2014; Markevych et al. 2014a, b).

A study from Finland reported that adolescents living in more natural areas with higher biodiversity had richer skin microbiota, which in turn was associated with lower risk of atopy through improved immunoregulation (Hanski et al. 2012). Similarly, higher surrounding greenness was related to fungi diversity and variation in house dust in Germany (Weikl et al. 2016), which in turn was associated with lower risk of wheezing in children (Tischer et al. 2016). Improved immunoregulation induced by an enriched environmental microbiome in green spaces has not only been suggested to reduce the risk of allergic conditions but has also been postulated to enhance brain development (Rook 2013). Few studies have proposed physical activity as another potential mechanism underlying the aforementioned associations (Banay et al. 2017). The potential mediatory role of other factors such as stress (Markevych et al. 2014a), noise and heat exposure and social contact are yet to be investigated.

6.2 Pregnancy and Childhood as Important Windows of Vulnerability

An accumulating body of evidence has documented the especial vulnerability of foetuses and infants to the effects of socio-environmental factors (Nieuwenhuijsen et al. 2013). Accordingly, pregnancy and childhood are increasingly recognised as particularly influential for shaping health over the course of life (Hines et al. 2009). The influence of exposures during these periods is not limited to reproductive and childhood outcomes and can extend over a lifetime, as stated by the Developmental Origins of Health and Diseases (DOHaD) concept (Barker 1995; Gluckman and Hanson 2006). DOHaD suggests that environmental exposures during the prenatal and early postnatal periods may permanently alter the body's physiology, metabolism and structure, and that such changes can promote disease long after the environmental exposure has ceased (Hanson et al. 2016). In this context, the ability of green spaces to promote health and development of foetuses and children and to mitigate adverse health effects of urban-related environmental hazards such as air pollution, noise and heat could have lifelong implications.

6.3 Pregnancy Outcomes and Complications

Among different pregnancy outcomes and complications that have been evaluated in relation to maternal exposure to green spaces, the association with foetal growth was the most consistent (Banay et al. 2017; Dzhambov et al. 2014). Higher greenness surrounding maternal residences has been associated with higher birth weight, higher head circumference, lower risk of low birth weight and lower risk of small-for-gestational age (Banay et al. 2017; Dadvand et al. 2012a, b, 2014b; Dzhambov et al. 2014). Although less consistently shown in the literature, green spaces have been associated with longer gestational age at delivery and lower risk of preterm birth (Banay et al. 2017). A limited body of evidence has associated green spaces with a lower risk of pregnancy complications such as pre-eclampsia, gestational diabetes and peripartum depression (Banay et al. 2017). These associations have been suggested to be stronger among women of lower socio-economic status (Banay et al. 2017). A study from England reported that while for Caucasian British mothers there was a beneficial association between residential green spaces and birth weight, there was no such association for British mothers of Pakistani origin

(Dadvand et al. 2014b). This highlights a potential role of ethnicity in the association between green spaces and foetal growth.

6.4 Brain Development

The Biophilia hypothesis suggests that humans have essential evolutionary bonds to nature (Kellert and Wilson 1993; Wilson 1984). Accordingly, contact with nature, including green spaces, has been postulated to be crucial for brain development in children (Kahn 1997; Kahn and Kellert 2002). The brain develops steadily during the prenatal and early postnatal periods, which are considered to be the most vulnerable windows for environmental influences (Grandjean and Landrigan 2014). Upbringing in urban areas where children often have limited access to green spaces has been associated with a higher risk of neurodevelopmental disorders such as attention deficit hyperactivity disorder (ADHD) (Skounti et al. 2007) and autism spectrum disorders (Williams et al. 2006). Green spaces, in contrast, have been associated with short-term improvements in different brain functions, as well as enhanced development of these functions in the long term.

Earlier studies on the potential effects of contact with green spaces on brain function were mainly experimental studies evaluating short-term 'therapeutic' effects in ADHD children (Kuo and Taylor 2004; Schutte et al. 2017; Taylor and Kuo 2009; Taylor et al. 2001; van den Berg and van den Berg 2011). They mainly compared the effects of playing in indoor environments or urban settings in comparison to green spaces, and showed that the latter could improve attentional function and reduce ADHD symptoms. Later cross-sectional epidemiological studies evaluated the long-term association between green spaces and behavioural and emotional problems among healthy children (Aggio et al. 2015; Amoly et al. 2014; Feng and Astell-Burt 2017; Markevych et al. 2014c; Younan et al. 2017; Zach et al. 2016). They mainly characterised behaviour using the Strengths and Difficulties Questionnaire (SDQ), and associated nearby green spaces or time spent in them to lower risk of behavioural problems such as hyperactivity/inattention, conduct problems, emotional symptoms, peer relationship problems and aggressive behaviour. One cross-sectional study reported improved self-discipline associated with better visual access to green spaces from home (Taylor et al. 2002). A recent ecological study in 543 elementary schools in the USA reported lower prevalence of autism in schools with more green spaces (Wu and Jackson 2017). Another similar ecological study reported that more green spaces at primary schools were associated with better performance of students in math and English exams (Wu et al. 2014). Recently, longitudinal epidemiological studies have prospectively evaluated the association between long-term contact with green spaces and cognitive development (Dadvand et al. 2015a, 2017). They used repeated computerised tests to characterise cognitive function, and reported that more green space surrounding the residential address or at school was associated with improved cognitive functions including working memory and attention. A very recent study utilised magnetic resonance imaging of brain structure to assess whether lifelong exposure to green space surrounding the residential address was associated with beneficial structural changes in the developing brain in 253 urban schoolchildren (Dadvand et al. 2018a). This study detected that such exposure was associated with an increase in grey matter volume in the prefrontal and premotor cortices and an increase in white matter volume in the prefrontal, premotor and cerebellar regions. These structural changes were in turn associated with improved working memory and reduced inattentiveness. These findings provide novel evidence that long-term contact with green spaces is associated with beneficial and potentially lasting changes in brain structure.

6.5 Respiratory and Allergic Conditions

The available evidence on the effects of green spaces on asthma and allergic conditions in children is inconsistent (Lambert et al. 2017). While a number of studies have reported a higher risk of allergic conditions and exacerbation of asthma in children in relation to green spaces (Dadvand et al. 2014a; DellaValle et al. 2012; Fuertes et al. 2016; Lovasi et al. 2013), others have shown no or even protective associations (Dadvand et al. 2014a; Fuertes et al. 2016; Hanski et al. 2012; Lovasi et al. 2008; Müller-Rompa et al. 2018; Pilat et al. 2012; Tischer et al. 2017, 2018). These inconsistencies reflect the potential conflicting functions of green spaces in relation to these health outcomes. For example, green spaces can increase the risk of asthma and allergic conditions through releasing allergic pollens (DellaValle et al. 2012; Lovasi et al. 2013) and fungal spores (Bartra et al. 2009; De Linares et al. 2010), or through pesticides or fertilisers used for green space maintenance (Corsini et al. 2012; see also Damialis et al. Chap. 3, this volume). On the other hand, green spaces can prevent these conditions through enriching environmental biodiversity, mitigating exposure to air pollution and, to a lesser extent, encouraging physical activity and reducing the risk of obesity (Hanski et al. 2012; Lovasi et al. 2008; Pilat et al. 2012). The heterogeneity in the available literature could also have been, in part, due to the poor metrics that did not take into account the differential allergenicity of different vegetation species or seasonal variation in their allergenic properties. Different types of green spaces (e.g. parks vs. forests) and different climates/settings could also be contributing factors to such a heterogeneity. For example, a study from Spain reported that residing close to urban parks was associated with a higher risk of concurrent asthma and allergic rhinoconjunctivitis, while residing close to natural green spaces (e.g. forests) was not (Dadvand et al. 2014a). Another study that evaluated the impacts of green spaces on respiratory outcomes reported different impacts across two bio-geographic regions in Spain (Tischer et al. 2017). In the Euro-Siberian region, characterised by a humid climate with water availability throughout the year, cold winters and maximum vegetation during summer months (Alcaraz-Segura et al. 2009), green spaces were negatively associated with wheezing. In the Mediterranean region, characterised by an arid climate with hot and dry summers, mild and rainy winters, and maximum vegetation between autumn and spring (Alcaraz-Segura et al. 2009), living closer to green spaces was associated with a reduced risk of bronchitis. Similarly, a study including seven birth cohorts from across Europe, Australia and Canada has reported heterogeneous associations for different regions (Fuertes et al. 2016). While the association between green spaces and allergic rhinitis was positive in Sweden and Southern Germany, it was negative in Northern Germany and the Netherlands. For the Australian and two Canadian cohorts, no associations were observed. A similar pattern was observed for aeroallergen sensitisation (Fuertes et al. 2016). Further research with more refined green space assessment is warranted in this field.

6.6 Cardiometabolic Risk Factors

Living in a green neighbourhood or close to green spaces has been postulated to increase physical activity or, in other terms, reduce sedentary behaviour (see Cook et al. Chap. 11, this volume). However, the available evidence is not conclusive and there are inconsistencies in the reported direction and strength of associations (Lachowycz and Jones 2011; Markevych et al. 2017; McGrath et al. 2015). The main reason for this inconsistency could be the fact that the majority of these studies have only focused on the mere presence of green spaces without taking into account their quality aspects. Aesthetics, walkability, biodiversity, availability of sport/play facilities, organised social events and perceived safety have all been suggested to affect the use of green spaces for physical activity (McCormack et al. 2010). For children and their parents, the perceived safety and crime rate in the neighborhood are main determinants of their outdoor physical activity (Sullivan et al. 2017). Moreover, most studies have relied on the mere presence of green spaces without taking into account whether they are actually accessible. Some green spaces are not open to the public at all or have restricted access. The methods with which physical activity was measured can be another source of the observed heterogeneity. While some studies have applied objective measures of physical activity (e.g. personal monitors), others have relied on questionnaires to obtain data on physical activity. Each of these methods has strengths and limitations.

In addition to the association between residential green spaces and physical activity, studies have also evaluated how active children were while in green spaces (McCrorie et al. 2014). These studies mainly relied on Global Positioning Systems and accelerometers to objectively characterise time-activity patterns and the locations. They revealed that children are more likely to engage in moderate-to-vigorous physical activity while they are in green spaces, and such an activity accounts for a notable part of the total moderate-to-vigorous physical activity that a child might perform (McCrorie et al. 2014).

Similar to physical activity, the available evidence on the association between green spaces and obesity is not conclusive yet (Gascon et al. 2016). For other cardiometabolic risk factors, the available evidence for a potential influence of green spaces is very scarce (Markevych et al. 2014b, 2016; Thiering et al. 2016). A cross-sectional study of 10-year-old children in Germany reported higher blood pressure in children living in less green areas (Markevych et al. 2014b). A longitudinal study following the same cohort of children for 5 years did not find any association between residential green spaces and blood lipids (Markevych et al. 2016). Very recently, a study of a population-based sample of around 4,000 school children in Iran found a beneficial association between time spent in green spaces and fasting blood glucose levels (Dadvand et al. 2018b). These findings were in line with those of an earlier German study that reported an inverse association between residential green spaces and insulin resistance (Thiering et al. 2016). Further studies are required to investigate the effects of green spaces on cardiometabolic risk factors such as sedentary behaviour, obesity, dyslipidemia, hyperglycaemia and hypertension.

6.7 Final Remarks

Currently, about half of the world's population lives in cities (UN Department of Economic and Social Affairs 2015). By 2050, almost two-thirds of the global population are projected to live in urban areas (UN Department of Economic and Social Affairs 2015). Urban dwellers often have higher exposure to environmental hazards, limited access to green spaces, and a more sedentary and stressful lifestyle. Not surprisingly, urban children have been reported to be more likely to suffer from neurodevelopmental problems such as ADHD and autism spectrum disorders than rural children (Skounti et al. 2007; Williams et al. 2006). An accumulating body of evidence supports the potential of green spaces for mitigating and buffering the adverse impacts of urban living on child health and development. So far, green spaces have been consistently associated with brain development and foetal growth. The available evidence for preterm birth, obesity, respiratory and allergic conditions has remained relatively inconsistent. Similarly, while there is heterogeneity in the reported associations between access to green spaces and physical activity, available studies suggest higher levels of physical activity while the children are in green spaces. Few studies exist for other outcomes such as dyslipidemia, hyperglycaemia, hypertension and pregnancy complications (e.g. pre-eclampsia or diabetes). Moreover, to date, the vast majority of the studies on the effects of green spaces on child health and development have been conducted in high-income countries. As ethnicity, climate and lifestyle might modify such effects, the generalisability of studies from these countries to the rest of the world could be limited. There is a need for more studies in low- and middle-income countries. Although further research is needed, all in all, the body of evidence on the effects of green spaces on child health and development highlights the importance of providing children with a natural and biodiverse environment, enabling them to better grow and thrive in our rapidly urbanising world.

References

Aggio D et al (2015) Mothers' perceived proximity to green space is associated with TV viewing time in children: the growing up in Scotland study. Prev Med 70:46–49

Alcaraz-Segura D et al (2009) Baseline characterization of major Iberian vegetation types based on the NDVI dynamics. Plant Ecol 202:13–29

Amoly E et al (2014) Green and blue spaces and behavioral development in Barcelona Schoolchildren: The BREATHE Project. Environ Health Perspect 122:1351–1358

Banay RF et al (2017) Residential greenness: current perspectives on its impact on maternal health and pregnancy outcomes. Int J Womens Health 9:133

Barker DJP (1995) Fetal origins of coronary heart disease. BMJ 311:171–174

Bartra et al (2009) Sensitization to Alternaria in patients with respiratory allergy. Front Biosci 14:3372–3379

Corsini et al (2012) Pesticide induced immunotoxicity in humans: a comprehensive review of the existing evidence. Toxicology. https://doi.org/10.1016/j.tox.2012.10.009

Dadvand P et al (2012) Surrounding greenness and exposure to air pollution during pregnancy: an analysis of personal monitoring data. Environ Health Perspect 120:1286–1290

Dadvand P et al (2012a) Green space, health inequality and pregnancy. Environ Int 40:110–115

Dadvand P et al (2012b) Surrounding greenness and pregnancy outcomes in four Spanish birth cohorts. Environ Health Perspect 120:1481–1487

Dadvand P et al (2014a) Risks and benefits of green spaces for children: a cross-sectional study of associations with sedentary behavior, obesity, asthma, and allergy. Environ Health Perspect 122:1329–1325

Dadvand P et al (2014b) Inequality, green spaces, and pregnant women: roles of ethnicity and individual and neighbourhood socioeconomic status. Environ Int 71:101–108

Dadvand P et al (2015a) Green spaces and cognitive development in primary schoolchildren. Proc Natl Acad Sci USA 112:7937–7942. https://doi.org/10.1073/pnas.1503402112

Dadvand P et al (2015b) The association between greenness and traffic-related air pollution at schools. Sci Total Environ 523:59–63

Dadvand P et al (2017) lifelong residential exposure to green space and attention: a population-based prospective study. Environ Health Perspect 125:097016

Dadvand P et al (2018a) The association between lifelong greenspace exposure and 3-dimensional brain magnetic resonance imaging in Barcelona schoolchildren. Environ Health Perspect 126:027012

Dadvand P et al (2018b) Use of green spaces and blood glucose in children; a population-based CASPIAN-V study. Environ Pollut 243(Pt B):1134–1140

De Linares C et al (2010) Dispersal patterns of *Alternaria conidia* in Spain. Agric For Meteorol 150:1491–1500

DellaValle et al (2012) Effects of ambient pollen concentrations on frequency and severity of asthma symptoms among asthmatic children. Epidemiology 23:55–63

Dzhambov AM et al (2014) Association between residential greenness and birth weight: Systematic review and meta-analysis. Urban For Urban Greening 13:621–629

Feng X, Astell-Burt T (2017) The relationship between Neighbourhood green space and child mental wellbeing depends upon whom you ask: multilevel evidence from 3083 children aged 12-13 years. Int J Environ Res Public Health 14:235

Fuertes E et al (2016) Residential greenness is differentially associated with childhood allergic rhinitis and aeroallergen sensitization in seven birth cohorts. Allergy. https://doi.org/10.1111/all.12915:n/a-n/a

Gascon M et al (2016) The built environment and child health: an overview of current evidence. Curr Environ Health Rep 3:250–257. https://doi.org/10.1007/s40572-016-0094-z

Gluckman PD, Hanson MA (2006) The developmental origins of health and disease. Cambridge University Press, Cambridge

Grandjean P, Landrigan PJ (2014) Neurobehavioural effects of developmental toxicity. Lancet Neurol 13:330–338

Hanski I et al (2012) Environmental biodiversity, human microbiota, and allergy are interrelated. Proc Natl Acad Sci USA 109:8334–8339

Hanson MA et al (2016) Developmental aspects of a life course approach to healthy ageing. J Physiol 594:2147–2160

Hines RN et al (2009) Approaches for assessing risks to sensitive populations: lessons learned from evaluating risks in the pediatric population. Toxicol Sci 113:4–26

Hystad P et al (2014) Residential greenness and birth outcomes: evaluating the influence of spatially correlated built-environment factors. Environ Health Perspect 122:1095–1102

Kahn PH (1997) Developmental psychology and the biophilia hypothesis: children's affiliation with nature. Dev Rev 17:1–61

Kahn PH, Kellert SR (2002) Children and nature: psychological, sociocultural, and evolutionary investigations. Massachusetts Institute of Technology, Cambridge

Kellert SR, Wilson EO (1993) The biophilia hypothesis. Island Press, Washington, DC

Kuo FE, Taylor AF (2004) A potential natural treatment for attention-deficit/hyperactivity disorder: evidence from a national study. Am J Public Health 94:1580–1586

Lachowycz K, Jones AP (2011) Greenspace and obesity: a systematic review of the evidence. Obes Rev 12:e183–e189

Lambert KA et al (2017) Residential greenness and allergic respiratory diseases in children and adolescents: a systematic review and meta-analysis. Environ Res 159:212–221

Lovasi GS et al (2008) Children living in areas with more street trees have lower prevalence of asthma. J Epidemiol Community Health 62:647–649. https://doi.org/10.1136/jech.2007.071894

Lovasi GS et al (2013) Urban tree canopy and asthma, wheeze, rhinitis, and allergic sensitization to tree pollen in a New York City birth cohort. Environ Health Perspect. https://doi.org/10.1289/ehp.1205513

Markevych I et al (2014a) Surrounding greenness and birth weight: results from the GINIplus and LISAplus birth cohorts in Munich. Health Place 26:39–46

Markevych I et al (2014b) A cross-sectional analysis of the effects of residential greenness on blood pressure in 10-year old children: results from the GINIplus and LISAplus studies. BMC Public Health 14:477. https://doi.org/10.1186/1471-2458-14-477

Markevych I et al (2014c) Access to urban green spaces and behavioural problems in children: results from the GINIplus and LISAplus studies. Environ Int 71:29–35

Markevych I, Standl M, Sugiri D, Harris C, Maier W, Berdel D, Heinrich J (2016) Residential greenness and blood lipids in children: a longitudinal analysis in GINIplus and LISAplus. Environ Res 151:168–173

Markevych I et al (2017) Exploring pathways linking greenspace to health: theoretical and methodological guidance. Environ Res 158:301–317

McCormack GR et al (2010) Characteristics of urban parks associated with park use and physical activity: a review of qualitative research. Health Place 16:712–726

McCrorie PRW et al (2014) Combining GPS, GIS, and accelerometry to explore the physical activity and environment relationship in children and young people – a review. Int J Behav Nutr Phys Act 11:93. https://doi.org/10.1186/s12966-014-0093-0

McGrath LJ et al (2015) Associations of objectively measured built-environment attributes with youth Moderate vigorous physical activity: a systematic review and meta-analysis. Sports Med 45:841–865. https://doi.org/10.1007/s40279-015-0301-3

Müller-Rompa SEK et al (2018) An approach to the asthma-protective farm effect by geocoding: good farms and better farms. Pediatr Allergy Immunol. https://doi.org/10.1111/pai.12861

Nieuwenhuijsen M et al (2013) Environmental risk factors of pregnancy outcomes: a summary of recent meta-analyses of epidemiological studies. Environ Health 12:6

Pilat MA et al (2012) The effect of tree cover and vegetation on incidence of childhood asthma in metropolitan statistical areas of texas. Hort Technol 22:631–637

Rook GAW (2013) Regulation of the immune system by biodiversity from the natural environment: an ecosystem service essential to health. Proc Natl Acad Sci USA 110:18360–18367

Schutte AR et al (2017) Impact of urban nature on executivefunctioning in early and middle childhood. Environ Behav 49:3–30. https://doi.org/10.1177/0013916515603095

Skounti M et al (2007) Variations in prevalence of attention deficit hyperactivity disorder worldwide. Eur J Pediatr 166:117–123

Sullivan SM et al (2017) Associations of neighborhood social environment attributes and physical activity among 11 year old children from 12 countries. Health Place 46:183–191

Taylor AF, Kuo FE (2009) Children with attention deficits concentrate better after walk in the park. J Atten Disord 12:402–409

Taylor AF et al (2001) Coping with ADD The surprising connection to green play settings. Environ Behav 33:54–77

Taylor AF et al (2002) Views of nature and self-discipline: evidence from inner city children. J Environ Psychol 22:49–63

Thiering E et al (2016) Associations of residential long-term air pollution exposures and satellite-derived greenness with insulin resistance in German adolescents. Environ Health Perspect 124:1291–1298

Tischer C et al (2016) Urban dust microbiome: impact on later atopy and wheezing. Environ Health Perspect 124:1919–1923

Tischer C et al (2017) Urban green and grey space in relation to respiratory health in children. Eur Respir J 49:1502112. https://doi.org/10.1183/13993003.02112-2015

Tischer C et al (2018) Urban upbringing and childhood respiratory and allergic conditions: a multi-country holistic study. Environ Res 161:276–283

UN Department of Economic and Social Affairs (2015) World urbanization prospects; The 2014 revision vol ST/ESA/SER.A/366. United Nations, New York

van den Berg AE, van den Berg CG (2011) A comparison of children with ADHD in a natural and built setting. Child Care Health Dev 37:430–439

Weikl F et al (2016) Fungal and bacterial communities in indoor dust follow different environmental determinants. PLOS ONE 11:e0154131

Williams JG, Higgins JPT, Brayne CEG (2006) Systematic review of prevalence studies of autism spectrum disorders. Arch Dis Child 91:8–15

Wilson EO (1984) Biophilia. Harvard University Press, Cambridge

Wu J, Jackson L (2017) Inverse relationship between urban green space and childhood autism in California elementary school districts. Environ Int 107:140–146

Wu C-D et al (2014) Linking student performance in Massachusetts elementary schools with the "greenness" of school surroundings using remote sensing. PLoS One 9:e108548

Younan D et al (2017) Environmental determinants of aggression in adolescents: role of urban neighborhood greenspace. J Am Acad Child Adolesc Psychiatry 55:591–601

Zach A et al (2016) Association of sociodemographic and environmental factors with the mental health status among preschool children results from a cross-sectional study in Bavaria, Germany. Int J Hyg Environ Health 219:458–467

Part II
Biodiversity, Mental Health and Spiritual Well-being

Chapter 7
Theoretical Foundations of Biodiversity and Mental Well-being Relationships

Melissa R. Marselle

Abstract This chapter briefly describes six frameworks that offer perspective on the relationships between biodiverse natural environments and mental well-being. The aim of this chapter is to provide an overview of these frameworks to enable theoretical grounding of future biodiversity and mental well-being studies. The frameworks are largely from the field of environmental psychology and represent the majority of theories used in biodiversity and health research (The Preference Matrix; fractal geometry; the Biophilia Hypothesis; Stress Reduction Theory; Attention Restoration Theory; and Ecosystem Service Cascade Model). A general overview of each framework discusses its conceptualisation of biodiversity and mental well-being outcomes, with supporting empirical research. The chapter then summarises the six frameworks with regard to their hypotheses for biodiversity and mental well-being.

Keywords Mental well-being · Biodiversity · Theory · Ecosystem services · Attention restoration theory · Stress reduction theory

Highlights

- Six frameworks provide perspective into biodiversity and mental well-being relationships.
- There is no single framework to describe biodiversity and mental well-being relationships.
- Further research is needed to test these frameworks using biodiverse environments or stimuli.

M. R. Marselle (✉)
Department of Ecosystem Services, Helmholtz Centre for Environmental Research – UFZ, Leipzig, Germany

German Centre for Integrative Biodiversity Research (iDiv) Halle-Jena-Leipzig, Leipzig, Germany
e-mail: melissa.marselle@ufz.de

M. R. Marselle et al. (eds.), *Biodiversity and Health in the Face of Climate Change*, https://doi.org/10.1007/978-3-030-02318-8_7

7.1 Introduction

Biodiversity affects human health and well-being in a variety of ways (Lindley et al. Chap. 2; Cook et al. Chap. 11, both in this volume). It supports the ecosystem services that help to preserve people's health through regulating clean air and water, and providing food, medicine, shelter, clothing and heat (Mace et al. 2012; World Health Organization and Secretariat of the Convention on Biological Diversity 2015). Biodiversity also helps to mitigate the negative effects of climate change on human health (see Lindley et al. Chap. 2, this volume). Yet, biodiversity (with climate change) can also harm human health by discharging pollen and increasing contact with organisms carrying diseases (Vaz et al. 2017; see also Damialis et al. Chap. 3 and Müller et al. Chap. 4 in this volume). In addition to these impacts of biodiversity on physical health, biodiverse environments also affect mental health (see de Vries & Snep, Chap. 8, Marsell et al. Chap 9 both in this volume) and spiritual well-being (see Irvine et al. Chap 10 this volume). Researchers working in this emerging interdisciplinary field use existing frameworks, often from the field of environmental psychology, to explain these associations. The aim of this chapter is to provide an overview of these frameworks to enable theoretical grounding of future biodiversity and mental health and well-being studies. This chapter briefly describes six of the most widely used frameworks that offer perspective on the relationships between biodiverse natural environments and mental health and well-being, and related empirical research. These frameworks include the Preference Matrix; fractal geometry; the Biophilia Hypothesis; Stress Reduction Theory; Attention Restoration Theory; and the Ecosystem Service Cascade Model. The final section summarises these six frameworks and discusses a way forward.

7.2 Environmental Preference

Liking or preferring one thing over another influences behaviours. For example, preference for one environment over another may influence where to have a picnic, which house to buy or whether one supports nature conservation. Environmental preference frameworks examine relationships between physical characteristics of a landscape (e.g. urban vs. natural, water, land use type, open spatial arrangement, spatial definition, tree size, tree density) and psychological judgements of preference or aesthetic value (Kaplan and Kaplan 1989; Hartig and Evans 1993). Whilst these frameworks do not consider links to health and well-being, they are nevertheless included here, as preference for a specific environment may indicate the potential that environment could have on well-being (Hartig and Evans 1993; Hartig et al. 2011).

7.2.1 Aesthetic Model of Preferences

Berlyne's (1960, 1974) aesthetic model states that aesthetic responses are a function of four properties of a visual stimulus and the behaviour evoked by those stimuli. Importantly for this chapter, one of those properties is *complexity*, which is the variety of components that make up the environment (Bell et al. 2001; Ulrich 1983). High complexity in a visual stimulus is characterised by a large number of elements and the dissimilarity among them (Ulrich 1983). According to Berlyne's aesthetic model, preference is related to complexity in an inverted U-shape (Berlyne 1960, 1974). Environments with moderate levels of complexity are hypothesised to be most preferred, whereas environments with high or low complexity would be less preferred (Bell et al. 2001; Ulrich 1983). Testing this hypothesis, Wohlwill (1968) found that preference was greatest for environments with intermediate levels of complexity.

7.2.2 Preference Matrix

The Preference Matrix (Kaplan and Kaplan 1989) is an informational model of environmental preference which posits that preferences for environments are based on information that the environment provides. According to this framework, the foundation of environmental preferences is the desire to obtain information from the environment. As such, environments that support rapid information processing, understanding and exploration will be preferred (Hartig and Evans 1993).

In the Preference Matrix, four informational qualities in a landscape are ordered by the visitor's need for information and the level of interpretation required to obtain that information (see Table 7.1). The *coherence* of the various stimuli in the environment, and how they all fit together, will support immediate understanding of an environment. Coherence provides a sense of order, which contributes to one's ability to quickly understand an environment; it can be enhanced through redundant features, such as repeating patterns or uniformity of texture (Kaplan and Kaplan 1989). Exploration of the immediate environment depends on the *complexity* of the stimuli: "the number of different visual elements in a scene; how intricate the scene is; its richness" (Kaplan and Kaplan 1989, p. 53). Complexity in this context refers to how much there is to look at and think about; too much complexity and the environment cannot be understood and is confusing, but too little complexity and the individual is bored and not motivated to explore. Making sense of an inferred or

Table 7.1 The preference matrix (Kaplan and Kaplan 1989)

	Informational needs	
Level of interpretation	Understanding	Exploration
Immediate	Coherence	Complexity
Inferred, predicted	Legibility	Mystery

predicted environment, one that is currently out of view, requires two information qualities. *Legibility* helps facilitate understanding of the environment. A legible environment is "easy to understand and to remember" (Kaplan and Kaplan 1989, p. 55) and suggests that one can proceed further into the environment without getting lost. Features of legibility include landmarks and trails. *Mystery* is the promise of additional information with a change of vantage point, the possibility of more information just around the corner. Mystery encourages future involvement (there is some partially hidden information) and continued exploration of the environment (to find out what it is, what is over there). Features of mystery include a bend in a path, partial obstruction of a view, or a modest change in environmental features (Kaplan and Kaplan 1989).

7.2.2.1 Connection to Biodiversity in the Preference Matrix

In the Preference Matrix, biodiversity is implicitly mentioned as complexity; Kaplan and Kaplan (1989, p. 53) discuss an environment's "diversity" and "richness" when describing this information quality. Van den Berg et al. (2016) investigated whether perceived complexity of natural and urban scenes would explain differences in viewing times and ratings of mental restoration (a composite measure assessing fascination, beauty, relaxation, positive affect) (see Sect. 7.3.2 for further discussion on these concepts). Perceived complexity in this study was assessed as the number of different elements to see in the environment. Participants rated natural scenes as more complex than urban scenes. Further, within the type of environment, viewing times and mental restoration differed according to the complexity of the environment. More complex natural scenes with "information-rich tree-tops and forest" were viewed longer and rated as more restorative, than less complex natural scenes with shrubs and fields (van den Berg et al. 2016, p. 400). The authors suggest that complexity may be an important indicator of a scene's restorative potential.

7.2.3 Fractal Geometry and Visual Fluency

The term fractal is used to describe shapes, processes or systems that contain repeating patterns that are reduced-size copies of the whole (Bourke 1991; Ibanez and Bockheim 2013). As such, the defining feature of fractals is self-similarity; a "shape is made of smaller copies of itself…same shape but different size" (Frame et al. n.d.). This self-similarity can be identified and quantified by the fractal dimension, D. The equation for fractal dimension, D, is $\log(N^R)/\log(1/S^R)$, where N equals the number of line segments in the pattern, S is the scale factor, and R is the number of recursions of the pattern (Bies et al. 2016). For example, a fractal line will have a fractal dimension D score that is between 1.0 and 2.0, whilst a fractal surface will have a D score between 2.0 and 3.0 (Hagerhall et al. 2004).

7.2.3.1 Connection to Biodiversity with Fractals

Benoit Mandelbrot's (1983) book the "The Fractal Geometry of Nature" applied fractal geometry to common natural phenomena, such as coastlines, rivers, trees, leaves and snowflakes. The book argues that fractals are an essential tool for understanding the natural world (Mandelbrot 1983). Mandlebrot (1983, p. 1) reasoned that "clouds are not spheres, mountains are not cones, coastlines are not circles, and bark is not smooth, nor does lightning travel in a straight line", but are rather comprised of fragmented, self-similar repeated patterns. Figure 7.1 shows examples of fractals that occur in nature.

Ecologists have used fractal geometry to determine the biodiversity of an environment (Tokeshi and Arakaki 2012). The fractal dimension, *D*, has been used to determine habitat quality (Imre and Bogaert 2004), landscape structure and composition (Pe'er et al. 2013), habitat complexity (Dibble and Thomaz 2009) and species richness (Stevens 2018). The relative lack of fractals has been used to identify man-made landscapes (Pe'er et al. 2013). Irme and Bogaert (2004) used fractals to determine the habitat quality of 49 pine tree (*Pinus sylvestris* L.) woodlots in Belgium. The authors hypothesised that if the woodlots were created due to habitat fragmentation – the process through which large habitats are broken up into small parcels – then the fractal dimensions of the boundaries of these habitats should all be similar (Imre and Bogaert 2004). Fractal similarity for the boundary shape of the woodlots was found, highlighting that the 49 patches of woodland were once one large pine forest and were created as a result of habitat fragmentation. Dibble and Thomaz (2009) examined whether fractal dimension *D* scores could quantitatively describe the complexity of 11 species of aquatic plants, and if the *D* score could be used to predict density of invertebrates found within these aquatic plants. *D* scores were a good predictor of plants' complexity; plant species with high numbers of finely dissected leaves or roots had higher *D* scores compared to plants with single leaves. Furthermore, a significant relationship was found between *D* score and density of invertebrates; more complex plants, as measured by *D* score, were associated with a greater number of invertebrates. Stevens (2018) investigated whether fractal dimensions of the tree silhouette of a habitat would differ based on the species richness of plants, animals and fungi in that habitat. There was a significant difference in *D* scores between high or low species rich habitats; *D* scores were higher in tree silhouettes of high species-rich habitats compared to tree silhouettes of low species-rich habitats.

7.2.3.2 Fractal Dimension and Preference

Could the fractal dimension *D* predict environmental preference? Initially, inconsistent results were found, with studies showing preference for fractal patterns with both high and low *D* scores (Taylor 2001). Thinking that perhaps this inconsistency was related to the source of the *D* scores, Spehar et al. (2003) investigated preference for fractals generated by nature (e.g. trees, mountains, clouds), human beings

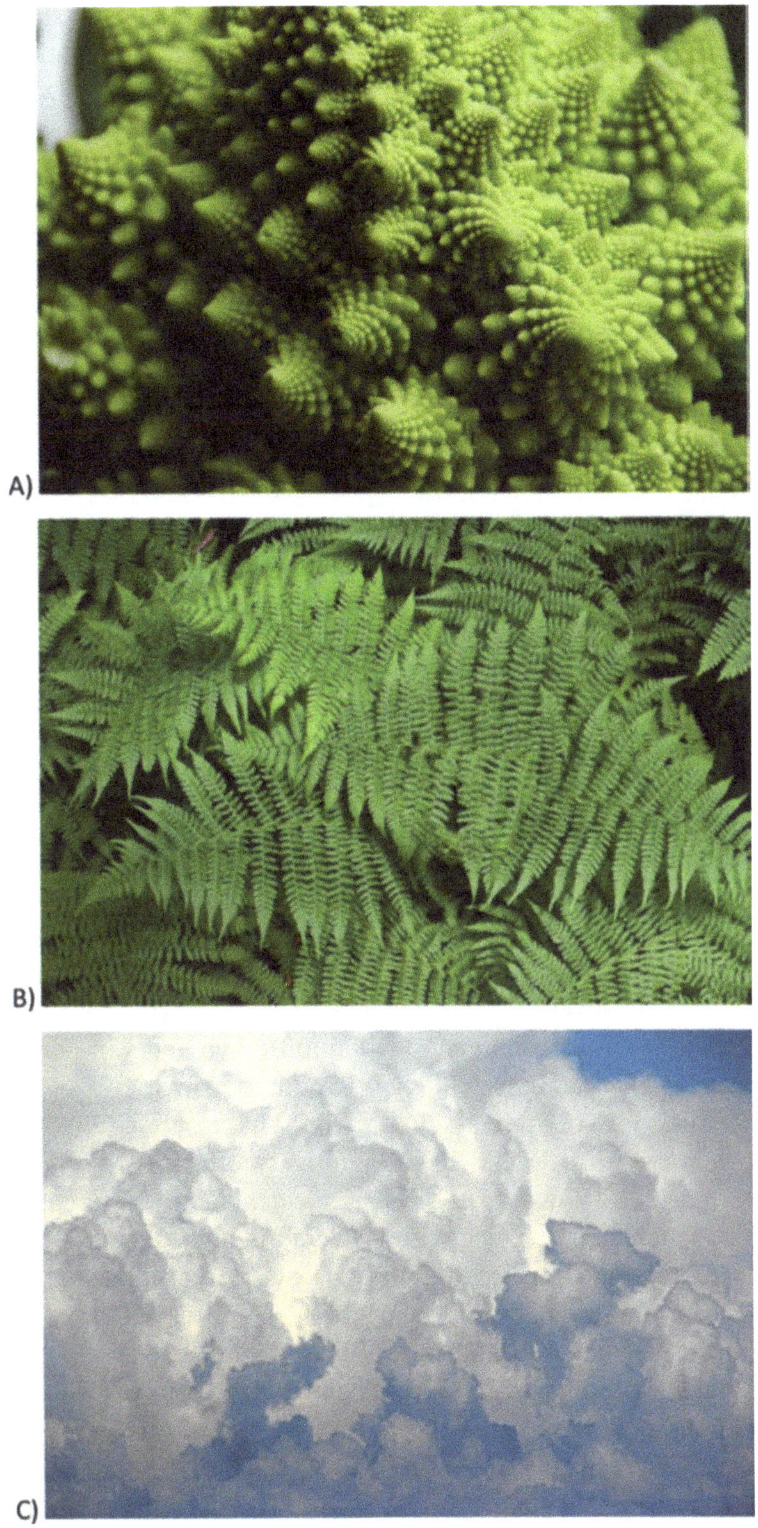

Fig. 7.1 Pictures of natural fractals, demonstrating self-similarity in which a repeated pattern is a reduced-size copy of the whole. (**a**) A Romanesco broccoli (by cyclonebill, CC BY-SA 2.0, https://commons.wikimedia.org/w/index.php?curid=8818018), (**b**) Lady Ferns (*Athyrium filix-femina*) (by Sanjay Ach, CC BY-SA 3.0, https://commons.wikimedia.org/w/index.php?curid=2169955) and (**c**) Clouds (by 3dman_eu, CC0, https://pixabay.com/en/clouds-sky-cloud-dark-clouds-1473311)

(e.g. a Jackson Pollock painting) or computer simulation. They found that fractal patterns with a mid-range *D* score around 1.3–1.5 were aesthetically preferred, irrespective of whether they were natural, human or computer generated (Spehar et al. 2003). Further support for preference for mid-range *D* scores was found in Bies et al.'s (2016) study investigating preferences for statistical (fractals that do not repeat exactly but have the same statistical qualities, like those found in nature) or exact (fractal patterns that repeat precisely, created by a computer programme) fractals. For statistical fractals mid-range *D* scores were preferred, whilst for exact fractals a higher *D* score was preferred (Bies et al. 2016). Interestingly, the mid-range *D* score of 1.3 is most prevalent in nature (Hagerhall et al. 2004, 2015), and found in species-rich habitats (Stevens 2018). These results fit with the environmental perception and preference theories that posit that intermediate levels of perceived visual complexity are most preferred (Kaplan and Kaplan 1989; Berlyne 1960, 1974; Wohlwill 1968) (see Sects. 7.2.1 and 7.2.2).

7.2.3.3 Fractal Dimension and Restorative Outcomes

One reason fractals are preferred could be due to perceptual fluency – the ease with which a specific visual stimulus is perceptually processed (Joye and van den Berg 2013). Fractal characteristics of visual stimuli contain redundant information, due to their self-similar repeating patterns, which could contribute to the experience of easy perceptual processing by the brain. This 'perceptual fluency' could result in restorative outcomes, such as attention restoration (Joye and van den Berg 2013) (see Sect. 7.3.2). Natural stimuli with fractal geometry may be processed more easily, resulting in lower cognitive resource demands of directed attention (Joye and van den Berg 2013) (see Sect. 7.3.2). This easier processing of natural stimuli may contribute to the restoration of directed attention (Joye and van den Berg 2013). Specifically testing the perceptual fluency hypothesis, Joye et al. (2016) investigated the effect that viewing fractal stimuli would have on cognitive performance. Participants were asked to complete a cognitively effortful task whilst viewing either high fractal or low fractal computer-generated (non-nature) stimuli. Participant's cognitive performance was better in the high fractal condition than in the low fractal condition (*D* scores were not assessed). Participants also perceived the cognitive tasks to be easier when looking at the high fractal stimuli, lending support to the perceptual fluency hypothesis.

Would fractals with a mid-range *D* score contribute to perceptual fluency? Juliani et al. (2016) found that people were best at navigating through virtual, computer-generated fractal landscapes with *D* scores between 1.1 and 1.3. Hagerhall et al. (2015) investigated participants' brain activity while viewing statistical or exact fractals. Participants' alpha brain waves were recorded as they looked at these fractal patterns. Alpha brain waves indicate a "wakefully relaxed state" and are commonly found when a person has their eyes closed and their attention directed inward on mental imagery (Hagerhall et al. 2015, p. 3). The authors found that the brain responded differently to statistical and exact fractals. Statistical fractals resulted in the highest alpha waves in the brain, suggesting that they attract effortless attention, enabling the mind to think about other things (Hagerhall et al. 2015). Taylor et al. (2011) tracked participants' eye movements with eye-tracking technology as they scanned a Jackson Pollock painting. The eye movement trajectories, themselves, had a *D* score of 1.4, and were not related to the *D* score of the Pollock painting being observed. The authors suggest that fractal patterns with mid-range *D* scores of 1.5 have a 'resonance' with the brain's own visual processing, which could contribute to the experience of perceptual fluency. This match between the fractal dimensions of the image and the brain's visual processing could account for aesthetic preference (Taylor et al. 2011).

7.2.4 Biophilia Hypothesis

Biophilia is "the innately emotional affiliation of human beings to other living organisms" (Wilson 1993, p. 31). This affiliation motivates humans to seek contact with animals, plants and landscapes (Sundli Tveit et al. 2013). The Biophilia Hypothesis emphasises human beings' positive response to nature, which can be manifest as a preference for specific animals, plants or environments (Hartig et al. 2011). Defining features of the Biophilia Hypothesis are highlighted in Box 7.1.

The Biophilia Hypothesis posits there is an innate, genetic basis for this affiliation with nature (Wilson 1984, 1993). Biological evolution is the process of continuous genetic adaptation to the environment; organisms that are better suited to the environment have a higher survival rate, which gives a genetic advantage compared to organisms that are less suited to their environment. As such, person-environment interactions that have an adaptive value will be genetically retained (Wilson 1984, 1993). Genetic adaptation to the environment arises from behaviours learned through human-nature interactions (Wilson 1993). Interacting with nature results in learnt emotional responses, which can range from attraction to aversion, from peacefulness to anxiety (Wilson 1993). Behavioural responses, such as approaching or avoiding a stimulus, result from these emotions (Wilson 1993).

Box 7.1: Defining Features of the Biophilia Hypothesis

- Humans have an innate, emotional connection to life and life-like processes
- This affinity motivates contact with animals, plants and natural landscapes
- Emphasises positive responses to nature, manifest as preference for nature

These emotional and behavioural responses to stimuli in the natural environment, such as the fear/avoidance response to snakes or to approach response to clean water sources, contribute to survival. This is called biologically prepared learning, in which, through evolution, humans have retained quick emotional and behavioural responses to specific natural stimuli (Ulrich 1993). These emotional outcomes and concomitant behavioural responses (approach vs. avoid) from natural stimuli are then transmitted through culture (e.g. the cultural symbolism of a snake as dangerous) (Wilson 1993). Biologically prepared learning to avoid certain natural stimuli is called biophobia (Ulrich 1993).

Criticisms of Biophilia exist (Kahn 1997; Joye and de Block 2011). First, the Biophilia Hypothesis is considered so general that *any* research studies on the relationship between human beings and natural environments – from human communication, cognitive and mental development, and aesthetic appreciation, to companion animals, learning survival skills, and environmental ethics – are considered as evidence for testing the Biophilia Hypothesis, even if the researcher is testing other theories (Kellert 1993, p. 22). Furthermore, the Biophilia Hypothesis is argued to be more of a general concept, rather than a theory with testable hypotheses (Joye and de Block 2011, p. 193); there is no model describing *how* connection to plants, animals and landscapes influences human communication, cognitive and mental development, and aesthetic appreciation. Whilst learning theory (Wilson 1993; Ulrich 1993) is proposed as a mechanism, it is unclear if learning theory can account for all outcomes, or if additional mediators are required. Additional criticisms are whether biophilia is innate (Kahn 1997; Joye and de Block 2011), and if biophobia contradicts the Biophilia Hypothesis (Kahn 1997).

7.2.4.1 Connection to Biodiversity in the Biophilia Hypothesis

The Biophilia Hypothesis emphasises human beings' positive response to nature, which can be manifest as a preference for animals, plants and natural landscapes. Furthermore, the Biophilia Hypothesis also considers the impacts to health and well-being due to biodiversity loss (Wilson 1993; Ulrich 1993). Unfortunately, the Biophilia Hypothesis does not specify *which* species or landscape types best fulfil people's biophilic needs (Sundli Tveit et al. 2013). The strongest work on Biophilia Hypothesis is on its converse, biophobia (Hartig et al. 2011).

Empirical support for Biophilia largely comes from studies investigating biodiversity and preference relationships. People prefer more biodiversity (Lindemann-Matthies et al. 2010). Hedblom et al. (2014) found preference was greater for birdsong from seven different species of birds than for birdsong from one bird species. Cracknell et al. (2017) found that people preferred viewing an aquarium with a high number of different species of fish/crustaceans, compared to the viewing an aquarium with a low number of different species. Johansson et al. (2014) explored the effect of three different levels of biodiversity (low, medium and high) in forest biotopes on preference ratings. An inverted U-shape was found for preference; the medium biotope was the most preferred followed by the high biotope and the low biotope (Johansson et al. 2014). This suggests that more biodiversity may be preferred up to a limit (see Sects. 7.2.1 and 7.2.2 for further discussion on why intermediate levels of biodiversity might be most preferred).

7.3 Theories of Restorative Environments

Restoration refers to the recovery of physiological or psychological resources that have been diminished through the demands of dealing with everyday life (Hartig et al. 2011). Physiological resources are the ability to mobilise energy toward a specific demand, such as running to catch a train home or working hard to meet a deadline. Psychological resources include the ability to focus attention in order to concentrate on a particular task. Without restoration of these resources, a person is unable to cope with new demands (imagine working to meet a *new* deadline with depleted physiological and psychological resources immediately after meeting the *last* deadline). Over time, lack of restoration of these resources can lead to mental and physical ill health (Hartig et al. 2011; von Lindern et al. 2016). Environments that facilitate the recovery and restoration of these depleted resources are called restorative environments. This section describes the two theories of restorative environments.

7.3.1 Stress Reduction Theory (SRT)

The Stress Reduction Theory (SRT) (Ulrich 1983; Ulrich et al. 1991) considers the physiological impact from viewing natural environments. Box 7.2 summarises the defining features of SRT. According to the theory, natural environments facilitate restoration from stress. Outcomes of restoration are reduced physiological arousal, psychological stress, and negative affect, and enhanced positive affect (Ulrich et al. 1991). Individuals who are stressed are most likely to experience reduced physiological arousal through contact with nature, whilst unstressed individuals are most likely to experience improved affect (Hartig and Evans 1993).

Box 7.2: Defining Features of the Stress Reduction Theory

- Natural environments benefit health by faciliating recovery from stress
- Stress recovery is manifest as reduced physiological arousal, psychological stress and negative affect, and enhanced positive affect
- Visual characteristics of restorative environments are: moderate complexity; moderate depth; a focal point; deflected vistas (e.g. path bending away); a ground surface conducive for movement; lack of threat; and water
- Biodiversity is considered to be a measure of an environment's complexity

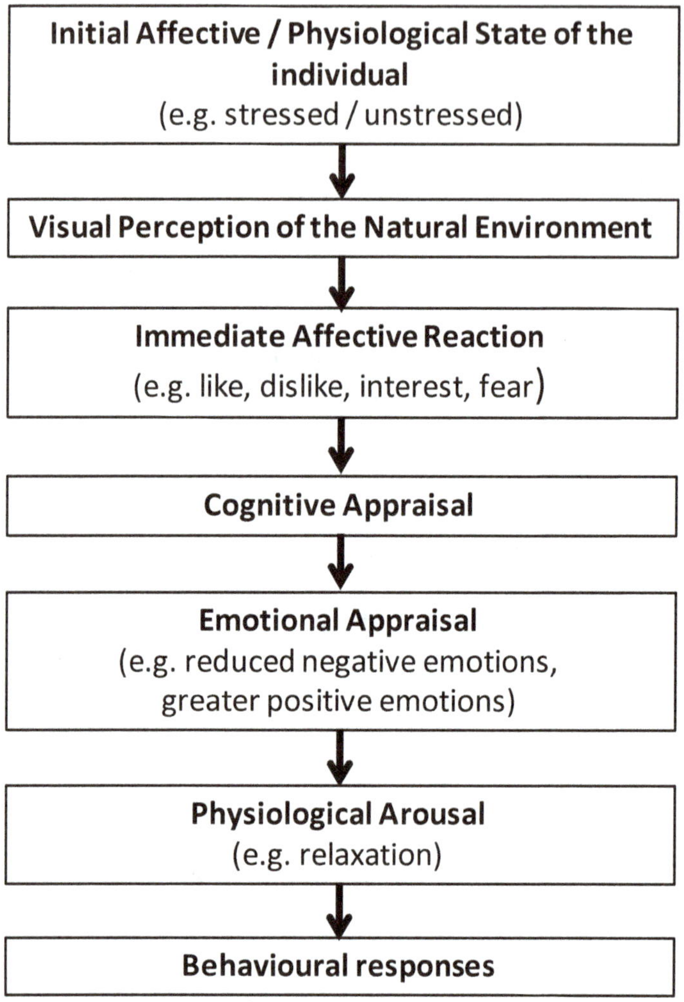

Fig. 7.2 Simplified version of the Stress Reduction Theory of affective/arousal response to a natural environment. (Based on Ulrich 1983)

The SRT details a sequential process in which viewing a natural scene has an effect on one's feelings and behaviour, largely through the autonomic nervous system (Irvine et al. 2013, p. 420) (see Fig. 7.2). The SRT starts with the individual's affective and physiological state (e.g. stressed/unstressed) prior to interacting with the natural environment. This initial state will determine what features of the environment are perceived (Ulrich 1983). According to the theory, visual perception of the natural environment will initiate an immediate, general affective reaction (e.g. like/dislike) and automatic approach-avoidance behavioural responses (Ulrich 1983). This immediate emotional reaction subsequently influences cognitive appraisals of the scene in terms of its significance for well-being and personal safety. This cognitive appraisal may modify the initial, general affective reaction and will produce additional emotional responses, which in turn will influence a change in physiological arousal, and behaviour (Ulrich 1983).

For example, an individual who is stressed spends time in a natural environment. This environment contains visual stimuli that facilitate a general positive affective reaction (i.e. like) and automatic behavioural responses (i.e. approach or stay). Cognitive appraisal assesses the setting for its significance for well-being. The cognitive appraisal is positive, which results in positive emotional responses, and a reduction in negative emotions. These emotions may result in a change in physiological arousal, which could foster feelings of relaxation. Behavioural responses are to approach, explore or continue with one's activities in this environment.

7.3.1.1 Connection to Biodiversity in the SRT

According to SRT, there are visual qualities of the natural environment that facilitate these restorative responses. These visual qualities are: moderate to high complexity (i.e. number of independently perceived elements in a setting); a focal point in the setting to attract or direct attention; moderate to high level of depth (or openness); a smooth and even ground surface that is conducive for movement; a lack of threat; and presence of a deflected vista (e.g. path bending away) and water (Ulrich 1983). Biodiversity can be considered as a measure of an environment's complexity (Ulrich 1983 p. 96). Based on Berlyne's aesthetic model (see Sect. 7.2.1), Ulrich (1983, p. 97) speculated that high (e.g. 'a thicket') and low levels (e.g. 'a flat, featureless open field') of complexity would not be preferred and generate an immediate emotional reaction of dislike and low interest. From this, it is reasonable to assume that environments with moderate levels of complexity would be restorative as they would be preferred, have an immediate emotional reaction of like and interest, and behavioural responses to stay or explore in the environment.

Researchers have investigated whether biodiverse environments could facilitate restorative outcomes associated with SRT. Inconsistent results have been found. Fractal dimensions of habitats with varying levels of species richness were negatively correlated with physiological arousal, suggesting that physiological arousal is related to the fractal dimension of a natural landscape (Stevens 2018) (see Sect. 7.2.3). Greater perceived species richness of animals/plants was associated with more positive mood and arousal, suggesting that higher perceived levels of biodiversity are associated with higher restorative outcomes related to SRT (White et al. 2017). In an experimental study, participants' positive affect, vitality and anxiety were assessed after viewing pictures of trees and birds with either low or high biodiversity (Wolf et al. 2017). Participants reported higher levels of positive affect, as well as lower levels of anxiety, in the high species-richness conditions of trees and birds, compared to low species-richness conditions; no effect was found for vitality between the high and low species-richness conditions of birds and trees. The level of biodiversity of fish and crustaceans in an aquarium had no effect on participants' heart rate, blood pressure and mood (Cracknell et al. 2016). In a separate study, pictures of fish and crustaceans with low or high species richness had no effect on happiness, when abundance of fish and crustaceans was held constant (Cracknell et al. 2017). Ensinger and von Lindern (2018) found that wilderness environments facilitated greater positive arousal, but no change in negative arousal, compared to other landscape types (see Box 7.4). See Korpela et al. (2018) for a deeper examination of studies investigating biodiversity and SRT outcomes.

7.3.2 Attention Restoration Theory (ART)

Attention restoration theory (ART) emphasises restoration of one's ability to concentrate or direct attention (Kaplan and Kaplan 1989; Kaplan 1995; Kaplan and Talbot 1983). Defining aspects of ART are highlighted in Box 7.3. Directed attention is important to human functioning because it is an executive cognitive function, which controls the ability to process information, working memory, inhibitory control, planning and problem solving (Kaplan 1995). The ability to direct attention is necessary for fulfilling a task (e.g. writing a report), and planning and managing behaviour (e.g. achieving life goals) (Kaplan 1995). However, the ability to direct attention is limited and can become fatigued due to continuous and prolonged use (Kaplan and Kaplan 1989). This depletion of the ability to concentrate is called directed attention fatigue. Consequences of directed attention fatigue include the inability to solve problems, impaired perception, impulsive behaviour, irritability with others and errors in one's work (Kaplan and Kaplan 1989; Kaplan 1995).

Restoration of directed attention fatigue requires person-environment transactions that can facilitate the experience of four experiential qualities: fascination, being away, coherence/extent and compatibility (Kaplan and Kaplan 1989; Kaplan 1995). In order to restore the ability to direct attention, a person needs to use a mode of attention that does not require any cognitive effort, called effortless attention. Environments with interesting stimuli that effortlessly attract one's attention will facilitate the experience of *fascination*. Examples of such fascinating stimuli are: "strange things, moving things, wild animals, bright things, pretty things…" (James 1892). Fascination can be sustained if the stimuli in the environment are organised in a coherent way and are rich enough to foster the experience of being in a whole other world (*coherence*). The theory also recognises that there needs to be a match between the environmental setting and one's purposes and inclinations; a compatible environment allows one to carry out his or her activities without struggle (*compatibility*). Finally, a restorative environment requires one to experience physical or psychological distance from everyday tasks or demands that draw upon directed attention (*being away*). Taken together, these four experiential qualities allow

Box 7.3: Defining Features of Attention Restoration Theory

- The ability to direct attention is an executive cognitive function that can become fatigued through overuse.
- The inability to concentrate or focus attention is a sign of directed attention fatigue.
- Restoration from directed attention fatigue requires an individual to experience a sense of being away, fascination, coherence and compatibility in a specific environment.
- Natural environments tend to afford an experience of these four restorative qualities.

people to rest and recover their ability to direct attention. Natural environments are theorised to be especially good environments for attention restoration, because natural environments have a high level of these four restorative qualities (Kaplan and Kaplan 1989; Kaplan 1995).

7.3.2.1 Connection to Biodiversity in the ART

Biodiversity was not a concept that was used in the original theoretical writings of the ART. However, using the theory, one could hypothesise that more biodiverse natural environments may be better environments for restoring directed attention as they may contain fascinating stimuli and afford the experience of being away. Indeed, the relationship between biodiverse environments and the four experiential restorative qualities of ART has been investigated. A significant, positive association between the objectively assessed level of biodiversity and all four qualities of a restorative environment has been found (Scopelliti et al. 2012). However, small urban green spaces rich in plant and animal species were found to be positively related to coherence, but negatively related to fascination, and not related to being away or compatibility (Peschardt and Stigsdotter 2013). Examing perceived biodiversity, Marselle et al. (2016) found perceived biodiversity of birds was positively associated with being away, fascination and compatibility, but not coherence (Marselle et al. 2016). Whereas, perceived biodiversity of plants/trees and butterflies were not related to any restorative qualities (Marselle et al. 2016). Foo (2016) investigated the mediating pathways between spending time in forest environments with low, medium or high levels of biodiversity, and mental health. Individuals who spent time in medium or high biodiverse forest environments experienced a sense of being away, which was positively associated with a change in mood, which then was related to improved mental health. This multiple mediation pathway was not found in the low biodiverse forest. Significant, positive associations between objectively assessed level of biodiversity and perceived restorativeness – a composite measure of all four experiential qualities – have also been found (Scopelliti et al. 2012; Carrus et al. 2015). Measuring biodiversity indirectly by investigating different landscape types in the Black Forest National Park, Ensinger and von Lindern (2018) found significantly greater fascination, being away and compatibility from walking in wilderness compared to other types of landscapes (see Box 7.4).

Researchers have also investigated whether biodiversity could facilitate restoration as an outcome – without investigating the specific four experiential qualities of ART. White et al. (2017) found greater perceived species richness of animals/plants was positively associated with perceived restorative potential. As the level of biodiversity perceived in the environment increased, more participants reported that the environment would be good for restoration. However, Cracknell et al. (2017) found that abundance of all fish/crustaceans, and not the number of species, influenced participants' perception of the scene as restorative. See Korpela et al. (2018) for further details of studies examining biodiversity and ART outcomes.

Box 7.4: Health Benefits of Experiencing Wilderness – Case Study in the Black Forest National Park

Kerstin Ensinger (✉)
Black Forest National Park, Seebach, Germany
e-mail: kerstin.ensinger@nlp.bwl.de

Eike von Lindern
Dialog N – Research and Communication for People, Environment and Nature, Zurich, Switzerland
e-mail: eike.von.lindern@dialog-n.ch

The Black Forest National Park is surrounded by densely populated areas, like the city of Stuttgart. It serves as both a refuge for wildlife and endangered species, and as a recreational area for the local population and tourists. Thus, its management objectives comprise both nature conservation and increasing human health and well-being via recreation opportunities. In 2016, the Black Forest National Park conducted an experimental study to explore the association between experiencing different types of natural landscapes and human health. Participants ($n = 111$) followed a pre-defined path that led through four landscape types: a cultivated spruce forest; a small trail with blueberry vegetation; open heathland; and a pristine forest (referred to as 'wilderness'). At designated stops within each of the different landscapes, participants reported their experience of the four restorative qualities of ART, and the SRT outcomes of positive and negative arousal (for details see Ensinger and von Lindern 2018).

While perceiving the landscape associated with 'wilderness', the participants experienced significantly more fascination compared to the other three landscapes. Ratings for being away and compatibility were stronger compared to the 'cultivated forest of spruce', but not significantly different from the 'small trail with blueberry vegetation' nor the 'open heathland'. Most striking, coherence was rated significantly lower in the wilderness setting compared to the other three landscapes (see Fig. 7.3).

Positive arousal was significantly higher in wilderness compared to the other three landscapes, but no differences emerged for negative arousal.

Among other results reported elsewhere (Ensinger and von Lindern 2018), the overall findings suggest that experiencing wilderness in National Parks and designated protected areas makes a unique and positive contribution to stronger restorative outcomes. Thus, the results can inform management plans that aim at complementing nature conservation with human health promotion.

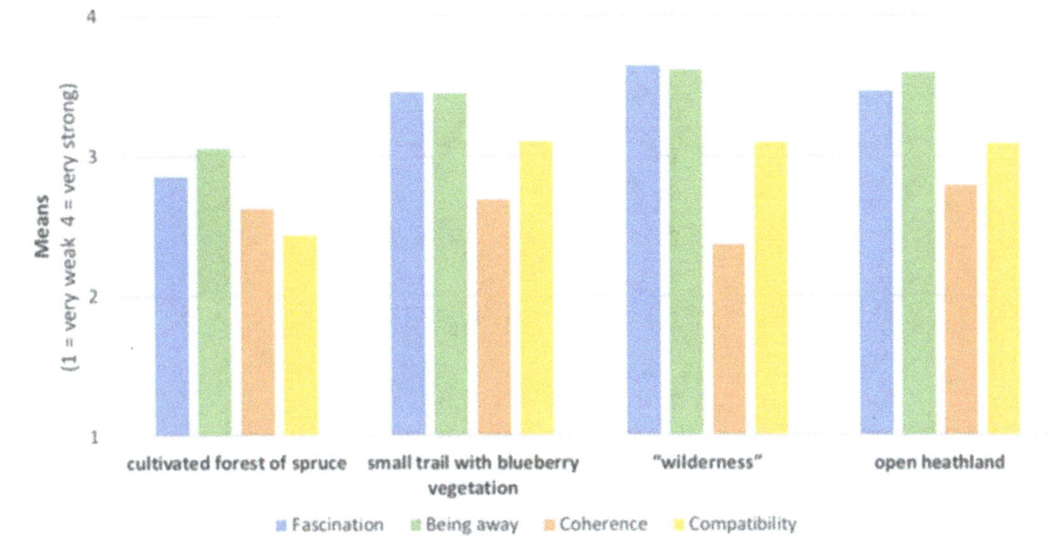

Fig. 7.3 Mean ratings for perception of restorative qualities for different types of landscape in the Black Forest National Park (n = 86)

7.4 Ecosystem Services Cascade Model

The Ecosystem Service Cascade Model details the links between biodiversity and human well-being (Haines-Young and Potschin 2010; Potschin and Haines-Young 2011). The model proposes causal pathways through which biodiversity benefits human well-being through ecosystem functions and services (Potschin and Haines-Young 2011) (see Fig. 7.4). These causal pathways are described as steps that cascade into one another. According to the Cascade Model, biophysical structures or processes are responsible for ecosystem functions, and ecosystem functions influence ecosystem services, which, in turn, result in ecosystem benefits.

The Ecosystem Service Cascade Model has an anthropocentric and utilitarian viewpoint of nature, meaning that an ecosystem service can only be a service *if* humans experience that service to be useful and beneficial (Haines-Young and Potschin 2010; Potschin and Haines-Young 2011). Thus, an ecosystem service is not a fundamental property of the ecosystem itself, but something that is useful to humans (Haines-Young and Potschin 2010). The Convention of Biological Diversity (United Nations Convention of Biological Diversity 1992) considers ecosystem services as a matter of societal choice in which different sectors of society may derive different economic, cultural and societal needs from ecosystems. Therefore, ecosystem services are not isolated from people's needs (Haines-Young and Potschin 2010) and are defined as "something that changes the level of [human] well-being" (Haines-Young and Potschin 2010, p. 117). An ecosystem benefit is "something that directly impacts on the welfare of the people" (Haines-Young and Potschin 2010, p. 117). Ecosystem benefits represent the many ways biodiversity can contribute to human well-being (Mace et al. 2012) through, for example, regulation of water quality for better drinking water, a more satisfying fishing trip (Haines-Young and Potschin 2010), improved human health (Sandifer et al. 2015) or increased feelings

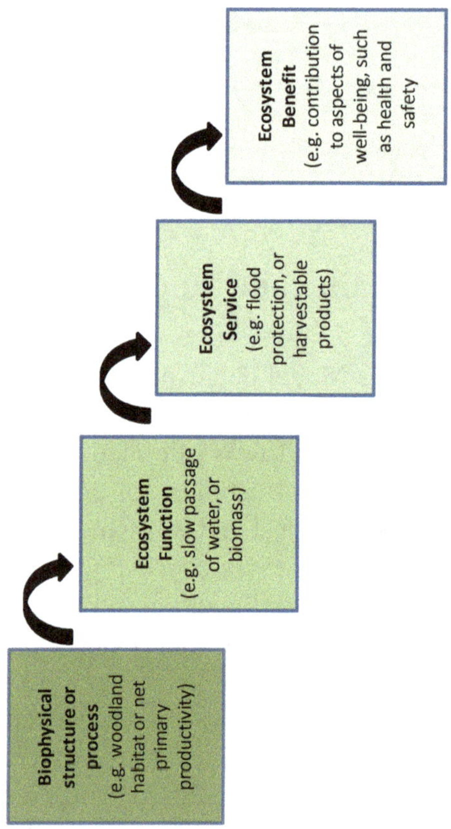

Fig. 7.4 Simplified version of the Ecosystem Service Cascade Model. (modified from Potschin and Haines-Young 2011)

of safety (Potschin and Haines-Young 2011). From this perspective, the cascade model can also work upstream, from the ecosystem benefit to its related ecosystem function. For example, if human beings receive a benefit from a nature-based solution for flood protection, then that flood protection measure is considered to be an ecosystem service, and its related function (e.g. slow passage of water) can be considered an ecosystem function (Potschin and Haines-Young 2011).

Importantly, biodiversity can have different roles in this cascade. Biodiversity can serve as a regulator of the underpinning ecosystem processes (e.g. through pollinating insects), as an ecosystem service (e.g. as a harvestable crop that provides food or timber) or as a benefit (e.g. an emblematic species that is valued for its aesthetics, and may be enjoyed through wildlife watching) (Mace et al. 2012). While mechanisms and linkages between biodiversity, ecosystem functions and ecosystem services are still being explored (Cardinale et al. 2012), and there has been a recent debate over the terminology and the utilitarian viewpoint of the ecosystem service approach (Díaz et al. 2018; Peterson et al. 2018), the Ecosystem Service Cascade Model still holds.

7.4.1 Connection to Health and Well-being in the Ecosystem Service Cascade Model

Human well-being is not explicitly discussed in the Ecosystem Service Cascade Model. Instead, the Model focuses on benefits derived from biodiversity and ecosystem services. Most of the research on the benefits of ecosystem services for human health and well-being focusses on the physical health benefits from provisioning and regulating ecosystem services (Sandifer et al. 2015). However, a developing area of literature investigates the mental well-being benefits from cultural ecosystem services (e.g. Bryce et al. 2016; Fish et al. 2016; Hegetschweiler et al. 2017; O'Brien et al. 2017). The exact casual pathways linking biodiversity to physical and mental health and well-being through the Cascade Model are little understood (Sandifer et al. 2015).

7.5 Discussion

Interest in the mental health and well-being benefits from biodiversity is growing (see Marselle et al. Chap. 9, this volume). This chapter presents a general description of six frameworks that can offer perspective on the relationships between biodiverse natural environments and mental well-being. The aim was to provide an overview of these frameworks to enable future researchers to theoretically ground their investigations of biodiversity and mental well-being relationships. The frameworks are largely from the field of environmental psychology and represent the majority of theories used in biodiversity and health research (Lovell et al. 2014). Table 7.2 provides a summary of these six frameworks.

Table 7.2 Summary of the six frameworks offering perspective on biodiversity and mental well-being relationships with descriptions of how biodiversity and mental well-being are conceptualised, and the mediating pathways that could explain biodiversity-health relationships

Framework	Description	Biodiversity conceptualisation	Mental well-being conceptualisation	Mediating pathways
Preference Matrix	Preferences for environments are based on information the environment provides	Four information qualities in a landscape are: complexity; coherence; legibility; and mystery. Biodiversity is implicitly considered as a measure of an environment's complexity, which refers to the 'richness' of a visual scene	Preference, or liking, for a specific environment or landscape	Informational needs of understanding and exploration
Fractal Geometry	Shapes, processes or systems that contain repeating patterns that are reduced-size copies of the whole	Natural phenomena, such as coastlines, rivers, trees, leaves and snowflakes, are fractal. Fractals have been used to determine biodiversity of an environment	Preference for, or liking, a specific visual landscape	Perceptual fluency – the ease with which a specific visual stimulus is perceptually processed. Fractals contain redundant information, due to their self-similar repeating patterns, which could contribute to the experience of easy perceptual processing by the brain
Biophilia Hypothesis	Humans have an innate, emotional connection to life and life-like processes, which motivates contact with animals, plants and natural landscapes	Posits that biodiversity and certain landscapes engender optimal human functioning. Does not specify which species or landscape types are best for Biophilia.	Preference for animals, plants or environments	Learning theory

(continued)

Table 7.2 (continued)

Framework	Description	Biodiversity conceptualisation	Mental well-being conceptualisation	Mediating pathways
Stress Reduction Theory (SRT)	Environments facilitate recovery from physiological arousal and psychological stress	Restorative environments are characterised by visual characteristics: moderate complexity; moderate depth; a focal point; deflected vistas (e.g. path bending away); a ground surface conducive for movement; lack of threat; and water. Biodiversity is considered to be a measure of an environment's complexity	Reduced physiological arousal, psychological stress and reduced negative affect, and enhanced positive affect	Autonomic nervous system
Attention Restoration Theory (ART)	Person-environment transactions in environments facilitate restoration from directed attention fatigue	A restorative environment is one that requires little cognitive effort. Natural environments are more likely to permit and promote restoration. Biodiversity is not explicitly considered	Ability to concentrate or direct attention. This is an executive cognitive function, required to process information, and inhibit and plan behaviour and problem solving	Experiential qualities between the person and the environment will help restore directed attention: fascination; coherence; compatibility and; being away
Ecosystem Service Cascade	Model details the links between biodiversity and human values through ecosystem services	Any biophysical structure or process. But biodiversity can also be part of an ecosystem function and ecosystem service	Ecosystem service benefit is described as "something that directly impacts on the welfare of people"	Ecosystem functions and ecosystem services

Which Theories Address Biodiversity? Biodiversity is explicitly considered in fractal geometry, the Biophilia Hypothesis, and the Ecosystem Service Cascade Model. Fractal dimensions have been used to determine habitat quality (Imre and Bogaert 2004), landscape structure and composition (Pe'er et al. 2013), habitat complexity (Dibble and Thomaz 2009) and species richness of an area (Stevens 2018). The Biophilia Hypothesis posits a preference for animals, plants and natural environments, but it does not specify which species or landscape types are best for fulfilling the biophilic need for connection to nature (Sundli Tveit et al. 2013). Further, the strongest work on the Biophilia Hypothesis is with its opposite, biophobia, the fear of specific animals and landscapes (Ulrich 1993). The Ecosystem

Service Cascade Model defines biodiversity as any biophysical structure or process (Potschin and Haines-Young 2011), and biodiversity can take on different roles in the cascade (Mace et al. 2012).

Biodiversity is not explicitly discussed in the Preference Matrix, SRT and ART. In both the Preference Matrix and SRT, the term 'complexity' is used, which could be considered as a proxy for biodiversity; both frameworks define complexity as the number of independently different visual elements in a setting (Kaplan and Kaplan 1989; Ulrich 1983). This suggests that a biodiverse environment could be a complex environment due to having a greater number of independently different stimuli (i.e. species; Korpela et al. 2018) and, indeed, Ulrich (1983) specifically states that biodiversity can be considered a measure of an environment's complexity. ART does not discuss biodiversity. As such, one has to hypothesise how biodiversity could be applied to the ART; for example, an environment with a greater number of different species may contain fascinating stimuli and afford the experience of being away (Marselle et al. 2016; Korpela et al. 2018). This hypothesis has empirical support (see Sect. 7.3.2.1).

Which Theories Address Mental Well-Being? Mental well-being is discussed in the ART and SRT. Both the ART and SRT are theories of restorative environments, which refer to the recovery of physiological or psychological resources that have been diminished through the demands of dealing with everyday life (Hartig et al. 2011; von Lindern et al. 2016). Over time, lack of restoration of these resources can lead to mental and physical ill health (Hartig et al. 2011; von Lindern et al. 2016). Health and well-being in the ART is the restoration of the ability to concentrate or direct attention. In SRT, health and well-being is considered as the recovery from psychological and physiological stress reactions.

Mental well-being is not explicitly discussed in the Preference Matrix, fractals, Biophilia Hypothesis and the Ecosystem Service Cascade Model. The first three of these frameworks are environmental preference models. Preference can signal that certain natural stimuli could possibly contribute to health or well-being (Hartig et al. 2011), but cannot in itself be considered a health or well-being outcome (Lovell et al. 2014). Recent studies on fractals are finding that visual fractal objects may contribute to attention restoration (Hagerhall et al. 2015) and physiological arousal (Stevens 2018). The Ecosystem Service Cascade Model discusses human health and well-being as benefits derived from biodiversity and ecosystem services (Haines-Young and Potschin 2010; Potschin and Haines-Young 2011), but little research links ecosystem services to human health and well-being (Sandifer et al. 2015).

Which Frameworks Discuss Mediating Pathways? All six frameworks detail the mediating pathways of the relationships between nature and health. These same mediating pathways could also account for biodiversity and mental well-being relationships. The Preference Matrix suggests that informational needs of understanding and exploration mediate the relationship between informational qualities (e.g. complexity) and preference. Frameworks on fractals in nature suggest that perceptual fluency, the ease of cognitively processing a visual stimulus, would explain relationships between fractals in nature and preference. This work on perceptual fluency can also contribute to the restorative outcomes discussed in the ART. The Biophilia Hypothesis proposes that the learning theory can explain preferences for certain animals and plants. The SRT posits that nature-health relationships are mediated through the autonomic nervous system. The ART states that experiencing four experiential, person-environment qualities (being away, fascination, coherence/extent and compatibility) are required for attention restoration. In the Ecosystem Service Cascade Model, the relationship between biodiversity properties and human benefit is mediated through biophysical structures or processes, ecosystem functions and ecosystem services in serial. But as biodiversity itself can occur in any stage of the Ecosystem Service Cascade Model, it is still unclear what are the exact casual pathways linking biodiversity to health and well-being (Sandifer et al. 2015).

Conclusion There does not appear to be a single, precise framework to describe biodiversity and mental well-being relationships, as none of the six frameworks discussed in this chapter fully describe either biodiversity or mental well-being outcomes. This is likely an artefact of the way in which the majority of these frameworks have been empirically tested, i.e. by comparing man-made and natural environments (Bowler et al. 2010; Thompson Coon et al. 2011). Natural environments, in these studies, are generally treated as uniform without consideration of their biological quality (Dallimer et al. 2012); in other words, the biodiversity of an environment was not explicitly investigated. Recently, a few researchers have started to test these frameworks using biodiverse environments or stimuli. However, issues still remain about using frameworks largely developed to describe differences in natural or built settings to examine biodiverse environments and specific species.

As this inter-disciplinary field develops, it is important for researchers to challenge these existing frameworks. Future researchers could empirically test these frameworks using environments with varying levels of species diversity. Such research can help determine which frameworks are fit for purpose for describing the inter-relationships between biodiversity and mental well-being. Only through this theoretically grounded research can the existing frameworks be ‘evolved’ to better fit biodiversity and mental well-being relationships.

Acknowledgements Thanks are due to Professor Aletta Bonn for her guidance on the Ecosystem Service Cascade Model and Dr. Katherine Irvine for her recommendations on shaping the chapter. I am grateful to the four peer reviewers and Eike von Lindern for their helpful suggestions.

References

Bell PA, Greene TC, Fisher JD, Baum A (2001) Environmental psychology. Harcourt, Fort Worth
Berlyne DE (1960) Conflict, arousal and curiosity. McGraw-Hill, New York
Berlyne DE (1974) Studies in the new experimental aesthetics: steps toward an objective psychology of aesthetic appreciation. Halsted Press, New York

Bies AJ, Blanc-Goldhammer DR, Boydston CR, Taylor RP, Sereno ME (2016) Aesthetic responses to exact fractals driven by physical complexity. Front Hum Neurosci 10:1. https://doi.org/10.3389/fnhum.2016.00210

Bourke P (1991) An introduction to fractals. http://paulbourkenet/fractals/fracintro/. Accessed 26 Feb 2018

Bowler DE, Buyung-Ali L, Knight T, Pullin AS (2010) A systematic review of evidence for the added benefits to health of exposure to natural environments. BMC Public Health 10:456. https://doi.org/10.1186/1471-2458-10-456

Bryce R, Irvine KN, Church A, Fish R et al (2016) Subjective Well-being indicators for large-scale assessment of cultural ecosystem services. Ecosyst Serv 21:258–269

Cardinale BJ, Duffy JE, Gonzalez A et al (2012) Biodiversity loss and its impact on humanity. Nature 486:59–67. https://doi.org/10.1038/nature11148

Carrus G, Scopelliti M, Lafortezza R et al (2015) Go greener, feel better? The positive effects of biodiversity on the Well-being of individuals visiting urban and peri-urban green areas. Landscape Urban Plan 134:221–228

Cracknell D, White MP, Pahl S, Nichols WJ, Depledge MH (2016) Marine biota and psychological Well-being: a preliminary examination of dose–response effects in an aquarium setting. Environ Behav 48(10):1242–1269. https://doi.org/10.1177/0013916515597512

Cracknell D, White MP, Pahl S, Depledge MH (2017) A preliminary investigation into the restorative potential of public aquaria exhibits: a UK student-based study. Landsc Res 42(1):18–32. https://doi.org/10.1080/01426397.2016.1243236

Dallimer M, Irvine KN, Skinner AMJ et al (2012) Biodiversity and the feel-good factor: understanding associations between self-reports human Well-being and species richness. Bioscience 62(1):47–55

Díaz S, Pascual U, Stenseke M et al (2018) Assessing nature's contributions to people. Science 359:270–272

Dibble ED, Thomaz SM (2009) Use of fractal dimension to assess habitat complexity and its influence on dominant invertebrates inhabiting tropical and temperate Macrophytes. J Freshw Ecol 24(1):93–102

Ensinger K, von Lindern E (2018) Wie wird Natur erlebt? Pilotstudie zum Naturerleben im Nationalpark Schwarzwald [How is nature perceived? Pilot-study regarding the experience of nature in the Black Forest National Park]. Black Forest National Park, Seebach

Fish R, Church A, Winter M (2016) Conceptualising cultural ecosystem services: a novel framework for research and critical engagement. Ecosyst Serv 21:208–217

Foo CH (2016) Linking forest naturalness and human wellbeing-a study on public's experiential connection to remnant forests within a highly urbanized region in Malaysia. Urban For Urban Green 16:13–24

Frame M, Mandelbrot B, Neger, N (n.d.) Introduction to fractals. In: Fractal geometry http://users.math.yale.edu/public_html/People/frame/Fractals/. Accessed 26 Feb 2018

Hagerhall CM, Purcell T, Taylor R (2004) Fractal dimension of landscape silhouette outlines as a predictor of landscape preference. J Environ Psychol 24(2):247–255

Hagerhall CM, Laike T, Küller M et al (2015) Human physiological benefits of viewing nature: EEG responses to exact and statistical fractal patterns. Nonlinear Dynamics Psychol Life Sci 19(1):1–12

Haines-Young R, Potschin M (2010) The links between biodiversity, ecosystem services and wellbeing. In: Raffaelli DG, Frid CLJ (eds) Ecosystem ecology: a new synthesis. Cambridge University Press, Cambridge, pp 110–139

Hartig T, Evans GW (1993) Psychological foundations of nature experience. In: Garling T, Golledge RG (eds) Advances in psychology. Vol 96: Behavior and environment: psychological and geographical approaches. New Holland, Amsterdam, pp 427–457

Hartig T, van den Berg AE, Hagerhall CM et al (2011) Health benefits of nature experience: psychological, social and cultural processes. In: Nilsson K, Sangster M, Gallis C et al (eds) Forests, trees and human health. Springer, Dordrecht, pp 127–168

Hedblom M, Heyman E, Antonsson H, Gunnarsson B (2014) Bird song diversity influences young people's appreciation of urban landscapes. Urban For Urban Green 13(3):469–474

Hegetschweiler KT, de Vries S, Arnberger A et al (2017) Linking demand and supply factors in identifying cultural ecosystem services of urban green infrastructures: a review of European studies. Urban For Urban Green 21:48–59

Ibanez JJ, Bockheim J (2013) Pedodiversity: state of the art and future challenges. CRC Press, Boca Raton

Imre AR, Bogaert J (2004) The fractal dimension as a measure of the quality of habitats. Acta Biotheor 52:41–56

Irvine KN, Warber SL, Devine-Wright P, Gaston KJ (2013) Understanding urban green space as a health resource: a qualitative comparison of visit motivation and derived effects among park users in Sheffield, UK. Int J Environ Res Public Health 10:417–442. https://doi.org/10.3390/ijerph10010417

James W (1892) Psychology: the briefer course. Holt, New York

Johansson M, Gyllin M, Witzell J, Küller M (2014) Does biological quality matter? Direct and reflected appraisal of biodiversity in temperate deciduous broad-leaf forest. Urban For Urban Green 13:28–37

Joye J, de Block A (2011) Nature and I are two': a critical examination of the Biophilia hypothesis. Environ Values 20(2):189–215. https://doi.org/10.3197/096327111X12997574391724

Joye Y, van den Berg A (2013) Restorative environments. In: Steg L, van den Berg AE, de JIM G (eds) Environmental psychology: an introduction. BPS Blackwell, West Sussex, pp 57–66

Joye Y, Steg L, Berfu Unal A, Pals R (2016) When complex is easy on the mind: internal repetition of visual information in complex objects is a source of perceptual fluency. J Exp Psychol Hum Percept Perform 42(1):103–114

Juliani AW, Bies AJ, Boydston CR et al (2016) Navigation performance in virtual environments varies with fractal dimension of landscape. J Environ Psychol 47:155–165

Kahn PJ (1997) Developmental psychology and the biophilia hypothesis: children's affiliation with nature. Dev Rev 17(1):1–61

Kaplan S (1995) The restorative benefits of nature: toward an integrative framework. J Environ Psychol 15(3):169–182

Kaplan R, Kaplan S (1989) The experience of nature: a psychological perspective. Cambridge University Press, Cambridge

Kaplan S, Talbot JF (1983) Psychological benefits of a wilderness experience. In: Altman I, Wohlwill JF (eds) Behavior and the natural environment. Plenum, New York, pp 163–203

Kellert SR (1993) Introduction. In: Kellert SR, Wilson EO (eds) The biophilia hypothesis. Island Press, Washington, DC, p 20

Korpela K, Pasanen T, Ratcliffe E (2018) Biodiversity and psychological well-being. In: Ossola A, Niemelä J (eds) Urban biodiversity. Routledge, New York, pp 134–149

Lindemann-Matthies P, Junge X, Matthies D (2010) The influence of plant diversity on people's perception and aesthetic appreciation of grassland vegetation. Biol Conserv 143:195–202

Lovell R, Wheeler BW, Higgins SL et al (2014) A systematic review of the health and wellbeing benefits of biodiverse environments. J Toxicol Environ Health B Crit Rev 17(1):1–20. https://doi.org/10.1080/10937404.2013.856361

Mace GM, Norris K, Fitter AH (2012) Biodiversity and ecosystem services: a multilayered relationship. Trends Ecol Evol 27:24–31

Mandelbrot B (1983) The fractal geometry of nature. W.H. Freeman, New York

Marselle MR, Irvine KN, Lorenzo-Arribas A, Warber SL (2016) Does perceived restorativeness mediate the effects of perceived biodiversity and perceived naturalness on emotional Well-being following group walks in nature? J Environ Psychol 46:217–232

O'Brien L, De Vreese R, Kern M et al (2017) Cultural ecosystem benefits of urban and peri-urban green infrastructure across different European countries. Urban For Urban Green 24:236–248

Pe'er G, Zurita GA, Schober L et al (2013) Simple process-based simulators for generating spatial patterns of habitat loss and fragmentation: a review and introduction to the *G-RaFFe* model. PLoS One 8(5):e64968. https://doi.org/10.1371/journal.pone.0064968

Peschardt KK, Stigsdotter UK (2013) Associations between park characteristics and perceived restorativeness of small public urban green spaces. Landscape Urban Plan 112:26–39

Peterson GD, Harmácková ZV, Meacham M et al (2018) Welcoming different perspectives in IPBES: "Nature's contributions to people" and "Ecosystem services". Ecol Soc 23(1):39. https://doi.org/10.5751/ES-10134-230139

Potschin MB, Haines-Young RH (2011) Ecosystem services: exploring a geographical perspective. Prog Phys Geogr 35:575–594

Sandifer PA, Sutton-Grier AE, Ward BP (2015) Exploring connections among nature, biodiversity, ecosystem services, and human health and Well-being: opportunities to enhance health and biodiversity conservation. Ecosyst Serv 12:1–15

Scopelliti M, Carrus G, Cini F et al (2012) Biodiversity, perceived Restorativeness and benefits of nature: a study on the psychological processes and outcomes of on-site experiences in urban and Peri-Urban Green areas in Italy. In: Kabisch S, Kunath A, Schweizer-Ries P, Steinführer A (eds) Vulnerability, risks and complexity: impacts of global change on human habitats. Hogrefe Publishing, Gottingen, p 255

Spehar B, Clifford CWG, Newell BR, Taylor RP (2003) Universal aesthetics of fractals. Comput Graph 27:813–820

Stevens P (2018) Fractal dimension links responses to a visual scene to its biodiversity. Ecopsychology. https://doi.org/10.1089/eco.2017.0049

Sundli Tveit M, Ode Sang A, Hagerhall CM (2013) Scenic beauty: visual landscape assessment and human landscape perception. In: Steg L, van den Berg AE, de Groot JIM (eds) Environmental psychology: an introduction. BPS Blackwell, West Sussex, pp 37–46

Taylor R (2001) Architect reaches for the clouds: how fractals may figure in our appreciation of a proposed new building. Nature 410:18. https://doi.org/10.1038/35065154

Taylor RP, Spehar B, van Donkelaar P, Hagerhall CM (2011) Perceptual and physiological responses to Jackson Pollock's fractals. Front Hum Neurosci 5. https://doi.org/10.3389/fnhum.2011.00060

Thompson Coon J, Boddy K, Stein K et al (2011) Does participating in physical activity in outdoor natural environments have a greater effect on physical and mental wellbeing than physical activity indoors? A systematic review. Environ Sci Technol 45(5):1761–1772. https://doi.org/10.1021/es102947t

Tokeshi M, Arakaki S (2012) Habitat complexity in aquatic systems: fractals and beyond. Hydrobiologia 685:27–47. https://doi.org/10.1007/s10750-011-0832-z

Ulrich R (1983) Aesthetic and affective response to natural environment. In: Altman I, Wohlwill J (eds) Human behavior and the natural environment. Plenum Press, New York, pp 85–125

Ulrich RS (1993) Biophilia, biophobia, and natural landscapes. In: Kellert SR, Wilson EO (eds) The biophilia hypothesis. Island Press, Washington, DC, p 73

Ulrich R, Simons R, Losito B et al (1991) Stress recovery during exposure to natural and urban environments. J Environ Psychol 11(3):201–230

United Nations Convention on Biological Diversity (1992) Convention on biological diversity. https://wwwcbdint/doc/legal/cbd-enpdf. Accessed 12 July 2018

van den Berg AE, Joye Y, Koole SL (2016) Why viewing nature is more fascinating and restorative than viewing buildings: a closer look at perceived complexity. Urban For Urban Green 20:397–401

Vaz AS, Kull CA, Kueffer C, Richardson DM, Vicente JR, Kühn I, Schröter M, Hauck J, Bonn A, Honrado JP (2017) Integrating ecosystem services and disservices: insights from plant invasions. Ecosyst Serv 23:94–107

von Lindern E, Lymeus F, Hartig T (2016) The restorative environment: a complementary concept for salutogenesis studies. In: Mittelmark MB, Sagy S, Eriksson M et al (eds) The handbook of Salutogenesis. Springer, New York, pp 181–195

White MP, Weeks A, Hooper T et al (2017) Marine wildlife as an important component of coastal visits: the role of perceived biodiversity and species behaviour. Mar Policy 78(80):89

Wilson EO (1984) Biophilia. Harvard University Press, Cambridge, MA

Wilson EO (1993) Biophilia and the conservation ethic. In: Kellert SR, Wilson EO (eds) The biophilia hypothesis. Island Press, Washington, DC, p 31
Wohlwill JF (1968) Amount of stimulus exploration and preference as differential functions of stimulus complexity. Percept Psychophys 4:307–312
Wolf LJ, zu Ermgassen S, Balmford A, White M Weinstein N (2017) Is variety the spice of life? An experimental investigation into the effects of species richness on self-reported mental Well-being. PLoS One 12(1):e0170225. https://doi.org/10.1371/journal.pone.0170225
World Health Organisation & Secretariat of the Convention on Biological Diversity (2015) Connecting global priorities: biodiversity and human health. A state of the knowledge review. http://www.who.int/globalchange/publications/biodiversity-human-health/en/

Chapter 8
Biodiversity in the Context of 'Biodiversity – Mental Health' Research

Sjerp de Vries and Robbert Snep

To measure is to know, but know what you measure.
(anonymous)

Abstract In this chapter the concept of biodiversity and its measurement and use in 'biodiversity – mental health' research is discussed, as well as access to and contact with biodiverse nature. It is pointed out that biodiversity is an ecological concept that originated in the context of nature conservation. It has evolved without consideration of its potential role in mental health promotion. In studying the latter, the concept of biodiversity is frequently adapted. Such adaptations are likely to occur at the expense of its relevance for nature conservation. Using the concept of biodiversity as originally intended may be fruitful for a different type of research question, focusing more on multi-functionality issues: can the same nature constitute a healthy, biodiverse ecosystem and enhance mental health simultaneously? By pointing out this and related issues, this chapter aims to support researchers and students in future research, and help both scientists and policy-makers to position and assess studies in this field.

Keywords Health promotion · Nature conservation · Functional biodiversity · Ecosystem health · Measurement · Multi-functionality

Highlights

- The concept 'biodiversity' is frequently adapted in studies on its health effects.
- Such adaptations tend to make these studies less relevant for nature conservation.
- Health promotion and nature conservation may have different requirements.

S. de Vries (✉) · R. Snep
Wageningen Environmental Research, Wageningen University & Research, Wageningen, The Netherlands
e-mail: sjerp.devries@wur.nl; robbert.snep@wur.nl

M. R. Marselle et al. (eds.), *Biodiversity and Health in the Face of Climate Change*, https://doi.org/10.1007/978-3-030-02318-8_8

8.1 Key Concepts

In this chapter we take a closer look at one of the central concepts of this book, biodiversity, and especially at the way it is defined. We do so because the definition of this concept has a bearing on what to measure, how best to measure it, and how to study its relationship to other concepts, such as mental health and well-being. The latter concepts are also discussed, but only briefly.

8.1.1 Biodiversity

These days, the term 'biodiversity' is often interpreted and used by conservationists, policy-makers and the general public as an alternative for the broader term 'nature', more or less suggesting that they are interchangeable (Kaphengst et al. 2014; for examples, see Wossink et al. 1997; Wall et al. 2016, Chap. 4). 'Biodiversity', however, originates from the scientific fields of ecology and nature conservation, and there it has a much stricter meaning. Here we start from this original meaning in which biodiversity – as defined by the Convention on Biological Diversity (CBD 1992) – is the variability among living organisms and the ecological complexes of which they are part. Sources of this variability include intra-species diversity (e.g. genetic variability), interspecies diversity (species diversity) and diversity in ecosystems (from biomes to biotopes). Although biodiversity encompasses these three levels of variability, in relationship to human health the species diversity level seems to be the most studied level thus far (Lovell et al. 2014; see also Marselle et al. Chap. 9, this volume). To confine the discussion, in this chapter we therefore focus on this level.

An initial question is whether species are required to be part of an ecological complex, and if so, what counts as such a complex. We equate the term 'ecological complex' with 'ecosystem', for which the CBD (1992) also has provided a definition: a dynamic complex of plant, animal and micro-organism communities and their non-living environment interacting as a functional unit. Some authors include humans as a possible species within an ecosystem. In this chapter, we do not. Given the requirement of interacting as a functional unit and the exclusion of humans, although a zoo contains many animal species, it can hardly be considered an ecosystem. The same holds true for a *hortus botanicus* or arboretum. With regard to species, Angermeier (1994) already made a distinction between biodiversity and artificial diversity.

To a lesser extent, urban parks and private gardens may also contain combinations of plants and animals that do not occur in that composition in a (natural) ecosystem, many of which may not be indigenous to the area. Non-indigenous plants include (wild) ornamental trees, shrubs, perennials and garden pond plants. Non-indigenous animals include (feral) cats, dogs, aviary birds and other pet species. The living nature that parks and gardens contain usually is not intended or allowed to interact as a functional unit. Therefore, most parks and gardens require constant human interference (maintenance and wild management) to remain in existence in their present (desired) state. Actually, human influence is virtually omnipresent, but the level of this influence differs. Consequently, it is a matter of choice how much human interference is deemed acceptable to still consider a collection of plants, animals, insects and micro-organisms a natural ecosystem, or an ecosystem at all.

Biodiversity – here limited to species diversity – has its primary focus on *variability* in the biotic part of nature, the living nature. But even the concept of variability may be interpreted differently. One interpretation is in terms of species richness, usually defined as the number of species in a certain area. This implies the notion that more (richer) is better. From an ecological perspective this interpretation has little value. Ecologists study communities that are linked to the ecosystem type present in the study area. Diversity here is seen more from a functional perspective. The question is to what extent the species diversity of an area contributes to the health of the ecosystem, with ecosystem health being defined in terms of sustainability and resilience (Costanza 2012). This leads to the following more specific questions: Is the species community complete, or are (key) species missing? Are population levels of the species above the viability level, so the species may expect to survive in the defined area in the long run? Are there sufficient species – and sufficient individuals per species – within a functional group (e.g. pollinators) to ensure functional traits (e.g. pollination) continue to be present, even under changing conditions (e.g. climate change)? Thus, desired diversity here is seen as a combination of species diversity (number of species, within each functional group) and species abundance (number of individuals per species). If key species are missing and population levels of existing species are below the viability level, one may define the ecosystem as degraded. If the diversity within a functional group is small, the ecosystem may be considered vulnerable. It is important to note that some ecosystems require a higher number of species to be present in order to be considered healthier than others. Adhering to a strict, functional definition of biodiversity would require that first the applicable ecosystem is determined, and only subsequently the level of biodiversity at the species diversity level of those ecosystems is assessed.

We already mentioned that the concept 'biodiversity' has its origin in ecology. *A priori*, there is no reason why it should be as relevant from a human health perspective as it is from a nature conservation perspective. It may be too specifically geared towards its ecological purpose, as well as too crude from a public health perspective. With regard to the latter, the composition of species that hides behind a certain level of biodiversity may be relevant with regard to its influence on mental health. This latter argument is similar to one made in a more advanced field of environmental epidemiology, that on air pollution. It is not only the level of air pollution that matters, but also the precise pollutants that make up the air pollution, with some being more harmful than others for human physical health. Also from an ecological perspective all animals are equal but some more than others: rare species tend to be more valued than very common species. But this does not necessarily mean that the presence of rare species will coincide with higher mental health benefits.

Thus, one may question whether the level of biodiversity, especially that in terms of functional species diversity, is a relevant factor with regard to the mental health benefits that a certain amount of nature or a natural area may generate. Given that nature conservation and mental health promotion are two separate goals, an appropriate first question might be whether successful nature conservation and efficient application of nature to promote mental health can go hand in hand. Are the requirements that nature conservation imposes compatible with those that the promotion of mental health imposes? Such a question fits in the context of multi-functional use of space, something that is particularly relevant in the urban domain. And yes, perhaps there are synergy benefits to be had by using the same area to accomplish both goals. But it is also possible that trade-offs have to be made. Some ecologically desirable species of animals or plants may be either considered too dangerous to expose people to, or too vulnerable to human presence or certain types of human activity in their habitat to allow people to access the area.

8.1.2 Mental Health and Well-Being

Although the focus of this chapter is on biodiversity, this is in the context of biodiversity – mental health research. Therefore, we discuss the concepts of mental health and mental well-being as well, although less extensively. Mental health is defined by the WHO as a state of well-being in which an individual realises his or her own abilities, can cope with the normal stresses of life, can work productively, and is able to make a contribution to his or her community (World Health Organization 2016). Although the WHO does not provide a definition of well-being, mental health is clearly not merely about the absence of mental disorders. For a definition of mental well-being, in this book the description proposed by Linton et al. (2016) is suggested: dimensions linked to the theme of mental well-being assess the psychological, cognitive and emotional quality of a person's life. This includes the thoughts and feelings that individuals have about the state of their life, and a person's experience of happiness.

A first comment regarding these definitions of mental health and mental well-being is that it is difficult to say where the one ends and the other begins. Furthermore, although the WHO definition of mental health talks about a state, this is not a very transient or momentary state. Mental health usually is not thought of as fluctuating over the course of a day. The time dimension of mental well-being is less clear. Happiness can be used to describe a very momentary state of affairs or be interpreted more in terms of life satisfaction: satisfaction with one's life when looking back over a longer period of time (Eid and Diener 2004). Linton et al. (2016) seem to focus on the latter, given their use of the term 'state of their life'. Furthermore, both life satisfaction and happiness may be thought of as having both a hedonistic (pleasurable) and a eudaimonic (meaningful/fulfilling) component (Ryan and Deci 2001). In the remainder of this chapter, when we use the term 'mental health', mental well-being is implied.

Yet another definitional issue is where to draw the line between a risk factor and mental health itself. Risk factors may act as mediators, with a high risk of increasing the likelihood of poor mental health or a specific mental disorder. However, if something is not to be considered a risk factor, but a specific form of poor mental health, then it becomes questionable to use it as a mediator at the same time.[1] A case in point is chronic stress. Whereas some authors suggest that chronic stress may cause poor mental (and physical) health (e.g. Marin et al. 2011), others see it as an expression of poor mental health in itself (e.g. Aszatalos et al. 2009).[2]

8.1.3 Linking Biodiversity to Mental Health: Research Questions and Conceptual Model

Methodological choices in doing research depend not only on the definition of the key concepts, but also on the question that the research is intended to answer. In the section on biodiversity, it was stated that biodiversity is predominantly an ecological concept, not evolved from theoretical notions on how contact with nature is thought to positively impact mental health. The section ended suggesting that a relevant first research question might be whether or not nature with a high level of biodiversity can go together with high mental health benefits resulting from contact with that same nature. This issue of compatibility does not yet look into possible causal relationships, whether the one leads to the other or not. However, the question, under which conditions a high level of biodiversity may go together with high mental health benefits, already necessitates insight into which characteristics of nature are important with regard to mental health. Of course, the level of biodiversity present within a certain amount of nature might still be one of those characteristics.

With regard to the level of biodiversity of a natural area actually being an instrumental factor in mental health promotion, it may be that the sheer (sustained) existence of a certain (highly biodiverse) natural area engenders mental health benefits, even though one never visits or otherwise comes in direct contact with it (van den Born et al. 2018). However, most theories focus on pathways requiring some sort of sensory contact with that nature for it to exert its positive influence on mental health (Markevych et al. 2017). Furthermore, more contact is usually assumed to lead to greater benefits, at least up to a certain point (Shanahan et al. 2016). This is likely to have consequences for what one may want to measure. In the remainder of this chapter, we limit ourselves to the latter type of pathways, requiring direct contact.

[1] It still can be used as a predictor of overall mental health, but such an analysis may also be interpreted as showing how important a component it is of overall mental health, more than as a causal factor.

[2] A similar argument can be made with regard to being seriously overweight and having bad physical health.

8.2 Measurement of Biodiversity

The choice of definition, in this case of biodiversity, has implications for (a) how to (objectively) measure the level of biodiversity and, as a consequence, (b) which environments will be considered high, and which ones will be considered low in biodiversity. For example, an arboretum may be considered an area with an extremely high biodiversity per acre, or it may be discarded completely, as not constituting an ecosystem.

8.2.1 Characteristics of Nature in General

It seems fair to say that most of the epidemiological research on nature and human health until now has focussed on access to or availability of nature, and has not paid much attention to its characteristics, including the level of biodiversity (Hartig et al. 2014). Moreover, in such studies nature usually translates to green space, greenery or vegetation, without much consideration for whether or not it may be considered a part of an ecosystem. For example, studies have been conducted looking at the amount of green space, including everything from urban parks to agricultural areas to forests (de Vries et al. 2003), the amount of greenery (Cohen-Cline et al. 2015), that of streetscape greenery (van Dillen et al. 2012) and even the number of street trees per kilometre of road (Taylor et al. 2015). Characterising the nature included in these amounts in meaningful ways with regard to its mental health impact may be considered an important next step in the research agenda (Hartig et al. 2014; Shanahan et al. 2015).

8.2.2 The Object to Be Assessed: The Biodiversity of What?

Another issue is the definition of the area or object of which the biodiversity is to be assessed. In experimental research on nature and human health, this area or object is usually well-defined, for example the biodiversity present in the landscape that is depicted on a screen (Wolf et al. 2017) or that is present in a large aquarium (Cracknell et al. 2016). In intervention studies, the focus is usually on a single green area, such as an urban park. For example, such a study may be about evaluating the impact of the redevelopment of a park or woodland (see e.g. Ward Thompson et al. 2013). In large-scale epidemiological studies, the area of choice is often the residential environment. Note that from an ecological perspective, the area that is assessed may not constitute an ecosystem in itself, but be a part of a larger ecosystem.[3] If so,

[3]This could be linked to the discussion on what constitutes the unit that provides a certain ecosystem service (see Andersson et al. 2015).

it is relevant to take the functional role of the area within that ecosystem into account. For example, the redevelopment of a park may either be beneficial or detrimental to this function.

We will focus on the residential environment for a moment. This environment is defined in very different ways. In some studies it is defined as an administrative unit, such as a census tract or postcode area. In other studies, the residential area is defined as a buffer around the resident's home. In the latter case, the buffer sizes that are used vary considerably, from 100 metres up to 3 km (Egorov et al. 2017; van den Berg et al. 2010). There are no clear rules for the most appropriate definition to use. However, using the boundaries of administrative units may be considered rather arbitrary from the perspective of a citizen's lived experience. A very nearby green area that is located just on the other side of an administrative boundary may be as relevant as a green area within one's own administrative area (which might even be located further away). Furthermore, administrative units may not all have the same size, which may introduce confounds.

As for using buffer sizes, it may be argued that the optimal size depends on the mobility of the population, or the population segment, at hand. For example, when focusing on physical activity during outdoor play without adult supervision by children below the age of 10 years, then in many contexts using a buffer size of 1 km or more does not seem very sensible; parents usually do not allow their young children to play that far away from home on their own. Using a 'wrong' buffer size is likely to lower the strength of associations. If too large, irrelevant natural areas or natural elements are included; if too small, relevant natural areas/elements are ignored.

8.2.3 How to Measure Distance?

With regard to the use of distance in buffer approaches, there is also the issue of whether this should be Euclidean distance or network distance. Accessibility depends more on network distance than on Euclidean distance, since in the latter case barriers may prevent people from travelling in a straight line. However, network distances depend on the mode of transport. The network for travelling by foot may be quite different from that for travelling by car. Stairs, lawns and small alleys may be accessible or crossed by foot, but not by car. Incomplete networks can easily lead to an overestimation of network distance for some people, and in this way introduce a source of error. Nowadays, some researchers also take vertical distance into account (Jim and Chen 2010). A person living on the 20th floor of a high-rise residential building first has to get to the ground level, before getting out of doors (except for balconies and roof gardens, of course). When small buffer sizes are considered appropriate, taking vertical distance into account may make a substantial difference.

8.2.4 Aggregating Biodiversity Across Different Areas

With regard to the level of biodiversity, an additional issue is how to arrive at an aggregated measure for the residential environment as a whole. One way might be to look at the biodiversity of each green area separately, and to calculate an average biodiversity level. This would allow for conclusions such as 'the green areas in this environment are highly biodiverse on average'. Another approach is to assess biodiversity at the level of the residential environment as a whole. That is, to pool all the species from the different green areas in the residential environment (and perhaps include isolated natural elements as well), and base the biodiversity score on the variety in this total pool. This would allow for conclusions such as 'there is a lot of biodiversity in this residential environment'.

Note that in extreme cases the two approaches may lead to quite different rankings of residential environments. A residential area with few urban parks, each with a rather high level of biodiversity in itself, but very similar to each other in species composition, may score high in the first approach. However, in the second approach it may be outscored by a residential environment with a larger number of smaller urban parks that each in themselves are not very biodiverse, but are complementary to each other in species composition. In the latter case there is more variety in the residential environment as a whole, but less variety in each individual park. Note that from an ecological perspective, one might also want to look at the functional links between the different green areas and natural elements that the inventoried area contains or their contribution to the larger ecosystem of which they are a part. In ecological studies, the Shannon Diversity index, which combines number of species and abundance of each species, is sometimes used to indicate functional diversity within a taxonomic group (Krebs 1989).[4]

8.2.5 Type of Access Metric

In the above, we focused on access to nature in terms of the availability or presence of nature within a certain area. Ekkel and de Vries (2017) have termed this a cumulative opportunity access metric, given that it takes all nature within that area into account. They distinguish the cumulative opportunity metric from another type of access metric, based on the distance to the nearest qualifying natural area. 'Qualifying' here refers to the area having at least a certain size and usually being open to the public as well. A minimum level of biodiversity could be added as another criterion in such an approach. A second option is not to use it as an additional criterion, but to look at it as a quality aspect of the otherwise qualifying natural area. The latter is more similar to the way access is handled in the cumulative

[4]Required abundance across taxonomic groups may differ by group, e.g. lower numbers for top predators than for prey animals.

opportunity approach. As for the merits and (implicit) assumptions behind the two types of access metrics, the reader is referred to Ekkel and de Vries (2017).

8.2.6 *Actual Versus Perceived Biodiversity*

Information on the level of biodiversity, in terms of species diversity, is not always readily available. Sometimes data are gathered on perceived biodiversity, as for example in terms of how survey respondents rate the species richness of a specific site, or the number of species present in their residential environment. It is not clear to what extent perceived biodiversity coincides with actual biodiversity, not even if the latter is defined in terms of species richness (see e.g. Fuller et al. 2007 and Dallimer et al. 2012 for contradictory findings).[5] Perceived biodiversity is likely to depend strongly on the visibility of the different species, and on the extent to which they are perceived as being different. For example, biodiversity in the aquatic domain may go largely unnoticed (with the exception of aquaria). The same may be the case for the variety in the insect world, and even more so for that of micro-organisms. On the other hand, the biodiversity as perceived may be more likely to influence mental health than the objectively defined actual biodiversity (Dallimer et al. 2012). To the extent that the two do not coincide, different things are measured.

Furthermore, there is the methodological issue of a potential single-source bias when both biodiversity and mental health information are provided by the same source. Actually, when people rate the level of biodiversity of the same area, and subsequently how this is associated with their mental health is analysed, it is solely the co-variation of individual differences in perception and those in mental health that is studied, and not that of the actual level of biodiversity, which in that case is the same for everyone. A potential solution for the single-source problem is not using perceptions at the individual level, but aggregating the ratings regarding the same object to an average score for that object. A more sophisticated method of aggregating individual level data to characterise an environment is the ecometric approach introduced by Raudenbush and Sampson (1999). In this approach, the number of informants sampled, as well as the intersubjective agreement among informants, is statistically taken into account. This ecometric approach does not seem to have been applied for perceived biodiversity specifically thus far (but see de Jong et al. 2011).

[5] Fuller et al. (2007) provide an example of a study in which objectively assessed and perceived species richness for three categories of species/taxonomic groups are compared. It may be pointed out that they selected rather easy to perceive species: plants, birds and butterflies. Moreover, they aggregated individual perceptions per site. This may have helped them to arrive at the conclusion that greenspace users can more or less accurately perceive species richness. Even so, Dallimer et al. (2012), using the same approach, did not observe a positive association between perceived and actual species richness for any of the three taxonomic groups. See Marselle et al. Chap. 9, this volume.

8.2.7 Access Versus Exposure, and Type of Contact

Earlier in this chapter, it was stated that most theories regarding pathways by which nature affects mental health assume that contact with that nature is required (see e.g. Hartig et al. 2014, on stress and social contact as mediators). Therefore, it is important to make a clear distinction between access to nature and actual contact with nature. According to these theories, only if access to nature leads to exposure to nature, will it be accompanied by mental health benefits. Although in some studies access is equated to exposure, the first is a proxy for the latter at best. Given the focus on biodiversity, exposure should be about the biodiversity with which an individual comes into contact. The level of biodiversity of a natural area might be hypothesised to increase the mental health effect of a visit to that area. It might also be hypothesised to make the area more attractive to visit (initially and subsequently), and thereby increase the frequency and/or duration of visits to that area.

It may be noted that a visit is a specific form of contact. People may also encounter nature, especially small natural elements such as street trees and those present in front gardens, while they are travelling to and from all kinds of destinations. Moreover, they may also have a window view of nature, allowing visual contact with outdoor nature while indoors. And even the latter has been shown to be related to mental health (Honold et al. 2016). It depends on the definition of biodiversity that is used whether or not such contacts should be included in the measure of the amount of biodiversity that a person comes into contact with over a certain period of time.

A focus on exposure implies that not only the residential environment is of interest, but also natural areas and elements that are encountered elsewhere, as in the work or school environment, as well as between such settings of ordinary activity. Nowadays, exposure measurement seems to head in the direction of the exposome: a comprehensive description of lifelong exposure history (Wild 2012; Kondo et al. 2018). The concept of 'exposome' is introduced as the environmental counterpart of the genome. Measuring actual total exposure is not easily achieved. For example, even when looking only at the number of visits to a specific type of nature, such as forests, retrospective self-reports tend to be rather inaccurate (Jensen 1999), though this presumably depends on the time frame for recall. To complicate matters further, the type of contact itself, ranging from indirect contact (e.g. looking at a nature documentary or looking at actual nature through a window), to being in a natural environment and actually interacting with nature (e.g. gardening or picking berries), may also have consequences for its mental health effects (Keniger et al. 2013).

8.2.8 Mediators, Confounders and Covariates

The level of biodiversity, in terms of species diversity, may go hand in hand with that of other characteristics of a natural area, such as its perceived naturalness. From studies on landscape appreciation it is well known that the perceived naturalness of an area tends to have a positive impact on its scenic beauty (Gobster et al. 2007), and therefore may be a relevant concept in itself. Although perceived naturalness is not a very well-defined concept, it is almost by definition negatively affected by the presence of buildings and other human artefacts, while this presence does not necessarily lower the level of biodiversity of an area. Also, a park may seem highly natural to a lay person, while it is completely artificial from an ecological perspective. Thus, although the two concepts are likely to be correlated, they are definitely not the same. This brings up the following question: if, whether by observation or experimentation, the level of biodiversity has been shown to be associated with mental health, is it really the level of biodiversity that is instrumental in these associations, either directly or indirectly, by way of its effect on perceived naturalness? Or does the level of biodiversity tend to co-vary with perceived naturalness, without actually influencing it? In other words, is perceived naturalness to be considered a mediator, or a confounder, when researching the effect of the level of biodiversity on mental health?

Besides perceived naturalness, there are other characteristics that might be considered, for example visual complexity in terms of the richness and diversity of elements in the landscape, including their shapes, and how these are arranged in space (Ode et al. 2010; see also Marselle, Chap. 7, this volume). This is also not the same as, but likely to co-vary with, the level of biodiversity, while at the same time it may be relevant for mental health in itself. Similar conceptual questions can be asked as those for perceived naturalness. Moreover, a specific causal path may involve more than one mediator, complicating matters further (Dzhambov et al. 2018).

Especially in epidemiological research, there are also confounders that are less directly linked to the level of biodiversity, but are likely to co-vary with it in real-life situations, even more so when it comes to availability and access. These are to a large extent the same variables that are also important covariates in research on the amount of nature, rather than on its variety in terms of the number of species. For example, one could think of noise level, air quality, socio-economic position and population density. In research focusing on biodiversity, it should be noted that an additional covariate is the amount of nature: one would like to make sure that the variety makes an independent contribution, and it is not solely the amount of nature that is present, or the size of the nature area, that drives the association or the effect.

8.3 Concluding Remarks

In this chapter, we focused on definitional and measurement issues with regard to access to and contact with nature, more specifically the biodiversity of that nature. We stated that biodiversity is originally an ecological concept, developed in the context of nature conservation. As we have illustrated, the concept has been adapted ('tweaked') to make it more relevant in the context of mental health. To begin with, frequently its functional aspect with regard to the sustainability and resilience of ecosystems is ignored. In addition to this, in several studies the measurement of biodiversity is limited to the parts that are perceivable and/or appreciated by lay persons. At the same time, such adaptations are likely to make the concept less relevant from a nature conservation perspective. So, much depends on the research question at hand.

We envision two lines of research. The first line has its focus on mental health promotion. In this line of research it makes perfect sense to look for qualities of nature that are likely to be conducive to produce (more or greater) mental health benefits. The concept of biodiversity may be adapted at will (preferably though based on theoretical arguments), but confusion may be reduced by (a) making clear that the concept has been adapted and (b) consistently labelling it differently (e.g. perceived species richness rather than biodiversity, without equating the both). The second line of research is about whether or which ecologically sound systems, requiring a certain amount of functional biodiversity, may go together with mental health promotion. Within this second line of research, focusing on multi-functional land use, adapting the concept of biodiversity seems less fruitful. To evaluate whether nature conservation and mental health promotion by contact with nature go well together, the success of each function, ecological and human health, needs to be assessed according to its own criteria.

Up till now, the first line of research seems to be more popular. That is, while there is a broad array of studies that refer to biodiversity and (mental) health, few of these studies address biodiversity in its ecological sense of functional species diversity. In fact, Dean et al. (2011) identified only one study, that of Fuller et al. (2007). We agree that the latter study provides one of the best examples of a rigorous measurement of species richness in the context of 'biodiversity – mental health' research. At the same time, even this study does not seem to put species richness in the context of the functional species diversity that is needed for a healthy ecosystem. The same argument can be made for the additional studies addressing species richness in the context of biodiversity and health that have been identified in more recent reviews (Lovell et al. 2014; Korpela et al. 2018; Marselle et al. Chap. 9, this volume). Also, in ecological science, where it is more likely that a stricter definition of biodiversity is adhered to, the compatibility of ecosystem health and human health also does not seem to be high on the agenda. Von Döhren and Haase (2015) conclude that in ecosystem services research possible negative effects, or ecosystem disservices, are an understudied subject.[6] Despite it not being a popular line of research, we strongly feel that research focusing on the combination of healthy ecosystems that help people keep mentally healthy is also worthwhile pursuing, not only from a nature conservation perspective (Bugter et al. 2018), but also from a long-term mental health, as well as an urban planning, perspective (Tzoulas et al. 2007).

References

Andersson E, McPhearson T, Kremer P et al (2015) Scale and context dependence of ecosystem service providing units. Ecosyst Serv 12:157–164

Angermeier P (1994) Does biodiversity include artificial diversity ? Conserv Biol 8(2):600–602

Aszatalos M, Wijndaele K, De Bourdeaudhuij I et al (2009) Specific associations between types of physical activity and components of mental health. J Sci Med Sport 12(4):468–474

Bugter R, Harrison P, Haslett J, Tinch R (2018) Making a better case for biodiversity conservation: the BESAFE project. Biodivers Conserv 27(7):1549–1560

CBD (1992) Convention on biological diversity. United Nations

Cohen-Cline H, Turkheimer E, Duncan GE (2015) Access to green space, physical activity and mental health: a twin study. J Epidemiol Community Health 69(6):523–529

Costanza R (2012) Ecosystem health and ecological engineering. Ecol Eng 45:24–29

Cracknell D, White MP, Pahl S, Nichols WJ, Depledge MH (2016) Marine biota and psychological well-being: a preliminary examination of dose–response effects in an aquarium setting. Environ Behav 48(10):1242–1269

Dallimer M, Irvine KN, Skinner AM et al (2012) Biodiversity and the feel-good factor: understanding associations between self-reported human well-being and species richness. Bioscience 62(1):47–55

de Jong K, Albin M, Skärbäck E et al (2011) Area-aggregated assessments of perceived environmental attributes may overcome single-source bias in studies of green environments and health: results from a cross-sectional survey in southern Sweden. Environ Health 10. https://doi.org/10.1186/1476-069X-10-4

de Vries S, Verheij RA, Groenewegen PP, Spreeuwenberg P (2003) Natural environments-healthy environments? An exploratory analysis of the relationship between greenspace and health. Env Plan A 35(10):1717–1731

Dean J, van Dooren K, Weinstein P (2011) Does biodiversity improve mental health in urban settings? Med Hypotheses 76(6):877–880

Dzhambov A, Hartig T, Markevych I, Tilov B, Dimitrova D (2018) Urban residential greenspace and mental health in youth: different approaches to testing multiple pathways yield different conclusions. Environ Res 160:47–59

Egorov AI, Griffin SM, Converse RR et al (2017) Vegetated land cover near residence is associated with reduced allostatic load and improved biomarkers of neuroendocrine, metabolic and immune functions. Environ Res 158:508–521

Eid M, Diener E (2004) Global judgments of subjective well-being: situational variability and long-term stability. Soc Indic Res 65(3):245–277

Ekkel ED, de Vries S (2017) Nearby green space and human health: evaluating accessibility metrics. Landsc Urban Plan 157:214–220

[6]This in contrast to the traditional focus of the environmental epidemiological branch of public health research, which focuses on the hazards that the environment may contain (Frumkin 2001).

Frumkin H (2001) Beyond toxicity 11. The full text of this article is available via AJPM Online at www.elsevier.com/locate/ajpmonline. Am J Prev Med 20(3):234–240

Fuller RA, Irvine KN, Devine-Wright P, Warren PH, Gaston KJ (2007) Psychological benefits of greenspace increase with biodiversity. Biol Lett 3(4):390–394

Gobster PH, Nassauer JI, Daniel TC, Fry G (2007) The shared landscape: what does aesthetics have to do with ecology? Landsc Ecol 22(7):959–972

Hartig T, Mitchell R, de Vries S, Frumkin H (2014) Nature and health. Annu Rev Public Health 35(1):207–228

Honold J, Lakes T, Beyer R, van der Meer E (2016) Restoration in urban spaces: nature views from home, greenways, and public parks. Environ Behav 48(6):796–825

Jensen FS (1999) Forest recreation in Denmark from the 1970s to the 1990s. Danish Forest and Landscape Research Institute, Hørsholm

Jim CY, Chen WY (2010) External effects of neighbourhood parks and landscape elements on high-rise residential value. Land Use Policy 27(2):662–670

Kaphengst T, Davis M, Gerstetter C et al (2014) Quality of life, wellbeing and biodiversity. Ecologic Institute, Berlin

Keniger LE, Gaston KJ, Irvine KN, Fuller RA (2013) What are the benefits of interacting with nature? Int J Environ Res Public Health 10(3):913–935

Kondo MC, Fluehr JM, McKeon T, Branas CC (2018) Urban green space and its impact on human health. Int J Environ Res Public Health 15. https://doi.org/10.3390/ijerph15030445

Korpela K, Pasanen T, Ratcliffe E (2018) Biodiversity and psychological well-being. In: Ossola A, Niemelä J (eds) Urban biodiversity. Routledge in association with GSE Research, pp 134–149

Krebs C (1989) Ecological methodology. HarperCollins, New York

Linton M, Dieppe P, Medina-Lara A (2016) Review of 99 self-report measures for assessing well-being in adults: exploring dimensions of well-being and developments over time. BMJ Open 6(7):e010641. https://doi.org/10.1136/bmjopen-2015-010641

Lovell R, Wheeler BW, Higgins SL, Irvine KN, Depledge MH (2014) A systematic review of the health and Well-being benefits of biodiverse environments. Journal of Toxicology and Environmental Health, Part B 17(1):1–20

Marin M-F, Lord C, Andrews J et al (2011) Chronic stress, cognitive functioning and mental health. Neurobiol Learn Mem 96(4):583–595

Markevych I, Schoierer J, Hartig T et al (2017) Exploring pathways linking greenspace to health: theoretical and methodological guidance. Environ Res 158:301–317. https://doi.org/10.1016/j.envres.2017.06.028

Ode Å, Hagerhall CM, Sang N (2010) Analysing visual landscape complexity: theory and application. Landsc Res 35(1):111–131

Raudenbush SW, Sampson RJ (1999) Ecometrics: toward a science of assessing ecological settings, with application to the systematic social observation of neighborhoods. Sociol Methodol 29(1):1–41

Ryan RM, Deci EL (2001) On happiness and human potentials: a review of research on hedonic and eudaimonic well-being. Annu Rev Psychol 52(1):141–166

Shanahan DF, Lin BB, Bush R et al (2015) Toward improved public health outcomes from urban nature. Am J Public Health 105(3):470–477

Shanahan DF, Bush R, Gaston KJ et al (2016) Health benefits from nature experiences depend on dose. Sci Rep 6. https://doi.org/10.1038/srep28551

Taylor MS, Wheeler BW, White MP, Economou T, Osborne NJ (2015) Research note: urban street tree density and antidepressant prescription rates—a cross-sectional study in London, UK. Landsc Urban Plan 136:174–179

Tzoulas K, Korpela K, Venn S et al (2007) Promoting ecosystem and human health in urban areas using Green Infrastructure: a literature review. Landsc Urban Plan 81(3):167–178

van den Berg AE, Maas J, Verheij RA, Groenewegen PP (2010) Green space as a buffer between stressful life events and health. Soc Sci Med 70(8):1203–1210

van den Born RJ, Arts B, Admiraal J et al (2018) The missing pillar: eudemonic values in the justification of nature conservation. J Environ Plan Manag 61(5–6):841–856 van Dillen SME, de Vries S, Groenewegen PP, Spreeuwenberg P (2012) Greenspace in urban neighbourhoods and residents' health: adding quality to quantity. J Epidemiol Community Health 66(6):e8–e8

von Döhren P, Haase D (2015) Ecosystem disservices research: a review of the state of the art with a focus on cities. Ecol Indic 52:490–497

Wall B, Derham J, O'Mahoney T (2016) Ireland's environment 2016; an assessment. Environmental Protection Agency, Ireland

Ward Thompson C, Roe J, Aspinall P (2013) Woodland improvements in deprived urban communities: what impact do they have on people's activities and quality of life? Landsc Urban Plan 118:79–89

Wild CP (2012) The exposome: from concept to utility. Int J Epidemiol 41(1):24–32

Wolf LJ, zu Ermgassen S, Balmford A, White M, Weinstein N (2017) Is variety the spice of life? An experimental investigation into the effects of species richness on self-reported mental well-being. PLoS One 12:e0170225. https://doi.org/10.1371/journal.pone.0170225

Wossink A, van Wenum J, Jurgens C, de Snoo G (1997) The what, how and where of nature conservation and agriculture: the co-ordination of ecological-economic, behaviourial and spatial aspects. In: Abstracts of the VIIIth Annual conference of the European Association of Environmental and Resource Economists (EAERE). Tilburg University, Tilburg

Chapter 9
Review of the Mental Health and Well-being Benefits of Biodiversity

Melissa R. Marselle, Dörte Martens, Martin Dallimer, and Katherine N. Irvine

Abstract Little is known about the contribution that biodiversity has on mental health and well-being. To date, only one systematic review has investigated the health and well-being benefits from contact with biodiversity (Lovell et al. J Toxicol Environ Health B Crit Rev 17(1):1–20, 2014). The number of research studies investigating the health and well-being effects of biodiversity has increased since this publication. Here, we provide an update, focusing on the impact of biodiversity on mental health and well-being. Our objectives are to: (i) identify and describe the literature published after 2012; and (ii) synthesise all results from Lovell et al. (J Toxicol Environ Health B Crit Rev 17(1):1–20, 2014) and the more recently published literature to assess whether biodiversity influences mental health and well-being. Sixteen recently published studies met the inclusion criteria. The literature is varied with different study designs, measures of biodiversity, mental health and well-being. The synthesis of results was drawn from 24 studies: nine from Lovell et al. (J Toxicol Environ Health B Crit Rev 17(1):1–20, 2014) and 15 identified by this chapter. There is some evidence to suggest that biodiversity promotes better

M. R. Marselle (✉)
Department of Ecosystem Services, Helmholtz Centre for Environmental Research – UFZ, Leipzig, Germany

German Centre for Integrative Biodiversity Research (iDiv) Halle-Jena-Leipzig, Leipzig, Germany
e-mail: melissa.marselle@ufz.de

D. Martens
Eberswalde University for Sustainable Development, Eberswalde, Germany
e-mail: d.martens@hnee.de

M. Dallimer
Sustainability Research Institute, School of Earth and Environment, University of Leeds, Leeds, UK
e-mail: m.dallimer@leeds.ac.uk

K. N. Irvine
Social, Economic and Geographical Sciences Research Group, The James Hutton Institute, Aberdeen, Scotland, UK
e-mail: katherine.irvine@hutton.ac.uk

M. R. Marselle et al. (eds.), *Biodiversity and Health in the Face of Climate Change*, https://doi.org/10.1007/978-3-030-02318-8_9

mental health and well-being. However, more studies reported non-significant results. The evidence is not yet of the extent necessary to characterise the role of biodiversity in relation to mental health or well-being. Future interdisciplinary research directions are discussed.

Keywords Mental health · Mental well-being · Biodiversity · Species richness · Synthesis · Review

Highlights

- Research into the health and well-being effects of biodiversity has grown since Lovell et al. (2014).
- We update Lovell et al. (2014) and focus on the impact of biodiversity on mental health and well-being.
- 16 recently published studies on biodiversity and mental health and well-being were identified.
- Synthesis of results found some evidence that biodiversity promotes better mental health and well-being.
- Overall, more studies reported non-significant effects.

9.1 Introduction

Contact with natural environments facilitates diverse health and well-being benefits (Bowler et al. 2010; Frumkin 2001; Hartig et al. 2014; Irvine and Warber 2002; Keniger et al. 2013). However, in this body of research the natural environment is often "treated as uniform" (Dallimer et al. 2012, p. 48), as studies commonly compare broad urban and natural environment categories (e.g. Hartig et al. 2003; Korpela et al. 2016) or analyse the amount of, or proximity to, green space (e.g. Groenewegen et al. 2012; Triguero-Mas et al. 2015). Whilst a substantial amount of literature investigates the impact of nature or green space on health and well-being, little is known about the contribution that different qualities of the natural environment, such as biodiversity, have on mental health and well-being.

Systematic reviews of the mental health or well-being benefits from contact with nature do not include studies that assess the biodiversity of the natural environment (e.g. Bowler et al. 2010; Dadvand et al. 2015; Thompson Coon et al. 2011). This same body of literature on the mental health or well-being effects of nature is also present in systematic reviews of the health benefits of biodiversity (e.g. Horwitz and Kretsch 2015; Hough 2014; Whitmee et al. 2015), resulting in a closed loop of examined literature. To date, only one systematic review has explicitly investigated the health and well-being benefits from contact with biodiversity (Lovell et al. 2014). While the authors found some evidence for a positive benefit from exposure to biodiversity, overall, the synthesis of 15 quantitative studies showed no clear pattern of results for the effects of biodiversity on human health and well-being.

Since the publication of Lovell et al. (2014), interest has grown in the potential contribution of biodiverse environments for health and well-being. Growth in this field is shown clearly by the increase in the number of related scientific publications. For example, a search in the Web of Science on just one term, 'biodiversity and health', yielded 0 hits for 1980–1989, 3 hits for 1990–1999, 2 hits for 2000–2009, 6 hits for 2010–2013, and 16 hits from 2014–2018. This coincides with increased interest from governments and international organisations on the mental health and well-being effects of biodiversity (Convention on Biological Diversity 2017a, b; EKLIPSE 2017; WBGU – German Advisory Council on Global Change 2016; World Health Organisation & Secretariat of the Convention on Biological Diversity 2015). Given this research expansion and increased interest, in this chapter we update the literature reviewed by Lovell et al. (2014). In particular, we focus on the relationships between biodiversity and mental health and mental well-being, as such an analysis has yet to be conducted. Box 9.1 details these definitions.

The aim of this chapter is to identify, summarise and synthesise research on the impact of biodiversity on mental health and well-being. There are two objectives:

1. Describe the state and nature of the body of evidence, published since the review by Lovell et al. (2014), relating biodiversity to mental health and well-being;
2. Provide a synthesis of results from Lovell et al. (2014) and the more recently published literature to assess whether biodiversity influences mental health and well-being.

Box 9.1: Definitions of Biodiversity, Health, Mental Health and Mental Well-being

- *Biodiversity* is "the variability among living organisms from all sources including, *inter alia*, terrestrial, marine and other aquatic ecosystems and the ecological complexes of which they are part; this includes diversity within species, between species and of ecosystems" (United Nations Convention on Biological Diversity 1992, p. 3).
- *Health* is "a state of complete physical, mental and social well-being and not merely the absence of disease or infirmity" (World Health Organization 1946).
- *Mental health* "a state of well-being in which an individual realises his or her own abilities, can cope with the normal stresses of life, can work productively and is able to make a contribution to his or her community" (World Health Organization 2016).
- *Mental well-being* is "the psychological, cognitive and emotional quality of a person's life. This includes the thoughts and feelings that individuals have about the state of their life, and a person's experience of happiness" (Linton et al. 2016, p. 12).

9.2 Methods

9.2.1 *Literature Review*

A systematic search strategy was used to identify published, peer-reviewed studies that specifically examined relationships between biodiversity and mental health or mental well-being outcomes. The literature search was conducted in October 2017, following a replicable procedure (Koricheva et al. 2013). Inclusion criteria (Box 9.2) was identical to those used by Lovell et al. (2014), except with a focus on literature published (i) between 2013 and September 2017, and (ii) in any language. Thus, we are building on, rather than replicating, the review by Lovell et al. (2014).

Literature was identified through structured searches of the Web of Science, which identified 189 articles (see the Appendix for the search terms). One reviewer [MM] initially screened titles and abstracts, with a second reviewer [DM] applying the inclusion criteria to articles that needed a second opinion. Nineteen articles were identified as eligible for full text review (see Fig. 9.1). Backward and forward reference searches (Cǒté et al. 2013) were conducted on these 19 articles. The resulting 1610 articles were first screened by year and title for eligibility, then abstracts were read. This method identified an additional four articles, all from forward citations. Backward and forward reference searches of these four articles resulted in an additional 242 references, which underwent a similar screening process. No new articles were identified. Twenty-three articles underwent full text screening (by MM and

Box 9.2: Study Inclusion Criteria (Adapted from Lovell et al. 2014)

1. Any peer-reviewed study, published between January 2013 and September 2017
2. Any recognised and reliable study design, with any population group, from any country and in any language
3. An explicit consideration of biodiversity, species richness and/or a setting protected because of its biodiversity, and
4. An explicit consideration of either a primary health-related outcome including any self-reported or objective measure of mental health or mental well-being, or a secondary health-related outcome including self-report or objective measures of physical activity or self-report social cohesion.

Exclusion criteria: Studies were excluded if they did not assess (i) biodiversity and (ii) mental health, mental well-being, physical activity and social cohesion related outcome measures. Studies assessing preferences, physiological outcomes, use/visitation, the amount of green space without specification of its biodiversity, or physical activity without identification of where it occurred were excluded. Studies not reporting primary research (e.g. review papers) were also excluded.

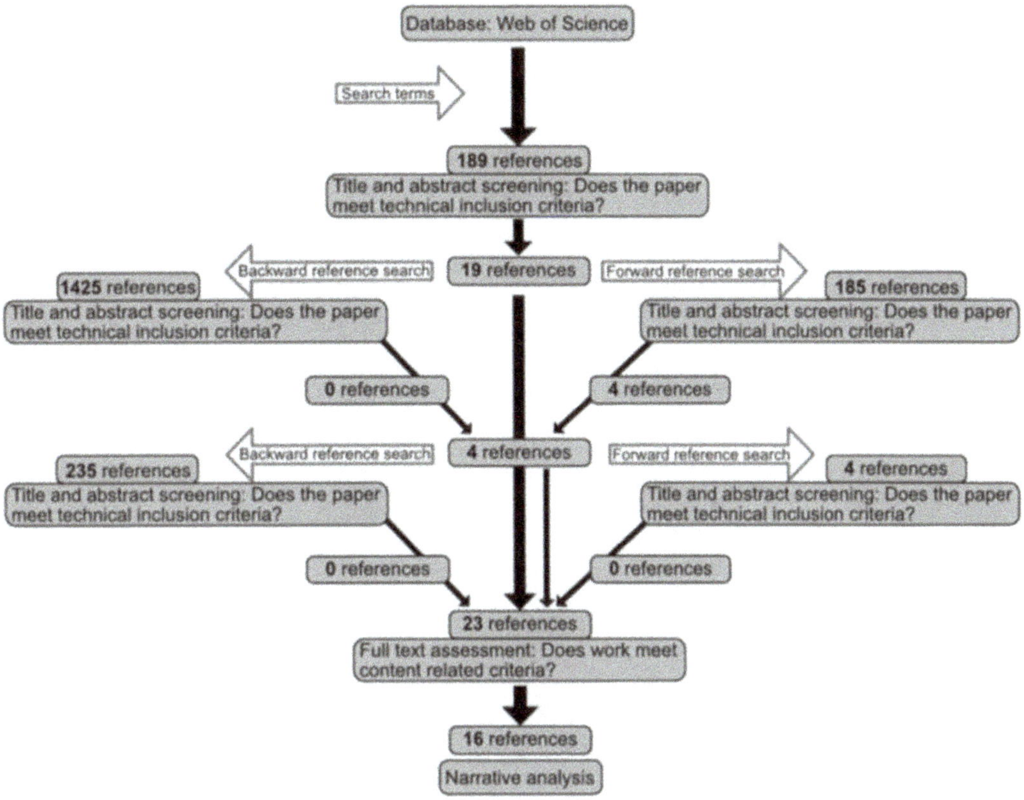

Fig. 9.1 Process of literature review and identified relevant articles

DM); seven were excluded primarily because they did not assess biodiversity, mental health, mental well-being, physical activity or social cohesion. In total, 16 articles were identified (see Table 9.1).

9.2.2 Characteristics of the Recent Literature

To describe the recently published literature on biodiversity and mental health and well-being, a standardised data extraction form was used to record relevant information from the 16 studies: country of origin, participants, theoretical position, biodiversity indicators, outcome measures, contact with biodiverse environment, moderators, mediators and results.

Biodiversity indicators were classified on the basis of biodiversity levels identified by Botzat et al. (2016) – namely, ecosystems/habitats (e.g. parks, forests); species communities (e.g. plants, birds, butterflies); or single species. Within the species community level, both species richness (e.g. the number of different bird species) and abundance of a specific taxonomic group irrespective of species (e.g. the number of all birds) were identified. Both variables have been shown to have differential effects (Hedblom et al. 2017). Abundance may be more important to mental health or mental well-being than the number of different species (Dallimer et al. 2012).

Table 9.1 Study characteristics of the 24 studies assessing biodiversity and mental health and well-being (9 studies identified from 1980 to 2012 (Lovell et al. 2014) and 16 studies identified from 2013 to September 2017 in this chapter)

Reference	Objectives	Biodiversity indicator	Contact with nature[a]	Health outcome (measure[b])	Population	General result
Experimental studies						
Jorgensen et al. (2010)[c]	Explored the impact of complexity of the environment on psychological restoration	Naturalness, biodiversity and structural complexity of 3 green spaces	Indirect, viewing videos	Self-report mood (Profile of Mood States)	UK, students from a single university, 47% female, *M* age = 22 (range 17–40), $n = 102$	No relationship – No difference in mood between 3 green spaces.
Wolf et al. (2017)	Explored the impact of species richness on mental health and well-being	Study 1: tree species richness (high, low)	Indirect, viewing videos	Self-report positive affect (PANAS); vitality (Subjective Vitality Scale); and anxiety (State Trait Anxiety Inventory)	Study 1: USA, 42% female, *M* age = 36 (range 18 and over), $n = 140$	Study 1: Positive – Reduced levels of anxiety in high tree species richness condition compared to low condition. Marginal difference between conditions on positive affect.
						Study 1: No relationship – No difference between high and low tree species richness conditions on vitality.
		Study 2: bird species richness (high, low)			Study 2: USA, 52% female, *M* age = 35 (range 18 and over), $n = 264$	Study 2: Positive – Enhanced levels of positive affect, and reduced anxiety in high bird species richness condition compared to low condition.
						Study 2: No relationship – No difference between high and low bird species richness conditions on vitality.

Quasi-experimental studies						
Cracknell et al. (2017), Study 2 only	Explored the effect of biodiversity of aquarium exhibit on affect	Species richness of marine fauna (high, low); abundance (high, low) of fish/crustaceans	Indirect, viewing photographs	Self-report happiness	UK, students from a single university, 67.5% female, *M* age = 20.8 (range 18–35), *n* = 40	Positive – Higher levels of happiness in high abundance, compared to low abundance condition, when species richness held constant.
						No relationship – No difference in high or low species richness conditions on happiness, when abundance is held constant.
Johansson et al. (2014)	Explored effect of different levels of biodiversity in forest biotopes on affect	Categorised 3 broad-leaf forest biotopes based on vegetation layer, species composition and vegetation type (high, medium, low)	Indirect, viewing photographs	Self-report affect (Basic Emotional Process)	Sweden, staff from a single university and their family and friends, 51% female, *M* age = 46; *n* = 35	Positive – Affect was greatest in the medium biotope, followed by the high and then the low biotopes.
White et al. (2017), Study A only	Explored the effect of perceived biodiversity on mental well-being	Perceived biodiversity (high, medium, low)	Indirect, viewing photographs	Self-report mood (valence, Feelings Scale); arousal (Felt Arousal Scale), and recovery	UK, 51% female, age range 18–80 (no mean given) *n* = 1,478	Positive – Greater perceived biodiversity associated with increase in positive valence, arousal and recovery.
Natural experiment						
Cracknell et al. (2016), Study 2 only	Explored the effect of restocking an aquarium with marine biota on affect	Species richness of fish/crustaceans (low, high)	Indirect, viewing nature in an aquarium	Self-report mood (valence, Feeling Scale; and arousal (Felt Arousal Scale)	UK, students from a single university, 76% female, *M* age = 24, *n* = 84	No relationship – No difference in mood between low and high biodiversity conditions.

(continued)

Table 9.1 (continued)

Reference	Objectives	Biodiversity indicator	Contact with nature[a]	Health outcome (measure[b])	Population	General result
Jones (2017)	Explored the impact of an invasive species on mental health and well-being	Presence of the invasive species Emerald ash borer (EAB) (*Agrilus planipennis*), which is responsible for the loss of North American ash trees (*Fraxinus* spp.)	Unspecified, assessments of EAB infestations in US counties	Self-report depression (single item from PHQ-12) and life satisfaction	USA, people who live in 189 counties with detected EAB infestations in 15 states, 61% female, M age = 53, n = 481,405	Positive – Biodiversity loss of ash trees, 5-years after EAB detection, associated with less life satisfaction and more depressive symptoms.
Longitudinal (cohort) studies						
Annerstedt et al. (2012)[c]	Explored the impact of the presence of environmental qualities on mental health over a 5-year period	Scania Green Score 'lush, rich in species': Perceived environmental dimensions identified using CORINE land cover data.	Unspecified, assessed diversity 300 m from participants' home	Self-report mental health (GHQ-12)	Sweden, Residents of rural and suburban areas who did not move house, gender % not given, M age women = 50, n = 7,549	No relationship – No effect of living in an environment that is 'rich in species' on mental health.
Annerstedt van den Bosch et al. (2015)	Explored if changes in neighbourhood nature, as an effect of moving home, are related to mental health	Scania Green Score 'lush, rich in species': Perceived environmental dimensions identified using CORINE land cover data.	Unspecified, assessed diversity 300 m from participants' home	Self-report mental health (GHQ-12)	Sweden, Residents of rural and suburban areas who moved house, 58% female, M age = 48, n = 1,419	No relationship – Moving to an environment that is more 'rich in species' had no effect on mental health.
Repeated measures studies						
Marselle et al. (2016)	Explored indirect effect of perceived biodiversity on affect through perceived restorativeness	Perceived species richness of: plants/trees; birds; and butterflies	Direct, walks outdoors	Self-report affect (PANAS) and happiness	UK, English residents who participate in group walks, 55% female, age range 55 and over (no mean given), n = 127	Positive – Perceived bird biodiversity indirectly influences affect and happiness via perceived restorativeness. No relationship – No indirect effect of perceived plants/trees and butterflies species richness on affect or happiness via perceived restorativeness.

Marselle et al. (2015)	Explored the direct effect of perceived biodiversity on affect	Perceived species richness of: plants/trees; birds; and butterflies	Direct, walks outdoors	Self-report affect (PANAS) and happiness	UK, English residents who participate in group walks, 55% female, age range 55 and over (no mean given), $n = 127$	No relationship – No association of perceived biodiversity on positive affect or happiness.
						Negative – Small increase in perceived bird species richness was related to more negative emotions.
Cross-sectional studies						
Bjork et al. (2008)[c]	Explored the impact of the presence of preferred environmental dimensions in promoting health and well-being	Scania Green Score 'lush, rich in species': Perceived environmental dimensions identified using CORINE land cover data.	Unspecified, assessed diversity 100 and 300 m from participants' home	Self-report physical and psychological health; and vitality (SF36)	Sweden, Residents of rural and suburban areas, 54% female, *M* age 50 (range 19–76), $n = 24,819$	No relationship – No effect of living near to a 'lush, rich in species' environment on health or vitality.
Carrus et al. (2015)	Explored the direct effect of level of biodiversity on physical and mental well-being, and indirect effect through perceived restorativeness	Categorised 4 green spaces based on structural complexity (low, high)	Direct, in-situ assessments of 4 green spaces	Self-report physical and mental well-being (composite measure)	Italy, users of green space, 52% female, *M* age = 41, $n = 568$	Positive – Greater physical and mental well-being in high biodiversity condition, compared to low condition.
						Positive – Indirect effect of biodiversity on physical and mental well-being via perceived restorativeness.
Cox et al. (2017)	Explored the association between neighbourhood nature and mental health	Bird abundance in the morning and afternoon; bird species richness in the morning and afternoon.	Unspecified, biodiversity assessed 250 m from centre of participants' postcode	Self-report mental health (Depression; Anxiety; Stress, DASS 21).	UK, residents in 3 towns in southern England, 56% female, age range 18 and over (no mean given), $n = 263$	Positive – Greater afternoon bird abundance associated with less depression, anxiety and stress.
						No relationship – No effect of morning bird abundance, and morning and afternoon bird species richness on mental health.

(continued)

Table 9.1 (continued)

Reference	Objectives	Biodiversity indicator	Contact with nature[a]	Health outcome (measure[b])	Population	General result
Dallimer et al. (2012)[c]	Explored the role of species richness in riverine environments in promoting psychological well-being	Species richness of: birds; butterflies; and plant/trees; bird abundance; Shannon Diversity Index of habitat types; tree cover; perceived species richness of: birds, butterflies and plant/trees	Direct, in-situ assessments of 34 green spaces	Self-report psychological well-being (reflection; continuity with the past; and attachment subscales)	UK, users of green space, 38% female, age range 16–70 (no mean given), $n = 1{,}108$	Positive – Greater bird abundance and bird species richness, tree cover, and perceived species richness of birds, butterflies and plants/trees positively associated with psychological well-being.
						Negative – Psychological well-being declined with greater plant species richness.
						No relationship – Butterfly biodiversity and Shannon Diversity Index had no effect on psychological well-being.
De Jong et al. (2012)[c]	Explored associations between environmental dimensions and general health	Scania Green Score 'lush, rich in species': Perceived environmental dimensions. CORINE land cover data.	Unspecified, assessed diversity 300 m from participants' home	Self-report general health (physical and mental health)	Sweden, Residents of rural and suburban areas, 55% female, age range 18–80 (no mean given), $n = 24{,}847$	No relationship – No effect of living near to a 'lush, rich in species' environment on health, after adjusting for covariates.
Duarte-Tagles et al. (2015)	Explored the association between biodiversity indicators and prevalence of depressive symptoms	Margalef Diversity index of eco-regions	Unspecified, biodiversity assessed at state level	Self-report mental health (based on DSM-IV criteria for depression)	Mexico, residents in all states, 78.7% female, M age 40.5 (range 20–65), $n = 4{,}777$	No relationship – More ecoregions in the state lowers the risk of depression. However, no effect when accounting for hierarchical quality of data.

Foo (2016)	Explored the mediating pathways between environment with different levels of naturalness and well-being	Three forests that vary on their species richness (low, medium, high)	Direct, *in situ* assessments of 3 forest environments	Self-report well-being; and mental health	Malaysia, Users of green space. No gender or age given, $n = 350$	No relationship – All three levels of forest diversity had a similar influence on well-being and mental health, but mediating pathways differed.
Fuller et al. (2007)[c]	Explored the effect of species richness in urban green space to psychological well-being	Species richness of: birds; butterflies; and plants; number of habitat types; and tree cover	Direct, in-situ assessments of 15 green spaces	Self-report psychological well-being (reflection; distinct identity; continuity with the past; and attachment subscales)	UK, users of green space, no gender or age given, $n = 312$	Positive – Greater bird and plant species richness, and number of habitat types positively associated with psychological well-being.
						No relationship – Butterfly species richness and tree cover were not associated with psychological well-being.
Grahn & Stigsdotter (2010)[c]	Attempted to identify the dimensions of nature people prefer and use for stress relief	Perceived environmental dimensions: 'rich in species' (precursor to Scania green score)	Not applicable	Self-report level of stress	Sweden, residents in central and southern urban areas, no gender or age given, $n = 733$	No relationship – Environments 'rich in species' not significantly correlated with stress level.
Huby et al. (2006)[c]	Explored the integration of natural and social sciences data to understand relationships between environment and society	Bird species richness	Unspecified, Lower Super Output Areas (LSOA)	Mental health deprivation indicator of English Indices of Deprivation	England, residents of rural areas, no gender, age or *n* given	Positive – Greater bird species richness associated with mental health.

(continued)

Table 9.1 (continued)

Reference	Objectives	Biodiversity indicator	Contact with nature[a]	Health outcome (measure[b])	Population	General result
Luck et al. (2011)[c]	Examined the relationships between biodiversity and residents' personal well-being, neighbourhood well-being, and connection to nature	Bird species richness; abundance of birds; amount of vegetation cover; and vegetation density	Unspecified, assessed diversity in the neighbourhood	Self-report life satisfaction	Australia, residents of New South Wales and Victoria, no gender or age given, n = 1,078	Positive – Life satisfaction positively associated with greater bird species richness and abundance and vegetation cover and density.
Rantakokko et al. (2018)	Explored the association between neighbourhood nature diversity and mental health and well-being	Shannon Diversity Index of land use types	Unspecified, assessed diversity 500 m from participants' home.	Self-report mental well-being (WHO QoL) and mental health (depression, CES-D)	Central Finland, older people, 62% female, M age = 80.6 (range 75–90), n = 848	Positive – Greater Shannon Diversity of land use types associated with greater quality of life. No relationship – No effect of Shannon Diversity of land use types on depressive symptoms.
Saw et al. (2015)	Explored the effect of access to different types of green space on well-being	Nature reserves (legally protected sites for wildlife, flora and fauna)	Indirect, access to nature reserves within 1.2 km from participants' home	Self-report mental well-being (composite measure of PANAS and Satisfaction with Life scale)	Singapore, students from a single university, 68% female, age range 18–35 (no mean given), n = 426	No relationship – Access to nature reserves had no relationship with mental well-being.

Wheeler et al. (2015)	Explored the association between type and quality of different natural environments and health	Shannon Diversity Index of land cover types; and bird species richness	Unspecified, biodiversity assessed at Lower Super Output Areas (LSOA)	Self-reported general health	UK, Residents of England aggregated at LSOA, no gender, age or *n* given	Positive – Greater Shannon Diversity of land cover associated with good health, and inverse associations with bad health. Bird species richness positive association with good health only.

Note. Biodiversity variables with a slash ('/') are a combined variable where investigator did not separate out the contribution of each taxon; two taxa are analysed together

[a]'Direct' and 'indirect' contact with nature categories based on Keniger et al. (2013)

[b]Measures are listed only when reported by the original authors

[c]Study from Lovell et al. (2014)

Contact with the biodiverse environment was coded as either indirect or direct following Keniger et al. (2013). Indirect contact "does not require a person to be physically present in nature" (Keniger et al. 2013, p. 916) and can include viewing nature through a window, and looking at photographs, paintings or motion pictures of nature. Direct contact with nature stipulates that nature, or natural elements, are physically present in the same space as the individual (Keniger et al. 2013).[1] Examples of direct contact include indoor plants, using urban green spaces for education purposes, reading or having a picnic in the park, doing sports or exercise in a natural setting, gardening and camping.

Moderating variables were categorised as either personal (e.g. age, gender, socio-economic status) or contextual (e.g. urbanicity, safety) (Hartig et al. 2014; Markevych et al. 2017). Mediators were classified as 'reducing harm', 'restoring capacities' or 'building capacities' according to Markevych et al. (2017). 'Reducing harm' considers the role of the natural environment to reduce exposure to environmental stressors like heat or noise pollution. 'Restoring capacities' mediators support renewal of adapted resources that have become depleted through everyday demands, such as attention restoration and stress recovery. 'Building capacities' mediators highlight the role of green spaces in strengthening an individual's capacity to acquire new adaptive resources like fostering physical activity and social cohesion.

9.2.3 Synthesis of Results

To provide a synthesis of results assessing the influence of biodiversity on mental health and well-being, a combined set of 24 studies, drawn from Lovell et al. (2014) and from our updated review, was utilised. Nine quantitative studies identified in Lovell et al. (2014) that assessed biodiversity and mental health and well-being relationships were included (Table 9.1). Consequently, 4 studies from Lovell et al. (2014) with physical health as the outcome were excluded (Huynen et al. 2004; Poudyal et al. 2009; Sieswerda et al. 2001; Tilt et al. 2007). Also excluded were 4 studies that, according to Lovell et al. (2014), did not directly assess biodiversity but were included in their analysis nevertheless (Barton et al. 2009; Curtin 2009; Lemieux et al. 2012; Pereira et al. 2005). In this sense our synthesis of results is more critical than Lovell et al.'s (2014) by including only those studies that consider the biodiversity of the environment in some way. Fifteen of the 16 articles identified in our updated search were included in the synthesis of results. Foo (2016) was excluded from the synthesis of results because it analysed the associations between use of the environment, individual differences in environmental experience, and perceived physical activity, well-being and mental health given a certain level of actual biodiversity instead of an investigation of the influence of biodiversity levels on mental health and well-being.

[1] This is a combination of Keniger et al. (2013) 'incidental' and 'intentional' interaction types as both describe being in the presence of nature.

Due to the heterogeneity of the selected articles in terms of research design, measures and participants, data were analysed using narrative synthesis (Popay et al. 2006). The purpose of narrative synthesis is to identify the factors that explain the differences in results in the body of literature (Popay et al. 2006). Patterns of results across all 24 studies were identified according to study design, measures of biodiversity and mental health or well-being. Vote counting (Popay et al. 2006) was used to describe the frequency of significant and non-significant results across the 24 quantitative studies. This analytical approach has been used previously (Lovell et al. 2014). While we acknowledge that vote counting has known deficiencies (e.g. giving equal weight to studies with different research designs, samples and effect sizes), it is a useful as a preliminary interpretation of results across studies (Popay et al. 2006). Our findings should thus be interpreted with caution.

9.3 Results

9.3.1 Characteristics of the Recent Literature, Published Since Lovell et al.'s (2014) Review, Relating Biodiversity to Mental Health and Well-being

The following describes the recent literature (n = 16), published since 2012, on biodiversity and mental health and well-being. See Lovell et al. (2014) for description of the body of evidence up to 2012.

All 16 studies examined, wholly or in part, the relationships between biodiversity and one or more mental health or well-being outcomes (see Table 9.1). Eleven studies were based in Western Europe, three in North America and two in Asia. Two studies were from emerging economies of Malaysia and Mexico. Six different study designs were used to examine the relationship between biodiversity and mental health and well-being (Fig. 9.2).

9.3.1.1 Spatial Scale

The spatial scale at which the relationships were examined ranged from the national (Duarte-Tagles et al. 2015; Wheeler et al. 2015) to the local (Carrus et al. 2015; Foo 2016; Marselle et al. 2015, 2016). Specifically, scales considered whole countries (England (Wheeler et al. 2015) and Mexico (Duarte-Tagles et al. 2015)), geographical regions within countries (England (Cox et al. 2017), Finland (Rantakokko et al. 2018), Sweden (Annerstedt van den Bosch et al. 2015), the USA (Jones 2017)) and specific places such as forests in the Klang Valley region of Malaysia (Foo 2016), protected nature reserves in Singapore (Saw et al. 2015) and green spaces in Italy (Carrus et al. 2015).

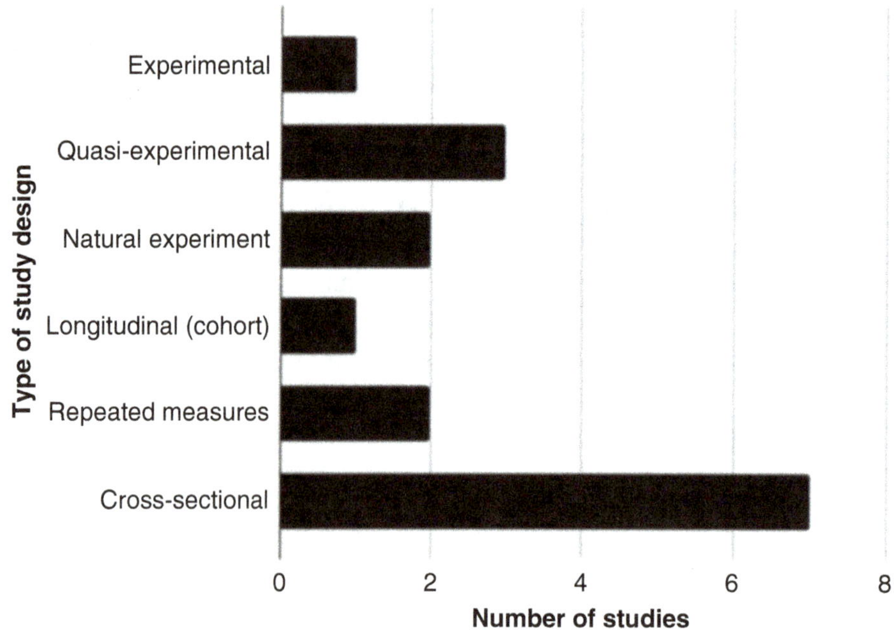

Fig. 9.2 Type of study design used to examine biodiversity and mental health and well-being relationships across the 16 studies published after 2012

9.3.1.2 Participants

The number of participants varied considerably among the recently published studies: ranging from 35 (Johansson et al. 2014) through to the millions (with the use of data from the national census, Wheeler et al. 2015). Participant type also differed, including university students (Cracknell et al. 2016, 2017; Saw et al. 2015) and staff (Johansson et al. 2014), adults participating over the internet (White et al. 2017; Wolf et al. 2017), group walkers over the age of 55 (Marselle et al. 2015; Marselle et al. 2016), park users (Carrus et al. 2015), visitors to forests (Foo 2016), and residents of specific countries or regions as previously detailed (Annerstedt van den Bosch 2015; Cox et al. 2017; Duarte-Tagles et al. 2015; Jones 2017; Rantakokko et al. 2018; Wheeler et al. 2015).

9.3.1.3 Theoretical Position

Where articulated, the theoretical underpinnings largely reflected the dominant understandings of environment-health linkages (for further discussion on biodiversity and health theories, see Marselle Chap. 7, this volume). Specifically, 9 studies (Annerstedt van den Bosch, et al. 2015; Cox et al. 2017; Cracknell et al. 2016, 2017; Foo 2016; Marselle et al. 2015, 2016; Saw et al. 2015; White et al. 2017) used the Attention Restoration Theory (Kaplan and Kaplan 1989; Kaplan 1995) and the Stress Reduction Theory (Ulrich 1983; Ulrich et al. 1991) to explain the effects of biodiversity on mental health and/or well-being. Additionally, the Biophilia hypothesis (Kellert and Wilson 1993) was also mentioned (Annerstedt van den Bosch et al.

2015; Carrus et al. 2015; Saw et al. 2015; Wolf et al. 2017), as was appraisal theory (Johansson et al. 2014). Four studies (Duarte-Tagles et al. 2015; Jones 2017; Rantakokko et al. 2018; Wheeler et al. 2015) did not articulate a theory for why or how biodiversity may be related to better health and well-being.

9.3.1.4 Biodiversity Assessment

There was considerable variation across the 16 studies on the organisational level at which biodiversity was studied, the data collection method used, and the type of environment/organism investigated (see Table 9.2). Seven studies assessed biodiversity at the ecosystem or habitat level. Measurement across these studies included use of secondary, geographically-referenced data to determine land cover and land use diversity using the Shannon Diversity Index (Rantakokko et al. 2018; Wheeler et al. 2015), eco-region diversity using the Margalef Diversity Index (Duarte-Tagles et al. 2015) and access to protected areas (Saw et al. 2015). Investigator categorisation of ecosystem/habitat biodiversity was used to classify environments into low, medium and high biodiversity biotopes (Johansson et al. 2014) or low vs. high biodiverse green spaces (Carrus et al. 2015). Participants' perception of habitats/ecosystem was used in one study; the Scania Green Score uses interpreted satellite imagery-derived land use data (i.e. mixed forest and marshes, beaches, sand plains and bare rock, biotopes and national parks) to map perceived biodiversity ('lush, rich in species') of an environment (Annerstedt van den Bosch et al. 2015). At the species community level, 6 studies assessed biodiversity in terms of species richness for various taxa (i.e. birds, butterflies, plants, trees, fish/crustaceans). Species richness was measured using standard ecological field survey techniques (Cox et al. 2017; Cracknell et al. 2016), secondary data (Wheeler et al. 2015) or investigator categorisation of species richness (e.g. low vs. high based on assessment of content in images or videos (Cracknell et al. 2017; Wolf et al. 2017)). Participants' perception of species richness was employed in 3 studies (Marselle et al. 2015, 2016; White et al. 2017). At the species community level, abundance of a specific taxonomic group (i.e. birds, fish/crustaceans) was also assessed in 2 studies using standard ecological survey techniques (Cox et al. 2017), and investigator categorisation of stimuli (i.e. low vs. high abundance; Cracknell et al. 2017). At the single species level, Jones (2017) investigated biodiversity loss and ecosystem health through the loss of North American ash trees (*Fraxinus* spp.) following the presence of the invasive species emerald ash borer (EAB) (*Agrilus planipennis*). This was assessed using secondary data.

9.3.1.5 Mental Health and Well-being Assessment

There was considerable variation in the outcomes considered and the measures used among the studies (Fig. 9.3). Mental health was assessed in 7 studies (Annerstedt van den Bosch et al. 2015; Cox et al. 2017; Duarte-Tagles et al. 2015; Foo 2016;

Table 9.2 Level of biodiversity investigated and data collection method used in the 16 studies published after 2012

	Data collection method			
Biodiversity level	Standard ecological survey	Secondary data	Investigator categorisation of biodiversity	Perceived biodiversity
Ecosystems/habitats				
		Margalef Diversity Index of eco-regions (Duarte-Tagles et al. 2015)	Forest biotopes (Johansson et al. 2014)	Scania Green Score (Annerstedt van den Bosch et al. 2015)[a]
		Protected area designation (Saw et al. 2015)	Green spaces (Carrus et al. 2015)	
		Shannon Diversity Index of land cover (Wheeler et al. 2015) and land use (Rantakokko et al. 2018)		
Species communities				
Species richness	Birds in the morning, and birds in the afternoon (Cox et al. 2017)	Birds (Wheeler et al. 2015)	Fish/crustaceans (Cracknell et al. 2017)	Animals/plants (White et al. 2017)
	Fish/crustaceans (Cracknell et al. 2016)		Plants, birds, mammals and reptiles/amphibians (Foo 2016)	Birds, butterflies and plants/trees (Marselle et al. 2016; Marselle et al. 2015)
			Trees and birds (Wolf et al. 2017)	
Abundance of a specific taxonomic group	Birds in the morning, and birds in the afternoon (Cox et al. 2017)		Fish/crustaceans (Cracknell et al. 2017)	
Single species				
		Emerald ash borer (EAB) (*Agrilus planipennis*), which is responsible for biodiversity loss of North American ash trees (*Fraxinus* spp.) (Jones 2017)		

Note. Biodiversity levels are based on Botzat et al. (2016). Data in the cells identifies the specific biodiversity variable assessed; no data in a cell means no studies investigated that biodiversity level using a specific data collection method. Biodiversity variables with a slash ('/') are a combined variable where the investigator did not separate out the contribution of each taxon; two taxa are analysed together

[a] 'Lush, rich in species' is a perceived biodiversity assessment that is then mapped using interpreted, secondary land cover data

Jones 2017; Rantakokko et al. 2018; Wolf et al. 2017). The majority of these assessed depression (Cox et al. 2017; Duarte-Tagles et al. 2015; Jones 2017; Rantakokko et al. 2018) using self-report standardised measures such as the DASS (Cox et al. 2017), CES-D (Rantakokko et al. 2018) and PHQ-12 (Jones 2017). Anxiety was assessed also through the use of standardised self-report measures: DASS (Cox et al. 2017) and the STAI (Wolf et al. 2017). The DASS was additionally used to assess perceived stress (Cox et al. 2017). General mental health was assessed by Foo (2016) who utilised scales specifically developed for the study.

Mental well-being was examined in 13 studies (Carrus et al. 2015; Cracknell et al. 2016, 2017; Foo 2016; Johansson et al. 2014; Jones 2017; Marselle et al. 2015, 2016; Rantakokko et al. 2018; Saw et al. 2015; Wheeler et al. 2015; White et al. 2017; Wolf et al. 2017). The majority assessed emotions (Cracknell et al. 2016, 2017; Johansson et al. 2014; Jones 2017; Marselle et al. 2015, 2016; White et al. 2017; Wolf et al. 2017) using standardised self-report measures such as the PANAS (Marselle et al. 2015, 2016; Wolf et al. 2017), the Feeling Scale and Felt Arousal Scale (Cracknell et al. 2016; White et al. 2017), and the Basic Emotional Process 12 (Johansson et al. 2014). Quality of life was assessed with the WHO QoL (Rantakokko et al. 2018). Four studies measured general well-being: 3 studies (Carrus et al. 2015; Foo 2016; Wheeler et al. 2015) did not separate physical from mental well-being, and 1 study (Saw et al. 2015) did not separate mood (a short-term, affective aspect of well-being) from life satisfaction (a long-term, cognitive aspect of well-being, Diener et al. 1985).

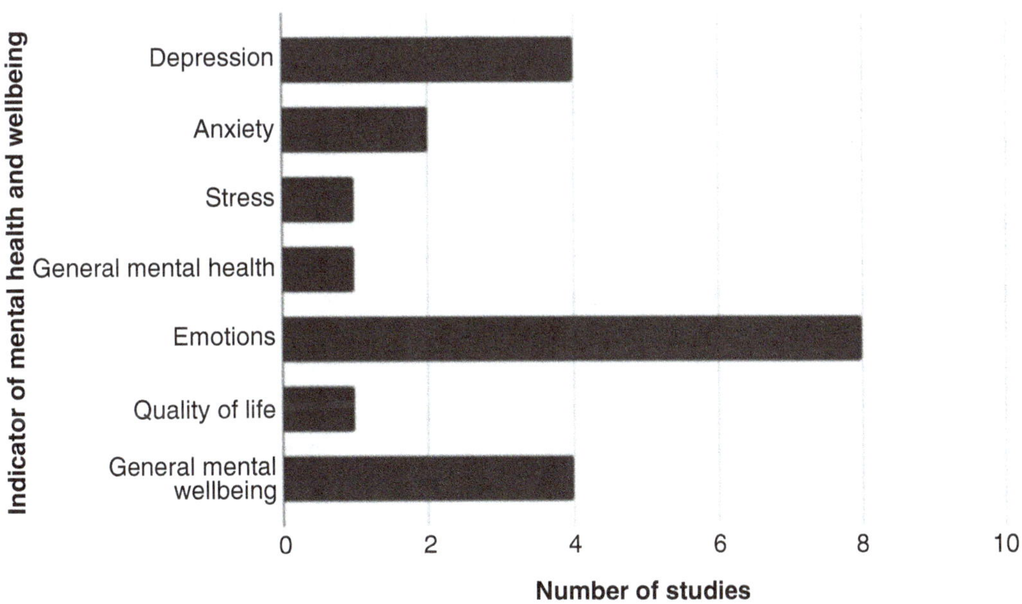

Fig. 9.3 Number of mental health and mental well-being variables used across the 16 studies published after 2012. The sum may exceed 100% because some studies address more than one mental health or well-being variable

9.3.1.6 Type of Contact with the Biodiverse Environment

Table 9.3 details the type of contact by biodiversity level. In general, authors hypothesised that direct or indirect contact with high biodiverse environments would have a positive effect on mental health and well-being. However, the majority of studies investigated the amount of biodiversity near to the home without specifying the type of contact (Annerstedt van den Bosch et al. 2015; Cox et al. 2017; Duarte-Tagles et al. 2015; Jones 2017; Rantakokko et al. 2018; Saw et al. 2015; Wheeler et al. 2015). Five studies, all experimental, considered indirect contact with biodiversity (Cracknell et al. 2016, 2017; Johansson et al. 2014; White et al. 2017; Wolf et al. 2017). In these studies, participants experienced biodiversity indirectly by viewing photographs (Cracknell et al. 2017; Johansson et al. 2014; White et al. 2017), videos (Wolf et al. 2017) or an aquarium exhibit (Cracknell et al. 2016). Four studies considered direct contact with biodiversity by assessing users who were in specific environments (Carrus et al. 2015; Foo 2016; Marselle et al. 2015, 2016). The impacts of changes in biodiversity on mental health and well-being were investigated in 2 studies. Annerstedt van den Bosch et al. (2015) assessed the relationship between mental health and moving to a neighbourhood that is perceived to be 'lush, rich in species'. Jones (2017) examined the mental health and well-being impact of biodiversity loss of North American ash trees due to the invasive species EAB. None of the studies investigated dose-response relationships of the effect of biodiversity on mental health or well-being.

9.3.1.7 Moderation Analyses

Moderation analyses were conducted in 4 studies (Carrus et al. 2015; Jones 2017; Wheeler et al. 2015; White et al. 2017). These were categorised as either personal (e.g. gender, age, socio-economic status) or contextual (e.g. urbanicity), based on previous research (Hartig et al. 2014; Markevych et al. 2017). Gender was found to moderate the influence of perceived biodiversity on positive affect and recovery; men reported greater positive affect and recovery from high (perceived) species rich environments (White et al. 2017). Age moderated the effect of perceived species richness on arousal (White et al. 2017), and biodiversity loss on life satisfaction (Jones 2017). People less than 35 years old reported more arousal from a perceived species rich environment, than those aged 35 and over (White et al. 2017). Whilst all age groups reported a reduction in life satisfaction from living in EAB infected areas, the largest (and only statistically significant) impact was for young adults aged 18–24 years old (Jones 2017). Socio-economic status was found to moderate the effect of biodiversity on health; the associations of Shannon Diversity of land cover types and bird species richness on health were the strongest for individuals who lived in the most socio-economically deprived neighbourhoods (Wheeler et al. 2015). Other personal variables such as being a member of an environmental organisation (White et al. 2017) had no moderating effect. The biodiversity-health relationship was also moderated by urbanicity. In Wheeler et al.'s (2015) study, Shannon Diversity of land cover types had the strongest association with good health for

Table 9.3 Level of biodiversity investigated by the type of contact with biodiversity investigated in the 16 studies published after 2012

	Type of contact with biodiversity		
Biodiversity levels	Direct	Indirect	Unspecified
Ecosystem/habitats			
	Green spaces (Carrus et al. 2015)	Forest biotopes (Johansson et al. 2014)	Margalef Diversity Index (Duarte-Tagles et al. 2015)
			Protected area designation (Saw et al. 2015)
			Scania Green Score (Annerstedt van den Bosch et al. 2015)
			Shannon Diversity Index (Wheeler et al. 2015; Rantakokko et al. 2018)
Species communities			
Species richness	Birds, plants/trees, and butterflies (Marselle et al. 2016; Marselle et al. 2015)	Animals/plants (White et al. 2017)	Birds in the morning, and birds in the afternoon (Cox et al. 2017)
	Plants, birds, mammals and reptiles/amphibians (Foo 2016)	Fish/crustaceans (Cracknell et al. 2016, 2017)	Birds (Wheeler et al. 2015)
		Trees and birds (Wolf et al. 2017)	
Abundance a specific taxonomic group		Fish/crustaceans (Cracknell et al. 2017)	Birds in the morning, and birds in the afternoon (Cox et al. 2017)
Single species			
			Emerald ash borer (*Agrilus planipennis*), which is responsible for biodiversity loss of North American ash trees (*Fraxinus* spp.) (Jones 2017)
Total	4	5	7

Note. 'Direct' and 'indirect' contact with nature categories based on Keniger et al. (2013). Biodiversity levels are based on Botzat et al. (2016). Data in the cells identifies the specific biodiversity variable assessed in each study; no data in a cell means no studies investigated that biodiversity level and type of contact with the biodiverse environment. Biodiversity variables with a slash ('/') are a combined variable where the investigator did not separate out the contribution of each taxon; two taxa are analysed together

individuals who lived in rural areas, whilst, conversely, bird species richness had the strongest positive effect on health for those who lived in urban areas. Carrus et al. (2015) found a high level of biodiversity was more strongly associated with well-being in urban green spaces than in peri-urban areas suggesting that higher biodiversity is more important in urban areas for well-being. Other contextual variables, such as living near to the coast (White et al. 2017), had no moderating effect.

9.3.1.8 Mediation Analyses

Mediators were explored in 3 studies (Carrus et al. 2015; Foo 2016; Marselle et al. 2016). Investigated mediators fell within two of the three domains mentioned by Markevych et al. (2017): 'restoring capacities' (perceived restorativeness (Carrus et al. 2015; Foo 2016; Marselle et al. 2016)) and 'building capacities' (physical activity and social interaction (Foo 2016)). 'Reducing harm' mediators were not investigated in these studies. Perceived restorativeness was found to mediate the relationship between biodiversity of green space and general well-being (Carrus et al. 2015), and between perceived bird species richness and positive affect, happiness and negative affect (Marselle et al. 2016). Perceived bird species richness also had an indirect effect on positive affect and happiness via the restorative components of being away, fascination and compatibility, and an indirect effect on negative affect via compatibility (Marselle et al. 2016). Foo (2016) conducted path analyses to determine how spending time in forest environments with different levels of biodiversity influenced mental health and general well-being. Multiple mediating pathways were found; time spent in a forest environment with intermediate or high biodiversity engendered a sense of being away, which was positively associated with a change in mood, which then was related to mental health. In only the high biodiverse forest was mental health related to general well-being. In the intermediate biodiverse forest, physical activity mediated the relationships between being away and mental health and general well-being. Social interaction did not mediate the effect of a forest environment on either outcome.

9.3.2 *Synthesis of the Results from the Combined Published Literature on Biodiversity and Mental Health and Well-being Relationships*

A combined set of 24 studies were included in the synthesis of results pertaining to the influence of biodiversity and mental health and well-being: 15 of the 16 recently published studies identified through our search process and nine of the 16 studies identified in Lovell et al. (2014). Fourteen of these 24 studies reported one or more positive associations between biodiversity and mental health or well-being outcomes (Carrus et al. 2015; Cox et al. 2017; Cracknell et al. 2017; Dallimer et al. 2012; Foo 2016; Fuller et al. 2007; Huby et al. 2006; Johansson et al. 2014; Jones 2017; Luck et al. 2011; Marselle et al. 2016; Rantakokko et al. 2018; Wheeler et al. 2015; White et al. 2017; Wolf et al. 2017) (see Table 9.4). Seventeen of the 24 studies reported one or more results with no significant relationship (Annerstedt van den Bosch et al. 2015; Annerstedt et al. 2012; Björk et al. 2008; Cox et al. 2017; Cracknell et al. 2016, 2017; Dallimer et al. 2012; de Jong et al. 2012; Duarte-Tagles et al. 2015; Fuller et al. 2007; Grahn and Stigsdotter 2010; Jorgensen et al. 2010; Marselle et al. 2015, 2016; Rantakokko et al. 2018; Saw et al. 2015; Wolf et al. 2017). Two studies reported one or more negative associations between biodiversity and mental health or well-being outcomes (Dallimer et al. 2012; Marselle et al. 2015) (Table 9.4).

Table 9.4 Trends of results by type of study design across all 24 studies

Study design	Positive; greater biodiversity associated with better health	No significant relationship	Negative; greater biodiversity associated with poorer health
Experimental	Wolf et al. (2017)	Jorgensen et al. (2010)[a]	
		Wolf et al. (2017)	
Quasi-experimental (no random assignment)	Cracknell et al. (2017)	Cracknell et al. (2017)	
	Johansson et al. (2014)[b]		
	White et al. (2017)		
Natural experiment	Jones (2017)[c]	Cracknell et al. (2016)	
Longitudinal cohort		Annerstedt et al. (2012)[a]	
		Annerstedt van den Bosch et al. (2015)	
Repeated measures	Marselle et al. (2016)[d]	Marselle et al. (2015)	Marselle et al. (2015)
		Marselle et al. (2016)[d]	
Cross-sectional	Carrus et al. (2015)[e]	Cox et al. (2017)	Dallimer et al. (2012)[a]
	Cox et al. (2017)	Dallimer et al. (2012)[a]	
	Dallimer et al. (2012)[a]	De Jong et al. (2012)[a]	
	Fuller et al. (2007)[a]	Duarte-Tagles et al. (2015)	
	Huby et al. (2006)[a]	Fuller et al. (2007)[a]	
	Luck et al. (2011)[a]	Grahn and Stigsdotter (2010)[a]	
	Rantakokko et al. (2018)	Rantakokko et al. (2018)	
	Wheeler et al. (2015)	Saw et al. (2015)	
		Wheeler et al. (2015)	
Total	14	17	2

Note. Papers may be included more than once, if variation in individual results
[a]Study from Lovell et al. (2014)
[b]Effect was greatest in the medium biotope, followed by the high and then the low biotopes
[c]Inverse relationship
[d]Mediation analysis only
[e]Mediation analysis also significant

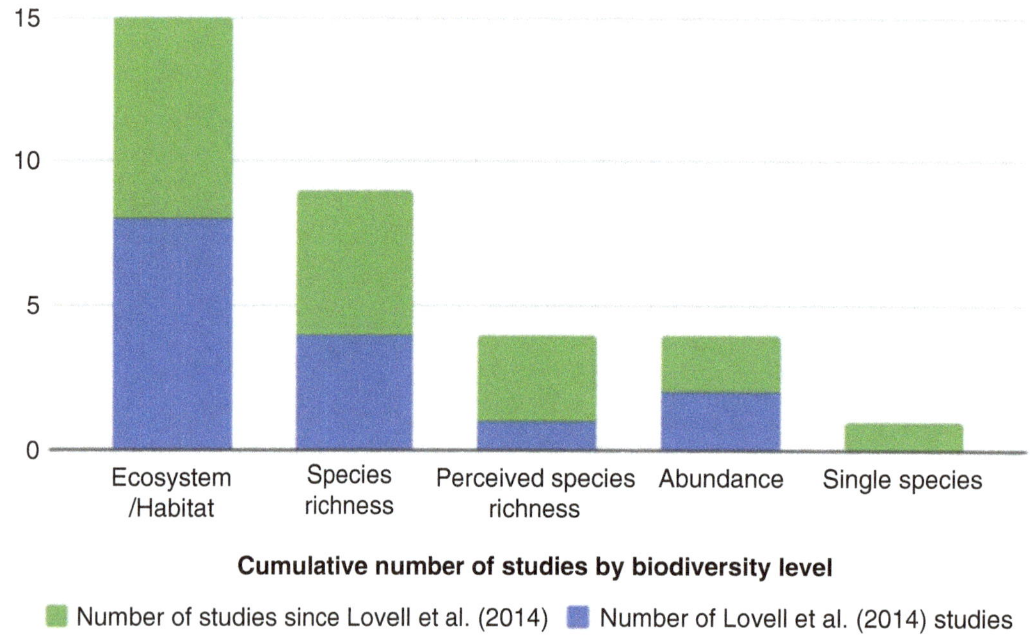

Fig. 9.4 Biodiversity levels addressed by the 24 studies on the mental health and well-being effects of biodiversity. The sum may exceed 100% because studies address more than one level of biodiversity

Biodiversity levels were not equally covered by the 24 studies (see Fig. 9.4). Fifteen studies assessed biodiversity at the ecosystem/habitat level, with clear decreases to the single species level. However, the number of studies investigating biodiversity at these other levels has increased since Lovell et al. (2014).

9.3.2.1 Pattern of Results

To identify patterns in the results, we examined studies by biodiversity level and mental health and well-being outcomes (Table 9.5). We also identified the specific biodiversity variable that was measured (e.g. habitat types, birds) next to each result. The purpose was to gain insight into when biodiversity influences mental health and well-being and when it does not.

Mental Health and Well-being Outcomes

We started by looking at the results by outcome measure to determine if either outcome was more influenced by biodiversity. Nine studies investigated mental health outcomes, the majority of which were published after 2012, demonstrating a growth area for the field since Lovell et al. (2014). Mental well-being was investigated in 19 of the 24 studies. Two-thirds of the results (65%) pertaining to the influence of

Table 9.5 Pattern of results by biodiversity levels and mental health and well-being indicator (n = 24 studies)

	Outcome variable	
Biodiversity levels	Mental health	Mental well-being
Ecosystems/habitats		
	Annerstedt van den Bosch et al. (2015) (o) Scania Green Score 'Lush, rich in species' Annerstedt et al. (2012)[a] (o) Scania Green Score 'Lush, rich in species' Duarte-Tagles et al. (2015) (o) Margalef Diversity of eco-regions Rantakokko et al. (2018) (o) Shannon Diversity of land use	Bjork et al. (2008)[a] (oo) Scania Green Score 'Lush, rich in species' Carrus et al. (2015) (++[b]) Green spaces Dallimer et al. (2012)[a] (ooo) Shannon Diversity of habitat types (+++) Tree cover De Jong et al. (2012)[a] (o) Scania Green Score 'Lush, rich in species' Fuller et al. (2007)[a] (+++o) Number of habitat types (oooo) Tree cover Grahn & Stigsdotter (2010)[a] (o) Scania Green Score 'Lush, rich in species' Johansson et al. (2014) (+) Forest biotopes[c] Jorgensen et al. (2010)[a] (o) Green spaces Luck et al. (2011)[a] (+) Vegetation cover (+) Vegetation density Rantakokko et al. (2018) (+) Shannon Diversity of land use Saw et al. (2015) (o) Protected areas Wheeler et al. (2015) (++) Shannon Diversity of land over

(continued)

Table 9.5 (continued)

	Outcome variable	
Biodiversity levels	Mental health	Mental well-being
Species communities		
Species richness	Cox et al. (2017) (ooo) Morning birds (ooo) Afternoon birds Huby et al. (2006)[a] (+) Birds Wolf et al. (2017) (+) Trees (+) Birds	Cracknell et al. (2016) (oo) Fish/crustaceans Cracknell et al. (2017) (o) Fish/crustaceans Dallimer et al. (2012)[a] (+++) Birds (– – –) Plants (ooo) Butterflies Fuller et al. (2007)[a] (++oo) Birds (++oo) Plants (oooo) Butterflies Luck et al. (2011)[a] (+) Birds Wheeler et al. (2015) (+o) Birds Wolf et al. (2017) (+o) Trees (+o) Birds
Perceived species richness		Dallimer et al. (2012)[a] (+++) Birds (+++) Plants/trees (+++) Butterflies Marselle et al. (2016) (+++) Birds[b] (ooo) Plants/trees[b] (ooo) Butterflies[b] Marselle et al. (2015) (–oo) Birds (ooo) Plants/trees (ooo) Butterflies White et al. (2017) (+++) Animals/plants
Abundance of a specific taxonomic group	Cox et al. (2017) (ooo) Morning birds (+++) Afternoon birds	Cracknell et al. (2017) (+) Fish/crustaceans Dallimer et al. (2012)[a] (+++) Birds Luck et al. (2011)[a] (+) Birds

(continued)

Table 9.5 (continued)

	Outcome variable	
Biodiversity levels	Mental health	Mental well-being
Single species		
	Jones (2017) (+)[d] Ash trees	Jones (2017) (+)[d] Ash trees

Note. Papers may be included more than once, if variation in individual results. Biodiversity levels are based on Botzat et al. (2016). Biodiversity variables with a slash ('/') are a combined variable where investigator did not separate out the contribution of each taxon; two taxa are analysed together. Each –, o or + symbol represents the direction of each individual result reported in the paper. – = significant negative relationship; o = non-significant relationship; + = significant positive relationship

[a]Study from Lovell et al. (2014)

[b]Mediation analysis

[c]Effect was greatest in the medium biotope, followed by the high and then the low biotopes

[d]Inverse relationship

biodiversity on mental health were non-significant. About half of the results (49%) showed non-significant relationships between biodiversity and mental well-being. These findings suggest that the results are equally ambiguous for both mental health and mental well-being.

Ecosystems/Habitats

Sixteen studies investigated the impact of biodiversity at the ecosystem/habitat level on mental health and well-being (Table 9.5). All 4 of the studies that assessed the influence of ecosystem/habitat biodiversity on mental health were non-significant (Annerstedt van den Bosch et al. 2015; Annerstedt et al. 2012; Duarte-Tagles et al. 2015; Rantakokko et al. 2018).

Results were mixed for the 12 studies that investigated the impact of biodiversity at the ecosystem/habitat level on mental well-being. Positive relationships were found for Shannon Diversity Index of land cover and land use, and mental well-being; more biodiverse ecosystems/habitats were positively associated with greater quality of life (Rantakokko et al. 2018) and good health (Wheeler et al. 2015), and negatively associated with poor health (Wheeler et al. 2015). Non-significant results for Shannon Diversity Index of habitat types were found (Dallimer et al. 2012). Greater vegetation cover and density of vegetation cover were associated with greater life satisfaction (Luck et al. 2011). Number of habitat types was associated with greater reflection and distinct identity (Fuller et al. 2007). Tree cover was positively associated with greater reflection, continuity with the past and attachment in Dallimer et al. (2012), but was non-significant in Fuller et al. (2007). A significant non-linear trend of forest biotope on positive affect was also found; intermediate biotope was rated the most positive followed by the high biotope and the low biotope (Johansson et al. 2014). Carrus et al. (2015) found biodiversity of different green spaces had a significant direct, and indirect, effect on general well-being. Individuals in the high biodiversity condition had greater general well-being scores than individuals in the low biodiversity condition, and perceived restorativeness mediated the relationship between biodiversity and well-being (Carrus et al. 2015). Studies assessing ecosystems/habitats by Scania Green Score 'lush, rich in species' (Björk et al. 2008; de Jong et al. 2012; Grahn and Stigsdotter 2010), protected areas (Saw et al. 2015) and green space types (Jorgensen et al. 2010) on mental well-being were all non-significant.

Species Richness

Ten studies examined the effect of species richness (Table 9.5). Three of these investigated the influence of species richness on mental health, with mixed results. Huby et al. (2006) found positive associations between mental health and greater bird species richness. Similarly, Wolf et al. (2017) found that participants in the high species rich conditions of trees and birds, reported less anxiety, compared to participants in the low species rich conditions. However, Cox et al. (2017) found no influence of morning and afternoon bird species richness on depression, anxiety or stress.

Across the 7 studies that measured mental well-being just over half of results (55%) were non-significant. Specifically, there was no difference in positive affect and arousal between low and high species richness conditions of fish/crustaceans (Cracknell et al. 2016). Additionally, species richness of fish/crustaceans had no effect on happiness, when species abundance was held constant (Cracknell et al. 2017). There was also no difference in vitality scores between the high and low species richness conditions of birds and trees (Wolf et al. 2017). However, for positive affect, participants reported higher levels in the high species richness conditions of trees, and birds, compared to low species richness conditions (Wolf et al. 2017). Bird species richness was positively associated with good health (Wheeler et al. 2015). However, the negative association between bird species richness and poor health did not hold when accounting for covariates (Wheeler et al. 2015). Butterfly species richness had no significant effect (Dallimer et al. 2012; Fuller et al. 2007), and plant species richness had a negative effect, on psychological well-being (Dallimer et al. 2012). Greater species richness of birds (Dallimer et al. 2012; Fuller et al. 2007; Luck et al. 2011) and plants (Fuller et al. 2007) were both associated with greater mental well-being.

Perceived Species Richness

No study investigated the effect of perceived richness on mental health (see Table 9.5). Four studies examined the influence of perceived species richness on mental well-being. Just over half of the results (53%) demonstrated a positive effect.

White et al. (2017) found that greater perceived species richness of animals/plants was associated with more positive mood, arousal and recovery. Dallimer et al. (2012) found positive associations between perceived species richness of birds, butterflies and plants/trees and psychological well-being (measured as reflection, continuity with the past and attachment). Using the same perceived species richness variables, Marselle et al. (2015, 2016) found no associations between perceived plant/tree and butterfly species richness and emotional well-being; perceived bird species richness had no influence on positive affect and happiness but was associated with an increase in negative affect (Marselle et al. 2015). An indirect effect of perceived bird species richness on positive affect, happiness and negative affect through perceived restorativeness was also found (Marselle et al. 2016). Bird biodiversity was associated with greater perceived restorativeness, which was in turn associated with greater positive affect and happiness, and reduced negative affect.

Abundance of Specific Taxonomic Groups

Abundance was investigated in 4 studies (see Table 9.5). One study examined the impact on mental health, with mixed results. Cox et al. (2017) found that afternoon, but not morning, bird abundance was associated with less depression, anxiety and stress. The reason for this difference for mental health, according to Cox et al. (2017), is that afternoon abundance is a measure of the number of birds that people are likely to experience, as opposed to a measure of the total number of birds that are actually there. Three studies investigated the influence of the abundance of specific taxonomic groups on mental well-being, all with positive results. Bird abundance was positively associated with reflection, continuity with the past and attachment (Dallimer et al. 2012) and life satisfaction (Luck et al. 2011). Greater abundance of fish/crustaceans, viewed in photographs, was related to greater reported happiness, when species richness was held constant (Cracknell et al. 2017). This suggests that it may be the quantity of fish/crustaceans, and not the number of species per se, that influences happiness.

Single Species

One study assessed the effect of biodiversity loss by investigating the decline of a single species, the North American ash tree following infestation by the invasive emerald ash borer, on mental health and well-being (Jones 2017). The loss of ash trees, 5 years after initial infestation, was associated with an increase in depression, as well as a decrease in life satisfaction. The results suggest the negative influence that biodiversity loss could have on mental health and well-being.

9.4 Discussion

This chapter identifies, summarises and synthesises research on the impact of biodiversity on mental health and mental well-being. This was done by identifying and describing the body of evidence, published since Lovell et al.'s (2014) systematic review, relating biodiversity to mental health and well-being, and by synthesising results from the studies identified by both Lovell et al. (2014) and in this chapter.

Sixteen primary research studies met our inclusion criteria. The assessment of biodiversity in these recently published studies has improved, compared to the studies reviewed in Lovell et al. (2014). Four studies in Lovell et al.'s (2014) review did not directly assess biodiversity (Barton et al. 2009; Curtin 2009; Lemieux et al. 2012; Pereira et al. 2005). The growing availability of biodiversity-focused studies meant that all 16 studies identified for our updated review considered the diversity of the environment in some way. Additionally, the recent body of literature investigates a greater variation of the biodiversity at the species community and single species levels. Further, the number of studies investigating mental health has grown since Lovell et al. (2014).

Our synthesis of the combined set of 24 studies (nine from Lovell et al. (2014) and 15 identified in this Chapter) was conducted to describe the body of literature focused on mental health and well-being as an outcome. There is some evidence to suggest that biodiverse natural environments may be associated with good mental health and well-being. Fourteen of these studies showed one or more positive relationships manifested as either better mental health or mental well-being. Positive relationships were found across all, but one, study designs. Positive relationships were most evident when assessing species abundance and mental well-being relationships. However, 17 of these studies reported one or more non-significant findings. Non-significant effects were found across all study designs, and were most evident when assessing impact of biodiversity at the ecosystem/habitat level on mental health. There was some evidence of negative relationships (in 2 of the 24 quantitative studies). Overall, the body of evidence across these 24 studies is not yet of the extent necessary to characterise the role of biodiversity in relation to mental health and/or mental well-being. Variation in the evidence may relate to the level at which biodiversity is investigated, how the biodiversity data are collected, and which taxonomic groups are explored. These raise issues for cross-study comparability.

The synthesis of results suggests that abundance of specific taxonomic groups may be an important variable. Abundance of a taxonomic group may be more noticeable by people than the number of species (Dallimer et al. 2012). As such, it may not be the number of different species (i.e. species richness) that matter, but the total number of animals, plants or birds (i.e. abundance). Indeed, Cracknell et al. (2017) found differential results between species richness and abundance on mental well-being; only abundance was related to happiness, but not species richness. Similar results were found elsewhere (Hedblom et al. 2017).

Clear gaps in the research were also found. None of the 24 studies investigated the effect of perceived species richness on mental health. Another possible area of investigation, not assessed in any of the 24 studies, is participants' perception of the abundance of a specific taxonomic group on mental health and/or mental well-being.

Lovell et al. (2014) provided a number of recommendations for future research, which were to improve study design, and specify the type of contact and frequency of exposure to biodiversity, and test for moderating and mediating variables. Most of the recently published studies were cross-sectional; a similar observation made by Lovell et al. (2014). However, the number of robust research designs (experimental, natural experimental, longitudinal), as well as quasi-experimental and before-and-after repeated measures studies has increased, reflecting the call for improved study designs. Additionally, 2 studies sought to examine impacts of changes in biodiversity on mental health and well-being outcomes, which is an increase from Lovell et al. (2014), which had no such studies. Regarding contact with biodiversity, more than half of the recently published studies explicitly investigated direct and indirect contact, thus heeding Lovell et al.'s (2014) call to investigate how type of contact with the biodiverse environment may influence outcomes. However, no studies have yet heeded Lovell et al.'s (2014) call for investigations of frequency of exposure to biodiversity. Four of the identified 16 studies investigated moderators that qualified the biodiversity and mental health and well-being relationship. Three of the recently published studies conducted mediation analyses to determine the mechanisms through which biodiversity affects mental health and/or well-being. These few moderator and mediator studies are nevertheless an increase from those reported in Lovell et al. (2014).

9.4.1 Concluding Observations

In conclusion, we provide some thoughts to guide future research:

Better Integration
By its nature, the questions considered within this field of inquiry are interdisciplinary and thus by necessity require integration of natural, social and health sciences. Future research should be interdisciplinary as this will improve measurement of biodiversity, mental health and well-being.

Research Design
We encourage researchers to consider more robust designs such as before-and-after comparison studies, as well as to take advantage of natural experiment situations, and to consider development of integrative mixed method studies. Experimental studies, which test short-term effects, are particularly suited for assessing changes in momentary mental well-being. Future reviews of the influence of biodiversity and health could include a statistical meta-analysis to address the limitations from vote-counting reported here and in Lovell et al. (2014). Qualitative research designs could help identify what aspects of biodiversity people attend to, and what experiences this creates. This information could help to unravel the process by which biodiversity affects mental health and well-being.

Biodiversity Assessment
We encourage future research to use well accepted approaches for measuring biodiversity in the field or from secondary data, such as those used in the ecological

literature. The synthesis presented here indicates that different metrics of biodiversity (e.g. species richness; abundance) could play a role and should, therefore, have their relationships with mental health and well-being assessed separately. Functional aspects of biodiversity, such as phenotypic diversity (colour of fish, height of trees) (Botzat et al. 2016) and charismatic species (Dallimer et al. 2012) could also be usefully explored. Further, studies should also measure the biodiversity that is experienced by people, as opposed to the objectively measured diversity in an environment. The bird hiding in a bush, or the nocturnal mammal, that is not seen nor heard, is unlikely to be experienced by humans, and unlikely to influence mental health or well-being (Bell et al. 2014; Cox et al. 2017). Assessments of the biodiversity that people perceive or experience can be captured with Global Positioning System (GPS) trackers, eye-tracking technology and mobile electroencephalography (EEG) devices. We also recognise that one's perception of biodiversity is important for health and well-being. The synthesis presented here demonstrated that perceived species richness is associated with mental well-being. Future studies could investigate perceived species richness-mental health relationships. Further, whilst not investigated in any of the studies reviewed here, perceived biodiversity could also be investigated to assess whether it mediates the effect of objectively measured biodiversity on mental health and/or well-being. See de Vries and Snep Chap. 8, this volume, for further discussion on biodiversity measurement considerations.

Mental Health and Well-being Assessment

To facilitate cross study comparison, we encourage future research to use validated scales of mental health and well-being that have been used previously in psychology and health.[2] As such, researchers may wish to consider the reliability of using a mental health or well-being measure for understanding the biodiversity-health relationship. When developing new measures, theoretically grounded outcome measures are essential.

Theory

Future studies should articulate the theoretical framework(s) they are using to hypothesise about biodiversity-health relationships (see also Marselle Chap. 7, this volume). Researchers should use theory to drive the selection of outcome measures and identify mediators, moderators and confounders. To our knowledge, no study has investigated the effect of biodiversity on attention restoration, and more studies could investigate stress as an outcome measure; both of which explicitly test theories of restorative environments. Additionally, theories on the relationship of natural environments on health, such as Attention Restoration Theory could be developed further, e.g. by differentiating general effects of natural environments, and specific aspects of biodiversity, on health aspects.

Mechanisms

Future studies should continue to investigate the mediators of biodiversity and mental health and well-being using the pathways identified in nature-health frameworks (Hartig et al. 2014; Markevych et al. 2017).

[2] Researchers may wish to see Linton et al. (2016) for a list of such measures.

Moderators
Future studies should continue to investigate personal and contextual factors as moderators (Markevych et al. 2017) of biodiversity-mental health and well-being relationships.

Dose-Response Relationships
None of the studies examined dose-response relationships of biodiversity on mental health and well-being. At present, we do not know how much biodiversity is required for an effect, how long before effects take place, or how long they last. For example, future studies could usefully investigate the amount of time spent in the biodiverse environment required for a change in mental health or well-being.

Acknowledgements Thanks are due to Professor Zoe Davies and Professor Aletta Bonn for their comments on an earlier draft of this manuscript, the three peer reviewers, and to Popay et al. (2006) for permission to use the ESRC-funded Narrative Synthesis guidance. Dr. Martens' involvement was supported through funding from the Federal Agency for Nature Conservation, Germany. Dr. Irvine's involvement was supported through funding from Rural & Environment Science & Analytical Services Division of the Scottish Government. Dr. Dallimer's involvement was supported by the UK government's Natural Environment Research Council (NERC) grant number NE/R002681/1.

Appendix: Search Terms Used in Web of Science

	Search terms used	Number of references found
#01	Biodiversity OR 'species richness' OR 'protected area*' AND 'mental health' OR 'mental well-being' OR 'social cohesion' OR 'social well-being' or 'physical activity' TS = (biodiversity OR 'species richness' or 'protected area*') AND TS = ('mental health' OR 'mental well-being' OR 'social cohesion' OR 'social well-being' or 'physical activity') AND DOCUMENT TYPES: (Article). Timespan: 2013–2017. Indexes: SCI-EXPANDED, SSCI, A&HCI, ESCI.	79
#02	biodiversity AND 'mental health'	23
#03	biodiversity AND 'mental well-being'	3
#04	'species richness' AND 'mental health'	5
#05	'species richness' AND 'mental well-being'	1
#06	'protected area' AND 'mental health'	1
#07	'protected area' AND 'mental well-being'	0
#08	biodiversity AND 'physical activity'	39
#09	'species richness' AND 'physical activity'	6
#10	'protected area' AND 'physical activity'	3
#11	'protected area' AND 'social cohesion'	4
#12	'protected area' AND 'social well-being'	2
#13	biodiversity AND 'social cohesion'	16
#14	'species richness' AND 'social cohesion'	0
#15	'species richness' AND 'social well-being'	0
#16	biodiversity AND 'social well-being'	4
	Total references	189

References

Annerstedt van den Bosch MA, Östergren P, Grahn P, Skärbäck E, Währborg P (2015) Moving to serene nature may prevent poor mental health-results from a swedish longitudinal cohort study. Int J Environ Res Public Health 12:7974–7989

Annerstedt M, Östergren P, Björk J, Grahn P, Skärbäck E, Währborg P (2012) Green qualities in the neighbourhood and mental health – results from a longitudinal cohort study in Southern Sweden. BMC Public Health 12:337

Barton J, Hine R, Pretty J (2009) The health benefits of walking in green spaces of high natural and heritage value. J Integr Environ Sci 6:261–278

Bell R, Irvine K, Wilson C, Warber S (2014) Dark nature: exploring potential benefits of nocturnal nature-based interaction for human and environmental health. Eur J Ecopsychol 5:1–15

Björk J, Albin M, Grahn P, Jacobsson H, Ardö J, Wadbro J, Östergren P, Skärbäck E (2008) Recreational values of the natural environment in relation to neighbourhood satisfaction, physical activity, obesity and wellbeing. J Epidemiol Community Health 62(4):e2. https://doi.org/10.1136/jech.2007.062414

Botzat A, Fischer LK, Kowarik I (2016) Unexploited opportunities in understanding liveable and biodiverse cities. A review on urban biodiversity perception and valuation. Glob Environ Chang 39:220–233

Bowler DE, Buyung-Ali L, Knight T, Pullin AS (2010) A systematic review of evidence for the added benefits to health of exposure to natural environments. BMC Public Health 10:456. https://doi.org/10.1186/1471-2458-10-456

Carrus G, Scopelliti M, Lafortezza R, Colangelo G, Ferrini F, Salbitano F, Agrimi M, Portoghesi L, Semenzato P, Sanesi G (2015) Go greener, feel better? The positive effects of biodiversity on the well-being of individuals visiting urban and peri-urban green areas. Landsc Urban Plan 134:221–228

Convention on Biological Diversity (2017a) Recommendation adopted by the subsidiary body on scientific, technical and technological advice. XXI/3. Health and biodiversity. Available: https://www.cbd.int/doc/recommendations/sbstta-21/sbstta-21-rec-03-en.pdf. Accessed 17 May 2018

Convention on Biological Diversity (2017b) Workshop on Biodiversity and Health for the European Region. Available via: https://www.cbd.int/health/european/default.shtml. Accessed 17 May 2018

Cŏté IM, Curtis PS, Rothstein HR, Steward GB (2013) Gathering data: searching literature and selection criteria. In: Koricheva J, Gurevitch J, Mengersen K (eds) Handbook of meta-analysis in ecology and evolution. Princeton University Press, Princeton, p 37

Cox DTC, Shanahan DF, Hudson HL, Plummer KE, Sirwardena GM, Fuller RA, Anderson K, Hancock S, Gaston KJ (2017) Doses of neighborhood nature: the benefits for mental health of living with nature. Bioscience 67:147–155. https://doi.org/10.1093/biosci/biw173

Cracknell D, White MP, Pahl S, Nichols WJ, Depledge MH (2016) Marine biota and psychological well-being: a preliminary examination of dose–response effects in an aquarium setting. Environ Behav 48(10):1242–1269. https://doi.org/10.1177/0013916515597512

Cracknell D, White MP, Pahl S Depledge MH (2017) A preliminary investigation into the restorative potential of public aquaria exhibits: a UK student-based study. Landsc Res 42(1):18–32. https://doi.org/10.1080/01426397.2016.1243236

Curtin S (2009) Wildlife tourism: the intangible, psychological benefits of human-wildlife encounters. Curr Issue Tour 12(451):474

Dadvand P, Nieuwenhuijsen MJ, Esnaola M et al (2015) Green spaces and cognitive development in primary schoolchildren. PNAS 112(26):7937–7942

Dallimer M, Irvine KN, Skinner AMJ et al (2012) Biodiversity and the feel-good factor: understand associations between self-reports human well-being and species richness. Bioscience 62(1):47–55 de Jong K, Albin M, Starback E et al (2012) Perceived green qualities were associated with neighborhood satisfaction, physical activity, and general health: results from a cross-sectional study in suburban and rural Scania, southern Sweden. Health Place 18:1374–1380

Diener E, Emmons R, Larsen R, Griffin S (1985) The satisfaction with life scale. J Pers Assess 49(1):71–75

Duarte-Tagles H, Salinas-Rodriguez A, Idrovo AJ et al (2015) Biodiversity and depressive symptoms in Mexican adults: exploration of beneficial environmental effects. Biomedica 35:46–57. https://doi.org/10.7705/biomedica.v35i0.2433

EKLIPSE (2017) Types and components of natural or man-made urban and suburban green and blue spaces affecting human mental health and mental well-being. Available via: http://www.eklipse-mechanism.eu/documents/32503/0/Final_DoW_Health_08092017.pdf/d5e269a2-da6b-4809-9458-fd9747ca383c. Accessed 15 Jan 2018

Foo CH (2016) Linking forest naturalness and human wellbeing-a study on public's experiential connection to remnant forests within a highly urbanized region in Malaysia. Urban For Urban Green 16:13–24

Frumkin H (2001) Beyond toxicity: human health and the natural environment. Am J Prev Med 20(3):234–240

Fuller RA, Irvine KN, Devine-Wright P et al (2007) Psychological benefits of greenspace increase with biodiversity. Biol Lett 3:390–394

Grahn P, Stigsdotter UK (2010) The relation between perceived sensory dimensions or urban green space and stress restoration. Landsc Urban Plan 94:264–275

Groenewegen PP, van den Berg AE, Maas J et al (2012) Is a green residential environment better for health? If so, why? Ann Assoc Am Geogr 102(5):996–1003. https://doi.org/10.1080/00045608.2012.674899

Hartig T, Evans GW, Jamner LD et al (2003) Tracking restoration in natural and urban field settings. J Environ Psychol 23(2):109–123

Hartig T, Mitchell R, de Vries S Frumkin H (2014) Nature and health. Annu Rev Public Health 35:207–228. https://doi.org/10.1146/annurev-publhealth-032013-182443

Hedblom M, Knez I, Gunnarsson B (2017) Bird diversity improves the well-being of city residents. In: Murgui E, Hedblom M (eds) Ecology and conservation of birds in urban environments. Springer, Cham, pp 287–306

Horwitz P, Kretsch C (2015) Contribution of biodiversity and green spaces to mental and physical fitness, and cultural dimensions of health. In: World Health Organisation, Secretariat of the Convention on Biological Diversity (eds) Connecting global priorities: biodiversity and human health. A state of the knowledge review. World Health Organization, Geneva, p 200

Hough RL (2014) Biodiversity and human health: evidence for causality? Biodivers Conserv 23:267–288

Huby M, Cinderby S, Crowe AM et al (2006) The association of natural, social and economic factors with bird species richness in rural England. J Agric Econ 57(2):295–312

Huynen M, Martens P, de Groot RS (2004) Linkages between biodiversity loss and human health: a global indicator analysis. Int J Environ Health Res 14:13–30

Irvine KN, Warber SL (2002) Greening healthcare: practicing as if the natural environment really mattered. Altern Ther Health Med 8(5):76–83

Johansson M, Gyllin M, Witzell J, Küller M (2014) Does biological quality matter? Direct and reflected appraisal of biodiversity in temperate deciduous broad-leaf forest. Urban For Urban Green 13:28–37

Jones B (2017) Invasive species impacts on human well-being using the life satisfaction index. Ecol Econ 134(250):257

Jorgensen A, Wilson E, van den Berg A (2010) Evaluating stress relief in urban green and open spaces: does perceived naturalness make a difference?

Kaplan S (1995) The restorative benefits of nature: toward an integrative framework. J Environ Psychol 15(3):169–182

Kaplan R, Kaplan S (1989) The experience of nature: a psychological perspective. Cambridge University Press, Cambridge

Kellert SR, Wilson EO (eds) (1993) The Biophilia hypothesis. Island Press, Washington, DC

Keniger LE, Gaston KJ, Irvine KN, Fuller RA (2013) What are the benefits of interacting with nature? Int J Environ Res Public Health 10:913. https://doi.org/10.3390/ijerph10030913

Koricheva J, Gurevitch J, Mengersen K (eds) (2013) Handbook of meta-analysis in ecology and evolution. Princeton University Press, Princeton

Korpela KM, Stengård E, Jussila P (2016) Nature walks as part of a therapeutic intervention for depression. Ecopsychology 8:8–15. https://doi.org/10.1089/eco.2015.0070

Lemieux CJ, Eagles PF, Slocombe DS et al (2012) Human health and wellbeing motivations and benefits associated with protected area experiences: an opportunity for transforming policy and management in Canada. Parks 18:71–86

Linton M, Dieppe P, Medina-Lara A (2016) Review of 99 self-report measures for assessing well-being in adults: exploring dimensions of well-being and developments over time. BMJ Open 6(7). https://doi.org/10.1136/bmjopen-2015-010641

Lovell R, Wheeler BW, Higgins SL et al (2014) A systematic review of the health and wellbeing benefits of biodiverse environments. J Toxicol Environ Health B Crit Rev 17(1):1–20. https://doi.org/10.1080/10937404.2013.856361

Luck GW, Davidson P, Boxall D, Smallbone L (2011) Relations between urban bird and plant communities and human well-being and connection to nature. Conserv Biol 25:816–826

Markevych I, Schoierer J, Hartig T et al (2017) Exploring pathways linking greenspace to health: theoretical and methodological guidance. Environ Res 158:301–317. https://doi.org/10.1016/j.envres.2017.06.028

Marselle MR, Irvine KN, Lorenzo-Arribas A, Warber SL (2015) Moving beyond green: exploring the relationship of environment type and indicators of perceived environmental quality on emotional well-being following group walks. Int J Environ Res Public Health 12(1):106. https://doi.org/10.3390/ijerph120100106

Marselle MR, Irvine KN, Lorenzo-Arribas A, Warber SL (2016) Does perceived restorativeness mediate the effects of perceived biodiversity and perceived naturalness on emotional well-being following group walks in nature? J Environ Psychol 46:217–232

Pereira E, Queiroz C, Pereira HM, Vicente L (2005) Ecosystem services and human well-being: a participatory study in a mountain community in Portugal. Ecol Soc 10(2):41–64

Popay J, Roberts H, Sowden A et al (eds) (2006) Guidance on the conduct of narrative synthesis in systematic reviews. ESRC Methods Programme, Lancaster

Poudyal NC, Hodges DG, Bowker JM, Cordell HK (2009) Evaluating natural resource amenities in a human life expectancy production function. Forest Policy Econ 11:253–259

Rantakokko M, Keskinen KE, Kokko K, Portegijs E (2018) Nature diversity and well-being in old age. Aging Clin Exp Res 30(5):527–532. https://doi.org/10.1007/s40520-017-0797-5

Saw LE, Lim FKS, Carrasco LR (2015) The relationship between natural park usage and happiness does not hold in a tropical city-state. PLoS One 10(7):e0133781. https://doi.org/10.1371/journal.pone.0133781

Sieswerda LE, Soskolne CL, Newman SC et al (2001) Toward measuring the impact of ecological disintegrity on human health. Epidemiology 12:28–32

Thompson Coon J, Boddy K, Stein K et al (2011) Does participating in physical activity in outdoor natural environments have a greater effect on physical and mental wellbeing than physical activity indoors? A systematic review. Environ Sci Technol 45(5):1761–1772. https://doi.org/10.1021/es102947t

Tilt J, Unfried T, Roca B (2007) Using objective and subjective measures of neighborhood greenness and accessible destinations for understanding walking trips and BMI in Seattle, Washington. Am J Health Promot 21:371–379

Triguero-Mas M, Dadvand P, Cirach M et al (2015) Natural outdoor environments and mental and physical health: relationships and mechanisms. Environ Int 77(35):41

Ulrich R (1983) Aesthetic and affective response to natural environment. In: Altman I, Wohlwill J (eds) Human behavior and the natural environment. Plenum Press, New York, pp 85–125

Ulrich R, Simons R, Losito B et al (1991) Stress recovery during exposure to natural and urban environments. J Environ Psychol 11(3):201–230

United Nations (1992) Convention on biological diversity. Available via: https://www.cbd.int/doc/legal/cbd-en.pdf. Accessed 17 May 2018

WBGU – German Advisory Council on Global Change (2016) Humanity on the move: unlocking the transformative power of cities. WBGU, Berlin

Wheeler BW, Lovell R, Higgins SL et al (2015) Beyond greenspace: an ecological study of population general health and indicators of natural environment type and quality. Int J Health Geogr 14(1):17. https://doi.org/10.1186/s12942-015-0009-5

White MP, Weeks A, Hooper T et al (2017) Marine wildlife as an important component of coastal visits: the role of perceived biodiversity and species behaviour. Mar Policy 78(80):89

Whitmee S, Haines A, Beyrer C et al (2015) Safeguarding human health in the Anthropocene epoch: report of The Rockefeller Foundation–*Lancet* Commission on planetary health. Lancet 386:1973–2018. https://doi.org/10.1016/S0140-6736(15)60901-1

Wolf LJ, zu Ermgassen S, Balmford A et al (2017) Is variety the spice of life? An experimental investigation into the effects of species richness on self-reported mental well-being. PloS ONE 12(1):e0170225. https://doi.org/10.1371/journal.pone.0170225

World Health Organisation & Secretariat of the Convention on Biological Diversity (2015) Connecting global priorities: biodiversity and human health. A state of the knowledge review. Available via: http://www.who.int/globalchange/publications/biodiversity-human-health/en/. Accessed 17 May 2017

World Health Organization (1946) Preamble to the Constitution of the World Health Organization as adopted by the International Health Conference, New York, 19 June – 22 July 1946; signed on 22 July 1946 by the representatives of 61 States (Official Records of the World Health Organization, no. 2, p. 100) and entered into force on 7 April 1948. The definition has not been amended since 1948. Available via: http://www.who.int/suggestions/faq/en/. Accessed 17 May 2018

World Health Organization (2016) Mental health: strengthening our response. Fact Sheet. Available via: http://www.who.int/mediacentre/factsheets/fs220/en/. Accessed 17 May 2018

Chapter 10
Biodiversity and Spiritual Well-being

Katherine N. Irvine, Dusty Hoesly, Rebecca Bell-Williams, and Sara L. Warber

Abstract Among government agencies, practitioners and researchers there is growing interest in the potential of natural environments for human health and well-being. In parallel, conserving biodiversity is seen as critical in this effort. Likewise, spiritual well-being is increasingly considered as an important dimension of human health. This chapter examines the inter-relationship between biodiversity and spiritual well-being. We first consider what spiritual well-being is. Then, based on a review of literature, we discuss four themes that illustrate biodiversity and spiritual well-being relationships, including: (i) influence of spiritual traditions on biodiversity; (ii) sacred places as repositories of biodiversity; (iii) the spiritual domain within ecosystems services; and (iv) the effects of biodiversity on spiritual well-being. We bring these strands together in a conceptual model and discussion of measurement issues that can inform future research.

Keywords Spiritual traditions · Sacred places · Ecosystem services · Connectedness · Conceptual model

K. N. Irvine (✉)
Social, Economic and Geographical Sciences Research Group, The James Hutton Institute, Aberdeen, Scotland, UK
e-mail: katherine.irvine@hutton.ac.uk

D. Hoesly
University of California, Santa Barbara, CA, USA
e-mail: hoesly@ucsb.edu

R. Bell-Williams
University of Nottingham, Nottingham, UK

S. L. Warber
Department of Family Medicine, University of Michigan, Ann Arbor, MI, USA

European Centre for Environment and Human Health, University of Exeter Medical School, Truro, Cornwall, UK
e-mail: swarber@umich.edu

M. R. Marselle et al. (eds.), *Biodiversity and Health in the Face of Climate Change*, https://doi.org/10.1007/978-3-030-02318-8_10

Highlights

- Spiritual well-being includes relations to self, community, environment and a transcendent other(s).
- Spiritual beliefs and practices can foster respect and action for biodiversity.
- Few studies empirically examine the effect of biodiversity on spiritual well-being.
- Research can benefit from appropriate measures of spiritual well-being and biodiversity.
- Research could use existing conceptual frameworks for how nature affects human health.

10.1 Introduction

Governments and practice-focused organisations are interested in natural environments as a resource for improving human health and well-being (e.g. World Health Organization [WHO] & Secretariat of the Convention on Biological Diversity [CBD] 2015). Conserving biodiversity is increasingly considered critical for this effort (e.g. Hough 2014; Sandifer et al. 2015; CBD 2017a, b). In tandem, scholars and practitioners recognise spiritual well-being as an important dimension of human health (e.g. Chuengsatiansup 2003; McKee and Chappel 1992). This chapter focuses specifically on the beneficial relationships between biodiversity and the spiritual domain of human health and well-being. Our aims are to: (i) examine definitions of spiritual well-being; (ii) provide an overview of relationships between biodiversity and spiritual aspects of well-being; and (iii) develop a conceptual model to inform future research into the effects of biodiversity on spiritual well-being.

10.1.1 Our Approach

We conducted a literature review, identifying articles through structured searches and authors' knowledge of their respective fields. Searches were conducted primarily through Scopus and Web of Science and were supplemented by targeted topical sources (ATLA, PsychInfo, SSCI) and commercially available compilations (SpringerLink, JSTOR) alongside Google Scholar. As a starting point, we used definitions of biodiversity, health and spiritual well-being as indicated in Box 10.1.

Search terms included combinations of biodiversity, ecology or environment with spirit*, relig*, sacred, faith, well-being, health, meaning, connection, indigenous or beliefs. Searches were limited by language (English) and publication year (1945–2017). We sought to identify empirical studies whenever possible. Titles and abstracts were reviewed to assess relevance and focus; because of our focus on spiritual well-being (rather than physical health) and relative expertise, we excluded from consideration literature focused on medicinal plants, microbial diversity, economic valuation and environmental justice. When available, we noted research

Box 10.1: Definitions of Biodiversity, Health, Spiritual Well-Being

- **Biodiversity** is "the variability among living organisms from all sources including, *inter alia*, terrestrial, marine and other aquatic ecosystems and the ecological complexes of which they are part; this includes diversity within species, between species and of ecosystems" (United Nations 1992, p. 3).
- **Health** is "a state of complete physical, mental and social well-being and not merely the absence of disease or infirmity" (WHO 1948).
- **Spiritual well-being** is "concerned with meaning, connection to something greater than oneself and, in some cases, a faith in a higher power" (Linton et al. 2016, p. 12).

design, measurement – of biodiversity, of spiritual well-being – mediating pathways and moderating variables. We undertook a thematic, narrative analysis of the literature. Findings were interpreted through the lens of four spiritual well-being domains identified through our examination of definitions of spiritual well-being (see Sect. 10.2).

10.1.2 Our Biases

Our approach to such a task has several biases that we think are important to delineate up front. First, the authors' different ways of knowing – academic researchers; disciplinary training in environmental psychology (KNI, RB-W), sociology and religious studies (DH); integrative family medicine (SLW); and Western worldview (USA, UK) – bring a certain perspective to the selection and interpretation of the literature. Second, while we recognise that aspects of religious traditions can have negative effects on biodiversity (e.g. White 1967) and that not all experiences of biodiversity or nature foster well-being (e.g. Dallimer et al. 2012, see pp. 52–53; Heintzman 2016, see pp. 394–395), this chapter focuses on beneficial aspects of the biodiversity/spiritual well-being nexus. Third, although this is a chapter about the relationship between biodiversity and spiritual well-being, our author team does not include an ecologist, which limits our interpretation of the biodiversity component within the selected literature.

10.1.3 Chapter Structure

In Sect. 10.2 we provide a contextualised understanding of the concept of spiritual well-being that is taken forward throughout the chapter. We discuss four themes from our assessment of the literature in Sect. 10.3: (i) influence of spiritual traditions on biodiversity; (ii) sacred places as repositories of biodiversity; (iii) spiritual domain within ecosystems services; and (iv) the effects of biodiversity on spiritual well-being. Section 10.4 considers future directions for research.

10.2 Defining Spiritual Well-Being

The World Health Organization's (WHO) (1948) definition of health emphasises physical, mental and social well-being (Box 10.1). While lauded as a holistic approach to health, the importance of considering the spiritual domain is increasingly being recognized as well. This can be found, for example, in the WHO's Health Promotion Glossary (1998) and discussions of health impact assessments (Chuengsatiansup 2003) as well as in medicine's expanded focus on a biopsychosocial-spiritual model of health (e.g. McKee and Chappel 1992). In debates about health and wellness, spiritual health is considered by some as a component of overall health or integral to holistic health (e.g. Greenberg 1985; Hawks 1994), and there is a rich body of research on its role in illness recovery and end-of-life care (e.g. McClain et al. 2003; Lin and Bauer-Wu 2003) as well as its effect on other dimensions of health (e.g. depression; Bekelman et al. 2007). Despite this growing interest, definitional debates over the meaning – and measurement – of the spiritual domain continue.

To understand these definitional challenges we first consider the wider context within which the notion of spiritual well-being sits. While the word 'spirituality' historically arises from a Christian milieu (Principe 1983), it has been applied to non-Christian religions (e.g. Buddhism) and to non-religious orientations such as 'secular spirituality' (Jespers 2011; van Ness 1996). Such applications inevitably raise questions about the concepts of 'religion' and 'spirituality' as well as 'religious' and 'spiritual' (Casey 2013) – terms that are themselves difficult to define, and for which varying, and sometimes overlapping, definitions exist. For example, while some scholars describe spirituality as a subset of religion (Streib and Hood 2011), others consider these concepts as independent yet complementary (e.g. Berghuijs et al. 2013; Zinnbauer et al. 1997). Typically, religiousness is described narrowly as "formally structured and identified with religious institutions and prescribed theology and rituals" (Zinnbauer et al. 1997, p. 551), whereas spirituality is considered more expansively as subjective, eclectic and individualised, with authority deriving from personal experience (Fuller 2001). In one cross-cultural study (Gall et al. 2011), survey respondents claimed that spirituality referred to core aspects of personal identity and experiences of transcendence – "defined traditionally as God or a higher power, or in more secular terms as unity with the greater world or mystery" (p. 158) – with religion seen as a pathway for accessing spirituality and community. These scholarly distinctions between religion and spirituality reflect the growing population of those who identify as "spiritual but not religious" (Saucier and Skrzypinksa 2006). Rican (2004) and Moberg (2010) provide useful overviews of these debates.

These conceptual difficulties and cultural transformations have proved problematic for efforts to define and measure spiritual well-being. Its meaning is also often confused by the use of similar concepts, including spiritual health (e.g. Bensley 1991) and spiritual wellness (e.g. Westgate 1996), with debate as to whether these are synonymous or distinct (e.g. Ingersoll 1998). Some scholars (Klein et al. 2016; Koenig 2008; Moreira-Almeida and Koenig 2006; Salander 2006; Tsuang et al. 2007) have argued that spiritual well-being conceptually overlaps too much with existential well-being, psychological well-being and mental health, suggesting that spiritual well-being may be insufficiently distinct to stand as a separate category in rigorous empirical research. Similar problems attend distinctions among psychological, emotional or mental well-being (Hird 2003; Veenhoven 2008). These disparities may be a corollary to the fact that discussions are undertaken across multiple fields of inquiry: sociology (e.g. Moberg 1971, 1979), psychology (e.g. Paloutzian and Ellison 1982; Ellison, C. 1983), palliative care (e.g. Lin and Bauer-Wu 2003), nursing (e.g. Buck 2006) and leisure studies (e.g. Jepson 2015), which may understand and use the terms differently.

The concept of 'spiritual well-being' originated in the sociology of aging and health (Moberg 1971); there, it referred to social and psychological adjustments that draw upon a person's "inner resources" and "central philosophy of life" to provide meaning, stability and coping (p. 10). Spiritual well-being was subsequently defined at the US-based National Interfaith Coalition on Aging (NICA) as "the affirmation of life in a relationship with God, self, community and the environment that nurtures and celebrates wholeness" (NICA 1975, as cited in Moberg 1984, p. 352). This definition provides some guidance for understanding the phrase "connection to something greater than oneself" in Linton et al.'s (2016) definition of spiritual well-being. J. Fisher (2011) has further developed the relational element, arguing that spiritual health is dependent on the "extent to which people are living in harmony within relationships" (p. 21), i.e. relation with self, relations with community, relation with the environment and relation with a transcendent other(s). Thus, for J. Fisher (2011), "when [these] relationships are not right, or are absent, we lack wholeness, or health" (p. 23).

Across multiple disciplines, conceptualisations of the spiritual aspect of well-being and health appear to share a number of consistent features (Table 10.1) including: meaning, intrinsic values, wholeness, community relationship and transcendence (Bensley 1991; Fisher, J. 2011; Hawks 1994; Hood-Morris 1996; Ingersoll 1994; Westgate 1996). J. Fisher's (2011) articulation of the environmental aspect of spiritual well-being suggests that a relationship with the environment can go "beyond care and nurture for the physical or biological, to a sense of awe and wonder" (p. 22) and, for some, a sense of unity with the environment and a feeling of connection to nature. This same sense of oneness with nature is identified in Hawks' (1994) spiritual health literature review, which also examined how a spiritually-well individual would outwardly act (e.g. altruism, compassion, service).

This section has examined the development of the concept of spiritual well-being, the health contexts in which it originated and the variety of meanings that have been applied to the term 'spiritual' over time. For the purposes of this chapter, we take

Table 10.1 Proposed features of spiritual well-being organised by four relational domains of self, others, environment and transcendent other(s) (Fisher, J. 2011). These domains and their proposed features are used to interpret the identified literature in terms of the relationships between biodiversity and spiritual well-being

Domains	Example references
1. Self	
Meaning – meaning and purpose in life	Hawks (1994), Linton et al. (2016), and Westgate (1996)
Intrinsic values – values and beliefs of community and self; concern and care for something greater than self	Bensley (1991) and Westgate (1996)
Wholeness – a sense of completeness in life; a sense of all well-being dimensions being met	Bensley (1991) and Fisher (2011)
2. Others	
Community relationship – connectedness with others; in-depth relationships	Bensley (1991), Ellison (1983), Fisher (2011), Hawks (1994), Ingersoll (1994), and Westgate (1996)
3. Environment	
Environment – connection with nature; oneness with nature	Fisher (2011) and Buck (2006)
4. Transcendent other	
Transcendence – beliefs relating to something beyond the human level; the human-spiritual interaction; unity with something beyond the material world	Bensley (1991), Ellison (1983), Fisher (2011), Hood-Morris (1996), and Westgate (1996)
Divine – a god-like force; conception of the divine	Bensley (1991) and Moberg (1971)

forward an expanded understanding of spiritual well-being that encompasses one's relationships with the self, the community, the environment and a transcendent other(s) inclusive of the different features identified in Table 10.1. In Sect. 10.4.2 we discuss challenges in measurement of spiritual well-being.

10.3 Themes Within the Literature

Few empirical studies were identified that specifically investigated the effect of biodiversity on spiritual well-being. The literature did contain a rich account of the multiple relationships among various spiritual traditions, ecology and biodiversity conservation, including spiritual aspects of well-being, which we considered important to delineate. The identified literature is clustered into four themes: the influence of different spiritual traditions on biodiversity; sacred places as repositories of biodiversity; the spiritual domain ecosystem services; and the effects of biodiversity on spiritual well-being. Figure 10.1 provides a visual representation of these biodiversity/spiritual well-being relationships.

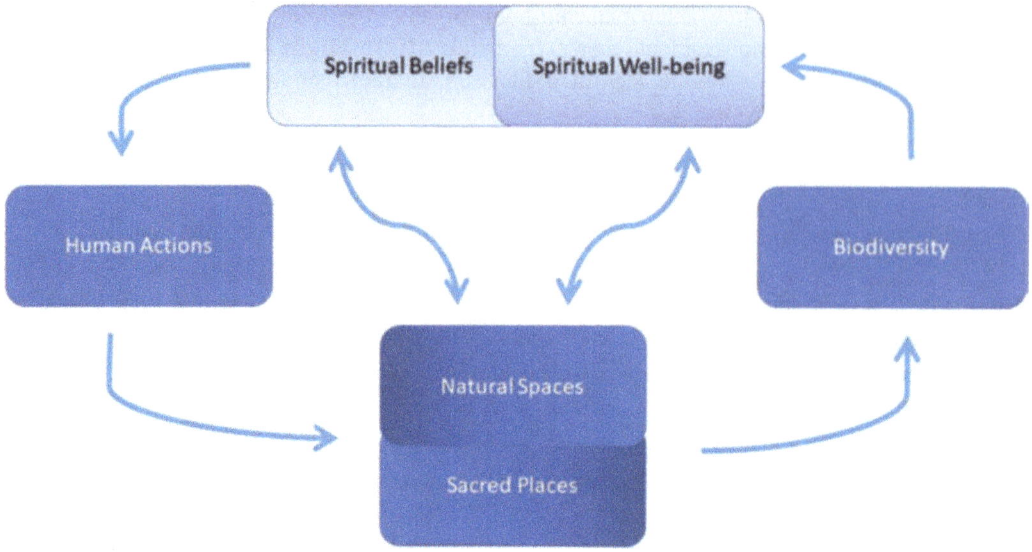

Fig. 10.1 Relationships among spiritual beliefs, nature, biodiversity and spiritual well-being. Our four themes are demonstrated in different sections of the diagram. The left side demonstrates how spiritual beliefs influence human actions and have influence on natural spaces (Sect. 10.3.1). The lower half of the diagram depicts how human actions (or protection from human actions) on sacred spaces affect biodiversity (Sect. 10.3.2). The center of the diagram demonstrates the bidirectional relations between spiritual beliefs, spiritual well-being, natural spaces and sacred places as reflected in ecosystem services literature (Sect. 10.3.3). The right side of diagram reflects the effects of nature and biodiversity on human spiritual well-being (Sect. 10.3.4). (Illustration by SL Warber and KN Irvine)

10.3.1 Influence of Spiritual Traditions on Biodiversity

The spirituality-nature connection has been explored across several academic disciplines and religious traditions, giving rise to a number of related topics, such as nature religion, nature spirituality, ecological spirituality, ecofeminist spirituality, eco-spirituality and ecotheology (see Kinsley 1995). Grim and Tucker (2014) and Kinsley (1995) outline how various indigenous traditions, 'world religions' and emerging spiritualities (e.g. Neopaganism) inspire ecological action and a deep relationship with the earth and all its beings. In an era of increased resource extraction and species extinction, it has been argued that such connections can foster conservation of biodiversity (Golliher 1999; Hamilton and Takeuchi 1993; Negi 2005).

10.3.1.1 Indigenous Spiritual Beliefs and Practices

Many indigenous cultures worldwide have spiritual beliefs, ethical values and/or traditional practices that directly link to the environment (Bodeker 1999; Posey 1999). For example, Gregory Cajete (Tewa), a Native North American educator, emphasises the importance of understanding and incorporating an indigenous worldview to achieve long-term sustainability. He repeats an admonishment from Tewa elders to "look to the mountain", that is, to think about the impact on future generations over thousands of years. He argues that "Indian kinship with the land, its climate, soil, water, mountains, lakes, forests, streams, plants, and animals has literally determined the expressions of an American Indian theology [of place]" (Cajete 1999, p. 3).

Grim (2001) asserts that most native peoples share a perception that non-human beings are equal in status with humans, that all life exists in familial relationships, and that these relationships are sustained in ritually prescribed ways that often conserve biodiversity. While "there is no one 'indigenous' view on religion and ecology… spiritual relationships established between native peoples and their homelands" often foster ecological commitments and activism, including biodiversity conservation (Grim 2001, p. xxxiv). For example, the indigenous Ifugao Igorots of the Philippines conduct rituals led by a native priest to control rice pests, thus preserving plant species on which the Igorots rely for food. Additionally, the Ifugao believe that "nature spirits" inhabit trees and stones in forests and watersheds, which are "centers of biodiversity," including over 200 plant varieties (Tauli-Corpuz 2001, p. 295).

Furthermore, indigenous groups value reciprocity. They care for the land, and thus their health, including spiritual well-being, is maintained. K. Wilson (2003) writes of the importance of tangible places for maintaining the physical, emotional, mental and spiritual health of individuals and communities among the Anishinabek (Ojibway and Odawa) living in northern Ontario, Canada. She summarises this as:

> Activities such as hunting and harvesting are not only of nutritional benefit, which supports physical health, they also allow individuals to connect spiritually with Mother Earth, the Creator and spirits while being on the land. This is important because it allows individuals to pursue simultaneously physical and spiritual connections to the land that are important for emotional and mental health (Wilson, K. 2003, p. 90).

Many native peoples have engaged – and continue to engage – in local ecological activism to preserve their lands, cultures and spiritual traditions, struggles that often preserve biodiversity. For example, in the 1970s the James Bay Cree in Quebec taught non-natives their spiritual worldview and formed a coalition to oppose a hydroelectric dam that threatened Cree hunting spaces and lifeways (Feit 2001). The dam threatened the destruction of many species on which the Cree rely for sustenance and cultural vitality as well as the ancestral homeland where Cree spirits live alongside them. More recently, Native Hawaiians protested the construction of a new telescope on Mauna Kea because it was to be located on a sacred mountain that is rich in biodiversity and home to important native deities. In Nigeria and other West African countries, native African religious traditions have blended with African Christian churches to support tree-planting projects, including developing "inter-religious rituals" that "tap salient aspects of indigenous knowledge" and add "conscious, proactive conservation" of biodiversity (Kalu 2001, p. 242).

Grim (2001) observes that native lifeways that stress the inter-relatedness of all beings do not necessarily result in ecological balance or harmony, and that romanticised notions of the "ecological Indian" could disempower native actors in their environments (p. xxxiv–xxxvii). Despite these caveats, the examples provided in this section illustrate the potential of indigenous worldviews to promote biodiversity conservation. The deep connection with the earth and reverence for nature and spirits that inhabit the natural world that are expressed through indigenous beliefs and practices echo themes of environmental connection and relations with a transcendent other(s) found in spiritual well-being definitions. Thus, indigenous biodiversity conservation can be a pathway from spiritual beliefs to spiritual well-being.

10.3.1.2 World Religions and Alternative Spiritualities

Ethical prescriptions and community practices that can promote ecological conservation are also present in various 'world religions' and alternative spiritualities. Whether the divine is seen as transcendent or immanent, dualistic or monistic, the range of beliefs and practices described in this section demonstrate increasing concern for biodiversity and engagement in specific actions to preserve it.

The Religions of the World and Ecology series from Harvard University Press illustrates the vitality of concern for ecological conservation within many 'world religions'. The series includes volumes on Buddhism, Christianity, Confucianism, Daoism, Hinduism, Indigenous Traditions, Islam, Jainism and Judaism. Similarly, various 'world religions' alongside other spiritual orientations are included in several scholarly handbooks on religion and ecology (e.g. Jenkins et al. 2017), at least one of which includes a chapter on biodiversity (Lovejoy 2017). In Hinduism, for example, natural objects such as rivers, trees, stones and animals can manifest the sacred as forms of divinity worthy of devotion and conservation. As one Hindu woman explains: "When I look into the face of the goddess on the tree, I feel a strong connection (*sambandha*) with this tree" (Haberman 2017, p. 40). Such an orientation can lead to environmental activism, for example, cleaning up the polluted Yamuna River in northern India or protecting sacred groves threatened with deforestation (Haberman 2017). Similarly, Buddhist environmentalists rely on Buddhist teachings about interdependence to support claims to oneness with nature and conservation. Joanna Macy, an eco-Buddhist activist, writes that in Buddhism the egotistical self is "replaced by wider constructs of identity and self-interest– by what you might call the ecological self or the eco-self, co-extensive with other beings and the life on our planet" (quoted in Ives 2017, p. 44). These religious perspectives, based on modern interpretations of ancient traditions, can spur people toward conservation of biodiversity.

Some Christian theologians and ethicists argue that since biodiversity is part of God's creation, it must be conserved (Jenkins 2003, 2013; McFague 1997; O'Brien 2010; S. Taylor 2007). They suggest that since God is present in all things, experiences of biodiversity are sacramental opportunities and that human-created species loss impoverishes the human connection to God. Catholic theologians have discussed how biodiversity gives rise to sacred feelings of enchantment and suggests the divine multiplicity of the Holy Trinity (Boff 1997). Pope Francis' environmentalist encyclical *Laudato Si'* (2015) includes a major section entitled "loss of biodiversity", lamenting species extinction caused by capitalist exploitation and calling on people of faith to protect all life. The pope claims biodiversity is important intrinsically but also for its potential for food, medicine and other factors: "Because of us, thousands of species will no longer give glory to God by their very existence, nor convey their message to us. We have no such right" (p. 25). Jewish leaders have also reinterpreted their tradition to provide a "foundation for a Jewish ethic of biodiversity" based on biblical texts that show "God creates, takes care of, and takes pleasure in the diversity of life in the world" (Troster 2008, p. 4 and 11). From this theocentric perspective, Creation provides an environmental "ethic of the inherent value of all species which would… demand the preservation of whole ecosystems… where all creation becomes a source of wonder" (Troster 2008, p. 16). Reinterpreting sacred texts in light of present environmental concerns has led religious leaders to advocate eco-activism and biodiversity conservation.

Indeed, a large-scale 'religious environmentalism' movement in America has challenged prior emphases on humanity's dominion over the earth, instead insisting on 'creation care' or 'stewardship' as a central religious principle (Ellingson 2015; Fowler 1995; Gottlieb 2006a). Early American impulses toward environmental preservation and conservation emerged from the idea that nature is God's creation and should be protected in all its diversity (Berry 2015; Stoll 2015). Similarly, some British Muslims have used Islamic principles to grow gardens in neglected public green spaces to preserve natural habitats, reduce mosque carbon footprints and build environmental sustainability organisations that have helped facilitate biodiversity conservation (Gilliat-Ray and Bryant 2011).

New Age and Neopagan spiritualities, including Wicca and Goddess worship, are also engaged in biodiversity conservation, in part because practitioners experience spiritual well-being through interaction with nature. These new religions draw on indigenous traditions, Asian religions and/or Western sources to create holistic spiritualities based on unity with nature and harmony with natural cycles. As Neopagan leader Starhawk writes: "The craft is earth religion, and our basic orientation is to the earth, to life, to nature.… All that lives (and all that is, lives), all that serves life, is Goddess" (1979, p. 263). Identification with nature in all its diverse manifestations impels Neopagans to protect nature through social engagement and religious practice. One survey study showed that members of such alternative spirituality movements view both experiences in nature and environmental actions as spiritual (Bloch 1998). One practitioner of this Gaia-centered spirituality said that "getting back to the earth" means to "give back and give thanks to the earth, and be more of that one community… [of] oneness" (Bloch 1998, p. 66). Based on these views and experiences with nature, many Neopagan and New Age people engage in ecological activism and preservation efforts, including "recycling, tree-planting, alternative energy strategies, petitions, and so forth" (Bloch 1998, p. 59).

10.3.1.3 Nature Spirituality

Apart from the discrete traditions discussed above, our review of the literature found voluminous sources on 'nature spirituality', which can be related to particular religious traditions or its own orientation (e.g. Gottlieb 2013). In his book on nature spirituality, B. Taylor (2009) defines 'dark green religion' as that "in which nature is sacred, has intrinsic value, and is therefore due reverent care" (p. 10). Contemporary nature spiritualities combine indigenous, Asian, Western and scientific sources to foster biophilic kinship, reverence and humility, and a metaphysics of interconnection and interdependence wherein biological diversity is intrinsically valuable and sacred, and thus worthy of defense (B. Taylor 2009, 2012). Related worldviews include deep ecology (Sessions 1995), eco-spirituality (Cummings 1991) and other earth-based spiritualities. Examples of biodiversity conservation actions rooted in nature spirituality include protecting endangered species, preserving natural habitats, supporting environmental regulations, and protesting polluters (B. Taylor 2012). These feelings of connection, humility and transcendence align with concepts of spiritual well-being outlined in Sect. 10.2.

Historian Michael P. Nelson claims that people commonly argue for wilderness preservation because nature is a "site for spiritual, mystical, or religious encounters: places to experience mystery, moral regeneration, spiritual revival, meaning, oneness, unity, wonder, awe, inspiration, or a sense of harmony with the rest of creation – all essential religious experiences" (quoted in Gottlieb 2006b, p. 15). This motive is amply demonstrated across a variety of religious and spiritual traditions, linking various spiritual ecologies (Sponsel 2012) with experiences of spiritual well-being and biodiversity conservation. The indigenous traditions, world religions, alternative spiritualities and nature spiritualities described in Sect. 10.3.1 promote a view of humans as interdependent and interrelated with the rest of the natural world, living in reverential humility with fellow natural beings, and thus inspiring ecological activism. These worldviews and their related practices can result in conservation of biodiversity and increased spiritual well-being, expressed through experiences of connection, meaning and transcendence in nature.

10.3.2 Sacred Places as Repositories of Biodiversity

In addition to spiritual beliefs and practices that can foster respect and action for biodiversity, we found ample sources on sacred natural sites as repositories of biodiversity. Spiritual values and taboos associated with sacred natural sites can help to preserve biodiversity (Dudley et al. 2009, 2010; Verschuure et al. 2010). In this context, sacred places are natural areas that have special significance for local communities, often linked to religious myths or rites. In their review of this topic, Dudley Higgins-Zogib and Mansourian (2009) conclude that sacred natural sites, which are often rich in biodiversity, "can contribute to biodiversity conservation strategies" due to the special precautions associated with them (p. 575). Additionally, conservation of these sites aids the preservation of local cultures and their traditional ecological knowledges.

Of particular interest amongst researchers in this area are sacred groves and sacred forests (e.g. Juhé-Beaulaton 2008; Ormsby and Bhagwat 2010; Sheridan and Nyamweru 2008; Sponsel 2012; Tomalin 2009). Sacred groves are patches of natural vegetation dedicated to local deities and protected by religious tenets and cultural traditions; they may also be tree-stands raised in honor of heroes and warriors and maintained by the local community (Ramanujam and Cyril 2003). Taboos against over-harvesting, harming particular sacred species or disrupting the ecological balance of sacred groves and forests can preserve species richness. For example, the Nkodurom and Pinkwae sacred groves in Ghana have been protected through traditional beliefs and taboos, resulting in preservation of threatened mollusk, turtle, monkey and heron species (Ntiamoa-Baidu 2008). In India, the number and spatial distribution of sacred groves creates a network that preserves "a sizable portion of the local biodiversity in areas where it would not be feasible to maintain large tracts of protected forests" (Bhagwat and Rutte 2006, p. 520). Local traditions that include worshipping trees in a sacred grove helped to preserve a rare bat species, and, in another area, spiritual beliefs about a hidden shrine within a sacred grove preserved riparian forests and streams (Bhagwat and Rutte 2006). In central Italy, local Catholic practices around pilgrimage sites have helped to conserve biodiversity through preserving relic habitats and vegetation assemblages, protecting old growth forests and tree species, and maintaining greater habitat heterogeneity due to sacred grottos and water sources (Frascaroli 2013). Reflecting on forest preservation by the official association of Shinto shrines in Japan, Rots (2015) observes: "The significance of these forests … extends well beyond ecology and nature conservation proper. Constituting continuity between the present and the ancestral past, they have come to be seen as local community centers that provide social cohesion and spiritual well-being" (p. 209).

Many studies of biodiversity at sacred sites have used standard ecological survey techniques of tree species diversity, tree species richness, regeneration status, floristic surveys of vegetation composition and ethnobotanical uses of species (Bharathi and Devi Prasad 2017; Hu et al. 2011; Khumbongmayum et al. 2005). An alternative approach was taken by Anderson et al. (2005) in documenting the biodiversity of sacred mountains in the Himalayas of Tibet. Existing vegetation maps and geographic information systems (GIS) were used to remotely assess species composition, diversity and frequency of useful and endemic plant species. Sacred mountains had significantly greater overall species diversity than surrounding areas. These studies highlight the various measures being used to document biodiversity preservation in sacred protected areas.

10.3.3 Spiritual Domain Within Ecosystem Services

A third way in which biodiversity and the spiritual domain of human health and well-being can be considered is through the lens of ecosystem services (ESS). The ESS concept broadly frames the relationship between people and nature in terms of benefits and services, i.e. the benefits people derive from the 'services' provided by ecosystems (Millennium Ecosystem Assessment [MEA] 2005). This framework has been used to try to incorporate the value – often in monetary terms – of these services for use in decision-making (Fisher, B. et al. 2009). The MEA (2005) structured ESS into four clusters: provisioning (the products obtained from ecosystems, e.g. food, water), regulating (benefits obtained from the regulation of ecosystems, e.g. water purification, pest control), supporting (processes necessary to produce other ESS, e.g. soil formation, photosynthesis) and cultural ("nonmaterial benefits that people obtain from ecosystems through spiritual enrichment, cognitive development, reflection, recreation and aesthetic experiences" [MEA 2005, p. 4]). There is ongoing debate over the concept of and categorisation of ESS, the relationship between and operationalisation of 'service' and 'benefit' – in particular those conceived of as 'cultural' – as well as the knowledge base that has informed such effort (see Daniel et al. 2012; Díaz et al. 2018). Our focus here is to understand how spiritual well-being is discussed and operationalised in relation to biodiversity in this literature.

The language within this literature refers to spirituality, spiritual enrichment, spiritual values, spiritual fulfilment and spiritual benefits (e.g. MEA 2005; WHO and CBD 2015; UK National Ecosystem Assessment Follow-on 2014). One of the few specific mentions of spiritual well-being is found within the framing of spiritual and religious values, described as:

> Sacred elements of the biota, worship of biota, kindness and gratitude toward biota together or individually make a contribution to spiritual well-being, and a sense of wholeness and being 'at one', everywhere and forever (connecting the present with the past and the future) (WHO and CBD 2015, p. 213).

This description implies that spiritual well-being – and aspects conceived in this chapter as features of spiritual well-being, i.e. wholeness and connectedness (Table 10.1) – could be indirectly related to biodiversity through incorporating elements of the natural world into religious/spiritual practices. For example, a ceremony dedicated to the jaguar in southern Mexico among the Nahuatl (Caballero et al. 1998, cited in Russell et al. 2013) demonstrates how a particular species could serve local communities' spiritual well-being. Another route through which one might experience spiritual well-being is through acts of 'kindness and gratitude', for example, through environmental conservation volunteering. The following examples illustrate ways in which researchers have sought to measure the spiritual dimension of ESS and integrate biodiversity to enhance understanding of the relationship.

Using the ESS framework, De Lacy and Shackleton (2017) conducted a socio-ecological study of sacred urban greenspaces (i.e. gardens associated with places of worship) in South Africa to investigate the contribution of biodiversity (measured using ecological surveys) to worshipers' spiritual and aesthetic experience (collected via questionnaires). Analysis found a positive association between woody plant basal area (an indicator of volume or the footprint of an area taken up by trunks and stems) and participants' spiritual and aesthetic experience. The aesthetic experience was also positively associated with woody plant species richness and abundance (number of woody plants).

Hunter and Brehm (2004) explore spiritual values in their qualitative study of rural residents living in proximity to a national forest in the USA previously identified as a 'hotspot' for vertebrate biodiversity. Spiritual values were expressed in terms of biophilic moralistic values, defined as "a spiritual reverence and ethical concern for nature" (Kellert 1996, as cited in Hunter and Brehm 2004, p. 14). Interview participants described a responsibility on the part of humans to be good stewards for the environment and an inter-reliance between people and wildlife. For a few, this moral value was expressed in terms of a spiritual connection, e.g. "... yeah, I think there is certainly a spiritual connection between me and the animals around me" (as quoted in Hunter and Brehm 2004, p. 21). Such statements are also illustrative of the spiritual well-being domain of connection with nature (Table 10.1).

Callicott et al. (2007) approach the integration of biodiversity and spirituality through the use of biocomplexity modelling, the simulation of coupled biodiverse environments and human systems. This modelling considers material connections (e.g. through food, building materials; a.k.a. provisioning ESS) and psycho-spiritual connections (e.g. through religiously significant sites, ethnic identity) to the natural environment. Through a case-study analysis of biocomplex sites, the researchers operationalise the psycho-spiritual through an examination of the cultural history of the place. In their South American case study, the psycho-spiritual connectivity focuses on the symbolic meaning, religious practices and cultural identity associated with the natural setting. They argue that such modelling "may reveal historic synergies and symbioses between human systems (human life ways and livelihoods) and natural systems that may be useful for future biodiversity conservation strategies" (Callicott et al. 2007, p. 323).

Delgado et al. (2010) consider a biocultural approach to the management of natural resources that includes sacred natural sites, biodiversity conservation, spiritual values and spiritual well-being of local indigenous peoples. Working with local community members and other stakeholders, a set of mutually agreed upon indicators and criteria of spiritual well-being were developed; these included teaching and revitalisation of spiritual knowledge and the extent to which sacred sites were used and considered valuable by the local community. To assess spiritual well-being over time, the approach measured the proportion of families who implement ritual practices. By linking these ritual practices with measures of biodiversity conservation, the authors conclude that "human well-being and biodiversity is intimately related in sacred natural sites and imbued with spiritual values" (Delgado et al. 2010,

p. 192). Other authors have drawn similar conclusions that, due to their importance for local environmental decision-making, "sacred natural sites support spiritual well-being that many people find in their relationship with nature" (e.g. Verschuuren 2010, p. 63; see also Sect. 10.3.2).

Emerging from both conceptual frameworks and empirical evidence, the above examples suggest that the relationship between biodiversity and the spiritual domain is strongly related to cultural beliefs and practices, both current and historical. Cooper et al. (2016) and Russell et al. (2013) have argued that much of the ESS literature on the spiritual dimension of ESS and spiritual well-being focuses on indigenous peoples. We observe that the language within this literature suffers from a conflation of spiritual beliefs (antecedents) and spiritual well-being (outcomes), as discussed previously. We would add that most studies produce associative findings and few studies directly measure the relational aspects of spiritual well-being as contained within Table 10.1.

10.3.4 *Effects of Biodiversity on Spiritual Well-Being*

The preceding sections examined how spiritual beliefs/practices may influence attitudes and actions towards biodiversity, and how sacred natural sites might aid biodiversity conservation. We saw that religious worldviews and practices regarding nature and biodiversity can foster meaning, connection with nature and feelings of transcendence, linking them at least implicitly with spiritual well-being. Likewise, these attributes of spiritual well-being can be found in sacred natural sites that conserve biodiversity, and within the ecosystem services literature there continues to be a focus on clarification, measurement and integration of the spiritual aspect of well-being in relation to the natural environment. In this section, our focus is on how biodiversity and biodiverse settings contribute to spiritual well-being. While no studies explicitly investigated biodiversity's effect on spiritual well-being, we examine this relationship through an interpretation of several strands of research using our derived categories of spiritual well-being (Table 10.1).

10.3.4.1 Spiritual Outcomes from Wilderness Recreation

Within the field of leisure studies, a body of research has specifically examined the spiritual experience of wilderness settings. Price (1996) identified wilderness recreational activities as a form of modern secular spirituality and developed a taxonomy that includes: adventurous (e.g. mountaineering, surfing); observational (e.g. whale-watching, sightseeing); blended adventurous and observational (e.g. fly-fishing, scuba diving); and educational, such as programmes that embed an individual within a wilderness setting to learn skills (e.g. Outward Bound). He asserts that these nature-focused activities, where one encounters the natural environment as wilderness, can provide transformative experiences of that which is totally 'other'. He notes:

> Each of these recreational activities offers an experience in nature that often provides the participants with a sense of wonder, awe, wholeness, harmony, ecstasy, transcendence, and solitude. … Each can transfix and transform. Each takes place in a natural arena where the trials of the heart and the tribulations of the soul can be overcome (Price 1996, p. 415).

Price suggests that "the reason for returning to nature…is to regain touch with the divine" (p. 440) and that "replenished spiritually by the experience, the participants hope to retain its joy, its serenity, … its harmony" (p. 441), elements Hawks (1994) associates with spiritual well-being.

Curtin's (2009) study of wildlife tourists examined observational recreational activities and psychological well-being. Drawing on interviews and ethnographic fieldwork of wildlife tours in locations with high levels of species richness (Spain – bird watching; California – whale and bird watching), Curtin's analysis identified feelings of wonder, awe and a sense of timelessness that emerged through an encounter with wildlife. Wonder was expressed in terms of the beauty of what was being seen (e.g. seabirds in flight), the intricacy of nature's design (e.g. diversity of species) and the sense of being part of – rather than separate from – the natural world. Participants also noted a temporal shift whereby, as Curtin writes, "linear… time slips away" and one is provided with "still and motionless time in which to marvel, contemplate and philosophise" (p. 470). Participants described these moments as points during which one can transcend the self and find meaning through connection with the wildlife and the wider natural world. Although Curtin did not label these experiences as contributing to spiritual well-being, such descriptions are in keeping with our dimensions that make up spiritual outcomes.

Mitchell's (2016) study of national public parks in the USA illustrates how, through park design and viewpoint placements, people can experience such moments of awe, humility and wonder before scenes of natural grandeur that visitors label as 'spiritual'. A former director of the US National Park Service called these parks an "investment in the physical, mental, and spiritual well-being of Americans as individuals" (quoted in Mitchell 2016, p. 34), and spiritual well-being has been identified as both a reason for and an important benefit of visiting protected areas in Canada (Lemieux et al. 2012). Given that such places can contribute to conservation of biodiversity, they are examples of how experiences of biodiversity can contribute to spiritual well-being.

10.3.4.2 Heintzman's Model Connecting Nature-Based Recreation and Spirituality

Drawing together qualitative and quantitative research on nature-based recreation and spirituality, Heintzman (2000, 2002, 2009, 2016; Heintzman and Mannell 2003) has identified four elements that contribute to this relationship. These include: antecedent conditions, setting components, recreation components and spiritual outcomes (Box 10.2). The spiritual outcomes are parsed into three aspects: spiritual

Box 10.2: Elements of Nature-Based Recreation and Spirituality (Heintzman 2009, 2016)

Antecedent Conditions: Person-related factors; things people bring to their outdoor recreation experience, e.g.

- Personal history (e.g. previous experiences in nature; previous spiritual experiences)
- Current circumstances (e.g. present-day issues and events)
- Motivation (e.g. seeking or escaping spiritual experience)
- Socio-demographic (e.g. gender, age, income)
- Spiritual tradition and background (e.g. religion)

Setting Components:

- Nature (e.g. wilderness)
- Being away, i.e. physically being away from one's day-to-day setting and constraints
- Place processes (e.g. emotional attachment)

Recreation Components:

- Activity, i.e. type of and challenge associated with the recreational activity (e.g. canoeing, hiking)
- Free time, i.e. availability of unstructured time
- Solitude, i.e. being alone
- Group experiences (e.g. discussion, group effort)
- Facilitation

Spiritual Outcomes:

- Spiritual experience (e.g. awe, wonder, connectedness, heightened senses, inner calm, peace, happiness, joy, elatedness)
- Spiritual well-being (Hawks 1994)
  - Internal Aspects (e.g. sense of purpose/meaning; oneness with nature; connectedness with others; commitment to something greater than self; sense of wholeness in life; strong beliefs, principles, ethics and values that may or may not be grounded in a specific religion; feelings of love, joy, peace, hope, fulfilment)
  - External Manifestation
    - Interaction with others is characterised by, e.g., trust, honesty, integrity, altruism, compassion, service
    - Regular community or personal relationship with a higher power or larger reality that transcends observable physical reality
- Spiritual coping: i.e. "ways that people receive help from spiritual resources (e.g. higher power, spiritual practices, faith community) during periods of life stress" (Heintzman 2009, p. 84).

experience – considered a short-term outcome; spiritual well-being, something that occurs over the longer term; and the use of leisure for coping with issues (e.g. job change, cancer) that can raise spiritual questions (e.g. meaning of life). Spiritual well-being is delineated in terms of Hawks' (1994) interpretation, which distinguishes between the internal experience and the outward manifestation of spiritual well-being (see Box 10.2).

10.3.4.3 Setting Component

In terms of our interest in the biodiversity-spiritual well-being relationship, the setting component of Heintzman's model is perhaps most relevant. Heintzman's (2009) discussion of why the natural dimension of nature-based recreation might contribute to spiritual-focused outcomes specifically highlights extent and fascination as relevant qualities, two characteristics of a restorative environment (e.g. Kaplan, S. 1995; see Marselle 2018). As Heintzman (2009) describes it:

> …nature settings are characterized by extent (i.e., natural ecosystems provide rich settings that captivate, foster exploration and connect people to a larger world). Second, nature settings allow for soft fascination or attention, which suggests that natural features (e.g. sunsets, clouds, mountain vistas) can be observed effortlessly leaving opportunity for reflection on spiritual matters. (p. 78)

The restorative environment features of 'being away' and 'compatibility' (Kaplan, S. 1995; see Marselle 2018) are also present in Heintzman's model. 'Being away' is embedded in the setting element; for many, being in nature is a physical change in location and a removal from everyday routine and responsibilities, which has been found to facilitate spiritual outcomes (e.g. Ellard et al. 2009, as cited in Heintzman 2009). Compatibility – the degree of 'fit' or congruence between an environment and one's purposes, inclinations or reasons for being there – is implicitly present in Heintzman's (2002, 2009) discussion of the setting. He more explicitly argues that the activity itself can be compatible – or not – with fostering spiritual well-being.

Biodiversity, e.g. richness of species, is hypothesised as something that could contribute to the fascination quality of a restorative environment (Ulrich 1983; see Marselle 2018). It could also contribute to a conceptual sense of 'being away', an additional dimension of this restorative environment feature (Kaplan, S. 1995). As Goodenough (1998) argues and Curtin (2009) illustrates empirically, biodiversity can inspire spiritual feelings of humility, communion, awe, wonder and inter-relatedness with nature. Goodenough suggests that: "The outpouring of biological diversity calls us to marvel at its fecundity. It also calls us to stand before its presence with deep, abiding humility" that she likens to religious reverence (1998, p. 86).

The empirical research into the spiritual dimension of outdoor recreation is primarily qualitative and largely situated in wilderness within the USA (e.g. Fredrickson and Anderson 1999; Kaplan, R. and Kaplan 1989), Australia (e.g. Williams and

Box 10.3: Stargazing as a Spiritual Experience (Bell et al. 2014)

Bell et al.'s (2014) mixed methods study explored the well-being effects of stargazing – an intentional nature-interaction activity (Keniger et al. 2013) or, as per Price's (1996) typology, an observational recreation activity. Nature connectedness (Mayer and Frantz 2004) was found to be higher among individuals who had been stargazing for more years and for those who reported seeing wildlife, such as birds and bat species along with other nocturnal ground-dwelling wildlife (e.g. foxes, badgers, hedgehogs), when stargazing.

In response to open-ended questions, participants reported experiencing spiritual aspects of well-being, with comments reflecting the spiritual or transcendent aspect of stargazing. Some comments reflected a consideration of one's place in the universe, including: "The sense of crushing smallness compared to the universe one feels" and "Realizing how small we are." Others identified "the peace and the intrigue" and "the beauty" of the experience. Some participants mentioned regular occurrence of emotions such as awe and wonder whilst stargazing. One individual stated "I feel in awe of nature and the natural world... A sense of wonder at it all!" whilst another reported "It relaxes me and reminds me of how precious life is...". Emotions of awe and wonder, peaceful feelings, and greater connectedness echo Heintzman's (2009, 2016) description of spiritual experiences, which, though short-term, may contribute to longer-term spiritual well-being.

Harvey 2001), New Zealand (Schmidt and Little 2007) and Canada (e.g. Heintzman 2012) thus representing specific environmental and socio-cultural contexts. Some exceptions are studies of recreational use of urban parks in the Netherlands (Chiesura 2004) and the UK (Irvine et al. 2013), and several studies of gardens as spaces for leisure amongst individuals experiencing life challenges such as a health crisis or loss of a loved one in the UK (Milligan et al. 2004), the USA (Heliker et al. 2000; Infantino 2004/2005) and Canada (Unruh and Hutchinson 2011). Bell et al. (2014) provide an example of the spiritual experiences associated with stargazing (Box 10.3).

Few studies directly examine the specific environmental elements of the setting that might contribute to spiritual outcomes. Williams and Harvey's (2001) questionnaire-based study of forests in Victoria, Australia is one exception; they sought to identify how different qualities of forests might influence such experiences. People who visit, live or work in forests associate spiritual feelings of insignificance and humility with forests that contain compelling features or powerful symbols of the natural environment, such as tall trees, extensive views or high waterfalls. By contrast, settings that were more open in character fostered what the authors described as a "deep flow" experience, e.g. feelings of connectedness and belonging.

A recent US-based study by Joye and Bolderdijk (2015) sought to experimentally test these effects. Using a between-subject design, participants viewed one of three slideshows online: extraordinary nature (e.g. dramatic mountains, landscapes dominated by phenomena such as sunsets, thunderstorms), mundane nature (e.g. lawns, foliage) or neutral (e.g. everyday objects such as a chair). Those who viewed the extraordinary nature images experienced greater levels of awe, fear and smallness compared to the other two conditions. Participants in both nature conditions felt more spiritual, caring and connected to others; those who viewed extraordinary nature scenes felt more 'other' oriented (as measured by social values orientation).

10.3.4.4 Parallel Measurement of Biodiversity and Spiritual Well-Being

The previous Sects. (10.3.4.1, 10.3.4.2 and 10.3.4.3) detail studies that do not explicitly incorporate measures of biodiversity. Two interdisciplinary mixed methods field-based studies of urban public parks in the UK, utilising ecological surveys alongside quantitative and qualitative social science methods, provide further insight into how biodiversity might relate to spiritual well-being (Fuller et al. 2007; Dallimer et al. 2012). Ecological surveys assessed species richness of plants, birds and butterflies (direct measures of biodiversity) along with diversity of habitats and tree cover (proxy measures of biodiversity). Self-report questionnaires conducted with users of the same study sites during the period of ecological sampling explored motivations for park use and well-being benefits. Well-being measures included place attachment, place identity and reflection, the former two are related to place processes (Altman and Low 1992; Twigger-Ross and Uzzell 1996) and the latter, interpreted as the ability to think about things (e.g. personal matters) and gain perspective (e.g. on life), a dimension of attention restoration theory (Kaplan, S. 1995; see Marselle 2018). Fuller et al. (2007) reported positive associations between tree species richness, habitat diversity and both reflection and place identity; bird species richness was positively associated with attachment. Dallimer et al. (2012) found that all aspects of well-being had positive associations with bird species richness and tree cover but a negative association with plant species richness.

These findings are suggestive that greater diversity could contribute to place processes and restoration. While these are not conceptually considered spiritual outcomes (see Table 10.1), they could be considered a mechanism through which spiritual well-being might be achieved. For example, given the centrality of meaning and purpose in definitions of spiritual well-being, having opportunities to "reflect on one's life, on one's priorities and possibilities, on one's actions and one's goals" can be considered a deeply restorative experience (Kaplan, R. and Kaplan 1989, p. 197). Indeed, as J.W. Fisher, Francis and Johnson (2000) argue, the "personal domain – wherein one intra-relates with oneself with regards to meaning, purpose and values in life" (p. 135) is an important component of spiritual well-being.

Irvine et al.'s (2013) qualitative analysis of open-ended responses from Fuller et al.'s (2007) park users, as to why they were using the park and how they felt after being there, identified numerous statements reflective of features of spiritual well-being. While motivations largely fell within the physical health domain (e.g. walk, eat) and nature-focused reasons (e.g. fresh air), a small number of comments can be considered as factors that might facilitate achieving spiritual well-being: wanting to think; wanting to take a break; the peace and quiet of the place. Spiritual well-being was identified as one of the effects of being in the park. This was expressed in terms of a sense of calm, peace, being at ease, feeling tranquil, serene and quiet. A second theme included feeling a connection to nature, a sense of being part of a larger reality.

In light of these qualitative findings, it is instructive to examine the closed-ended statements that formed the reflection measure in Fuller et al. (2007) and Dallimer et al. (2012). Fuller et al. (2007 [data supplement]) included the statement "being here makes me feel more connected to nature", found within discussion and definitions of spiritual well-being. In Dallimer et al. (2012 [Supplementary Data]), the items "I feel peaceful", "I feel part of something that is greater than myself" and "I do not feel calm" were added in an effort to further explore spiritual outcomes. Future studies could usefully expand the reflection measure and develop appropriate close-ended statements, drawing from qualitative insight, to measure spiritual well-being.

In summary, few studies directly investigated biodiversity's effect on spiritual well-being. Literature on wilderness-based recreation provides some insight into the potential contribution that biodiverse settings could make to spiritual well-being. Fuller et al.'s (2007), Dallimer et al.'s (2012) and Irvine et al.'s (2013) socio-ecological studies identify outcomes (e.g. reflection, place processes) that could act as mediators for the effect of biodiversity on spiritual well-being outcomes and provide insight into quantitative measure construction for future studies. Heintzman (2009, 2016) provides one of the few conceptual models that specifically explores relationships between nature settings, recreational interaction and spiritual well-being.

10.4 Discussion

In this chapter we have sought to provide insight into the spiritual dimension of human health and explore its relationship with biodiversity. The body of literature identified contained few empirical studies that directly assessed the effects of biodiversity on spiritual well-being. The literature does, however, paint a holistic account of the wider suite of connections with respect to the interplay between biodiversity and spiritual well-being. We considered these connections in terms of four narratives which focused on the influence of spiritual traditions on biodiversity, sacred places as repositories for biodiversity, the spiritual domain within ecosystem services and the effects of biodiversity on spiritual well-being. Here we consider how one might parse these relationships for research investigation, measurement issues related to both spiritual well-being and biodiversity, and potential future directions.

10.4.1 Conceptualising Relationships

Our review has stimulated an awareness of the challenges inherent in understanding these aspects of nature and human health. We began with a simple model (Fig. 10.1) of the overlapping relationship between spiritual well-being and spiritual beliefs and considered how these constructs might relate to behaviour, nature and biodiversity.

There is suggestive, but not robust, evidence about specific elements of nature, including biodiversity, that appear to contribute to spiritual outcomes or to potential mediators for the relationship. Species diversity (trees/birds), habitat diversity and tree cover are associated with place processes and reflection; the same parks provided tranquility and connection with nature. Extraordinary nature, with beauty and grandeur, such as mountains, sunsets or big waterfalls, are associated with awe, humility and inspiration. Wilderness contributes to a sense of solitude, timelessness, transcendence, putting people in touch with the divine and experiencing serenity or harmony. Open nature scenes are associated with feelings of deep flow, wholeness and belonging, while ordinary nature, such as lawns or parks, tends one towards spiritual caring and connections to others. These findings highlight a need to measure both biodiversity and the composite type of environment of interest.

Another challenge uncovered is the lack of clarity as to whether or how spiritual well-being is different from spirituality/spiritual beliefs. Some conceptualise differences; some overlap or conflate them. Table 10.1 synthesised elements from across these concepts, structured by four relational aspects of spiritual well-being, i.e. relation with self, community, the environment and transcendent Other(s), that create wholeness.

What is clear is the fundamental and growing intersection of spiritual beliefs with the natural environment, whether among indigenous groups, world religions or new eco-spiritual practices. These beliefs and values are associated with actions or practices that may preserve biodiversity, a link noted in many models of environmental behaviour (e.g. Stern 2000). Additionally, such beliefs and values may predispose one to experience spiritual well-being within nature. Incorporating both spiritual beliefs and spiritual well-being measures will thus be important.

An overarching challenge is how to parse relationships between spiritual beliefs/well-being and nature/biodiversity. Studies investigating nature and spiritual well-being are largely qualitative; few account for the biodiversity of the setting. The evidence is almost exclusively correlational, which leads to a circularity of associative relationships, and causality is difficult, if not impossible, to ascribe. A way forward is to take what we have learned here and map it onto existing causal models of how nature may affect human health and well-being. In Fig. 10.2 we propose such a model. Structured using the four relational elements of spiritual well-being, it overlays Heintzman's nature-spirituality model (Box 10.2) onto Hartig et al.'s (2014) nature-health model while also incorporating insights from others (Irvine et al. 2013; Marselle et al. 2016; Shanahan et al. 2016; Yeh et al. 2016). This model is framed in terms of public health notions of an exposure (that affects health) and

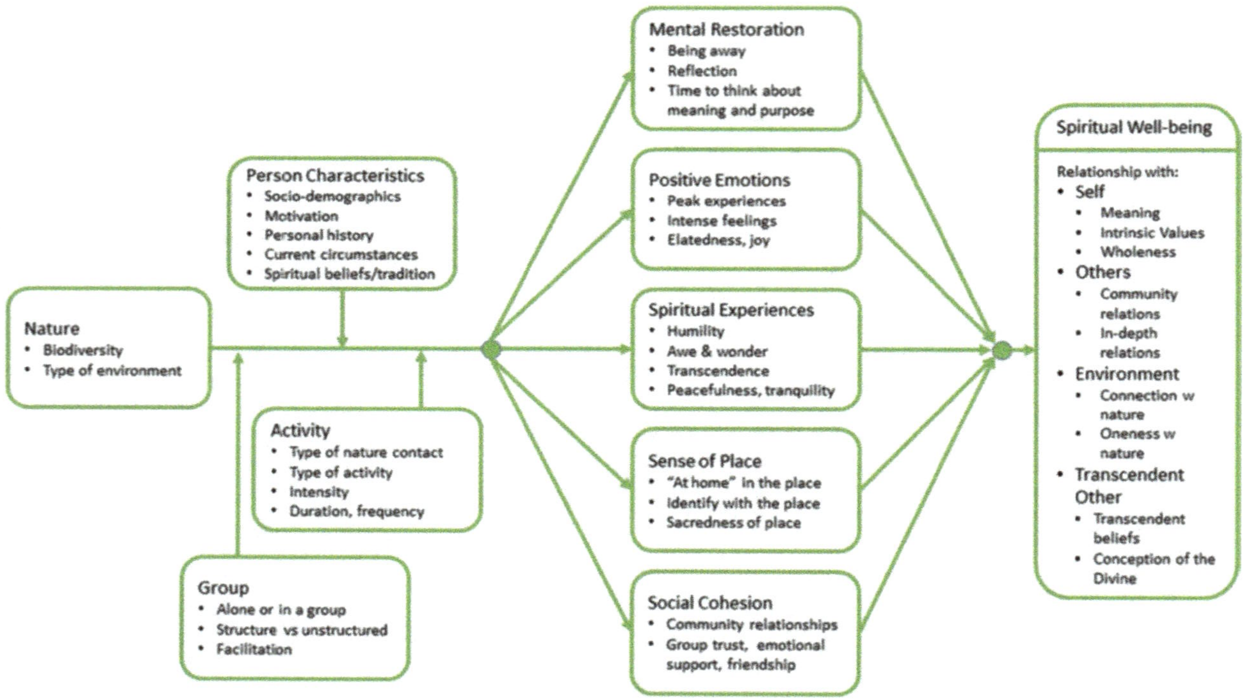

Fig. 10.2 Conceptual model of aspects to consider measuring and their relationships in order to assess the effects of biodiversity on spiritual well-being (developed from Irvine et al. 2013; Fisher, J. 2011; Hartig et al. 2014; Heintzman 2009, 2016; Marselle et al. 2016; Shanahan et al. 2016; Yeh et al. 2016). The model includes the exposure of interest (nature), potential moderators of effects (personal characteristics, activity and group processes), possible mediators (mental, emotional, spiritual, place and social) and the outcome of interest, spiritual well-being (see also Table 10.1). (Illustration by SL Warber and KN Irvine)

takes the positivist stance that we can quantitatively measure exposure, moderators, mediators and outcomes in meaningful ways. Below we explain our decision-making in the development of the model.

Exposure: Nature – The exposure of interest is the natural environment, particularly as measured by biodiversity. The literature reinforces the need to also consider the composite type of environment (see Marselle et al. 2013).

Moderators: Personal Characteristics, Activity, Group – The effects of any exposure or intervention will necessarily be moderated by the antecedent factors that the unique individuals bring to the situation. Socio-demographics are a well-known example in health literature, but Heintzman (2009, 2016) identifies additional features that are relevant for spiritual outcomes, including motivation, history, current circumstances and spiritual beliefs/traditions. Heintzman (2009, 2016) and Yeh et al. (2016), respectively writing in the leisure studies and sports medicine literature, identify various elements of the activity in nature as an important part of the exposure that will impact health. Additionally, Heintzman recognises that being alone or with a group, whether the group is structured or unstructured, and the type of group facilitation has a further impact on whether or not spiritual experiences are appreciated. Other authors have highlighted the importance of intensity, duration and frequency of a nature-based activity as being of relevance (e.g. Marselle et al. 2016).

Mediators/Pathways: Mental, Emotional, Spiritual, Place, Social – Hartig et al. (2014) posited several mediators or pathways through which nature might affect health. Based on the literature around spiritual well-being as an outcome, we have made modifications to their model: excluding physical activity and air quality; parsing stress into subcomponents of mental restoration and positive emotions. This latter change enables greater specificity in accommodating aspects of the nature experience associated with spiritual well-being. Heintzman (2009) proposes spiritual experiences as a short-term outcome, but other authors suggest that these experiences are what produce spiritual well-being which has informed our placement of spiritual experiences as a mediator. Heintzman also identifies place processes as important; here we subsume them under sense of place, including identification with, and attachment to, special places but also the sacred dimension of place that is clearly relevant (see Sects. 10.3.1 and 10.3.2). Social aspects of nature experiences have also been recognised as important by many authors, however measurement of relevant constructs is complicated. Heintzman's description of the literature and others' qualitative findings suggest that social cohesion is potentially critical for the development of spiritual well-being.

Outcome: Spiritual Well-being – Here we follow the synthesis presented in Sect. 10.2 and Table 10.1 that someone who has spiritual well-being has significant beneficial relationships with self, others, the environment and some type of transcendent Other(s) that confer wholeness. In Fig. 10.2 we identify possible constructs to measure as part of spiritual well-being.

In putting forth this model, we recognise that others may suggest placement of various constructs in different positions. We emphasise, however, that this model is a set of hypotheses to be tested. We also recognise that testing them all in one study is unlikely to be feasible; researchers will necessarily need to choose pieces of the model to investigate and may test various constructs as moderators, mediators or short-term outcomes.

10.4.2 Measurement of Key Constructs

Figure 10.2 provides insight into important elements and relationships of biodiversity and spiritual well-being. Here we consider the measurement of the two key constructs.

10.4.2.1 Spiritual Well-Being

Measurement of spiritual well-being has proved challenging and may be seen as aiming to "measure the immeasurable" (Moberg 2010, p. 99). Although few spiritual well-being measures have been applied in nature-health research, more than 300 scales to measure spiritual well-being, spirituality or similar constructs have been developed (see Fisher, J.W. 2015). The majority utilise closed-ended Likert scale measurements (e.g. Delaney 2005; Ellison, C. 1983; Elkins et al. 1988; Reker 2003) and often concentrate on specific aspects of spiritual well-being such as existential well-being (life meaning, purpose, values) or religious well-being (relationship with higher power) (see, e.g., Ellison, L. 2006; Peterman et al. 2002). In health-care settings, existential well-being, but not religious well-being, has been predictive of better quality of life, mental health or physical health (e.g. Edmondson et al. 2008). Spiritual well-being scales also have been critiqued for an overreliance on correlates of traditional Western religiosity, such as institutional affiliation and belief in God or a higher power (e.g. Klein et al. 2016). Such faith- or religious-focused content may alienate individuals who experience spiritual well-being but do not think of themselves as religious (Moreira-Almeida and Koenig 2006). Spiritual beliefs and well-being are culturally specific and need to be measured using language and ideas that fit the particular group of respondents under study. For example, Dominguez et al. (2010) created a Saint's Belief Index to explore the association of traditional beliefs in local Islamic Saints and new agro-pastoral practices that had previously been linked to biodiversity loss.

Few existing scales cover our four relational domains of spiritual well-being (see Table 10.1) evenly, with the relationship to the environment or to community often neglected. However, researchers have utilised qualitative methods effectively to explore the meanings and lived experience behind the concept of spiritual well-being and its presence in and through interaction with the natural environment (e.g. Bell-Williams 2016; Fredrickson and Anderson, 1999; Unruh and Hutchinson 2011). We favour measuring J. Fisher's (2011) four domains of spiritual well-being as the outcome of interest in studies of the effects of being in/living with biodiverse, extraordinary and ordinary nature, because of the explicit inclusion of the domains of relationship to environment and community. J. Fisher has published several scales that may be useful. For example, in the Spiritual Health and Life Orientation Measure (SHALOM)-generic (Fisher, J.W. 2014) participants select language for the 'transcendent Other(s)' to fit their own beliefs. This scale has been administered worldwide with adults. Similar scales for secondary school students (Gomez and Fisher 2003) and primary school children (Fisher, J. 2004) are also available.

10.4.2.2 Measuring Biodiversity

Appropriate measures of biodiversity also need to be incorporated into studies that purport to examine how biodiversity affects spiritual well-being. In our review, we encountered several approaches including field-based assessment (e.g. surveying species richness or abundance), use of secondary data (e.g. GIS) and categorisation of natural setting (e.g. wilderness). Within the field of ecology, numerous types of counts can be made. Dallimer et al. (2012) suggest that the number of animals or plants (i.e. species abundance) may be easiest for humans to recognise as representative of biodiversity. Other aspects of biological complexity which may be important to consider include species composition, functional organisation, relative abundance and species numbers (see also de Vries & Snep 2018; Marselle et al. 2018).

10.4.3 Future Directions for Research on Biodiversity's Effect on Spiritual Well-Being

There are continuous calls for upping the science bar, hence the examination here of how the relationship between nature (biodiversity) and health/well-being (spiritual) has been investigated in the literature. As noted in Sect. 10.4.1 and by others (Lovell et al. 2014; Marselle et al. 2018), most studies are cross-sectional and yield only associative results. We recommend taking a public health perspective and selecting research designs to more clearly investigate causal relationships. We would argue that activities in nature constitute complex interventions or exposures, including physical activity and group organisational effects, and recommend following suggestions about how to think about such interventions (Clark 2013) and the UK Medical Research Council guidance on how to study them (Craig et al. 2008). There is also a need for mixed methods research that integrates findings from qualitative and quantitative research methods (Fetters et al. 2013) to unpack the various components of both exposures and outcomes. Quantitative study designs could be improved by using natural experiments, quasi-experimental and before-and-after repeated measures designs as well as long-term longitudinal studies. Complex analyses are also needed, for example, structural equation modelling that allows identification of significant pathways or analyses that test various constructs as moderators, mediators or outcomes (see also commentary in Sect. 10.4.1). Given the complexity of both nature and health, illuminating research will necessitate interdisciplinary teams comfortably working across epistemologies (Diaz et al. 2018) and able to work with community groups and policy-makers to gather relevant data (CBD 2017c).

10.5 Implications and Conclusions

There is increasing international recognition of the role of biodiversity in human health and the relevance of considering the spiritual domain. Using a broad set of search terms, we identified an extensive body of scholarship that could provide important insights into the complexity of the relationship between biodiversity and spiritual well-being. We have identified and explained four themes from this literature: (i) influence of spiritual traditions on biodiversity; (ii) sacred places as repositories of biodiversity; (iii) the spiritual domain of ecosystems services; and (iv) effects of biodiversity on spiritual well-being. We have brought these strands together into a conceptual model and discussion of measurement issues that can inform future research. Research into spiritual well-being benefits from the natural environment needs to incorporate more detailed assessments of the environment, such as measures of biodiversity. The identified sacred places literature primarily focuses on measuring biodiversity; adding culturally-appropriate measures of spiritual well-being into these studies would address calls for interdisciplinary work and would help fill the gap of evidence on biodiversity and spiritual well-being. Within the ecosystem services rhetoric, the spiritual domain seems to be largely associated with indigenous peoples who hold monistic worldviews. Yet there are important emerging spiritualities as well as existing world religions that also have sacred beliefs about the importance of the natural environment. We need to embrace these as well. Additionally, given the availability of spiritual well-being scales that consider the relationship with the environment, these could be incorporated into research.

Lastly, we come to the question of 'so what'? The non-communicable diseases that the world currently faces – obesity, heart disease, depression – would suggest a need to focus on physical and mental well-being, thus raising the question of what an understanding of biodiversity and spiritual well-being would bring to such discussions. Yet the literature identified through our review, in particular the qualitative studies, illustrates an important additional dimension that can answer the question posed by E.O. Wilson in 1993 of "what service [do species bring] to the human spirit?" (p. 37). Given the role of biodiversity in health and the numerous ways in which biodiversity is related to spiritual well-being, the spiritual domain is clearly an important aspect of how nature influences us. Perhaps it is time to embrace this ethereal, enigmatic aspect of human culture and bring it into the mutually beneficial service of biodiversity conservation.

Acknowledgements The authors would like to thank the three anonymous reviewers for their valuable and insightful comments on an earlier draft of this chapter. Dr. Irvine's involvement was funded by the Rural and Environment Science and Analytical Services Division of the Scottish Government.

References

Altman I, Low SM (1992) Place attachment: human behavior and environment. Plenum Press, New York

Anderson DM, Salick J, Moseley RK, Ou XK (2005) Conserving the sacred medicine mountains: a vegetation analysis of Tibetan sacred sites in Northwest Yunnan. Biodivers Conserv 14(13):3065–3091

Bekelman DB, Dy SM, Becker DM, Wittstein IS, Hendricks DE, Yamashita TE, Gottlieb SH (2007) Spiritual well-being and depression in patients with heart failure. J Gen Intern Med 22(4):470–477

Bell R, Irvine KN, Wilson C, Warber SL (2014) Dark nature: exploring potential benefits of nocturnal nature-based interaction for human and environmental health. Eur J Ecopsychol 5(1):1–15

Bell-Williams R (2016) Spiritual wellbeing and the human-nature relationship: an exploration of the spiritual wellbeing experiences of home and community gardeners. Doctoral dissertation, De Montfort University, Leicester, UK

Bensley RJ (1991) Defining spiritual health: a review of the literature. J Health Educ 22(5):287–290

Berghuijs J, Pieper J, Bakker C (2013) Being 'spiritual' and being 'religious' in Europe: diverging life orientations. J Contemp Relig 28(1):15–32

Berry E (2015) Devoted to nature: the religious roots of American environmentalism. University of California Press, Berkeley

Bhagwat SA, Rutte C (2006) Sacred groves: potential for biodiversity management. Front Ecol Environ 4(10):519–524

Bharathi S, Devi Prasad AG (2017) Diversity, population structure and regeneration status of arboreal species in the four sacred groves of Kushalnagar, Karnataka. J For Res 28(2):357–370

Bloch JP (1998) Alternative spirituality and environmentalism. Rev Relig Res 40(1):55–73

Bodeker G (1999) Valuing biodiversity for human health and well-being: traditional health systems. In: Posey DA (ed) Cultural and spiritual values of biodiversity. United Nations Environment Programme, London, pp 261–284

Boff L (1997) Cry of the earth, cry of the poor. Maryknoll, Orbis, New York

Buck HG (2006) Spirituality: concept analysis and model development. Holist Nurs Pract 20(6):288–292

Cajete G (ed) (1999) A people's ecology: explorations in sustainable living. Clear Light Publishers, Santa Fe

Callicott JB, Rozzi R, Delgado L, Monticino M, Acevedo M, Harcombe P (2007) Biocomplexity and conservation of biodiversity hotspots: three case studies from the Americas. Philos Trans R Soc Lond Ser B Biol Sci 362(1478):321–333

Casey P (2013) 'I'm spiritual but not religious': implications for research and practice. In: Cook C (ed) Spirituality, theology and mental health: interdisciplinary perspectives. SCM Press, Norfolk, pp 20–40

Chiesura A (2004) The role of urban parks for the sustainable city. Landsc Urban Plan 68(1):129–138

Chuengsatiansup K (2003) Spirituality and health: an initial proposal to incorporate spiritual health in health impact assessment. Environ Impact Assess Rev 23(1):3–15

Clark AM (2013) What are the components of complex interventions in healthcare? Theorizing approaches to parts, powers and the whole intervention. Soc Sci Med 93:185–193

Convention on Biological Diversity (2017a) Recommendation adopted by the subsidiary body on scientific, technical and technological advice at its fourteenth meeting. Viewed on 6 July 2018, https://www.cbd.int/doc/recommendations/sbstta-21/sbstta-21-rec-03-en.pdf

Convention on Biological Diversity (2017b) Workshop on biodiversity and health for the European region. Viewed on 6 July 2018, https://www.cbd.int/health/european/default.shtml

Convention on Biological Diversity (2017c) Biodiversity and human health – note by the Executive Secretary for the 21st meeting 11–14 Dec 2017. Viewed on 6 July 2018, https://www.cbd.int/doc/c/72d6/b5bb/9244e977048688ec45735d2c/sbstta-21-04-en.pdf

Cooper N, Brady E, Steen H, Bryce R (2016) Aesthetic and spiritual values of ecosystems: recognising the ontological and axiological plurality of cultural ecosystem 'services'. Ecosyst Serv 21:218–229

Craig P, Dieppe P, Macintyre S, Michie S, Nazareth I, Petticrew M (2008) Developing and evaluating complex interventions: the new medical research council guidance. BMJ 337:979–983

Cummings C (1991) Eco-spirituality: toward a reverent life. Paulist, New York

Curtin S (2009) Wildlife tourism: the intangible, psychological benefits of human-wildlife encounters. Curr Issue Tour 12(5–6):451–474

Dallimer M, Irvine KN, Skinner A, Davies ZG, Armsworth P, Rouquette J et al (2012) Biodiversity and the feel-good factor: understanding associations between self-reported human well-being and species richness [Supplementary data]. Bioscience 62(1):47–55. https://academic.oup.com/bioscience/article/62/1/47/295411

Daniel TC, Muhar A, Arnberger A, Aznar O, Boyd JW, Chan KM et al (2012) Contributions of cultural services to the ecosystem services agenda. Proc Natl Acad Sci 109(23):8812–8819

De Lacy P, Shackleton C (2017) Aesthetic and spiritual ecosystem services provided by urban sacred sites. Sustainability 9(9):1–14

de Vries S, Snep R (2018) Biodiversity in the context of 'biodiversity – mental health' research. In: Marselle MR, Stadler J, Korn H, Irvine KN, Bonn A (eds) Biodiversity and health in the face of climate change. Springer, Cham

Delaney C (2005) The spirituality scale development and psychometric testing of a holistic instrument to assess the human spiritual dimension. J Holist Nurs 23(2):145–167

Delgado F, Escobar C, Verschuuren B, Hiemstra W (2010) Sacred natural sites, biodiversity, and well-being: the role of sacred sites in endogenous development in the COMPAS network. In: Verschuuren B, Wild R, McNeeley JA, Oviedo G (eds) Sacred natural sites: conserving nature and culture. Earthscan, London, pp 188–197

Díaz S, Pascual U, Stenseke M, Martín-López B, Watson RT, Molnár Z et al (2018) Assessing nature's contributions to people. Science 359(6373):270–272

Dominguez P, Zorondo-Rodriguez F, Reyes-Garcia V (2010) Relationship between religious beliefs and mountain pasture uses: a case study in the high Atlas mountains of Marrakech, Morocco. Hum Ecol 38(3):351–362

Dudley N, Higgins-Zogib L, Mansourian S (2009) The links between protected areas, faiths and sacred natural sites. Conserv Biol 23(3):568–577

Dudley N, Bhagwat S, Higgins-Zogib L, Lassen B, Verschuuren B, Wild R (2010) Conservation of biodiversity in sacred natural sites in Asia and Africa: a review of the scientific literature. In: Verschuuren B, Wild R, McNeeley JA, Oviedo G (eds) Sacred natural sites: conserving nature and culture. Earthscan, London, pp 19–32

Edmondson D, Park CL, Blank TO, Fenster JR, Mills MA (2008) Deconstructing spiritual well-being: existential well-being and HRQOL in cancer survivors. Psycho-Oncology 17(2):161–169

Elkins DN, Hedstrom LJ, Hughes LL, Leaf JA, Saunders C (1988) Toward a humanistic-phenomenological spirituality: definition, description, and measurement. J Humanist Psychol 28(4):5–18

Ellingson S (2015) To care for creation: the emergence of the religious environmental movement. University of Chicago Press, Chicago

Ellison CW (1983) Spiritual well-being: conceptualization and measurement. J Psychol Theol 11(4):330–340

Ellison LL (2006) The spiritual well-being scale. [Online] Marshall University. Viewed on 6 July 2018, http://mds.marshall.edu/cgi/viewcontent.cgi?article=1008&context=co_faculty

Feit HA (2001) Hunting, nature, and metaphor: political and discursive strategies in James Bay Cree resistance and autonomy. In: Grim JA (ed) Indigenous traditions and ecology: the interbeing of cosmology and community. Harvard University Press, Cambridge, MA, pp 411–452

Fetters MD, Curry LA, Creswell JW (2013) Achieving integration in mixed methods designs: principles and practices. Health Serv Res 48(6 Pt 2):2134–2156

Fisher J (2004) Feeling good, living life: a spiritual health measure for young children. J Beliefs Values 25(3):307–315

Fisher J (2011) The four domains model: connecting spirituality, health and well-being. Religion 2(1):17–28

Fisher JW (2014) Comparing the influence of God and other transcendents on spiritual well-being. Relig Educ J Aust 30(2):9–15

Fisher JW (2015) A critique of quantitative measures for assessing spirituality and spiritual well-being. In: Roberts EC (ed) Spirituality, global practices, societal attitudes and effects on health. Nova Science Publishers Inc, New York, pp 91–131

Fisher JW, Francis LJ, Johnson P (2000) Assessing spiritual health via four domains of spiritual wellbeing: the SH4DI. Pastor Psychol 49(2):133–145

Fisher B, Turner K, Morling P (2009) Defining and classifying ecosystem services for decision making. Ecol Econ 68(3):643–653

Fowler RB (1995) The greening of protestant thought. University of North Carolina Press, Chapel Hill

Francis P (2015) Laudato Si. Vatican Press, Vatican City

Frascaroli F (2013) Catholicism and conservation: the potential of sacred natural sites for biodiversity management in Central Italy. Hum Ecol 41(4):587–601

Fredrickson LM, Anderson DH (1999) A qualitative exploration of the wilderness experience as a source of spiritual inspiration. J Environ Psychol 19(1):21–39

Fuller RC (2001) Spiritual, but not religious: understanding unchurched America. Oxford University Press, New York

Fuller RA, Irvine KN, Devine-Wright P, Warren PH, Gaston KJ (2007) Psychological benefits of greenspace increase with biodiversity [data supplement]. Biol Lett 3(4):390–394. http://rsbl.royalsocietypublishing.org/content/3/4/390.figures-only

Gall TL, Malette J, Guirguis-Younger M (2011) Spirituality and religiousness: a diversity of definitions. J Spiritual Ment Health 13(3):158–181

Gilliat-Ray S, Bryant M (2011) Are British Muslims green? An overview of environmental activism among Muslims in Britain. J Stud Relig Nat Cult 5(3):284–306

Golliher J (1999) Ethical, moral, and religious concerns. In: Posey DA (ed) Cultural and spiritual values of biodiversity. United Nations Environment Programme, London, pp 435–502

Gomez R, Fisher JW (2003) Domains of spiritual well-being and development and validation of the spiritual well-being questionnaire. Personal Individ Differ 35(8):1975–1991

Goodenough U (1998) The sacred depths of nature. Oxford University Press, New York

Gottlieb RS (2006a) A greener faith: religious environmentalism and our planet's future. Oxford University Press, New York

Gottlieb RS (2006b) Introduction: religion and ecology – what is the connection and why does it matter? In: Gottlieb RS (ed) The Oxford handbook of religion and ecology. Oxford University Press, New York, pp 3–21

Gottlieb RS (2013) Spirituality: what it is and why it matters. Oxford University Press, New York

Greenberg JS (1985) Health and wellness: a conceptual differentiation. J Sch Health 55(10):403–406

Grim JA (ed) (2001) Indigenous traditions and ecology: the interbeing of cosmology and community. Harvard University Press, Cambridge, MA

Grim J, Tucker ME (2014) Ecology and religion. Island Press, Washington, DC

Haberman DL (2017) Hinduism: devotional love of the world. In: Jenkins W, Tucker ME, Grim J (eds) Routledge handbook of religion and ecology. Routledge, New York, pp 35–42

Hamilton LS, Takeuchi HF (eds) (1993) Ethics, religion, and biodiversity: relations between conservation and cultural values. White Horse Press, Cambridge

Hartig T, Mitchell R, de Vries S, Frumkin H (2014) Nature and health. Annu Rev Public Health 35(1):207–228

Hawks S (1994) Spiritual health: definition and theory. Wellness Perspect 10(4):3–3

Heintzman P (2000) Leisure and spiritual well-being relationships: a qualitative study. Soc Leisure 23(1):41–69

Heintzman P (2002) A conceptual model of leisure and spiritual well-being. J Park Recreat Adm 20(4):147–169

Heintzman P (2009) Nature-based recreation and spirituality: a complex relationship. Leis Sci 32(1):72–89

Heintzman P (2012) The spiritual dimension of campers' park experience: management implications. Manag Leis 17(4):291–310

Heintzman P (2016) Spirituality and the outdoors. In: Humberstone B, Prince H, Henderson KA (eds) Routledge international handbook of outdoor studies. Routledge, New York, pp 388–397

Heintzman P, Mannell R (2003) Spiritual functions of leisure and spiritual well-being: coping with time pressure. Leis Sci 25(2–3):207–230

Heliker D, Chadwick A, O'Connell T (2000) The meaning of gardening and the effects on perceived well-being of a gardening project on diverse populations of elders. Act Adapt Aging 24(3):35–56

Hird S (2003) What is well-being? A brief review of current literature and concepts. NHS Scotland

Hood-Morris LE (1996) A spiritual well-being model: use with older women who experience depression. Issues Ment Health Nurs 17(5):439–455

Hough RL (2014) Biodiversity and human health: evidence for causality? Biodivers Conserv 23(2):267–288

Hunter LM, Brehm JM (2004) A qualitative examination of value orientations toward wildlife and biodiversity by rural residents of the intermountain region. Hum Ecol Rev 11(1):13–26

Infantino M (2004/2005) Gardening: a strategy for health promotion in older women. J NY State Nurses Assoc 35(2):10–17

Ingersoll RE (1994) Spirituality, religion, and counseling: dimensions and relationships. Couns Values 38(2):98–111

Ingersoll RE (1998) Refining dimensions of spiritual wellness: a cross-traditional approach. Couns Values 42(3):156–165

Irvine KN, Warber SL, Devine-Wright P, Gaston KJ (2013) Understanding urban green space as a health resource: a qualitative comparison of visit motivation and derived effects among park users in Sheffield, U.K. Int J Environ Res Public Health 10(1):417–442

Ives C (2017) Buddhism: a mixed dharmic bag: debates about Buddhism and ecology. In: Jenkins W, Tucker ME, Grim J (eds) Routledge handbook of religion and ecology. Routledge, New York, pp 43–51

Jenkins W (2003) Biodiversity and salvation: thomistic roots for environmental ethics. J Relig 83(3):401–420

Jenkins W (2013) The future of ethics: sustainability, social justice, and religious creativity. Georgetown University Press, Washington, DC

Jenkins W, Tucker ME, Grim J (2017) Routledge handbook of religion and ecology. Routledge, New York

Jepson D (2015) The lure of the countryside: the spiritual dimension of rural spaces of leisure. In: Gammon S, Elkington S (eds) Landscapes of leisure: leisure studies in a global era. Palgrave Macmillan, London, pp 202–219

Jespers F (2011) The scientific study of religious and secular spiritualities. J Relig Eur 4(2):328–354

Joye Y, Bolderdijk JW (2015) An exploratory study into the effects of extraordinary nature on emotions, mood and prosociality. Front Psychol 5:1–9

Juhé-Beaulaton D (2008) Sacred forests and the global challenge of biodiversity conservation: the case of Benin and Togo. J Stu Relig Nat Cult 2(3):351–372

Kalu OU (2001) The sacred egg: worldview, ecology, and development in West Africa. In: Grim JA (ed) Indigenous traditions and ecology: the interbeing of cosmology and community. Harvard University Press, Cambridge, MA, pp 225–248

Kaplan S (1995) The restorative benefits of nature: toward an integrative framework. J Environ Psychol 15(3):169–182

Kaplan R, Kaplan S (1989) The experience of nature: a psychological perspective. Cambridge University Press, Cambridge

Keniger LE, Gaston KJ, Irvine KN, Fuller RA (2013) What are the benefits of interacting with nature? Int J Environ Res Public Health 10(3):913–935

Khumbongmayum A, Khan M, Tripathi R (2005) Sacred groves of Manipur, Northeast India: biodiversity value, status and strategies for their conservation. Biodivers Conserv 14(7):1541–1582

Kinsley D (1995) Ecology and religion: ecological spirituality in cross-cultural perspective. Prentice Hall, Englewood Cliffs

Klein C, Keller B, Silver CF, Hood RW Jr, Streib H (2016) Positive adult development and 'spirituality': psychological well-being, generativity, and emotional stability. In: Streib H, Hood RW Jr (eds) Semantics and psychology of spirituality: a cross-cultural analysis. Springer, New York, pp 401–436

Koenig HG (2008) Concerns about measuring 'spirituality' in research. J Nerv Ment Dis 196(5):349–355

Lemieux CJ, Eagles PFJ, Slocombe DS, Doherty ST, Elliot SJ, Mock SE (2012) Human health and well-being motivations and benefits associated with protected area experiences: an opportunity for transforming policy and management in Canada. Parks Int J Prot Area Conserv 18(1):71–85

Lin HR, Bauer-Wu SM (2003) Psycho-spiritual well-being in patients with advanced cancer: an integrative review of the literature. J Adv Nurs 44(1):69–80

Linton MJ, Dieppe P, Medina-Lara A (2016) Review of 99 self-report measures for assessing wellbeing in adults: exploring dimensions of well-being and developments over time. BMJ Open 6(7):1–16

Lovejoy TE (2017) Biodiversity: an inordinate fondness for living things. In: Jenkins W, Tucker ME, Grim J (eds) Routledge handbook of religion and ecology. Routledge, New York, pp 249–256

Lovell R, Wheeler BW, Higgins SL, Irvine KN, Depledge MH (2014) A systematic review of the health and well-being benefits of biodiverse environments. J Toxicol Environ Health B Crit Rev 17(1):1–20

Marselle MR (2018) Theoretical foundations of biodiversity & mental wellbeing relationships. In: Marselle MR, Stadler J, Korn H, Irvine KN, Bonn A (eds) Biodiversity and health in the face of climate change. Springer, Cham

Marselle MR, Irvine KN, Warber SL (2013) Walking for well-being: are group walks in certain types of natural environments better for well-being that group walks in urban environments? Int J Environ Res Public Health 10(11):5603–5628

Marselle MR, Irvine KN, Lorenzo-Arribas A, Warber SL (2016) Does perceived restorativeness mediate the effects of perceived biodiversity and perceived naturalness on emotional well-being following group walks in nature? J Environ Psychol 46:217–232

Marselle MR, Martens D, Dallimer M, Irvine KN (2018) Review of the mental health and well-being benefits of biodiversity. In: Marselle MR, Stadler J, Korn H, Irvine KN, Bonn A (eds) Biodiversity and health in the face of climate change. Springer, Cham

Mayer FS, Frantz CM (2004) The connectedness to nature scale: a measure of individuals' feeling in community with nature. J Environ Psychol 24(4):503–515

McClain CS, Rosenfeld B, Breitbart W (2003) Effect of spiritual well-being on end-of-life despair in terminally-ill cancer patients. Lancet 361(9369):1603–1607

McFague S (1997) Super, natural Christians: how we should love nature. Fortress Press, Minneapolis

McKee DD, Chappel JN (1992) Spirituality and medical practice. J Fam Pract 35(2):201, 205–201, 208

Millennium Ecosystem Assessment (2005) Ecosystems and human well-being: synthesis. Island Press, Washington, DC

Milligan C, Gatrell A, Bingley A (2004) Cultivating health: therapeutic landscapes and older people in Northern England. Soc Sci Med 58(9):1781–1793

Mitchell K (2016) Spirituality and the state: managing nature and experience at America's national parks. New York University Press, New York

Moberg DO (1971) Spiritual well-being: background [and] issues. White House conference on aging

Moberg DO (ed) (1979) Spiritual well-being: sociological perspectives. University Press of America, Washington, DC

Moberg DO (1984) Subjective measures of spiritual well-being. Rev Relig Res 25(4):351–364

Moberg DO (2010) Spirituality research: measuring the immeasurable? Perspect Sci Christ Faith 62(2):99–114

Moreira-Almeida A, Koenig HG (2006) Retaining the meaning of the words religiousness and spirituality: a commentary on the WHOQOL SRPB group's "a cross-cultural study of spirituality, religion, and personal beliefs as components of quality of life". Soc Sci Med 63(4):843–845

Negi CS (2005) Religion and biodiversity conservation: not a mere analogy. Int J Biodivers Sci Manag 1(2):85–96

Ntiamoa-Baidu Y (2008) Indigenous beliefs and biodiversity conservation: the effectiveness of sacred groves, taboos and totems in Ghana for habitat and species conservation. J Stu Relig Nat Cult 2(3):309–326

O'Brien KJ (2010) An ethics of biodiversity: Christianity, ecology, and the variety of life. Georgetown University Press, Washington, DC

Ormsby AA, Bhagwat S (2010) Sacred forests of India: a strong tradition of community-based natural resource management. Environ Conserv 37(3):320–326

Paloutzian RF, Ellison CW (1982) Loneliness, spiritual well-being, and quality of life. In: Peplau LA, Perlman D (eds) Loneliness: a sourcebook of current theory, research, and therapy. Wiley-Interscience, New York, pp 224–237

Peterman AH, Fitchett G, Brady MJ, Hernandez L, Cella D (2002) Measuring spiritual well-being in people with cancer: the functional assessment of chronic illness therapy – spiritual well-being scale (FACIT-Sp). Ann Behav Med 24(1):49–58

Posey DA (ed) (1999) Cultural and spiritual values of biodiversity. United Nations Environment Programme, London

Price JL (1996) Naturalistic recreations. In: van Ness PH (ed) Spirituality and the secular quest. Crossroad, New York, pp 414–444

Principe W (1983) Toward defining spirituality. Sci Relig/Stud Relig 12(2):127–141

Ramanujam M, Cyril K (2003) Woody plant species diversity of four sacred groves in the Pondicherry region of South India. Biodivers Conserv 12(2):289–299

Reker GT (2003) Provisional manual of the spiritual transcendence scale. Student Psychologists Press, Ontario

Rican PR (2004) Spirituality: the story of a concept in the psychology of religion. Arch Psychol Relig 26:135–156

Rots AP (2015) Sacred forests, sacred nation: the Shinto environmentalist paradigm and the rediscovery of 'Chinju no Mori. Jpn J Relig Stud 42(2):205–233

Russell R, Guerry AD, Balvanera P, Gould RK, Basurto X, Chan KM et al (2013) Humans and nature: how knowing and experiencing nature affect well-being. Annu Rev Environ Resour 38:473–502

Salander P (2006) Who needs the concept of 'spirituality'? Psycho-Oncology 15:647–649

Sandifer PA, Sutton-Grieb AE, Ward BP (2015) Exploring connections among nature, biodiversity, ecosystem services and human health and well-being: opportunities to enhance health and biodiversity conservation. Ecosyst Serv 12:1–15

Saucier G, Skrzypinksa K (2006) Spiritual but not religious? Evidence for two independent positions. J Pers 74(5):1257–1292
Schmidt C, Little DE (2007) Qualitative insights into leisure as a spiritual experience. J Leis Res 39(2):222–247
Sessions G (ed) (1995) Deep ecology for the 21st century: readings on the philosophy and practice of the new environmentalism. Shambala, Boston
Shanahan DF, Bush R, Gaston KJ, Lin BB, Dean J, Barber E, Fuller RA (2016) Health benefits from nature experiences depend on dose. Sci Rep 6(28551):1–10
Sheridan MJ, Nyamweru C (2008) African sacred groves: ecological dynamics & social change. Ohio University Press, Athens
Sponsel LE (2012) Spiritual ecology: a quiet revolution. Oxford University Press, New York
Starhawk (1979) Witchcraft and women's culture. In: Christ CP, Plaskow J (eds) Womanspirit rising: a feminist reader in religion. Harper & Row, San Francisco, pp 259–268
Stern PC (2000) Towards a coherent theory of environmentally significant behavior. J Soc Issues 56(3):407–424
Stoll M (2015) Inherit the holy mountain: religion and the rise of American environmentalism. Oxford University Press, New York
Streib H, Hood RW (2011) 'Spirituality' as privatized experience-oriented religion: empirical and conceptual perspectives. Implicit Relig 14(4):433–453
Tauli-Corpuz V (2001) Interface between traditional religion and ecology among the Igorots. In: Grim JA (ed) Indigenous traditions and ecology: the interbeing of cosmology and community. Harvard University Press, Cambridge, MA, pp 281–302
Taylor SM (2007) Green sisters: a spiritual ecology. Harvard University Press, Cambridge, MA
Taylor B (2009) Dark green religion: nature spirituality and the planetary future. University of California Press, Berkeley
Taylor B (2012) Wilderness, spirituality, and biodiversity in North America – tracing an environmental history from occidental roots to earth day. In: Feldt L (ed) Wilderness in mythology and religion. De Gruyter, Boston, pp 293–324
Tomalin E (2009) Biodivinity and biodiversity: the limits to religious environmentalism. Routledge, New York
Troster L (2008) God must love beetles: a Jewish view of biodiversity and the extinction of species. Conserv Jud 60(3):3–21
Tsuang MT, Simpson JC, Koenen KC, Kremen WS, Lyons MJ (2007) Spiritual well-being and health. J Nerv Ment Dis 195(8):673–680
Twigger-Ross CL, Uzzell DL (1996) Place and identity processes. J Environ Psychol 16:205–220
UK National Ecosystem Assessment Follow-on (2014) Synthesis of the key findings. WCMC, Cambridge
Ulrich R (1983) Aesthetic and affective responses to natural environment. In: Altman I, Wohlwill J (eds) Human behavior and the natural environment. Plenum Press, New York, pp 85–125
United Nations (1992) Convention on biological diversity. Viewed on 6 July 2018, https://www.cbd.int/doc/legal/cbd-en.pdf
Unruh A, Hutchinson S (2011) Embedded spirituality: gardening in daily life and stressful experiences. Scand J Caring Sci 25(3):567–574
van Ness PH (ed) (1996) Spirituality and the secular quest. Crossroad, New York
Veenhoven R (2008) Sociological theories of subjective well-being. In: Eid M, Larsen RJ (eds) The science of subjective well-being. Guilford Press, New York, pp 44–61
Verschuuren B (2010) Arguments for developing biocultural conservation approaches for sacred natural sites. In: Verschuuren B, Wild R, McNeeley JA, Oviedo G (eds) Sacred natural sites: conserving nature and culture. Earthscan, London, pp 62–72
Verschuuren B, Wild R, McNeely JA, Oviedo G (eds) (2010) Sacred natural sites: conserving nature and culture. Earthscan, London
Westgate CE (1996) Spiritual wellness and depression. J Couns Dev 75(1):26–35
White L Jr (1967) The historical roots of our ecological crisis. Science 155(3767):1203–1207

Williams K, Harvey D (2001) Transcendent experience in forest environments. J Environ Psychol 21(3):249–260

Wilson EO (1993) Biophilia and the conservation ethic. In: Kellert SR, Wilson EO (eds) The biophilia hypothesis. Island Press, Washington, DC, pp 31–41

Wilson K (2003) Therapeutic landscapes and first nations peoples: an exploration of culture, health and place. Health Place 9(2):83–93

World Health Organisation (1948) Precis of discussion. [Online] World Health Organisation. Viewed on 6 July 2018, http://www.nes.scot.nhs.uk/media/3723/spiritualcaremattersfinal.pdf

World Health Organisation (1998) Health promotion glossary. [Online] World Health Organisation. Viewed on 6 July 2018, http://www.who.int/healthpromotion/about/HPR%20Glossary%201998.pdf

World Health Organisation & Secretariat of the Convention on Biological Diversity (2015) Connecting global priorities: biodiversity and human health. A state of the knowledge review. Retrieved from http://www.who.int/globalchange/publications/biodiversity-human-health/en/

Yeh HP, Stone JA, Churchill SM, Wheat JS, Brymer E, Davids K (2016) Physical, psychological and emotional benefits of green physical activity: an ecological dynamics perspective. Sports Med 46(7):947–953

Zinnbauer BJ, Pargament KI, Cole B, Rye MS, Butter EM, Belavich TG, Kadar JL (1997) Religion and spirituality: unfuzzying the fuzzy. J Sci Study Relig 36(4):549–564

Part III
Implications of the Biodiversity and Health Relationship

Chapter 11
Biodiversity and Health in the Face of Climate Change: Implications for Public Health

Penny A. Cook, Michelle Howarth, and C. Philip Wheater

Abstract A biodiverse natural environment is a health-promoting resource. A given habitat can simultaneously provide multiple ecosystem (and therefore health) benefits, both directly through, for example, flood risk mitigation and cooling, and indirectly as a resource for cultural and physical activities. The single biggest priority for public health is to work across governments and countries to protect biodiverse natural resources and introduce measures to stem climate change. At a more local level, public health professionals are responsible for devising strategies to promote sustainable lifestyles and facilitate access to natural environments. Modern public health emphasises the reduction of avoidable differences in ill health between the most and least well-off in society. Such strategies therefore need to target those from socio-economically deprived areas, who are most at risk of ill health. Schemes such as nature-based social prescribing or community referral give local commissioners of health services the opportunity to bring people into contact with nature. Those with responsibility for the provision of nature-based schemes should be encouraged to use interventions that bring people into active, rather than passive, contact with nature. Further, targeting such interventions towards exposure to environments with the greatest biodiversity is likely to offer the greatest benefits for human health.

Keywords Public health, biodiversity, climate change · Socio-economic status · Health inequalities · Nature-based social prescribing · Green care · Salutogenesis · Community referral · Asset based approach

P. A. Cook (✉) · M. Howarth
School of Health and Society, University of Salford, Salford, UK
e-mail: p.a.cook@salford.ac.uk; M.L.Howarth2@salford.ac.uk

C. P. Wheater
Faculty of Science and Engineering, Manchester Metropolitan University, Manchester, UK
e-mail: p.wheater@mmu.ac.uk

M. R. Marselle et al. (eds.), *Biodiversity and Health in the Face of Climate Change*, https://doi.org/10.1007/978-3-030-02318-8_11

Highlights

- We consider the breadth of public health domains that are influenced by biodiversity.
- Existing models of greenspace and health are extended to look at the impact of biodiversity.
- Recommendations are provided for health professionals working from local to international levels.
- Nature-based social prescriptions or community referrals could maximise exposure to biodiversity.
- Case studies of health and biodiversity interventions for human and planetary health are presented.

11.1 Introduction

Public health is "the art and science of preventing disease, prolonging life and promoting health through the organised efforts of society" (Acheson 1988), and it focuses on the entire spectrum of health and well-being, not only the eradication of diseases. Public health activities can be targeted at both the population and the individual levels. Population-level interventions include those applied generally, such as a health campaign to increase knowledge and awareness of health risks or fluoridation of water supplies to reduce tooth decay, to those aiming to address the social, economic and environmental conditions that cause ill health, such as an urban regeneration project. Individual-level public health activities include personal services such as vaccinations, behavioural counselling and health advice. Non-medical interventions to individuals, which take place outside the clinical setting, and have a positive impact on health and well-being, also fall within the remit of public health. Such interventions include those promoting exposure to biodiverse environments.

Modern public health emphasises reducing avoidable differences in ill health between the most and least well-off in society (Acheson 1998; Marmot 2010). Morbidity and mortality rates are consistently and starkly higher among those with lower socio-economic status (SES) – typically 5–10 years' reduced life expectancy compared to those who are relatively more affluent (Marmot 2013; Elo 2009). Individuals of lower SES tend to live and work in less healthy environments and have higher exposure to disease risk factors; these are "social determinants of health" (Marmot and Wilkinson 2005). Moreover, lower SES is independently associated with a further 2-year reduction in life expectancy even after accounting for other risk factors for mortality, such as cardiovascular risk factors (Stringhini et al. 2017). The traditional approach to preventing disease – that is, counselling to reduce unhealthy behaviours – does not effectively address this phenomenon, because social and physical environments and circumstances mitigate behaviour change. Such inequalities are high on the political agenda (Marmot 2010, 2013; Marmot et al. 2008; Stringhini et al. 2017), and addressing the social determinants of health is an important and emerging area of clinical and public health practice (Axelson et al. 2018; Andermann 2016).

Reducing unhealthy behaviours requires the construction of supportive environments that facilitate healthier lifestyles. A biodiverse natural environment is a health-promoting resource (Lovell et al. 2014). More fundamentally, biodiverse environments are a foundation for human well-being and health, helping to sustain ecosystems that provide human health benefits, including within nutrition and medicine. A number of suggested conceptual and practical frameworks have been described that link ecosystem health and biodiversity with human health and well-being (Keune et al. 2013; Tzoulas et al. 2007, Fig. 11.1).

Biological diversity (biodiversity) is "the variability among living organisms from all sources including, *inter alia*, terrestrial, marine and other aquatic ecosystems and the ecological complexes of which they are part; this includes diversity within species, between species and of ecosystems" (United Nations Convention on

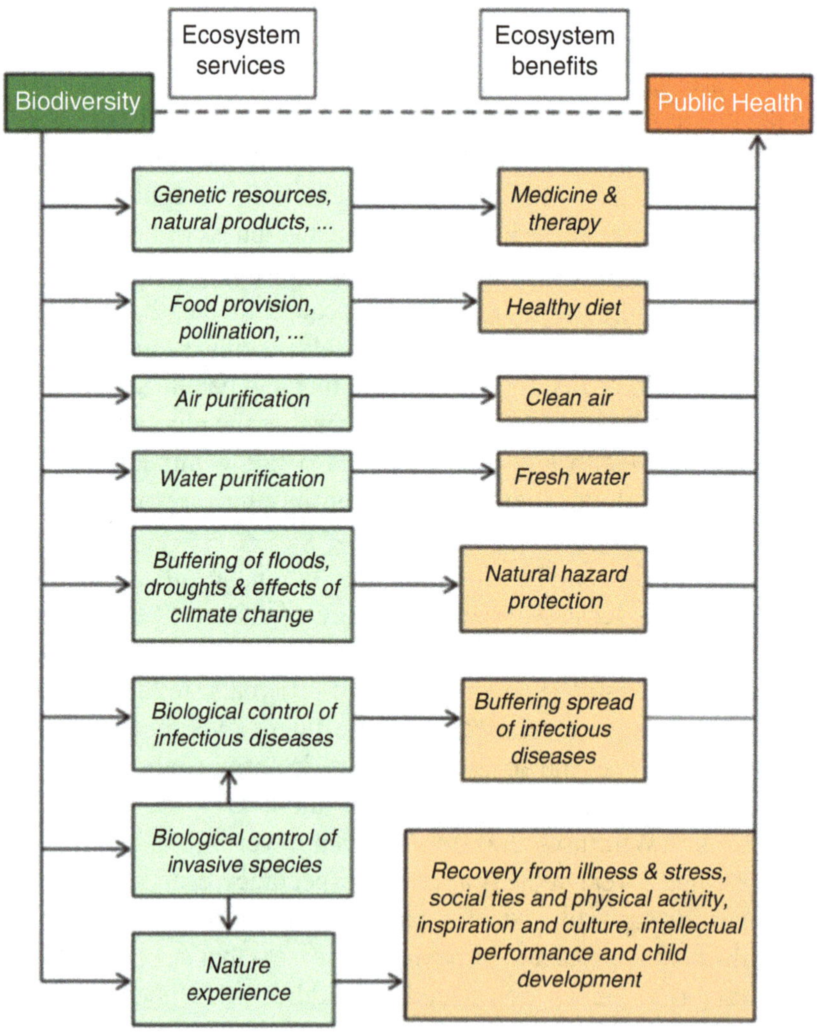

Fig. 11.1 Overview of the relationship between biodiversity and public health. (Source Keune et al. 2013)

Biological Diversity 1992). Consequently, biodiversity can be categorised in many ways. Genetic diversity, although often not apparent visually, is arguably the fundamental level of biodiversity that underpins all the others. Where genetic variation is low, wildlife and agricultural populations tend to be less resilient to environmental changes including disease, pollution and the impacts of climate change. Within a single species, underlying genetic variation can be crucial in providing phenotypic (i.e. observable) differences. For example, the single species *Canis lupus familiaris* (domestic dog) provides a range of valuable attributes to benefit humans, including support for hearing, seeing, disease detection and companionship. Within species, there are less visible genetic differences; for example, individual street trees have differing levels of tolerance to pollution. Genetic diversity can also be important in providing sustainable crops and in moderating disease pathogens. For most people, morpho-species (organisms that look different from others) provide the basis for perceived species richness. The number, type and mixture of species (community structures) provide useful measures of richness at a fairly basic level.

At a broader level of diversity, organisms live in habitats that may form distinct entities, usually described in terms of their vegetation or physical characteristics (e.g. woodlands, grasslands, ponds, rivers). Habitats may be complex, featuring gradual horizontal transitions between different types (tall herbaceous vegetation merging into scrub and then becoming denser and taller woodland; open areas of water, becoming vegetated at the edges, merging into marshy areas and then wet grassland). Complexity is also increased by the vertical layers found within them (woodlands may feature ground vegetation, herbaceous layers, scrub, lower canopies of saplings, full canopies of mature trees and emergent trees that poke beyond the canopy).

11.1.1 Chapter Overview

Having introduced some key concepts, we summarise the linkages between public health and biodiversity then discuss two spheres of public health influence. First, we discuss the role (and duty) of those working in public health to lobby for measures to tackle climate change and other threats to biodiversity. The second sphere of influence exploits the local links between access to biodiverse environments and public health, and the chapter examines how people (especially urban dwellers) can be encouraged to engage with such environments. This includes a critical look at the evidence for interventions that bring humans into health-promoting biodiverse environments, and we summarise the literature in a model. We explicate how a range of nature-based activities (including 'green care') within the nature, health and well-being sector can be used as environmentally biodiverse interventions to promote well-being, and we include two case studies on how organisations can enable communities to access and sustain biodiverse environments for the benefit of human and planetary health. Finally, we evaluate how access to biodiverse greenspace can fulfil the public health objective of reducing inequalities in health that are linked to socio-economic status.

11.2 Overview of Associations Between Public Health and Biodiversity

Some ecosystem benefits in Fig. 11.1 rely on explicit exploitation of biodiversity (e.g. for food, medicine). There is abundant evidence that biodiversity is required for the basic needs of life (e.g. food, clean water). However, for 'nature experience', biodiversity could have an impact on human health via multiple pathways, and these could operate differently depending on whether the nature experience is 'passive' or 'active'. A more biodiverse environment may offer greater opportunities for active participation, whereby the pathways to health outcomes could include physical activity and a reduction in social isolation. There are a number of theories proposed by which passive exposure to nature improves well-being, including Wilson's (1984) Biophilia hypothesis, Ulrich et al.'s (1991) Stress Recovery Theory, and Kaplan and Kaplan's (1989) Attention Restoration Theory (see Marselle Chap. 7, this volume, for further discussion of these theories). Specifically, greater biodiversity may offer greater scope for 'soft fascination' (passive interaction, entered into almost involuntarily, catching and holding one's attention), a feature of Attention Restoration Theory. Greater biodiversity would also be more likely to trigger the innate response predicted by the Biophilia Hypothesis.

A given habitat can simultaneously provide multiple ecosystem (and therefore health) benefits. For example, tree canopies and open water provide shade and cooling in urban areas, providing physical benefits to human physiological systems, and can elicit aesthetic and spiritual benefits, thereby reducing stress, mental fatigue and exhaustion. Exposure to greenspace has been linked to a range of health benefits (Maas et al. 2006; Nieuwenhuijsen et al. 2017), and more naturalistic (and therefore possibly more biodiverse) environments have been postulated as being best suited to promoting such benefits (e.g. Tyrvainen et al. 2014). There is little empirical evidence that biodiversity specifically (rather than natural environments in general) contributes directly to human health and well-being. Lovell et al.'s (2014) systematic review identified only 17 studies that included an explicit consideration of biodiversity and a health outcome, ten of which suggested an association. In the wider literature, there is some expectation that habitats found to provide health and well-being benefits may also be biodiverse; for example, Park et al. (2011) reported mood changes, including in depression, when comparing forest to urban settings. One major work that does explicitly link human health with biodiversity in an urban context is Fuller et al. (2007), who found an increase in psychological well-being with exposure to sites of high biodiversity (species richness). Luck et al. (2011) also described associations between well-being and biodiversity (especially of vegetation). Much other research in this area provides evidence of (mainly positive) links between people's perception of biodiversity and health and well-being benefits. From the wider literature, we can postulate some specific components of biodiversity that link to aspects of public health. Figure 11.2 presents a summary of our review of the links between levels of biodiversity (rows) and domains of public health (columns). The body of the table gives our assessment of the state of the evidence for links between the domains and levels of biodiversity. In general, the evidence for a direct link between biodiversity

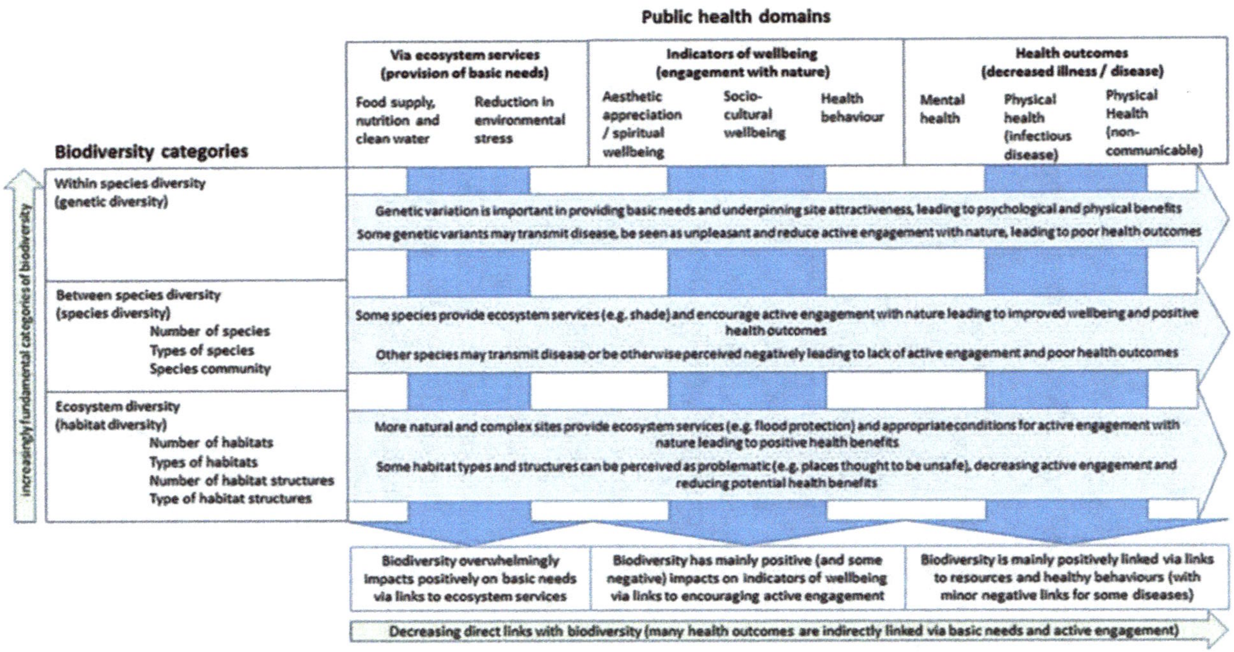

Fig. 11.2 Interaction of levels of biodiversity and domains of public health based on our assessment of the strength of the literature supporting the plausible links between biodiversity and health. Reductions in environmental stress includes flood risk, thermal comfort, pollution control, dust, atmospheric pollution

and health outcomes (the column on the right of Fig. 11.2) is less clear since the evidence of a causal relationship is less well established. However, there are plausible indirect links via the provision of the basic needs of life, which links to well-being and mental and physical health outcomes. There are also plausible (but unproven) direct relationships between exposure to biodiversity and mental and physical health outcomes. The following subheadings take each public health domain in turn and provide some selected examples to illustrate a public health viewpoint. A comprehensive review is beyond the scope of this chapter.

11.2.1 Food, Nutrition and Clean Water Supply

Biodiversity at all levels is linked to access to clean water and food of good nutritional value, which are fundamental for healthy populations. Urbanisation increases the distances that food travels and increases the challenges of maintaining clean water supplies. Public and environmental health initiatives are important in mitigating such problems. Increasing urbanisation has been followed by agricultural intensification to supply growing populations, which often leads to a reduction in biodiversity (e.g. Fahrig et al. 2015). However, conserving and enhancing the biodiversity of agricultural areas need not reduce crop productivity; for example, enhanced biodiversity reduces pest infestation, thus reducing the necessity for the use of pesticides (Petit et al. 2015). In addition, providing food across different environmental conditions (including those resulting from climate change) means that maintaining genetic and species diversity may be important in the development of food crops for the future (e.g. Bernstein 2014). There is a growing movement of urban-based food production and the biodiversity of such systems is often greater than those of other areas of greenspace (Lin et al. 2015). The supply of clean water for many cities worldwide relies on (often highly biodiverse) forest environments within the watershed (Dudley and Stolton 2003), although some land uses (including for livestock) may increase the likelihood of microbial contamination of water supplies, for example, with *Giardia lamblia* and *Cryptosporidium* species (Schreiber et al. 2015).

11.2.2 Environmental Stress

Urban environments tend to have poorer air and water quality, increased noise, decreased thermal comfort and increased stress (World Health Organisation 2016; Wheater 1999). Extreme temperatures in cities via the 'urban heat island' effect is a substantial threat to public health (World Health Organisation 2016). The most vulnerable in society (i.e. with the lowest SES) suffer disproportionately from these stresses (Diaz et al. 2006). Biodiversity can provide ecosystem services that buffer communities from environmental stress (Haines-Young and Potschin 2010), which may become especially important in the context of climate change. For example, different species and varieties of trees differ in the extent to which they provide shade, reduce particulate and other pollution, and buffer noise, humidity and temperature, as well as disrupting gusty wind flow through city streets (Wheater 1999). Therefore, a diverse tree community fulfils more of these functions. Higher habitat diversity provides even greater benefits on city cooling than does the presence of greenspace alone (Kong et al. 2014). Flood risk is increasingly important, causing disruption, risk of death from drowning and physical injury, as well as increasing the incidence of diseases (de Man et al. 2014). Biodiverse environments within the watersheds surrounding an urban area can help moderate flood risk (Carter et al. 2017). See Lindley et al. Chap. 2, this volume, for further discussion on the effects of climate change on health, and the use of biodiversity for climate change mitigation.

11.2.3 Aesthetic Appreciation and Spiritual Well-being

People have a range of preferences for different observable diversity at the genetic, species, communities of species and habitat levels. Whether viewing nature, experiencing it, or actively engaging with it, certain plants and animals and types of habitats may elicit appreciation or disgust, engagement or rejection. For example, many people feed squirrels in the park but not rats in the back streets (species preferences); others will take walks through open parkland but not dense scrub (habitat preferences). Such preferences may be age- and culture-specific (Bjerke et al. 2006). It is not only the type of species that may be attractive; the number (richness) of species and type of species community also affect aesthetic appreciation. Large populations and communities of birds, wildflowers and trees tend to be perceived as more attractive than swarms of insects or other invertebrates (e.g. Shwartz et al. 2014). Colourful wildflower meadows are usually preferred over sparsely vegetated brownfield sites (even where these contain many of the same species). Southon et al. (2017) identified that more biodiverse meadows increased people's appreciation of sites, and Sang et al. (2016) found that higher perceived naturalness was linked to higher aesthetic appreciation and more active engagement with urban greenspace. In urban greenspace, the presence of scrub may be off-putting if it is perceived as providing cover for criminal activity (Hough 2014).

Some studies have sought to investigate whether well-being is related to conscious perception of biodiversity. People's perception of the level of biodiversity often does not equate to actual biodiversity values. For example, although Southon et al. (2018) did find an alignment between perceived and actual biodiversity for some habitats, Dallimer et al. (2012) suggested that people may not be good at assessing actual biodiversity despite finding a link between perceived species biodiversity and well-being. Lindberg (2012) established that people will distinguish between spaces of differing quality but do not necessarily align these with actual biodiversity. Shwartz et al. (2014) found that people underestimated biodiversity in manipulated plots and were biased towards the biodiversity of particular groups (plants) over others (birds, trees and especially insects). Marselle et al. (2016) found a link between perceived bird biodiversity (but not perceived butterfly or plant/tree biodiversity) and restorativeness. The constructs of human health, human well-being and biodiversity are multi-dimensional and can be difficult to define and quantify (Naeem et al. 2016).

There appear to be strong links between the aesthetic and spiritual appreciation of nature, with mental health benefits and engagement with outdoor activities. These provide public health professionals with further opportunities to provide advice and interventions for improving the health of vulnerable communities. Interestingly, De Lacy and Shackleton (2017) reported that greenspace associated with urban sacred sites enhanced the spiritual experience of visitors. Nature is deeply embedded into a number of religions, therefore spending time in nature enhances a sense of belonging and the spiritual experience (Lindgren et al. 2018). See Irvine et al. Chap. 10, this volume, for a more indepth discussion about biodiversity and spiritual well-being.

11.2.4 Socio-cultural Well-being

Social isolation is linked to increased risk of overall mortality (Holt-Lunstad et al. 2015) and diseases such as coronary heart disease and stroke (Valtorta et al. 2016). Promoting social interaction is a key public health priority; one that could be facilitated by access to natural environments (World Health Organisation 2016). The Social Finance Report conveys the positive impact of biodiverse environments on older people and suggests that physical activity in the outdoor environment reduces social isolation, which in turn can reduce GP attendance and A&E admissions (Social Finance 2015). Access to nature and nature-based approaches such as green care can have a positive influence on an individual's social activation (Gonzalez et al. 2009). However, there are differences in how urban greenspace is used by different ages, genders and cultures (e.g. Bjerke et al. 2006; Maas et al. 2008), which may influence how planning takes place for public health purposes (e.g. Sang et al. 2016). See Kabisch Chap. 5, this volume, for more about the role of socio-demographic factors in greenspace and health effects.

11.2.5 Health Behaviour Including the Promotion of Physical Activity

Creating opportunities for engaging with physical activity and other healthy behaviours is important in public health practice. Research demonstrates that a sedentary lifestyle contributes to increases in coronary heart disease, diabetes and obesity (Wilmot et al. 2012). Studies have shown that people living nearer to parks were more likely to use them for physical activity (World Health Organization 2016) and were less likely to be overweight or obese (Coombes et al. 2010). Levels of physical activity were higher in greener neighbourhoods and, in those with over 15% greenspace, cardiovascular disease risk was reduced (Richardson et al. 2013). However, the biodiversity of habitats preferred for physical activity may vary with the activity involved, and the age group of the participants (e.g. Ward Thompson 2013). For example, playing (informal) football requires a large amount of open space with significant buffer zones separating the activity from other uses (Golicnik and Ward Thompson 2010). Such space would not tend to be particularly biodiverse. Runners and cyclists may prefer more open environments, whilst walkers may select more structured habitats. Site management may exploit such preferences to avoid conflicts (and even collisions) on shared tracks (Santos et al. 2016). People report greater enjoyment of outdoor exercise compared to equivalent exercise performed indoors (Thompson Coon et al. 2011). However, Shanahan et al. (2016) identify a knowledge gap in understanding which characteristics of nature are important in promoting physical activity. Exercise also benefits the immune system (Pedersen et al. 2007): general exercise releases myokines, and this effect is greater in colder environments, such as when exercising outdoors in a temperate climate. Myokines induce an inflammatory/pro-inflammatory response control, influencing the function of chronic inflammation, and can positively affect cognition, reduce depression and reduce inflammatory responses associated with osteoporotic disease (Kaji 2016). For a detailed discussion on green space interventions to promote physical activity, see Hunter et al. Chap. 17, this volume.

11.2.6 Mental Health

While the direct association between appreciation of different levels of biodiversity and well-being are clear, this is less so for mental health (as measured by the absence of mental disorders such as anxiety or depression). However, there is a clear link between access to natural environments and mental health (World Health Organization 2016). Bragg and Atkins (2016) suggest that three key components (being in the environment, meaningful activities within the environment, and the social context) can positively influence mental health. Both active participation in greenspace and observable greenspace are significant in achieving mental health benefits (Nutsford et al. 2013), and horticultural activities programmes for older people lead to reduced levels of depression and improved life satisfaction (Masuya et al. 2014). There is some evidence that exposure to 'beautiful' nature (potentially equating to perceived biodiversity) promotes socially desirable behaviours (Zhang et al. 2014). Beyer et al. (2014) suggested that greening could be useful within a population mental health strategy. For a more in-depth discussion on mental health and biodiversity, see de Vries and Snep Chap.8, this volume, and Marselle et al. Chap. 9, this volume.

11.2.7 Physical Health – Infectious Disease (Disease/Pathogen Reduction)

The links between biodiversity and infectious disease are complex. Although Bernstein (2014) suggested a possible swamping of disease transmission agents by larger species diversity, Wood et al. (2014) identified no such reduction for many diseases, suggesting that if such links were important then biodiversity may increase disease. Conversely, Keesing et al. (2010) found that, although areas of high biodiversity can be a source pool for new pathogens, there was increasing evidence that biodiversity loss can increase disease transmission. They suggested that preserving areas with endemic biodiversity should generally reduce infectious disease prevalence.

Sandifer et al. (2015) examined the links between microbial biodiversity, allergic reactions and respiratory diseases, arguing that exposure to microbial diversity can improve health, for example, reducing allergens that may also influence the management of some respiratory conditions. This reinforces aspects of the 'hygiene hypothesis', which proposes that exposure to microbes at an early age can enhance inflammatory responses and thus heighten human resilience to allergens (Hanski et al. 2012). This point was also reported by Ege et al. (2011), who identified that children raised on a farm were less likely to suffer from asthma. See Damialis et al. Chap. 3, this volume, for further discussion on allergenic responses, and Müller et al. Chap. 4, this volume, for more information about vector borne disease.

11.2.8 Physical Health – Non-Communicable Disease

Systematic review-level evidence demonstrates that proximity to greenspace is linked to a reduction in mortality due to all causes (van den Berg et al. 2015). Cross-sectional studies show increased neighbourhood greenspace is linked to lower levels of type 2 diabetes (Bodicoat et al. 2014). When specifically considering the role of biodiversity, the effects on physical health outcomes are likely to be indirect, via nutrition, protection from stressors, positive effects on personal and socio-cultural well-being, and creation of desirable natural areas for healthy behaviour. Epidemiological studies have been useful in providing evidence of a link between exposure to greenspace and health outcomes measurable at an area and population level (Mitchell and Popham 2008; de Vries et al. 2003). However, fully making the case for the health benefits of biodiverse environments will require further work on the type and nature of the greenspace and its links to health. Much work at the area level has tended to use crude measures of exposure to biodiversity; for example, the percentage of greenspace in the local environment. Recently, Dennis et al. (2018) have developed a sophisticated land-cover model that incorporates socio-demographics for an urban city area. Early findings suggest that the strength of the health–greenspace relationship depends on the nature of the greenspace, with lower diversity greenscapes (recreational grassland) having a less strong relationship with good health compared to areas with more complex greenspace (e.g. shrubs and trees).

Access to greenspace in general has been suggested to be beneficial in the management of long-term conditions such as obesity, cardiovascular disease and diabetes. Moreover, when people exercise in the natural environment, the impact of the two protective factors, exercise and greenspace, acting together may be greater than simply summing the positive effects (i.e. may be synergistic: Shanahan et al. 2016). The protective effect of greenspace begins early in life: among children, those with access to gardens and greenspace were less likely to be obese at age 7 years (Schalkwijk et al.

2018). For more on the effect of greenspace on children's health, see Dadvand et al. Chap 6, this volume. Chen and Janke (2012) reported that older people who garden suffer from fewer falls, possibly due to improved gait and balance.

11.3 The Role of Public Health in Lobbying for Protecting Biodiversity

Human societies increasingly place species and natural habitats (especially biodiverse habitats) under considerable pressure (Lawton et al. 2010). Threats to biodiversity include urbanisation, intensive agriculture, increased pollution and impacts of climate change. Whilst the first three threats can be managed locally, regionally or nationally, climate change requires international cooperation. The role and responsibility of public health experts to campaign on climate change and other threats to biodiversity are given forcefully in the 2015 Lancet Commission on Health and Climate Change (Watts et al. 2015). It has become vital for health departments of governments not to operate in isolation; health professionals need to ensure that climate-health-related considerations are integrated into government-wide strategies. One example of cross-governmental working can be seen in the recent UK Environment Strategy, in which health features as a major section (DEFRA 2018). In addition to averting biodiversity loss (e.g. preventing deforestation), climate-related topics requiring cross-governmental thinking also impact directly on public health (e.g. phasing out coal as an energy source will protect cardiovascular and respiratory health). Initiatives to support lifestyles that are healthy for both humans and the environment will also help to provide resilience in the face of the health risks posed by climate change. See Keune et al. Chap 15, this volume, for further information on international and national nature-health initiatives.

Public health professionals need to ensure investment in health systems that can respond to climate change-induced threats to human health. For example, urban flooding can be a significant risk to human health both directly (through the risk of drowning) and through exposure to pathogenic microbes (Jørgensen et al. 2016). Similarly, changes in extreme temperatures in cities (including in Europe) are contributing to significant increases in heat-related mortality levels (Mitchell et al. 2016). Drought conditions can also exacerbate risks to health, for example, from microorganisms in the plumes from cooling towers (Pagnier et al. 2009), since water drawn from rivers containing municipal waste may become more concentrated during droughts.

The appropriate policy for maintaining and developing greenspaces of appropriate size and accessibility for public health has long been debated. In 1929, for London (UK), Unwin recommended 7 acres (2.83 ha) of greenspace be allocated per 1,000 people as playing fields (first report of the Greater London Regional Planning Committee in 1933, cited by Turner 1992). Later work for English Nature recommended an Accessible Natural Greenspace Standards model with (*inter alia*) at least 2 ha of natural greenspace within 300 m of all residents and at least 2 ha of Local Nature Reserve per 1,000 people (Harrison et al. 1995). It was recognised that such guidance was not being implemented by all local authorities and Pauleit et al. (2003) recommended the standards become flexible to address local contexts. Whilst greenspace standards may be appropriate to promote human health and well-being, these may need to be revised if greenspace is to mitigate the impacts of climate change on urban centres. For additional discussion about how human health is addressed in planning legislation, see Heiland et al. Chap. 20, this volume.

The International Convention on Biodiversity (2017) suggested that there is already sufficient evidence to justify several actions to protect human health, including integrating biodiverse greenspaces in urban development. It identified the need to address the drivers of ill health and biodiversity loss together (for further discussion on policies linking biodiversity, health and climate change, see Korn et al. Chap. 14, this volume). Governments should invest in research and monitoring, including quantifying the savings from reduced health-care costs and the enhanced productivity that would accompany climate change mitigation (Convention on Biodiversity 2017; Watts et al. 2015). Internationally, governments must support countries to become low carbon economies as a global endeavour (Watts et al. 2015), since consumption in wealthier countries drives carbon use in less wealthy countries. Public health professionals need to engage the public as well (Corner et al. 2014): framing climate change concerns around health and well-being may be more powerful than arguing to conserve the environment without an explicit link to human health (Myers et al. 2012).

11.4 Public Health Action at a Local Level

Locally, a public health-informed system would encourage cities to support lifestyles that benefit both humans and the environment. Steps to achieve this include the development of highly energy-efficient sustainable housing; available low-cost active transportation; and increased access to greenspaces. These measures would promote more resilience in human health, whilst also reducing urban pollution, greenhouse gas emissions, rates of diseases associated with poor air quality (Watts et al. 2015) and diseases associated with a sedentary lifestyle (e.g. cardiovascular disease, cancer, obesity, diabetes). Whilst we acknowledge that all such actions are vital to the public health professional's role, here we focus on access to biodiverse greenspaces.

Although cities are places where the benefits of nature have been historically disregarded in favour of clean and hygienic space (Keune et al. 2013), the concept of greenspace as a resource for public health is long-standing. Access to, and immersion with, nature was first championed in 1772 by the English politician, Joseph Addison and later by the founder of nursing, Florence Nightingale (1860). Many Victorian public parks were created as a public health resource (Wheater et al. 2007). Historically, the visual experiences of rural landscapes as a source of refreshment and renewal of physical, mental and spiritual health was thought to complement medical approaches, and this belief influenced the location of asylums in the 19th century (Hickman 2009). The tradition of therapeutic landscapes was suggested in 1992 by Wilbert Gesler (Bell et al. 2018), who described these as natural environments, which interact with the social environment, to provide spaces of healing.

A complex set of transactions between accessing greenspace and participating in greenspace led Bell et al. (2018) to develop "palettes of place" from macro-scale areas (countryside, coasts and seaside), through meso-scale (urban parks and riversides) to micro-scale palettes (hospitals, clinic gardens, woods and allotments). Pauleit et al. (2003) make the point that greenspace needs not only to be accessible, but also of good quality. Quality influences the way nature is perceived, and the extent to which people participate in and use nature (Kaplan and Kaplan 1989; Pretty et al. 2005). The modern shift to engage nature has emerged from an ambition to use biodiversity to nurture human health. Hence, the appetite to determine the effect of a mere view of nature has evoked research in a range of settings, populations and activities to illustrate the therapeutic influence of the landscape. For example, Ulrich's (1984) seminal work exploring the restorative influence of views from windows on post-operative recovery of patients following cholecystectomy was one of the first influential studies to demonstrate the positive effects a view of nature can have on recovery. Ulrich reported that patients with a view of trees spent less time in hospital and required less analgesic than those without such views. It is worth noting that behaviour and cognition may also be moderated by naturalistic views: Kuo and Sullivan (2001) recorded reduced aggression associated with mental fatigue for residents in greener (nature-based) buildings, and Taylor et al. (2002) identified increased self-discipline (in girls at least) with increased natural views from home.

The ways in which exposure and engagement with nature for well-being has diffused into contemporary public health intervention strategies has been described in a series of models, which we have integrated and reformulated to incorporate the potential for biodiversity enhancement (Fig. 11.3). As a starting point, three distinct ways in which individuals engage with nature are described (Haubenhofer et al. 2010): (i) through outdoor activities such as walking as part of everyday life activities; (ii) through recreational activities such as the use of cycle paths and structured outdoor activities that could promote health; and (iii) nature being used as a therapeutic intervention within a 'green-care' context (left to right in Fig. 11.3). The latter includes, for example, those "nature-based therapy or treatment interventions — specifically designed, structured and facilitated for individuals with a defined need" (Bragg and Atkins 2016: 18). Hence the 'nature, health and well-being sector' is a term used to describe green care and health promotion services. The levels of nature and extent to which nature can be used to support well-being is depicted from top to bottom of Fig. 11.3 as earlier described by Pretty et al. (2005), who note that at one level ("viewing nature"), an individual is simply exposed to an environment through vistas; a second level ("being in the presence of nature") involves greater participation in nature through activities such as walking or gardening (referred to as green exercise). The final level ("active participation in nature") is based on a more prescribed approach where activities are considered as "therapies", with an intention to treat, heal or alleviate through experiencing and interacting with nature. Since none of the existing models explicitly consider biodiversity, we have added consideration of how biodiversity links with each of the levels of engagement and how this may be enhanced to improve actual (as well as perceived) biodiversity. The intensity of the

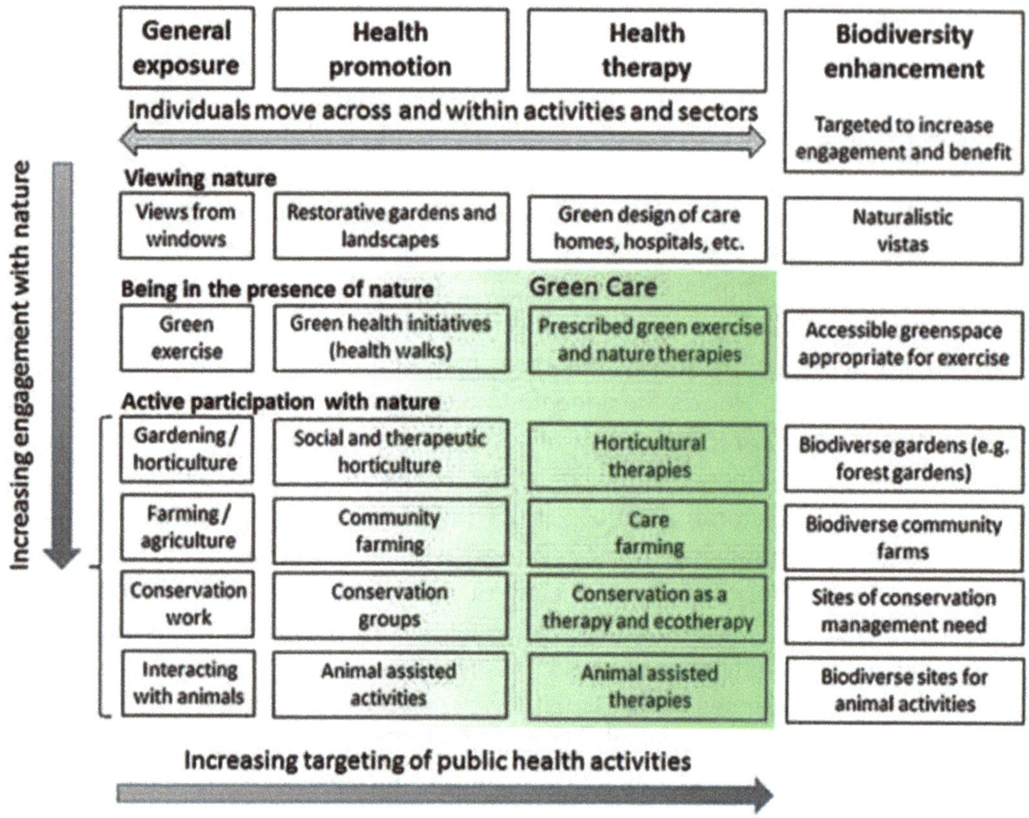

Fig. 11.3 Model of the interactions between level of engagement with nature, level of public health targeting (combining the models of Pretty et al. 2005; Haubenhofer et al. 2010; Annerstedt and Währborg 2011; Bragg and Leck 2017) with the additions of potential benefits due to enhanced biodiversity. Green care (shaded area) covers a range of targeted activities that overlap those developed through health promotion as well as specific health therapies

exposure to biodiversity varies depending on activity, and is likely to be higher when the participation is more active. For example, conservation volunteering may involve handling plant-life and soil, which brings people intimately in touch with biodiversity (soils can be extremely biodiverse even if they are not always perceived that way). Therapeutic gardens could be biodiverse, for example, through the variety in species required in the creation of a sensory garden. As per the Bragg and Leck (2017) extension to the existing models, well-being and the promotion of health are not static, and individuals often move across and within the nature, health and well-being sector (i.e. horizontally between health promotion and health therapy, and diagonally between different activities and therapies).

Box 11.1 is a case study that illustrates the variety of activities that can be supported in a community forest. This suggests multiple beneficial opportunities to access, engage with and, where prescribed, undertake as a therapy. Active participation probably has greater health benefits (Collins and O'Callaghan 2008), and more biodiverse environments can increase the therapeutic effects on humans (Annerstedt and Währborg 2011). Interventions that encourage people to support biodiversity, for example through choice of species when gardening, have the potential to simul-

Box 11.1: Case Study

City of Trees
***Jessica Thompson**, Health and Well-being Lead, City of Trees, UK*

The City of Trees (City of Trees 2018) movement based in Greater Manchester is one of the UK's Community Forestry (England's Community Forests 2018) organisations and forms part of the Northern Forest concept (Braby 2018). City of Trees represents urban forestry, a term widely used in the USA and Northern Europe to define the 'art, science and technology' in relation to trees and plants that exist within an urban setting as well as the "physiological, sociological, economic, and aesthetic benefits trees provide society" (Konijnendijk et al. 2006). In its physical form, the urban forest includes all aspects of green infrastructure found within the urban setting at varying spatial scales, e.g. the mosaic of street trees, woodlands, parks, orchards, gardens, incidental greenspaces, etc. City of Trees advocates a natural capital approach to the benefits of green infrastructure, described as ecosystem services (Natural England 2009), such as biodiversity, climate change adaptation, recreation, health and well-being.

City of Trees strives to be a public facing movement. A team delivers campaigns and community engagement programmes, such as Green Streets (a neighbourhood-greening programme that facilitates community-based street tree planting, Fig. 11.4), community orchard creation and pocket woodland

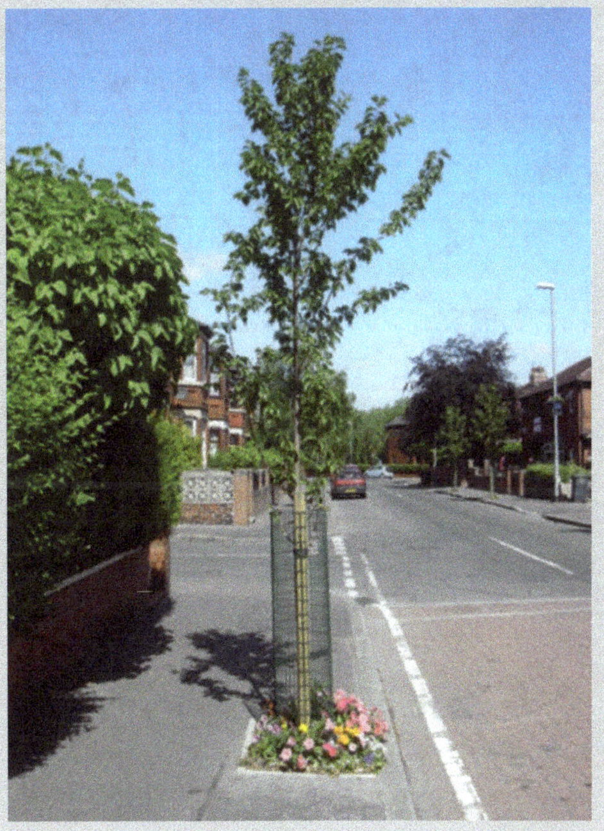

Fig. 11.4 A neighbourhood greening programme that facilitates community-based street planting. (Photo credit: City of Trees)

(continued)

Box 11.1 (continued)

planting, giving people the power to bring nature, biodiversity and food growing to their neighbourhoods. Outreach initiatives such as Woodland Futures and Dementia Naturally Active aim to connect people to nature (Fig. 11.5) as well as tackle issues around social isolation, by providing nature-based activities for therapeutic and vocational rehabilitation. Green infrastructure gives people the opportunity to become stewards of ecosystem services (Andersson et al. 2014), and City of Trees aims to inspire social inclusion through its volunteer initiative, Citizen Forester, encouraging a wide range of audiences to take part in tree planting, woodland habitat management and citizen science recording of tree species. City of Trees also works strategically to strive for an environmental justice approach to developing high-quality green infrastructure, to encourage utility and recreational walking and cycling in support of healthier lifestyles. The work and outcomes of City of Trees has implications for public health priorities on prevention, self-care and early intervention to improve population health and health inequalities.

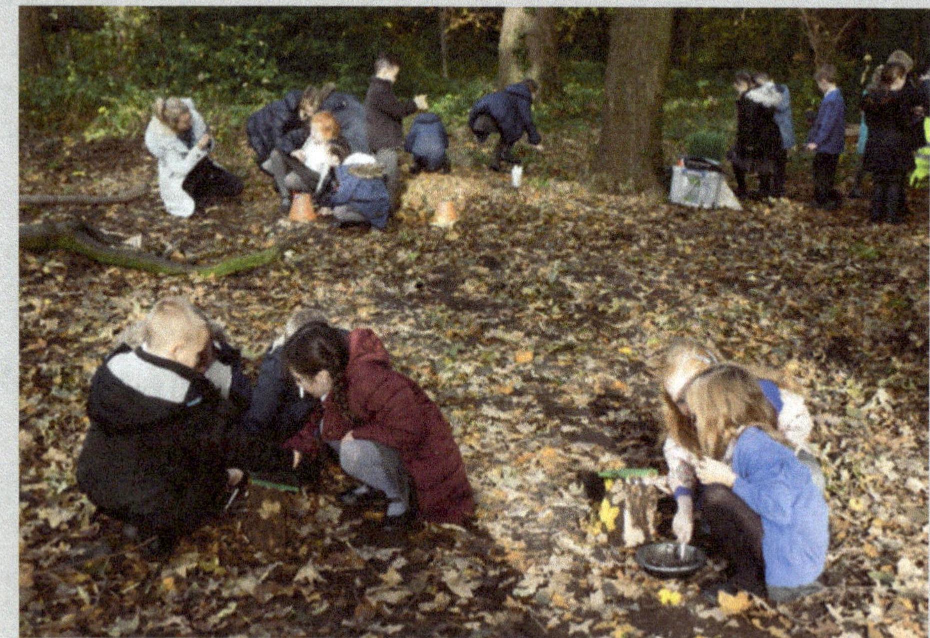

Fig. 11.5 Outreach work with schools connects young people with nature. (Photo credit: City of Trees)

Box 11.2: Case Study

Royal Horticultural Society: Plants for Bugs

***Alistair Griffiths**, Director of Science and Collections, Royal Horticultural Society, UK*

The Royal Horticultural Society (RHS) has identified that the UK's garden plants, gardeners and the 27 million gardens play a significant role in supporting biodiversity. They concluded that the best strategy for gardeners wanting to support pollinating insects in gardens is to plant a mix of flowering plants from different countries and regions. They also suggest that emphasis is given to plants native to the UK and the northern hemisphere (though exotic plants from the southern hemisphere can be used to extend the season). In addition, regardless of plant origin (native or non-native), the more flowers a garden can offer throughout the year, the greater the number of bees, hoverflies and other pollinating insects it will attract and support (Salisbury et al. 2015, 2017).

The RHS translated this research knowledge so as to reconnect people back with nature and encourage more people to put garden plants that attract wildlife into their gardens. An intervention such as this, which encourages people to support biodiversity through choice of species when gardening, has the potential to simultaneously improve both human health (by increasing exposure to biodiverse environments) and the health of the natural environment. The RHS worked with the UK horticultural industry and with the UK Government's National Pollinator Strategy and produced information for gardeners in the form of bulletins on-line (Royal Horticultural Society 2015).

The research findings were also used and disseminated through the RHS networks such as: through the Campaign for School Gardening with 34,000 schools; Britain in Bloom with 300,000 volunteers; and through shows, gardens, and retail, in order to help safeguard nature. The Plants for Bugs work (Fig. 11.6) showcases how scientific research and development, industry, gardeners and government can join together to inspire people to choose and grow garden plants for pollinator and biodiversity benefit. This creates a new ecosystem-service product line, which in turn increases plant sales and the economic bottom line for the horticulture industry, whilst encouraging and supporting biodiversity.

Pollination is a key ecosystem service that substantially contributes to the global food supply and human nutrition (Fig. 11.7). The RHS Pollinator plant lists have been widely adopted by the horticulture industry, and the government's National Pollinator Strategy (England) launched in November 2014 endorses RHS Plants for Pollinators and encourages gardeners to choose plants that provide resources for pollinators.

(continued)

Box 11.2 (continued)

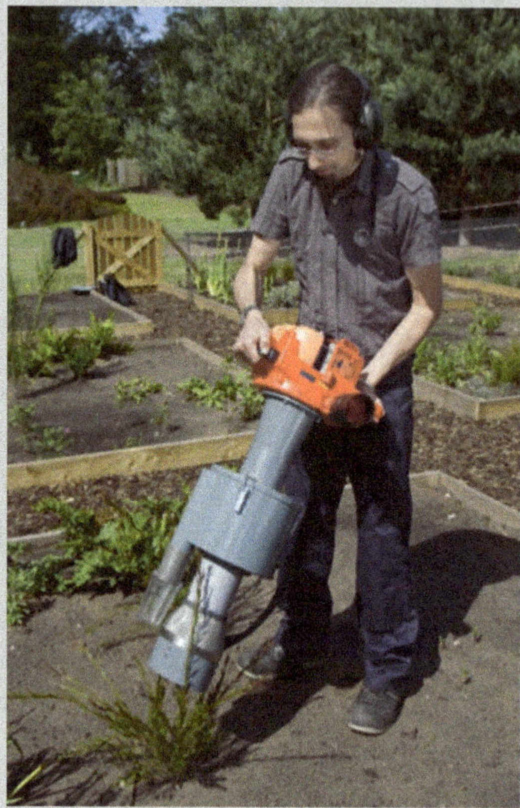

Fig. 11.6 Royal Horticultural Society Entomologist Andrew Salisbury using the Vortis bug sampler on the Plants for Bugs experimental plots at the Royal Horticultural Society Wisley Garden. (Photo credit: Royal Horticultural Society)

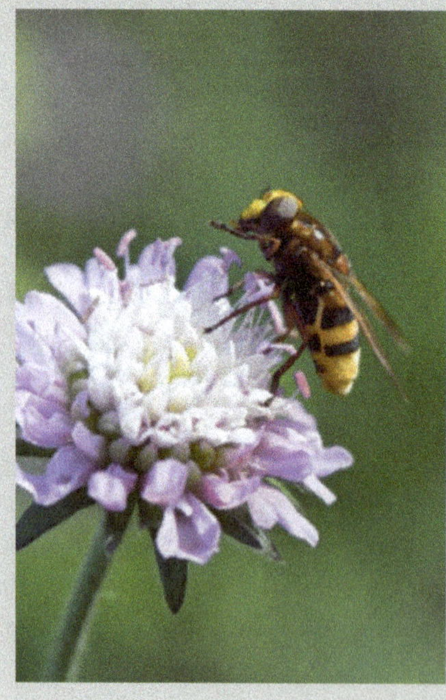

Fig. 11.7 Female hoverfly (*Volucella zonaria*) on field scabious (*Knautia arvensis*) on the Plants for Bugs experimental plot. (Photo credit: Royal Horticultural Society)

taneously improve both human health and the health of the semi-natural environment (see Box 11.2).

Research over the last 20 years describes a range of nature-based activities that constitute green care and, crucially, the positive impact on health and well-being for people who may be vulnerable or socially excluded (Berget et al. 2012). The increased interest in such innovative approaches to well-being has led to a proliferation of terms used to denote nature-based work; consequently, the terms *green care* and *nature-based interventions* are often used interchangeably (Bragg and Atkins 2016). The spectrum of nature-based activities includes gardening, vistas and walking, food growing, community gardens, prescribed (for example, an imposed or recommended regimen) exposure to nature, nature-based activity or structured green care activities (Green Care Coalition 2017). Thus, social prescriptions using outdoor nature-based approaches, as available within the nature, health and well-being sectors, provide one way in which health professionals with a public health role might facilitate individuals to access biodiverse greenspace.

11.4.1 Towards an Emerging Salutogenic Paradigm?

Salutogensis focuses on factors that support human health and well-being, rather than on those that cause disease (i.e. pathogenesis) (Antonovsky 1979). Predicated on the paradigm that health is a positive state of well-being rather than just "being well" and deterring ill health, salutogenesis originated through Antonovsky's (1979) asset-based approach, which endorses the skills, attributes and resources of individuals and communities to develop resilience and a sense of purpose. Hence, a salutogenic approach has influenced the move away from more medical, pathogenic models to provide a sense of coherence between health and illness.

The lack of proof of causality in the evidence base for biodiversity and human well-being has straitjacketed public health policy. This is because evidence-based commissioning, the process by which health interventions are funded on the basis of their proven effectiveness, requires strong evidence that the intervention (e.g. a green-care intervention) has a causal relationship with health (i.e. disease reduction). This is predicated on a medical evidence hierarchy in which a positivist paradigm prevails. Hence, commissioners may be reluctant to support services lacking experimentally-derived evidence and have been slow to embed salutogenic approaches within health-care policy. However, taking a more proactive and structured approach to the use of nature-based interventions, particularly those involving biodiverse environments, has the potential to influence public health discourse and morph into an emerging salutogenic paradigm. Such interventions may be cost effective by reducing the economic burden on health-care systems; however, in order to demonstrate this, it is essential to develop evaluation methods that can adequately define these health and economic benefits. Evaluation methods need to engage with the complexity rather than attempt to reduce it to measurable outcomes, as is recognised by the UK Medical Research Council's guidance on evaluating complex interventions (Craig et al. 2011). Such methods might include natural experiments/quasi-experiments analysed using stepped wedge or interrupted time-series analyses (Hu 2015), and should include a process evaluation to take into account the varying contexts in which the intervention takes place (Moore et al. 2015).

The shift from a medical model has encouraged a rethink of care and care provision and has latterly become established within a 'Social Prescribing' movement. As a non-medical approach, social prescribing interventions promote person-centred and asset-based approaches for people with diverse needs (Polley et al. 2017). Social prescribing can support communities and individuals by placing the "individual or service user in the driving seat so it creates the opportunity for real and lasting behaviour change because it involves learning and making choices" (Jackson 2016: 14). Also referred to as community referral or asset-based, person-centred approaches, there is no agreed single term used to describe social prescribing. Significantly, its definition may be difficult to hone as it is part of a larger social movement, initiated by the UK National Endowment for Science, Technology and the Arts (NESTA), based on 'people-powered health' designed to help reduce health inequalities, as highlighted in the influential UK Marmot Report (2010).

A social prescription enables a health professional to collaborate with a link worker or community navigator who facilitates a person-centred conversation to design the participant's own solutions to well-being (Bertotti et al. 2018). This well-being conversation can prevent unnecessary GP attendance, reduce hospital emergency admissions, reduce social isolation, and help support individuals with a range of conditions (Kimberlee et al. 2014; Chatterjee et al. 2017). Approaches to social prescribing range from long-term condition management to volunteer opportunities with a focus on well-being through supported activities (Dayson et al. 2015). Since 2013, four models of social prescribing have emerged: (i) signposting; (ii) linking with specific projects; (iii) joint partnerships; and (iv) holistic referrals (Kimberlee 2013). This includes, but is not exclusive to, therapeutic horticulture- and arts-based approaches. The ways in which these activities occur are diverse and reflect the contemporary public health approach adopted mainly within third-sector organisations, community groups and charities, rather than commissioned health services.

Examples of nature-based social prescribing interventions range from arranged walks in forests to conservation volunteering and more structured 'green-care' activities such as those observed within therapeutic gardens, all of which fit within the frameworks summarised in Fig. 11.3. Since the more active one becomes with nature, the more likely the exposure to biodiversity, health professionals should work with appropriate bodies to maximise biodiversity enhancement of nature-based social prescriptions. The case study in Box 11.2 explicitly brings people into contact with biodiversity for the benefit of the health of participants and the planet.

11.5 Use of Biodiverse Natural Environments to Reduce Inequalities in Health

A major drawback in using greenspace to improve public health is that those who are socially disadvantaged are least likely to have access to good quality greenspace. The health benefits from biodiverse environments tend to be disproportionately experienced by the most advantaged sectors of society (Diaz et al. 2006). This is a social justice issue: the wealthy have less need of the health benefit; they tend to already possess greenspace by having the financial resources to live in greener areas and to own private greenspace; they may travel more extensively to areas of natural beauty; they are more likely to exercise/make use of the greenspace; and finally, they are more likely to displace less advantaged communities from newly greened, previously brownfield sites (i.e. in a process of gentrification).

Estimates of health impacts due to SES can be made at a geographical area level, where for a given area the average SES status is known and health data are available. At such geographical areas (carried out at the neighbourhood level, approximately 1,500 persons), it is also possible to measure aspects of the natural environment using geographical information system databases. These area-level analyses show that greenspace is positively associated with health, even after accounting for SES, e.g. in Holland (de Vries et al. 2003) and the UK (Mitchell and Popham 2008; Dennis et al. 2018). Indeed, the impact of greenspace on health is greater for those in the most deprived neighbourhoods (de Vries et al. 2003; Mitchell and Popham 2008). Specifically, Mitchell and Popham (2008) demonstrated that proximity to greenspace reduced health inequalities, and that this effect was stronger in the neighbourhoods with the lowest SES (Fig. 11.8).

Good access to greenspace in the local environment can disrupt the expected link between relative poverty and ill health (Mitchell et al. 2015). However, Wolch et al. (2014) warn that policies promoting greening of areas for those community areas most in need of such a disruption of health inequality may lead to gentrification and a displacement of the very people most in need. They advocate a balance of greening "just enough" to provide benefits without too great a disruption to planning and development. More research will be needed to determine whether this is appropriate, feasible and at what level it should be implemented.

Residing near to greenspace may not guarantee the full benefits of the natural environment, and in areas where greenspace is more fragmented a more targeted approach might be needed to bring people into contact with nature. This is where the nature, health and well-being sector could target those in socially-deprived neighbourhoods (by using social prescriptions for nature-based interventions) to fit within a public health strategy that aims to reduce inequalities in health.

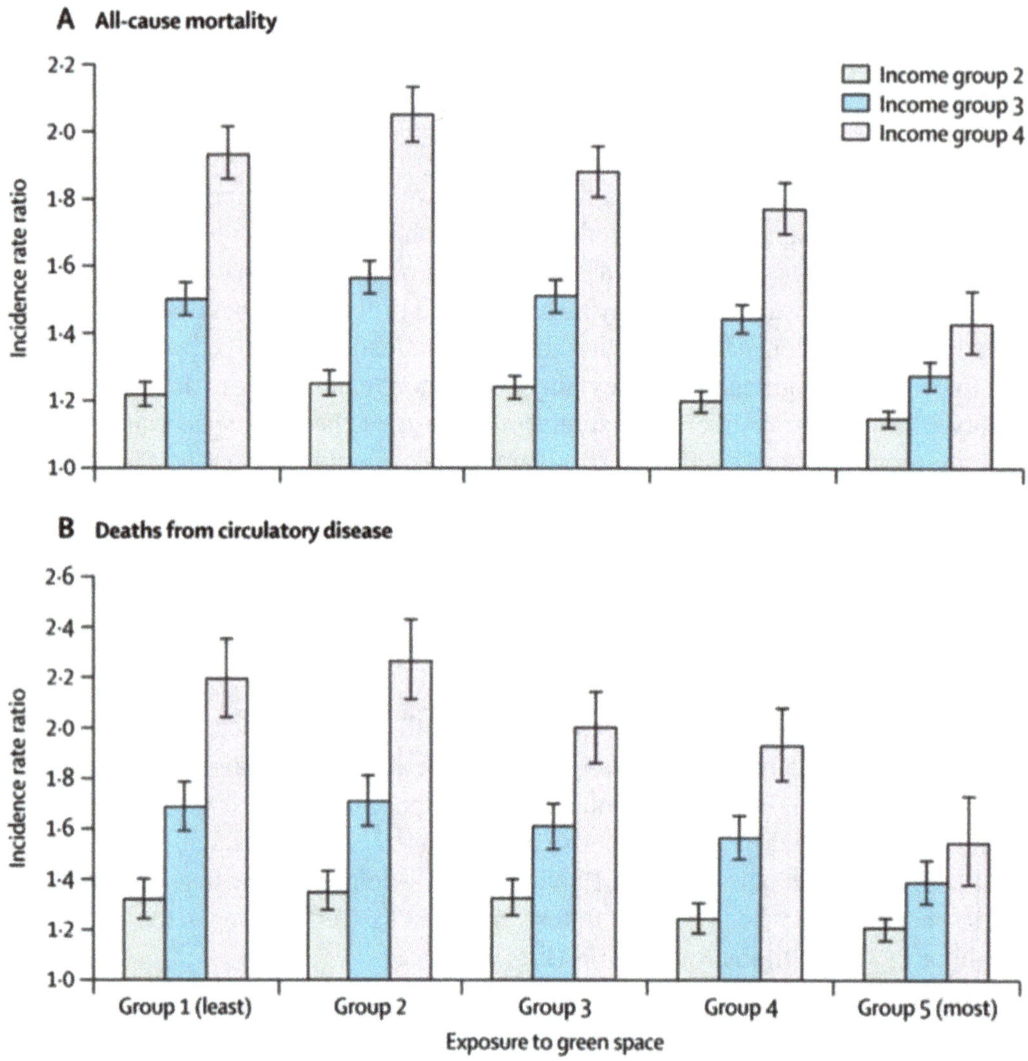

Fig. 11.8 Incidence rate ratios for all-cause mortality (**a**) and deaths from circulatory disease (**b**) in income-deprivation quartiles 2–4, relative to income deprivation quartile 1 (least deprived), stratified by exposure to green space. Bars are grouped according to population exposure to green space. Error bars indicate 95% CIs. The total mortality and deaths from cardiovascular disease decreases with increasing greenspace in the environment. In each category of greenspace, relative to the most wealthy (incidence ratio of 1), there is increasing mortality with decreasing income. However, this disparity is far less apparent in the greenest areas, with the least well off group appearing to benefit the most. (Source: Mitchell and Popham 2008)

11.6 Conclusion

Human health is intricately linked with the natural environment. Preservation of the variety of life on the planet is essential to maintain the complex interdependencies between ecosystems and human life. Biodiversity, because of its fundamental relationship with ecosystems services, helps to mitigate the effects of climate change, but is itself at risk of loss due to climate change. Arguably the single biggest priority for public health at a strategic international level is to work across governments and countries to protect biodiverse natural resources and introduce measures to stem climate change. Moreover, public support for such an endeavour is likely to be higher if the enormous impact on the health of the human population is emphasised as the outcome of a successful strategy to protect biodiversity and tackle climate change.

Public health professionals need to work on a large scale to support maintenance, enhancement and development of accessible, biodiverse greenspace. Public health leaders should work within governments to ensure that health considerations are incorporated into environment and sustainability strategies, and vice versa. Such strategies should be cognisant of the fact that populations that suffer from poverty and ill health are disproportionately more likely to also suffer from a lack of biodiverse natural environments. While these populations are a priority target for interventions to improve biodiversity, care should be taken that these efforts, by making the environment more pleasant, healthy and desirable, do not cause poorer populations to be displaced.

Public health practitioners are responsible for devising strategies to promote sustainable lifestyles and facilitate access to natural environments. Access to natural environments should be targeted at those most in need. There is an urgent need to embrace the fact that the natural environment is salutogenic, i.e. health giving. There is an equally urgent need to relax the usual positivistic standards of evidence of effectiveness required in medical intervention, and to utilise more suitable methods to evaluate nature-based solutions, for example, using quasi-experimental or mixed methodologies. This will allow more confident investment in schemes that prioritise access to nature over medical intervention. A significant driver for local decision-makers is the anticipated reduction in health-care costs, since improved outcomes will prevent costly use of doctors and hospitals. Such schemes, including nature-based social prescribing, give local commissioners of services the opportunity to target those from socio-economically deprived areas. Those with responsibility for social prescribing should be encouraged to use prescriptions that bring people into contact with nature, preferably where that engagement is active rather than passive. Further, it is likely that interventions resulting in exposure to environments with greater biodiversity will offer the greatest benefits for human health.

Whatever the scale, biodiversity has a fundamental role to play in human health and well-being. Public health professionals need to embrace biodiversity as a resource and be willing to fight to protect it. In so doing, they can target vulnerable populations and reduce inequalities in health between the richest and the poorest in our society.

References

Acheson D (1988) Public health in England. The report of the Committee of Inquiry into the future development of the public health function. HMSO, London

Acheson D (1998) Inequalities in health – report on inequalities in health did give priority for steps to be tackled. Br Med J 317(7173):1659–1659. https://doi.org/10.1136/bmj.317.7173.1659

Andermann A (2016) Taking action on the social determinants of health in clinical practice: a framework for health professionals. Can Med Assoc J 188(17–18):E474–E483. https://doi.org/10.1503/cmaj.160177

Andersson E, Barthel S, Borgström S, Colding J, Elmqvist T, Folke C, Gren Å (2014) Reconnecting cities to the biosphere: stewardship of green infrastructure and urban ecosystem services. Ambio 43(4):445–453. https://doi.org/10.1007/s13280-014-0506-y

Annerstedt M, Währborg P (2011) Nature-assisted therapy: systematic review of controlled and observational studies. Scand J Public Health 39(4):371–388. https://doi.org/10.1177/1403494810396400

Antonovsky A (1979) Health, stress, and coping, Jossey-Bass social and behavioral science series. Jossey-Bass, San Francisco

Axelson DJ, Stull MJ, Coates WC (2018) Social determinants of health: a missing link in emergency medicine training. AEM Educ Train 2(1):66–68. https://doi.org/10.1002/aet2.10056

Bell SL, Foley R, Houghton F, Maddrell A, Williams AM (2018) From therapeutic landscapes to healthy spaces, places and practices: a scoping review. Soc Sci Med 196:123–130. https://doi.org/10.1016/j.socscimed.2017.11.035

Berget B, Lidfors L, Palsdottir A, Soini K, Thodberg T (2012) Green care in the Nordic countries – a research field in progress. Report from the Nordic research workshop on green care in Trondheim. Health UMB, Norwegian University of Life Sciences

Bernstein AS (2014) Biological diversity and public health. Annu Rev Public Health 35:153–167. https://doi.org/10.1146/annurev-publhealth-032013-182348

Bertotti M, Frostick C, Hutt P, Sohanpal R, Carnes D (2018) A realist evaluation of social prescribing: an exploration into the context and mechanisms underpinning a pathway linking primary care with the voluntary sector. Prim Health Care Res Dev 19(3):232–245. https://doi.org/10.1017/s1463423617000706

Beyer KMM, Kaltenbach A, Szabo A, Bogar S, Nieto FJ, Malecki KM (2014) Exposure to neighborhood green space and mental health: evidence from the survey of the health of Wisconsin. Int J Environ Res Public Health 11(3):3453–3472. https://doi.org/10.3390/ijerph110303453

Bjerke T, Østdahl T, Thrane C, Strumse E (2006) Vegetation density of urban parks and perceived appropriateness for recreation. Urban For Urban Gree 5(1):35–44. https://doi.org/10.1016/j.ufug.2006.01.006

Bodicoat DH, Donovan G, Dalton AM, Gray LJ, Yates T, Edwardson C, Hill S, Webb DR, Khunti K, Davies MJ, Jones AP (2014) The association between neighbourhood greenspace and type 2 diabetes in a large cross-sectional study. BMJ Open 4(12):e006076

Braby A (2018) A new Northern Forest – beyond the headlines. Woodland Trust https://www.woodlandtrust.org.uk/blog/2018/01/a-new-northern-forest-beyond-the-headlines/, accessed 14/02/2019

Bragg R, Atkins G (2016) A review of nature-based interventions for mental health care. London. http://publications.naturalengland.org.uk/publication/4513819616346112

Bragg R, Leck C (2017) Good practice in social prescribing for mental health: the role of nature-based interventions. York

Carter JG, Handley J, Butlin T, Gill S (2017) Adapting cities to climate change – exploring the flood risk management role of green infrastructure landscapes. J Environ Plan Manag:1–18. https://doi.org/10.1080/09640568.2017.1355777

Chatterjee HJ, Camic PM, Lockyer B, Thomson LJM (2017) Non-clinical community interventions: a systematised review of social prescribing schemes. Art Health:1–27. https://doi.org/10.1080/17533015.2017.1334002

Chen TY, Janke MC (2012) Gardening as a potential activity to reduce falls in older adults. J Aging Phys Activ 20(1):15–31. https://doi.org/10.1123/Japa.20.1.15

City of Trees (2018) Growing more trees for Greater Manchester. http://www.cityoftrees.org.uk/. Accessed 26 June 2018

Collins CC, O'Callaghan AM (2008) The impact on health of horticultural responsibility indicators and quality of life in assisted living. HortTechnology 18(4):611–618

Convention on Biodiversity (2017) Biodiversity and human health. Paper presented at the twenty-first meeting of the subsidiary body on Scientific, Technical and Technological Advice, Canada, 11–14 December 2017

Coombes E, Jones AP, Hillsdon M (2010) The relationship of physical activity and overweight to objectively measured green space accessibility and use. Soc Sci Med 70(6):816–822. https://doi.org/10.1016/j.socscimed.2009.11.020

Corner A, Markowitz E, Pidgeon N (2014) Public engagement with climate change: the role of human values. Wiley Interdiscip Rev Clim Chang 5(3):411–422. https://doi.org/10.1002/wcc.269

Craig P, Cooper C, Gunnell D, Haw S, Lawson K, Macintyre S, Ogilvie D, Petticrew M, Reeves B, Sutton M, Thompson S (2011) Using natural experiments to evaluate population health interventions: guidance for producers and users of evidence. Medical Research Council. https://www.mrc.ac.uk/documents/pdf/natural-experiments-guidance/

Dallimer M, Irvine KN, Skinner AMJ, Davies ZG, Rouquette JR, Maltby LL, Warren PH, Armsworth PR, Gaston KJ (2012) Biodiversity and the feel-good factor: understanding associations between self-reported human well-being and species richness. Bioscience 62(1):47–55. https://doi.org/10.1525/bio.2012.62.1.9

Dayson C, Bashir H, Bennett E, Sanderson E (2015) The Rotherham social prescribing service for people with long-term health conditions. Annual evaluation report. Sheffield Hallam University Centre for regional, social and economic research

De Lacy P, Shackleton C (2017) Aesthetic and spiritual ecosystem services provided by urban sacred sites. Sustainability 9(9):Artn 1628. https://doi.org/10.3390/Su9091628

de Man H, van den Berg HHJL, Leenen EJTM, Schijven JF, Schets FM, van der Vliet JC, van Knapen F, de Roda Husman AM (2014) Quantitative assessment of infection risk from exposure to waterborne pathogens in urban floodwater. Water Res 48:90–99. https://doi.org/10.1016/j.watres.2013.09.022

de Vries S, Verheij RA, Groenewegen PP, Spreeuwenberg P (2003) Natural environments—healthy environments? An exploratory analysis of the relationship between greenspace and health. Environ Plan A 35(10):1717–1731. https://doi.org/10.1068/a35111

DEFRA (2018) A green future: our 25 year plan to improve the environment. OGL, London

Dennis M, Barlow D, Cavan G, Cook P, Gilchrist A, Handley J, James P, Thompson J, Tzoulas K, Wheater P, Lindley S (2018) Mapping urban green infrastructure: a novel landscape-based approach to incorporating land use and land cover in the mapping of human-dominated systems. Land 7(1):17

Diaz S, Fargione J, Chapin FS, Tilman D (2006) Biodiversity loss threatens human well-being. PLoS Biol 4(8):1300–1305. ARTN e277. https://doi.org/10.1371/journal.pbio.0040277

Dudley N, Stolton S (2003) Running Pure: the importance of forest protected areas to drinking water. World Bank/WWF Alliance for Forest Conservation and Sustainable Use

Ege MJ, Mayer M, Normand AC, Genuneit J, Cookson WO, Braun-Fahrlander C, Heederik D, Piarroux R, von Mutius E (2011) Exposure to environmental microorganisms and childhood asthma. N Engl J Med 364(8):701–709. https://doi.org/10.1056/NEJMoa1007302

Elo IT (2009) Social class differentials in health and mortality: patterns and explanations in comparative perspective. Annu Rev Sociol 35:553–572. https://doi.org/10.1146/annurev-soc-070308-115929

England's Community Forests (2018) About England's community forests. http://www.communityforest.org.uk/aboutenglandsforests.htm. Accessed 18 June 2018

Fahrig L, Girard J, Duro D, Pasher J, Smith A, Javorek S, King D, Lindsay KF, Mitchell S, Tischendorf L (2015) Farmlands with smaller crop fields have higher within-field biodiversity. Agric Ecosyst Environ 200:219–234. https://doi.org/10.1016/j.agee.2014.11.018

Fuller RA, Irvine KN, Devine-Wright P, Warren PH, Gaston KJ (2007) Psychological benefits of greenspace increase with biodiversity. Biol Lett 3(4):390–394. https://doi.org/10.1098/rsbl.2007.0149

Golicnik B, Ward Thompson C (2010) Emerging relationships between design and use of urban park spaces. Landsc Urban Plan 94(1):38–53. https://doi.org/10.1016/j.landurbplan.2009.07.016

Gonzalez MT, Hartig T, Patil GG, Martinsen EW, Kirkevold M (2009) Therapeutic horticulture in clinical depression: a prospective study. Res Theory Nurs Pract 23(4):312–328

Green Care Coalition (2017) How does it differ from other nature-based activities? https://greencarecoalition.org.uk/About/How-Does-Green-Care-Differ-From-Other-Nature-Based-Activities/, Accessed 14/02/2019

Haines-Young R, Potschin M (2010) The links between biodiversity, ecosystem services and human well-being. In: Raffaelli DCF (ed) Ecosystem ecology: a new synthesis, BES Ecological Reviews Series. Cambridge University Press, Cambridge

Hanski I, von Hertzen L, Fyhrquist N, Koskinen K, Torppa K, Laatikainen T, Karisola P, Auvinen P, Paulin L, Mäkelä MJ, Vartiainen E, Kosunen TU, Alenius H, Haahtela T (2012) Environmental biodiversity, human microbiota, and allergy are interrelated. Proc Natl Acad Sci 109(21):8334

Harrison C, Burgess J, Allison M, Gerald D (1995) Accessible natural greenspace in towns and cities: a review of appropriate size and distance criteria. No. I53 – English Nature Research Reports, Peterborough

Haubenhofer DK, Elings M, Hassink J, Hine RE (2010) The development of green care in western European countries. Explore 6(2):106–111. https://doi.org/10.1016/j.explore.2009.12.002

Hickman C (2009) Cheerful prospects and tranquil restoration: the visual experience of landscape as part of the therapeutic regime of the British asylum, 1800-60. Hist Psychiatry 20(80 Pt 4):425–441. https://doi.org/10.1177/0957154x08338335

Holt-Lunstad J, Smith TB, Baker M, Harris T, Stephenson D (2015) Loneliness and social isolation as risk factors for mortality: a meta-analytic review. Perspect Psychol Sci 10(2):227–237. https://doi.org/10.1177/1745691614568352

Hough RL (2014) Biodiversity and human health: evidence for causality? Biodivers Conserv 23(2):267–288. https://doi.org/10.1007/s10531-013-0614-1

Hu Y (2015) Stepped wedge, natural experiments and interrupted time series analysis designs. In: Richards DA, Hallberg IR (eds) Complex interventions in health: an overview of research methods. Routledge, Abingdon

Jackson G (2016) Social prescribing at a glance North West England: a scoping report of activity for the North West. Health Education England, Manchester

Jørgensen C, Erichsen A, Mark O, Domingo N, Heinicke G, Hammond M (2016) Dynamic modelling of health risks during wastewater influenced urban flooding. NOVATECH

Kaji H (2016) Effects of myokines on bone. Bonekey Rep 5:Artn 826. https://doi.org/10.1038/Bonekey.2016.48

Kaplan R, Kaplan S (1989) The experience of nature: a psychological perspective. Cambridge University Press, Cambridge

Keesing F, Belden LK, Daszak P, Dobson A, Harvell CD, Holt RD, Hudson P, Jolles A, Jones KE, Mitchell CE, Myers SS, Bogich T, Ostfeld RS (2010) Impacts of biodiversity on the emergence and transmission of infectious diseases. Nature 468(7324):647–652. https://doi.org/10.1038/nature09575

Keune H, Martens P, Kretsch C, Prieur-Richard A-h (2013) Chapter 16 - the natural relation between biodiversity and public health: an ecosystem services perspective. In: Ecosystem services. Elsevier, Boston, pp 181–189. https://doi.org/10.1016/B978-0-12-419964-4.00016-0

Kimberlee R (2013) Developing a social prescribing approach for Bristol. Project Report. University of the West of England, Bristol. http://eprints.uwe.ac.uk/23221/1/Social%20Prescribing%20Report-final.pdf

Kimberlee R, Ward R, Jones M, Powell J (2014) Measuring the economic impact of Wellspring Healthy Living Centre's Social Prescribing Wellbeing Programme for low level mental health issues encountered by GP services. University West of England

Kong FH, Yin HW, James P, Hutyra LR, He HS (2014) Effects of spatial pattern of greenspace on urban cooling in a large metropolitan area of eastern China. Landsc Urban Plan 128:35–47. https://doi.org/10.1016/j.landurbplan.2014.04.018

Konijnendijk CC, Ricard RM, Kenney A, Randrup TB (2006) Defining urban forestry – a comparative perspective of North America and Europe. Urban For Urban Gree 4(3):93–103. https://doi.org/10.1016/j.ufug.2005.11.003

Kuo FE, Sullivan WC (2001) Aggression and violence in the Inner City: effects of environment via mental fatigue. Environ Behav 33(4):543–571. https://doi.org/10.1177/00139160121973124

Lawton JH, Brotherton PNM, Brown VK, Elphick C, Fitter AH, Forshaw J, Haddow RW, Hilborner S, Leafe RN, Mace GM, Southgate MP, Sutherland WJ, Tew TE, Varley J, Wynne GR (2010) Making space for nature: a review of England's wildlife sites and ecological network. London

Lin BB, Philpott SM, Jha S (2015) The future of urban agriculture and biodiversity-ecosystem services: challenges and next steps. Basic Appl Ecol 16(3):189–201. https://doi.org/10.1016/j.baae.2015.01.005

Lindberg S (2012) Is biodiversity attractive? On-site perception of recreational and biodiversity values in urban green space. Swedish University of Agricultural Sciences

Lindgren E, Almqvist MS, Elmqvist T (2018) Ecosystem services and health benefits an urban perspective. In: van den Bosch M, Bird W (eds) Oxford textbook of nature and public health: the role of nature in improving the health of a population. Oxford University Press, Oxford

Lovell R, Wheeler BW, Higgins SL, Irvine KN, Depledge MH (2014) A systematic review of the health and Well-being benefits of biodiverse environments. J Toxicol Environ Health Part B 17(1):1–20. https://doi.org/10.1080/10937404.2013.856361

Luck GW, Davidson P, Boxall D, Smallbone L (2011) Relations between urban bird and plant communities and human Well-being and connection to nature. Conserv Biol 25(4):816–826. https://doi.org/10.1111/j.1523-1739.2011.01685.x

Maas J, Verheij RA, Groenewegen PP, de Vries S, Spreeuwenberg P (2006) Green space, urbanity, and health: how strong is the relation? J Epidemiol Community Health 60(7):587–592. https://doi.org/10.1136/jech.2005.043125

Maas J, Verheij RA, Spreeuwenberg P, Groenewegen PP (2008) Physical activity as a possible mechanism behind the relationship between green space and health: a multilevel analysis. BMC Public Health 8. Artn 206 https://doi.org/10.1186/1471-2458-8-206

Marmot M (2010) Fair society healthy lives. UCL Institute of Health Equity. http://www.instituteofhealthequity.org/projects/fair-society-healthy-lives-the-marmot-review

Marmot M (2013) Review of social determinants and the health divide in the WHO European Region: final report. World Health Organisation, Copenhagen

Marmot M, Wilkinson RG (2005) Social determinants of health, 2nd edn. Oxford University Press, Oxford

Marmot M, Friel S, Bell R, Houweling TAJ, Taylor S (2008) Closing the gap in a generation: health equity through action on the social determinants of health. Lancet 372(9650):1661–1669. https://doi.org/10.1016/S0140-6736(08)61690-6

Marselle MR, Irvine KN, Lorenzo-Arribas A, Warber SL (2016) Does perceived restorativeness mediate the effects of perceived biodiversity and perceived naturalness on emotional well-being following group walks in nature? J Environ Psychol 46:217–232. https://doi.org/10.1016/j.jenvp.2016.04.008

Masuya J, Ota K, Mashida Y (2014) The effect of a horticultural activities program on the psychologic, physical, and cognitive function and quality of life of elderly people living in nursing homes. Int J Nurs Clin Pract 1:109. https://doi.org/10.15344/2394-4978/2014/109

Mitchell R, Popham F (2008) Effect of exposure to natural environment on health inequalities: an observational population study. Lancet 372(9650):1655–1660. https://doi.org/10.1016/S0140-6736(08)61689-X

Mitchell RJ, Richardson EA, Shortt NK, Pearce JR (2015) Neighborhood environments and socioeconomic inequalities in mental well-being. Am J Prev Med 49(1):80–84. https://doi.org/10.1016/j.amepre.2015.01.017

Mitchell D, Heaviside C, Vardoulakis S, Huntingford C, Masato G, Guillod BP, Frumhoff P, Bowery A, Wallom D, Allen M (2016) Attributing human mortality during extreme heat waves to anthropogenic climate change. Environ Res Lett 11(7):Artn 074006. https://doi.org/10.1088/1748-9326/11/7/074006

Moore GF, Audrey S, Barker M, Bond L, Bonell C, Hardeman W, Moore L, O'Cathain A, Tinati T, Wight D, Baird J (2015) Process evaluation of complex interventions: Medical Research Council guidance. BMJ 350:ARTN h1258. https://doi.org/10.1136/bmj.h1258

Myers TA, Nisbet MC, Maibach EW, Leiserowitz AA (2012) A public health frame arouses hopeful emotions about climate change. Clim Chang 113(3):1105–1112. https://doi.org/10.1007/s10584-012-0513-6

Naeem S, Chazdon R, Duffy JE, Prager C, Worm B (2016) Biodiversity and human well-being: an essential link for sustainable development. Proc R Soc B 283(1844):Artn 20162091. https://doi.org/10.1098/Rspb.2016.2091

Natural England (2009) Natural England's green infrastructure guidance (NE176). Natural England, Peterborough. http://publications.naturalengland.org.uk/publication/35033

Nieuwenhuijsen MJ, Khreis H, Triguero-Mas M, Gascon M, Dadvand P (2017) Fifty shades of green pathway to healthy urban living. Epidemiology 28(1):63–71. https://doi.org/10.1097/Ede.0000000000000549

Nightingale F (1860) Notes on nursing: what it is, and what it is not. D. Appleton and Co, New York

Nutsford D, Pearson AL, Kingham S (2013) An ecological study investigating the association between access to urban green space and mental health. Public Health 127(11):1005–1011. https://doi.org/10.1016/j.puhe.2013.08.016

Pagnier I, Merchat M, La Scola B (2009) Potentially pathogenic amoeba-associated microorganisms in cooling towers and their control. Future Microbiol 4(5):615–629. https://doi.org/10.2217/Fmb.09.25

Park BJ, Furuya K, Kasetani T, Takayama N, Kagawa T, Miyazaki Y (2011) Relationship between psychological responses and physical environments in forest settings. Landsc Urban Plan 102(1):24–32. https://doi.org/10.1016/j.landurbplan.2011.03.005

Pauleit S, Slinn P, Handley J, Lindley S (2003) Promoting the natural greenstructure of towns and cities: English nature's "accessible natural greenspace standards" model. Built Environ 29(2):157–170.

Pedersen BK, Åkerström TCA, Nielsen AR, Fischer CP (2007) Role of myokines in exercise and metabolism. J Appl Physiol 103(3):1093–1098. https://doi.org/10.1152/japplphysiol.00080.2007

Petit S, Munier-Jolain N, Bretagnolle V, Bockstaller C, Gaba S, Cordeau S, Lechenet M, Meziere D, Colbach N (2015) Ecological intensification through pesticide reduction: weed control, weed biodiversity and sustainability in arable farming. Environ Manag 56(5):1078–1090. https://doi.org/10.1007/s00267-015-0554-5

Polley M, Bertotti M, Kimberlee R, Pilkington K, Refsum C (2017) A review of the evidence assessing impact of social prescribing on healthcare demand and cost implications. University of Westminster

Pretty J, Peacock J, Sellens M, Griffin M (2005) The mental and physical health outcomes of green exercise. Int J Environ Health Res 15(5):319–337. https://doi.org/10.1080/09603120500155963

Richardson EA, Pearce J, Mitchell R, Kingham S (2013) Role of physical activity in the relationship between urban green space and health. Public Health 127(4):318–324. https://doi.org/10.1016/j.puhe.2013.01.004

Royal Horticultural Society (2015) Plants for Bugs results. https://www.rhs.org.uk/science/conservation-biodiversity/plants-for-bugs/plants-for-bugs-results, Accessed 14/02/2019

Salisbury A, Armitage J, Bostock H, Perry J, Tatchell M, Thompson K (2015) Enhancing gardens as habitats for flower-visiting aerial insects (pollinators): should we plant native or exotic species. J Appl Ecol 52(5):1156–1164. https://doi.org/10.1111/1365-2664.12499

Salisbury A, Al-Beidh S, Armitage J, Bird S, Bostock H, Platoni A, Tatchell M, Thompson K, Perry J (2017) Enhancing gardens as habitats for plant-associated invertebrates: should we plant native or exotic species? Biodivers Conserv 26(11):2657–2673. https://doi.org/10.1007/s10531-017-1377-x

Sandifer PA, Sutton-Grier AE, Ward BP (2015) Exploring connections among nature, biodiversity, ecosystem services, and human health and well-being: opportunities to enhance health and biodiversity conservation. Ecosyst Serv 12:1–15. https://doi.org/10.1016/j.ecoser.2014.12.007

Sang AO, Knez I, Gunnarsson B, Hedblom M (2016) The effects of naturalness, gender, and age on how urban green space is perceived and used. Urban For Urban Gree 18:268–276. https://doi.org/10.1016/j.ufug.2016.06.008

Santos T, Mendes RN, Vasco A (2016) Recreational activities in urban parks: spatial interactions among users. J Outdoor Recreat Tour 15:1–9. https://doi.org/10.1016/j.jort.2016.06.001

Schalkwijk AAH, van der Zwaard BC, Nijpels G, Elders PJM, Platt L (2018) The impact of greenspace and condition of the neighbourhood on child overweight. Eur J Pub Health 28(1):88–94. https://doi.org/10.1093/eurpub/ckx037

Schreiber C, Rechenburg A, Rind E, Kistemann T (2015) The impact of land use on microbial surface water pollution. Int J Hyg Environ Health 218(2):181–187. https://doi.org/10.1016/j.ijheh.2014.09.006

Shanahan DF, Franco L, Lin BB, Gaston KJ, Fuller RA (2016) The benefits of natural environments for physical activity. Sports Med 46(7):989–995. https://doi.org/10.1007/s40279-016-0502-4

Shwartz A, Turbe A, Simon L, Julliard R (2014) Enhancing urban biodiversity and its influence on city-dwellers: an experiment. Biol Conserv 171:82–90. https://doi.org/10.1016/j.biocon.2014.01.009

Social Finance (2015) Investigating to Tackle Loneliness; A Discussion Paper. London. https://www.socialfinance.org.uk/sites/default/files/publications/investing_to_tackle_loneliness.pdf

Southon GE, Jorgensen A, Dunnett N, Hoyle H, Evans KL (2017) Biodiverse perennial meadows have aesthetic value and increase residents' perceptions of site quality in urban green-space. Landsc Urban Plan 158:105–118. https://doi.org/10.1016/j.landurbplan.2016.08.003

Southon GE, Jorgensen A, Dunnett N, Hoyle H, Evans KL (2018) Perceived species-richness in urban green spaces: cues, accuracy and Well-being impacts. Landsc Urban Plan 172:1–10. https://doi.org/10.1016/j.landurbplan.2017.12.002

Stringhini S, Carmeli C, Jokela M, Avendaño M, Muennig P, Guida F, Ricceri F, d'Errico A, Barros H, Bochud M, Chadeau-Hyam M, Clavel-Chapelon F, Costa G, Delpierre C, Fraga S, Goldberg M, Giles GG, Krogh V, Kelly-Irving M, Layte R, Lasserre AM, Marmot MG, Preisig M, Shipley MJ, Vollenweider P, Zins M, Kawachi I, Steptoe A, Mackenbach JP, Vineis P, Kivimäki M (2017) Socioeconomic status and the 25 × 25 risk factors as determinants of premature mortality: a multicohort study and meta-analysis of 1·7 million men and women. Lancet 389(10075):1229–1237. https://doi.org/10.1016/S0140-6736(16)32380-7

Taylor AF, Kuo FE, Sullivan WC (2002) Views of nature and self-discipline: evidence from inner city children. J Environ Psychol 22(1):49–63. https://doi.org/10.1006/jevp.2001.0241

Thompson Coon J, Boddy K, Stein K, Whear R, Barton J, Depledge MH (2011) Does participating in physical activity in outdoor natural environments have a greater effect on physical and mental wellbeing than physical activity indoors? A systematic review. Environ Sci Technol 45(5):1761–1772. https://doi.org/10.1021/es102947t

Turner T (1992) Open space planning in London: from standards per 1000 to green strategy. Town Plan Rev 63(4):365–386

Tyrvainen L, Ojala A, Korpela K, Lanki T, Tsunetsugu Y, Kagawa T (2014) The influence of urban green environments on stress relief measures: a field experiment. J Environ Psychol 38:1–9. https://doi.org/10.1016/j.jenvp.2013.12.005

Tzoulas K, Korpela K, Venn S, Yli-Pelkonen V, Kazmierczak A, Niemela J, James P (2007) Promoting ecosystem and human health in urban areas using green infrastructure: a literature review. Landsc Urban Plan 81(3):167–178. https://doi.org/10.1016/j.landurbplan.2007.02.001

Ulrich RS (1984) View through a window may influence recovery from surgery. Science 224(4647):420–421

Ulrich RS, Simons RF, Losito BD, Fiorito E, Miles MA, Zelson M (1991) Stress recovery during exposure to natural and urban environments. J Environ Psychol 11(3):201–230. https://doi.org/10.1016/S0272-4944(05)80184-7

United Nations (1992) Convention on biological diversity. United Nations, Rio de Janeiro. https://www.cbd.int/doc/legal/cbd-en.pdf

Valtorta NK, Kanaan M, Gilbody S, Ronzi S, Hanratty B (2016) Loneliness and social isolation as risk factors for coronary heart disease and stroke: systematic review and meta-analysis of longitudinal observational studies. Heart 102(13):1009–1016. https://doi.org/10.1136/heartjnl-2015-308790

van den Berg M, Wendel-Vos W, van Poppel M, Kemper H, van Mechelen W, Maas J (2015) Health benefits of green spaces in the living environment: a systematic review of epidemiological studies. Urban For Urban Gree 14(4):806–816. https://doi.org/10.1016/j.ufug.2015.07.008

Ward Thompson C (2013) Activity, exercise and the planning and design of outdoor spaces. J Environ Psychol 34:79–96. https://doi.org/10.1016/j.jenvp.2013.01.003

Watts N, Adger WN, Agnolucci P, Blackstock J, Byass P, Cai W, Chaytor S, Colbourn T, Collins M, Cooper A, Cox PM, Depledge J, Drummond P, Ekins P, Galaz V, Grace D, Graham H, Grubb M, Haines A, Hamilton I, Hunter A, Jiang X, Li M, Kelman I, Liang L, Lott M, Lowe R, Luo Y, Mace G, Maslin M, Nilsson M, Oreszczyn T, Pye S, Quinn T, Svensdotter M, Venevsky S, Warner K, Xu B, Yang J, Yin Y, Yu C, Zhang Q, Gong P, Montgomery H, Costello A (2015) Health and climate change: policy responses to protect public health. Lancet 386(10006):1861–1914. https://doi.org/10.1016/S0140-6736(15)60854-6

Wheater CP (1999) Urban habitats. Habitat guides. Routledge, London

Wheater CP, Potts E, Shaw EM, Perkins C, Smith H, Casstles H, Cook PA, Bellis MA (2007) Urban parks and public health: exploiting a resource for healthy minds and bodies. Liverpool John Moores University. http://www.cph.org.uk/wp-content/uploads/2012/08/urban-parks-and-public-health-exploiting-a-resource-for-healthy-minds-and-bodies.pdf

Wilmot EG, Edwardson CL, Achana FA, Davies MJ, Gorely T, Gray LJ, Khunti K, Yates T, Biddle SJH (2012) Sedentary time in adults and the association with diabetes, cardiovascular disease and death: systematic review and meta-analysis. Diabetologia 55(11):2895–2905. https://doi.org/10.1007/s00125-012-2677-z

Wilson EO (1984) Biophilia. Harvard University Press, Cambridge

Wolch JR, Byrne J, Newell JP (2014) Urban green space, public health, and environmental justice: the challenge of making cities 'just green enough'. Landsc Urban Plan 125:234–244. https://doi.org/10.1016/j.landurbplan.2014.01.017

Wood CL, Lafferty KD, DeLeo G, Young HS, Hudson PJ, Kuris AM (2014) Does biodiversity protect humans against infectious disease? Ecology 95(4):817–832. https://doi.org/10.1890/13-1041.1

World Health Organisation (2016) Urban green spaces and health: a review of evidence. World Health Organisation Regional Office for Europe, Copenhagen

Zhang JW, Piff PK, Iyer R, Koleva S, Keltner D (2014) An occasion for unselfing: beautiful nature leads to prosociality. J Environ Psychol 37:61–72. https://doi.org/10.1016/j.jenvp.2013.11.008

Chapter 12
Biodiversity and Health: Implications for Conservation

Zoe G. Davies, Martin Dallimer, Jessica C. Fisher, and Richard A. Fuller

Abstract The human health and well-being benefits of contact with nature are becoming increasingly recognised and well understood, yet the implications of nature experiences for biodiversity conservation are far less clear. Theoretically, there are two plausible pathways that could lead to positive conservation outcomes. The first is a direct win-win scenario where biodiverse areas of high conservation value are also disproportionately beneficial to human health and well-being, meaning that the two sets of objectives can be simultaneously and directly achieved, as long as such green spaces are safeguarded appropriately. The second is that experiencing nature can stimulate people's interest in biodiversity, concern for its fate, and willingness to take action to protect it, therefore generating conservation gains indirectly. To date, the two pathways have rarely been distinguished and scarcely studied. Here we consider how they may potentially operate in practice, while acknowledging that the mechanisms by which biodiversity might underpin human health and well-being benefits are still being determined.

Keywords Extinction of experience · Green space · Human-wildlife interaction · Nature connectedness · Protected areas · Well-being

---

Z. G. Davies (✉) · J. C. Fisher
Durrell Institute of Conservation and Ecology (DICE), School of Anthropology and Conservation, University of Kent, Canterbury, Kent, UK
e-mail: z.g.davies@kent.ac.uk; jcf22@kent.ac.uk

M. Dallimer
Sustainability Research Institute, School of Earth and Environment, University of Leeds, Leeds, UK
e-mail: m.dallimer@leeds.ac.uk

R. A. Fuller
School of Biological Sciences, University of Queensland, St Lucia, QLD, Australia
e-mail: r.fuller@uq.edu.au

M. R. Marselle et al. (eds.), *Biodiversity and Health in the Face of Climate Change*, https://doi.org/10.1007/978-3-030-02318-8_12

Highlights

- Green spaces vary in their conservation value, depending on the biodiversity present.
- Very few are designed and/or managed to deliver synergistic conservation and health benefits.
- Evidence suggests health might be related to specific, complex natural environments.
- These green spaces might be of greater conservation value.
- To maximise health, biodiversity must be in the right places for the right people.

12.1 Green Spaces Managed Primarily for People

Green spaces may support dramatically different levels of biodiversity, depending on their location, history, purpose and use by people. At one end of the spectrum are the green spaces that have been designed with human health and well-being primarily in mind. Historically, these areas were planned to provide inhabitants with relief from the unsanitary conditions that prevailed in overcrowded industrialised cities (Rayner and Lang 2012) and, while constructed from nature in the form of vegetation, there was no explicit consideration of whether these areas provided valuable habitats for species. Indeed, this anthropocentric view of managing natural resources for the benefit of people has re-emerged over the past two decades, with an emphasis on finding nature-based solutions to issues such as heat mitigation, pollution reduction and storm water protection (e.g. MA 2005; TEEB 2010; European Commission 2011; European Commission Horizon 2020 Expert Group 2015). This is particularly true for urban areas where the majority of the human population across the world live, and improving the health and well-being of these city dwellers is a priority in many national and international policy agendas (European Commission Horizon 2020 Expert Group 2015).

Urban areas are often characterised from a conservation perspective by the negative impacts they have on the ecosystems they replace and abut (e.g. see the discussion in Gaston 2010). Green spaces within cities are often considered too small and isolated from one another to sustain viable species populations (Goddard et al. 2010), requiring a collaborative effort on the part of different stakeholders to redress the lack of connectivity (Davies et al. 2009; Dearborn and Kark 2010). One legacy associated with green spaces intended to deliver aesthetic and recreational benefits is the simplification of habitats as a consequence of frequent management (e.g. mowing, pruning of trees and shrubs, removal of deadwood; Aronson et al. 2017). Likewise, the desire to maximise the multi-functionality of green spaces and infrastructure (e.g. green roofs, sustainable urban drainage systems) has perpetuated this problem further through the planting of horticultural cultivars rather than native species (Haase et al. 2017). While some of these initiatives can support biodiversity (e.g. non-native flowering species can be beneficial for some bees; MacIvor and

Ksiazek 2015; Salisbury et al. 2015), the use of horticultural cultivars has been linked to a reduction in the forage value of planting for pollinators in general (Bates et al. 2011; Salisbury et al. 2015). Moreover, the spread of alien invasive species from gardens and parks is another significant issue in many parts of the world (Reichard and White 2001; Russo et al. 2017). The conservation value of green spaces that are popular with people can also be limited by significant levels of disturbance and degradation, which prevent native species from colonising and persisting (Brown and Grant 2005), and result in assemblages dominated by adaptable generalists (Kowarik 2011) and the homogenisation of urban biodiversity (McKinney 2006). Even for human-nature interactions that people perceive as being good for wildlife, such as the supplementary feeding of wild birds, we have little evidence as to whether they deliver biodiversity conservation benefits (Fuller et al. 2008; Robb et al. 2008; Jones 2018).

Despite this, suitable habitat within urban areas can support threatened and specialist species, and warrant conservation attention (Baldock et al. 2015; Ives et al. 2016). In developed regions, where intensive use of the wider landscape, particularly through agriculture, has resulted in species declines, urban areas have become important for sustaining regional abundances of some species. Substantial proportions of the populations of some previously widespread and common species now occur in urban green spaces (e.g. Beebee 1997; Gregory and Baillie 1998; Mason 2000; Bland et al. 2004; Peach et al. 2004; Speak et al. 2015; Ives et al. 2016; Tryjanowski et al. 2017). For instance, over 600 species have been recorded in Weißensee Jewish Cemetery in Berlin. It supports 25 plants, five bats and nine birds that are species of conservation concern, and one of the lichens (*Aloxyria ochrocheila*) present on the site is considered very rare across the wider region. The cemetery therefore acts as an unintended refuge for a wide range of taxa (Buchholz et al. 2016).

12.2 Green Spaces Managed Primarily for Biodiversity

At the other end of the green space continuum are formal protected areas, now interpreted as a global conservation network, where the objective is to maintain and enhance biodiversity (see MacKinnon et al. Chap. 16, this volume). Currently, there are more than 200,000 protected areas globally, after a huge expansion of the network over the past few decades (Watson et al. 2014, Butchart et al. 2015). Some of the earliest protected areas were preferentially designated in locations used heavily for recreation (Pressey 1994), and some protected areas are still managed with access and use by people as a primary management goal, such as many of the National Parks in the UK (Smith 2013). However, this is usually the exception rather than the rule for three inter-related reasons.

First, protected areas have overwhelmingly been established in areas not needed for economic activity (Pressey 1994), so they are often sited at higher elevations, on steep slopes, on relatively unfertile soils and far away from cities and productive agricultural land (Pressey et al. 2002; Joppa and Pfaff 2009). Typically, the human population density is low in these areas and, as such, they are shielded from use by people by default. Indeed, the physical distance between human settlements and the location of protected areas can impose a substantial barrier to their recreational use (Kareiva 2008). Protected areas that are close to or within towns and cities tend to be smaller, more fragmented and in poorer ecological condition than those in remote locations (Jones et al. 2018).

Second, there has been a growing emphasis in recent years on proactive conservation strategies, such as those that aim to safeguard the last of the world's major wilderness areas (Sanderson et al. 2002; Mittermeier et al. 2003; Watson et al. 2017). This is based on the recognition that the predominant threats to biodiversity spread contagiously across landscapes (Boakes et al. 2010), suggesting that if an area can be protected while it is still intact, the risk of eventual habitat clearance or degradation is much lower (Klein et al. 2009). By definition, the absence of a high density of people, and the pressure they bring to bear on landscapes, is a key component of wilderness quality (Venter et al. 2016), thus further building a case for protected area designation in places away from human settlements.

Finally, there is often tension among management agencies about permitting recreation inside protected areas that have been designated for biodiversity conservation, with many viewing the two things as incompatible and preferring that people are actively excluded (Smith 2013). A prime example of this is mountain biking where, arguably, the impact on biodiversity is usually minimal, but is perceived as being much greater by managers and other types of green space user (Hardiman and Burgin 2013). A further complicating factor is that funds for managing protected areas for recreation are often derived from different sources to those centred on biodiversity (Miller et al. 2009). This means that interagency cooperation might be needed to effectively provide facilities for human use, or zoning configurations that minimise recreational pressures (Stigner et al. 2016). This can require substantial investment to deliver and be complex to achieve.

In spite of the historical bias where most protected areas are located away from regions of intense human activity, there is some evidence that new protected areas are now being established in closer proximity to towns and cities. Global biodiversity targets mandate protecting threatened species and landscapes that currently lack formal designation (Butchart et al. 2015), and many of the remaining high conservation value areas occur in fragmented landscapes nearer to human settlements (Brooks et al. 2006; McDonald et al. 2008). For example, recently established Australian protected areas are being preferentially sited in places with high human population density and large numbers of threatened species (Barr et al. 2016). Likewise, 32 cities within the European Union contain Natura 2000 sites (ten Brink et al. 2016).

Some protected areas have successfully integrated human health and well-being objectives into their remit more proactively. For instance, Secovlje Salina Nature Park in Slovenia hosts the Lepa Vida Spa, which has generated jobs and income in both the tourism and health sectors. In turn, this has provided better public access to the park for 50,000 annual visitors, and the habitat quality of the protected area, which is important for supporting migratory birds, has been improved (ten Brink et al. 2016). Similarly, Medvednica Nature Park in Zagreb attracts over a million visitors annually, while also being home to over 20% of Croatia's entire vascular flora, including more than 90 strictly protected species. Additionally, the park plays a role in improving air quality and mitigating urban air temperatures in neighbouring city suburbs (ten Brink et al. 2016).

12.3 Moving Forward with Green Spaces Planned for Both People and Biodiversity

Presently, although there are few sites explicitly designed and managed to deliver conservation and human health gains in tandem, the potential for synergistic benefits could be substantial. The opportunities to adopt such a strategy are considerable, given the rapid rates of urbanisation globally and that many regions are yet to be developed (Nilon et al. 2017). Urbanisation will not be geographically homogenous, chiefly taking place in small cities comprising less than 500,000 inhabitants across the Global South (United Nations 2015). This vast conversion of land to built infrastructure will undoubtedly pose a threat to biodiversity, not least because most of it will occur in extremely biodiverse regions such as the Brazilian Atlantic Forest and Guinean Forests of West Africa (Seto et al. 2012). Formal conservation protection is therefore imperative to prevent extinctions (Cincotta et al. 2000; Brooks et al. 2006; Venter et al. 2014). Justifying the need to protect natural environments in and around where people live to deliver a multi-faceted suite of objectives is more likely to be persuasive to decision-makers than a rationale based solely on conservation. In already established towns and cities, green spaces can be 'retrofitted' to provide complementary conservation and human health gains (for further information, see Hunter et al. Chap. 17, and Heiland et al. Chap. 19, both this volume). For example, initiatives such as the Biophilic Cities network (http://biophiliccities.org/) promote biodiversity as a central tenet of urban planning and management, so that improvements in human health and well-being arise from co-existence (Beatley and van den Bosch 2018). Metrics related to levels of biodiversity, wildness, tree cover and green space accessibility are included as indicators against which the performance of individual cities can be gauged.

Although not studied extensively thus far, there is evidence to suggest that positive human health and well-being outcomes might be related to specific and often complex natural environments, which could be of conservation value. For instance, people enjoy forests because of their quiet atmosphere, scenery and fresh air, which helps with stress management and relaxation (Li and Bell 2018). In Zurich, Sihlwald Forest is a major recreation area for the city. Formerly a timber concession, the ecosystem is now left to function with minimal human intervention and, therefore, offers residents a different sort of nature experience to more manicured green spaces (Seeland et al. 2002; Konijnendijk 2008).

The decisions regarding where green spaces should be located and how they are managed are complex, with conservation value being one of many factors that must be taken into consideration. Inevitably, biodiversity will be traded off against other economic and societal goals (Nilon et al. 2017). However, maximising the size of green spaces planned for both people and biodiversity is likely to be important for their success. While it is widely accepted that larger areas are likely to sustain more species (Beninde et al. 2015), evidence is growing to suggest that the same might be true for the supply of human health and well-being benefits. For instance, larger forested areas are preferred for outdoor activities (Tyrväinen et al. 2007).

Another core challenge associated with maximising the human health outcomes derived from experiencing nature is making sure that biodiversity is in the right locations for the right people. This is critical because the likelihood of someone visiting a site drops dramatically with distance, with only the fraction of the population that is already strongly connected to nature willing to travel to experience it (Shanahan et al. 2015). Indeed, cities are often characterised by a wide array of inequalities, with those living in deprived communities having the most to gain from using nearby green spaces (Mitchell and Popham 2008; Kabisch Chap. 5, this volume; Cook et al. Chap. 11, this volume). If the health and well-being of all urban residents were prioritised, then one would expect publicly owned green spaces to be more or less evenly distributed across the spatial extent of towns and cities (Boone et al. 2009; Landry and Chakroborty 2009; Pham et al. 2012). On the other hand, if green spaces were being used actively as an intervention to promote better human health and well-being, their placement would mostly likely be adjacent to communities characterised by a high prevalence of health disorders, such as depression and obesity (Lin et al. 2014). However, either is rarely the case, as individuals from ethnic/racial minorities (Heynen et al. 2006; Landry and Chakroborty 2009; Wolch et al. 2013) and/or lower socio-economic status (Vaughan et al. 2013) have comparatively worse access to high-quality green space than the rest of the population. It is therefore vital to ensure that the health benefits that might be derived from conservation initiatives are not just confined to societal groups that have the financial and/or social means to access them (Wolch et al. 2014).

12.4 Experiencing Nature to Promote Conservation

It is commonly asserted that urbanisation has led to the human population becoming progressively disconnected from the natural world (Wilson 1984; Pyle 2003; Miller 2005), a phenomenon that has variously been referred to as the 'extinction of experience' (Miller 2005), 'nature deficit disorder' (Louv 2008) and 'ecological boredom' (Monbiot 2013). By exposing people to nature, it is thought that these experiences can enhance an individual's connection with nature and, in turn, promote conservation concern and pro-environmental behaviours (see Soga and Gaston

2016; De Young Chap. 13, this volume). For instance, Rogerson et al. (2017) found relationships between people experiencing nature and positive environmental behaviour, such as volunteering with conservation organisations. Likewise, childhood experiences of nature have been linked to connectedness to nature in a study of French adults (Colléony et al. 2017), and individuals who grew up in rural areas demonstrated a greater preference for gardens containing more flowers and woodland species than urbanities (Shwartz et al. 2013). Nonetheless, the evidence underlying the relationship between nature experience and positive attitudes/behaviours remains scant and is yet to be fully established (Soga and Gaston 2016).

Individuals may not need to experience biodiversity to want to conserve it (termed 'existence value') (Cooper et al. 2016). This has been shown for coastal ecosystems on Vancouver Island, Canada (Klain and Chan 2012) and marine protected areas in the UK (Kenter et al. 2016), and can be a potential mediator between nature connectedness and well-being (Cleary et al. 2017). Additionally, it is difficult to draw meaningful lessons from studies due to the level of inconsistency between the definitions of what constitutes an experience, what comprises nature, and what attitude or perception is being measured (Clayton et al. 2017; Ives et al. 2017). Moreover, the 'extinction of experience' concept is considered oversimplified because it fails to acknowledge the multi-dimensionality of people's experiences of biodiversity (Clayton et al. 2017), and that some interactions with species can be negative, frightening or uncomfortable (Bixler and Floyd 1997). Relationships with nature are likely to be highly specific to individuals, with cultural contexts and norms also being important and variable across societies (Voigt and Wurster 2014). For example, feeding wild birds is a very popular human-biodiversity interaction in both the UK and the USA (Freyfogle 2003; Defra 2011), but negative associations with birds in Europe may inhibit a connectedness to nature for some individuals (Ratcliffe et al. 2013). Similarly, a fear of birds (known as 'ornithophobia') in Honduras has been reported to occur where birds are perceived as either pest species or as negative spiritual symbols (Bonta 2008). This is a fundamental consideration when designing and maintaining green spaces, as synergistic human health and conservation benefits will not be delivered successfully if the residents are intolerant of the biodiversity they support.

12.5 Conclusion

While very few green spaces are implemented explicitly with both conservation and human health and well-being in mind, the potential for delivering win-win outcomes is considerable. This is particularly apposite, given the rate and distribution of future urbanisation predicted across the highly biodiverse regions of the Global South. However, the rapidly growing body of research examining nature-related health benefits has yet to tease apart the relative value of green spaces that support different levels of biodiversity and ecosystem complexity. This knowledge gap needs to be addressed, so a strong evidence-base is in place to inform effective policy and practice.

Acknowledgements We are grateful to our respective funders: ZGD is supported by the European Research Council (ERC) Consolidator Grant 726104; MD is supported by the UK Natural Environment Research Council (NERC) grant NE/R002681/1; JCF is supported by the UK Economic and Social Research Council (ESRC) scholarship ES/J500148/1; and, RAF is supported by an Australian Research Council Future Fellowship.

References

Aronson MF, Lepczyk CA, Evans KL, Goddard MA, Lerman SB, MacIvor JS, Nilon CH, Vargo T (2017) Biodiversity in the city: key challenges for urban green space management. Front Ecol Environ 15:1–8

Baldock KCR, Goddard MA, Hicks DM, Kunin WE, Mitschunas N, Osgathorpe LM, Potts SG, Robertson KM, Scott AV, Stone GN, Vaughan IP, Memmott J (2015) Where is the UK's pollinator biodiversity? The importance of urban areas for flower-visiting insects. Proc R Soc B Biol Sci 282:20142849

Barr LM, Watson JEM, Possingham HP, Iwamura T, Fuller RA (2016) Progress in improving the protection of species and habitats in Australia. Biol Conserv 200:184–191

Bates AJ, Sadler JP, Fairbrass AJ, Falk SJ, Hale JD, Matthews TJ (2011) Changing bee and hoverfly pollinator assemblages along an urban-rural gradient. PLoS One 6:e23459

Beatley T, van den Bosch KC (2018) Urban landscapes and public health. In: van den Bosch M, Bird W (eds) Nature and Public Health. Oxford University Press, Oxford

Beebee TJC (1997) Changes in dewpond numbers and amphibian diversity over 20 years on chalk downland in Sussex, England. Biol Conserv 81:215–219

Beninde J, Veith M, Hochkirch A (2015) Biodiversity in cities needs space: a meta-analysis of factors determining intra-urban biodiversity variation. Ecol Lett 18:581–592

Bixler RD, Floyd MF (1997) Nature is scary, disgusting, and uncomfortable. Environ Behav 29:443–467

Bland RL, Tully J, Greenwood JJD (2004) Birds breeding in British gardens: an underestimated population? Bird Study 51:96–106

Boakes EH, Mace GM, McGowan PJK, Fuller RA (2010) Extreme contagion in global habitat clearance. Proc R Soc B Biol Sci 277:1081–1085

Bonta M (2008) Valorizing the relationships between people and birds: experiences and lessons from Honduras. Ornitol Neotropical 19:595–604

Boone GC, Buckley GL, Grove MJ, Sister C (2009) Parks and people: an environmental justice inquiry in Baltimore, Maryland. Assoc Am Geogr 99:767–787

Brooks TM, Mittermeier RA, da Fonseca GAB, Gerlach J, Hoffmann M, Lamoreux JF, Mittermeier CG, Pilgrim JD, Rodrigues ASL (2006) Global biodiversity conservation priorities. Science 313:58–61

Brown C, Grant M (2005) Biodiversity and human health: what role for nature in healthy urban planning? Built Environ 31:326–338

Buchholz S, Blick T, Hannig K, Kowarik I, Lemke A, Otte V, Scharon J, Schonhofer A, Teige T, von der Lippe M, Seitz B (2016) Biological richness of a large urban cemetery in Berlin: results of a multi-taxon approach. Biodivers Data J 4:e7057

Butchart SHM, Clarke M, Smith RJ, Sykes RE, Scharlemann JPW, Harfoot M, Buchanan GM, Angulo A, Balmford A, Bertzky B, Brooks TM, Carpenter KE, Comeros-Raynal MT, Cornell J, Francesco Ficetola G, Fishpool LDC, Fuller RA, Geldmann J, Harwell H, Hilton-Taylor C, Hoffmann M, Joolia A, Joppa L, Kingston N, May I, Milam A, Polidoro B, Ralph G, Richman

N, Rondinini C, Segan D, Skolnik B, Spalding M, Stuart SN, Symes A, Taylor J, Visconti P, Watson J, Wood L, Burgess ND (2015) Shortfalls and solutions for meeting national and global conservation area targets. Conserv Lett 8:329–337

Cincotta RP, Wisnewski J, Engelman R (2000) Human population in the biodiversity hotspots. Nature 404:990–992

Clayton S, Coll A, Conversy P, Maclouf E, Martin L, Torres A, Truong M, Prevot A (2017) Transformation of experience: toward a new relationship with nature. Conserv Lett 10:645–651

Cleary A, Fielding KS, Bell SL, Murray Z, Roiko A (2017) Exploring potential mechanisms involved in the relationship between eudaimonic wellbeing and nature connection. Landsc Urban Plan 158:119–128

Colléony A, Prévot A-C, Saint Jalme M, Clayton S (2017) What kind of landscape management can counteract the extinction of experience? Landsc Urban Plan 159:23–31

Cooper N, Brady E, Steen H, Bryce R (2016) Aesthetic and spiritual values of ecosystems: recognising the ontological and axiological plurality of cultural ecosystem 'services'. Ecosyst Serv 21:218–229

Dallimer M, Irvine KN, Skinner AMJ, Davies ZG, Rouquette JR, Maltby LL, Warren PH, Armsworth PR, Gaston KJ (2012) Biodiversity and the feel-good factor: understanding associations between self-reported human well-being and species richness. Bioscience 62:47–55

Davies ZG, Fuller RA, Loram A, Irvine KN, Sims V, Gaston KJ (2009) A national scale inventory of resource provision for biodiversity within domestic gardens. Biol Conserv 142:761–771

Dearborn DC, Kark S (2010) Motivations for conserving urban biodiversity. Conserv Biol 24:432–440

Defra (2011) A biodiversity strategy for England. Measuring progress: 2010 assessment. Department for Environment, Food and Rural Affairs, London

European Commission (2011) Our life insurance, our natural capital: an EU biodiversity strategy to 2020. European Commission, Brussels

European Commission Horizon 2020 Expert Group (2015) Towards an EU research and innovation policy agenda for nature-based solutions and re-naturing cities. A report for the European Commission. European Commission, Brussels

Freyfogle ET (2003) Conservation and the culture war. Conserv Biol 17:354–355

Fuller RA, Irvine KN, Devine-Wright P, Warren PH, Gaston KJ (2007) Psychological benefits of greenspace increase with biodiversity. Biol Lett 3:390–394

Fuller RA, Warren PH, Armsworth PR, Barbosa O, Gaston KJ (2008) Garden bird feeding predicts the structure of urban avian assemblages. Divers Distrib 14:131–137

Gaston KJ (2010) Urban ecology. Cambridge University Press, Cambridge

Goddard MA, Dougill AJ, Benton TG (2010) Scaling up from gardens: biodiversity conservation in urban environments. Trends Ecol Evol 25:90–98

Gregory RD, Baillie SR (1998) Large-scale habitat use of some declining British birds. J Appl Ecol 35:785–799

Haase D, Kabisch S, Haase A, Andersson E, Banzhaf E, Baró F, Brenck M, Fischer LK, Frantzeskaki N, Kabisch N, Krellenberg K (2017) Greening cities – To be socially inclusive? About the alleged paradox of society and ecology in cities. Habitat Int 64:41–48

Hardiman N, Burgin S (2013) Mountain biking: downhill for the environment or chance to up a gear? Int J Environ Stud 70:976–986

Heynen N, Perkins HA, Roy P (2006) The political ecology of uneven urban green space. The impact of political economy on race and ethnicity in producing environmental inequality in Milwaukee. Urban Aff Rev 42:3–25

Ives CD, Lentini PE, Threlfall CG, Ikin K, Shanahan DF, Garrard GE, Bekessy SA, Fuller RA, Mumaw L, Rayner L, Rowe R, Valentine LE, Kendal D (2016) Cities are hotspots for threatened species. Glob Ecol Biogeogr 25:117–126

Ives CD, Giusti M, Fischer J, Abson DJ, Klaniecki K, Dorninger C, Laudan J, Barthel S, Abernethy P, Martín-López B, Raymond CM, Kendal D, von Wahrden H (2017) Human–nature connection: a multidisciplinary review. Curr Opin Environ Sustain 26–27:106–113

Jones D (2018) The birds at my table: why we feed wild birds and why it matters. Cornell University Press, Ithaca

Jones KR, Venter O, Fuller RA, Allan JR, Maxwell SL, Negret PJ, Watson JEM (2018) One-third of global protected land is under intense human pressure. Science 360:788–791

Joppa LN, Pfaff A (2009) High and far: biases in the location of protected areas. PLoS One 4:e8273

Kareiva P (2008) Ominous trends in nature recreation. Proc Natl Acad Sci U S A 105:2757–2758

Kenter JO, Jobstvogt N, Watson V, Irvine KN, Christie M, Bryce R (2016) The impact of information, value-deliberation and group-based decision-making on values for ecosystem services: integrating deliberative monetary valuation and storytelling. Ecosyst Serv 21:270–290

Klain S, Chan K (2012) Navigating coastal values: participatory mapping of ecosystem services for spatial planning. Ecol Econ 82:104–113

Klein CJ, Wilson KA, Watts M, Stein J, Carwardine J, Mackey B, Possingham HP (2009) Spatial conservation prioritization inclusive of wilderness quality: a case study of Australia's biodiversity. Biol Conserv 142:1282–1290

Konijnendijk CC (2008) The forest and the city – The cultural landscape of urban woodland. Springer, Berlin

Kowarik I (2011) Novel urban ecosystems, biodiversity, and conservation. Environ Pollut 159:1974–1983

Landry SM, Chakraborty J (2009) Street trees and equity: evaluating the spatial distribution of an urban amenity. Environ Plan A 41:2651–2670

Li Q, Bell S (2018) The great outdoors: forests, wilderness and public health. In: van den Bosch M, Bird W (eds) Nature and public health. Oxford University Press, Oxford

Lin BB, Fuller RA, Bush R, Gaston KJ, Shanahan DF (2014) Opportunity or orientation? Who uses urban parks and why. PLoS One 9:e87422

Louv R (2008) Last child in the woods: saving our children from nature-deficit disorder. Atlantic Books, London

MA (2005) Millennium ecosystem assessment – ecosystems and human well-being. Island Press, Washington DC

MacIvor S, Ksiazek K (2015) Invertebrates on green roofs. In: Sutton R (ed) Green roof ecosystems. Springer, Cham

Mason CF (2000) Thrushes now largely restricted to the built environment in eastern England. Divers Distrib 6:189–194

McDonald RI, Kareiva P, Formana RTT (2008) The implications of current and future urbanization for global protected areas and biodiversity conservation. Biol Conserv 141:1695–1703

McKinney ML (2006) Urbanization as a major cause of biotic homogenization. Biol Conserv 127:247–260

Miller JR (2005) Biodiversity conservation and the extinction of experience. Trends Ecol Evol 20:430–434

Miller JR, Groom M, Hess GR, Steelman T, Stokes DL, Thompson J, Bowman T, Fricke L, King B, Marquardt R (2009) Biodiversity conservation in local planning. Conserv Biol 23:53–63

Mills JG, Weinstein P, Gellie NJC, Weyrich LS, Lowe AJ, Breed MF (2017) Urban habitat restoration provides a human health benefit through microbiome rewilding: the Microbiome rewilding hypothesis. Restor Ecol 25:866–872

Mitchell R, Popham F (2008) Effect of exposure to natural environment on health inequalities: an observational population study. Lancet 372:1655–1660

Mittermeier RA, Mittermeier CG, Brooks TM, Pilgrim JD, Konstant WR, da Fonseca GAB, Kormos C (2003) Wilderness and biodiversity conservation. Proc Natl Acad Sci U S A 100:10309–10313

Monbiot G (2013) Feral: searching for enchantment on the frontiers of rewilding. Allen Lane, Penguin Press, London

Nilon CH, Aronson MFJ, Cilliers SS, Dobbs C, Frazee LJ, Goddard MA, O'Neill KM, Roberts D, Stander EK, Werner P, Winter M, Yocom KP (2017) Planning for the future of urban biodiversity: a global review of city-scale initiatives. Bioscience 67:332–342

Peach WJ, Denny M, Cotton PA, Hill IF, Gruar D, Barritt D, Impet A, Mallord J (2004) Habitat selection by song thrushes in stable and declining farmland populations. J Appl Ecol 41:275–293

Pett TJ, Shwartz A, Irvine KN, Dallimer M, Davies ZG (2016) Unpacking the people–biodiversity paradox: a conceptual framework. Bioscience 66:576–583

Pham TTH, Apparicio P, Séguin AM, Landry S, Gagnon M (2012) Spatial distribution of vegetation in Montreal: an uneven distribution or environmental inequity? Landsc Urban Plan 107:214–224

Pressey RL (1994) Ad hoc reservations: forward or backward steps in developing representative reserve systems? Conserv Biol 8:662–668

Pressey RL, Whish GL, Barrett TW, Watts ME (2002) Effectiveness of protected areas in northeastern New South Wales: recent trends in six measures. Biol Conserv 106:57–69

Pyle RM (2003) Nature matrix: reconnecting people and nature. Oryx 37:206–214

Ratcliffe E, Gatersleben P, Sowden PT (2013) Bird sounds and their contributions to perceived attention restoration and stress recovery. J Environ Psychol 36:221–228

Rayner G, Lang T (2012) Ecological public health: reshaping the conditions for good health. Routledge, Abingdon

Reichard SH, White P (2001) Horticulture as pathways of plant introductions in the United States. Bioscience 51:103–113

Robb GN, McDonald RA, Chamberlain DE, Bearhop S (2008) Food for thought: supplementary feeding as a driver of ecological change in avian populations. Front Ecol Environ 6:476–484

Rogerson M, Barton J, Bragg R, Pretty J (2017) The health and wellbeing impacts of volunteering with the wildlife trusts. University of Essex, Colchester

Russo A, Escobedo FJ, Cirella GT, Zerbe S (2017) Edible green infrastructure: an approach and review of provisioning ecosystem services and disservices in urban environments. Agric Ecosyst Environ 242:53–66

Salisbury A, Armitage J, Bostock H, Perry J, Tatchell M, Thompson K (2015) Enhancing gardens as habitats for flower-visiting aerial insects (pollinators): should we plant native or exotic species? J Appl Ecol 52:1156–1164

Sanderson EW, Jaiteh M, Levy MA, Redford KH, Wannebo AV, Woolmer G (2002) The human footprint and the last of the wild. Bioscience 52:891–904

Schwarz N, Moretti M, Bugalho MN, Davies ZG, Haase D, Hack J, Hof A, Melero Y, Pett TJ, Knapp S (2017) Understanding biodiversity-ecosystem service relationships in urban areas: a comprehensive literature review. Ecosyst Serv 27:161–171

Seeland K, Moser K, Scheutle H, Kaiser FG (2002) Public acceptance of restrictions imposed on recreational activities in the per-urban Sihlwald Nature Reserve, Sihlwald, Switzerland. Urban For Urban Green 1:49–57

Seto KC, Güneralp B, Hutyra LR (2012) Global forecasts of urban expansion to 2030 and direct impacts on biodiversity and carbon pools. Proc Natl Acad Sci U S A 109:16083–16088

Shanahan DF, Lin BB, Gaston KJ, Bush R, Fuller RA (2015) What is the role of trees and remnant vegetation in attracting people to urban parks? Landsc Ecol 30:153–165

Shwartz A, Cheval H, Simon L, Julliard R (2013) Virtual garden computer program for use in exploring the elements of biodiversity people want in cities. Conserv Biol 27:876–886

Smith J (2013) Protected areas: Origins, criticisms and contemporary issues for outdoor recreation. Centre for environment and society research. Working paper series no. 15. Birmingham City University, Birmingham

Soga M, Gaston KJ (2016) Extinction of experience: the loss of human-nature interactions. Front Ecol Environ 14:94–101

Speak AF, Mizgajski A, Borysiak J (2015) Allotment gardens and parks: provision of ecosystem services with an emphasis on biodiversity. Urban For Urban Green 14:772–781

Stigner MG, Beyer HL, Klein CJ, Fuller RA (2016) Reconciling recreational use and conservation values in a coastal protected area. J Appl Ecol 53:1206–1214

TEEB (2010) The economics of ecosystems and biodiversity: mainstreaming the economics of nature: a synthesis of the approach, conclusions and recommendations of TEEB. Progress Press, Malta

ten Brink P, Mutafoglu K, Schweitzer J-P, Kettunen M, Twigger-Ross C, Baker J, Kuipers Y, Emonts M, Tyrväinen L, Hujala T & Ojala A (2016) The Health and Social Benefits of Nature and Biodiversity Protection. A report for the European Commission. Institute for European Environmental Policy, London/Brussels

Tryjanowski P, Morelli F, Mikula P, Krištín A, Indykiewicz P, Grzywaczewski G, Kronenberg J, Jerzak L (2017) Bird diversity in urban green space: a large-scale analysis of differences between parks and cemeteries in Central Europe. Urban For Urban Green 27:264–271

Tyrväinen L, Mäkinen K, Schipperijn J (2007) Tools for mapping social values of urban woodlands and other green areas. Landsc Urban Plan 79:5–19

United Nations (2015) World urbanization prospects, the 2014 revision. United Nations, New York

Vaughan KB, Kaczynski AT, Wilhelm Stanis SA, Besenyi GM, Bergstrom R, Heinrich KM (2013) Exploring the distribution of park availability, features, and quality across Kansas City, Missouri by income and race/ethnicity: an environmental justice investigation. Ann Behav Med 45:S28–S38

Venter O, Fuller RA, Segan DB, Carwardine J, Brooks T, Butchart SHM, Di Marco M, Iwamura T, Joseph L, O'Grady D, Possingham HP, Rondinini C, Smith RJ, Venter M, Watson JEM (2014) Targeting global protected area expansion for imperiled biodiversity. PLoS Biol 12:e101891

Venter O, Sanderson EW, Magrach A, Allan JR, Beher J, Jones KR, Possingham HP, Laurance WF, Wood P, Fekete PM, Levy MA, Watson JEM (2016) Sixteen years of change in the global terrestrial human footprint and implications for biodiversity conservation. Nat Commun 7:12558

Voigt A, Wurster D (2014) Does diversity matter? The experience of urban nature's diversity: case study and cultural concept. Ecosyst Serv 12:200–208

Watson JEM, Dudley N, Segan DB, Hockings M (2014) The performance and potential of protected areas. Nature 515:67–73

Watson JEM, Shanahan DF, Di Marco M, Allan J, Laurance WF, Sanderson EW, Mackey B, Venter O (2017) Catastrophic declines in wilderness areas undermine global environment targets. Curr Biol 26:2929–2934

Wilson EO (1984) Biophilia. Harvard University Press, Massachusetts

Wolch JR, Wilson JP, Fehrenbach J (2013) Parks and park funding in Los Angeles: an equity-mapping analysis. Urban Geogr 26:4–35

Wolch JR, Byrne J, Newell JP (2014) Urban green space, public health, and environmental justice: the challenge of making cities 'just green enough'. Landsc Urban Plan 125:234–244

Chapter 13
Supporting Behavioural Entrepreneurs: Using the Biodiversity-Health Relationship to Help Citizens Self-Initiate Sustainability Behaviour

Raymond De Young

Abstract Techno-industrial societies face biophysical limits and the consequences of disrupting Earth's ecosystems. This creates a new behavioural context with an unmistakable demand: Citizens of such societies must turn from seeking new resources to crafting new living patterns that function well within finite ecosystems. This coming transition is inevitable, but our response is not preordained. Indeed, given the complex, multi-decade-long context, the required pro-environmental behaviours cannot be fully known in advance. Furthermore, the urgency to respond will necessitate that whole clusters of behaviour be adopted; incremental and serial change will not suffice. Thus, a culture of small experiments must be nurtured. The process of change will seriously tax social, emotional and attentional capacities. Thus, priority is placed on emotional stability and clear-headedness, maintaining social relationships while stressed, pro-actively managing behaviour and a willingness to reskill. These aspects of coping share a common foundation: the maintenance of attentional vitality and psychological well-being. Changes also must occur in how pro-environmental behaviours are promoted. We must move beyond interventions that are expert-driven, modest in request, serial in implementation and short-term in horizon. New interventions must create the conditions under which citizens become behavioural entrepreneurs, themselves creating, managing and sharing successful approaches to behaviour change.

Keywords Behavioural entrepreneurs · Behavioural aesthetics · Biophysical limits · Behaviour change · Energy descent · Mental vitality

Highlights

- Biophysical limits and climate disruption have created a new behavioural context.

R. De Young (✉)
School for Environment and Sustainability, University of Michigan, Ann Arbor, MI, USA
e-mail: rdeyoung@umich.edu

M. R. Marselle et al. (eds.), *Biodiversity and Health in the Face of Climate Change*, https://doi.org/10.1007/978-3-030-02318-8_13

- Environmental behaviours needed later this century cannot be fully known in advance.
- Attentional vitality and psychological equipoise are needed for behaviour change.
- Clusters of behaviour must be adopted; serial, incremental change will not suffice.
- Conditions can be created under which citizens become behavioural entrepreneurs.

13.1 Introduction

How ever vast were the resources used to create techno-industrial society, they were never limitless. And how ever massive was the waste sink that these societies made out of the atmosphere, it is no longer able to absorb their wastes. Biophysical limits and the consequences of having disrupted the Earth's ecosystems lead to an unmistakable outcome: starting this century, citizens of these societies will consume fewer resources and live more simply. Unfortunately, their current worldviews, goals and behaviours are not prepared for this new reality.

Certainly, it is possible to live at a dramatically lower energy and material flux. Indeed, almost all of human history occurred within a pre-industrial low-energy context, and such an existence is commonplace for much of the current global population. However, the comforts and conveniences of techno-industrial society are unlikely to be possible under the new biophysical context outlined below. Thus, the focus of this chapter is on helping the citizens of such a society weather their inevitable transition to a more frugal existence, and it is the experiences and behaviours of those individuals to whom this chapter will refer.

A decline in resource availability occurring alongside a need to respond to climate disruption will upend life patterns and is not welcomed by reasonable individuals. Nonetheless, this looming reality is as well documented as it is stark. Consider that, near the end of this century, addressing climate disruption alone requires that we produce below a tenth of current greenhouse gas emissions, and probably requires a comparable reduction in consumption of energy and materials. The environmental community has long argued for significant reductions in consumption and emissions, but never have order-of-magnitude changes been envisioned.

Our species' adaptive, entrepreneurial nature suggests that we might respond well to this new reality under certain conditions. The needed changes will place a priority on clear-headedness, the ability to thoughtfully plan and manage behaviour and a willingness to continuously build new competencies. These capacities, in turn, depend on mental well-being (see Part II, this volume). After introducing how the new biophysical context has created a new behavioural context, this chapter suggests how to help people to respond well to this new reality.

13.2 New Biophysical Context

Numerous vulnerabilities have been uncovered within the techno-industrial development approach adopted in many parts of the globe (Meadows et al. 1972, 2004). Tainter (1988) evaluated 11 ways that societies might succumb to constraints and, in the process, identified a new vulnerability. Tainter's concept, the risk of diminishing marginal returns from increasing social complexity, is a social version of the economic principle of diminishing returns. In essence, societies solve the problems they face through an increasing investment in social and/or political complexity. However, this approach eventually becomes too costly to maintain and the society adopting that problem-solving approach becomes unsustainable.

Without providing an exhaustive account of all vulnerabilities, it is nonetheless possible to establish our predicament by considering a basic idea. Like all living systems, techno-industrial civilisation has a metabolism: resources are consumed, work done and waste products discharged. It is sufficient for the purpose here to follow just one of many metabolites, hydrocarbons, starting as a source of energy, consumed in the creation and support of social services and eventually becoming a waste. On the input side, the system vulnerabilities are from limits-to-growth (Jackson and Webster 2016; Turner 2008, 2012), a notion that has lingered on the fringe of environmental discourse. Most reactions to the fact of biophysical limits to material growth have varied within a narrow range between dismissive and derisive. However, an expected end to energy-fueled growth is receiving renewed attention from both ecologists and economists (Bardi 2014, 2011; Daly and Farley 2010; Hall and Day 2009). One aspect of hydrocarbon-based limits-to-growth, that of declining net energy, is particularly troublesome and discussed below. On the output side, the waste involves carbon-based emissions that create the well-documented disruptions to the climate system (Hansen et al. 2017). Taken together, these highlight a radically changed biophysical reality where, as McKibben (2010) contends, the planet onto which we were born has been so altered that it is not the world on which we now live.

13.2.1 Surplus Energy Decline

Social systems voraciously consume energy in the course of doing their work. Thus, for social services (e.g. infrastructure, manufacturing, maintenance, provisioning, education, governance, health-care, travel, tourism, entertainment) to continue functioning, there must be a net surplus of energy generated elsewhere. Maintaining a sufficient surplus is becoming increasingly difficult. The issue here has many technical aspects but is also commonsense; it takes energy to get energy and transform it into socially usable forms. Prosperity in techno-industrial society derives from there being a significant surplus available after deducting from the total energy extracted, the amount used to get it (Morgan 2016). One concern that highlights the new biophysical context is a decline in energy-returned-on-energy-invested (EROEI), which is one way to measure surplus energy. EROEI was first studied by Odum (1973); it is a foundation of biophysical economics (Cleveland et al. 1984) and energy analysis (Cleveland 2005; Hall 2011, 2012; Hall and Klitgaard 2011), and is proving useful in macroeconomic analysis (Fagnart and Germain 2016). The low-hanging fruit metaphor explains EROEI. Initially, extraction occurs at more attractive locations containing high-quality resources that are easy to extract, process and deliver. Later, resources are found at inhospitable sites, are of lower thermodynamic quality and are harder to recover, refine and transport. Harder here ultimately means consuming ever-greater amounts of energy in order to extract energy. This is a logical pattern – pursue the easiest to get first – but results in a decline over time in surplus energy (Murphy 2014).

Early on, a massive surplus of energy misled us with the false promise of endless physical growth. False because, although it largely went unnoticed, surplus energy was on an unrelenting decline (Hall 2012, 2017; Heinberg and Fridley 2016; Morgan 2016). The minimum EROEI needed to support a techno-industrial society is being explored by Hall and his colleagues (Hall 2011, 2012; Hall et al. 2009; Guilford et al. 2011). In their analysis, it matters enormously what social services are deemed necessary. As the features included in the definition increase, so too does the EROEI ratio needed to support that society. Historically, EROEI was calculated at the energy source – the wellhead – and included only the energy consumed by the hydrocarbon exploration and production industry. In order to make this concept useful for social decision-making, Hall et al. (2009) developed an analysis that accounts for the many indirect energy costs experienced when providing any particular service to society. This is the surplus energy needed by citizens, organisations or communities pursuing their everyday activities and is reported as the extended-EROEI ratio. This research is still maturing but its general conclusions are firm. Declining surplus energy at the societal level is bringing ever closer the day when the resources at our disposal will be insufficient to maintain growth in, and perhaps the full maintenance of, the personal, social and urban systems to which we have become accustomed.

Thus, considering just one aspect of one input to techno-industrial society's metabolism reveals a significant vulnerability. All is well so long as there is a significant surplus of energy. However, over time that surplus is getting smaller.

13.2.2 Climate Disruption

Climate disruption, a consequence of the rapacious use of hydrocarbon-based fuels, is empirically established and settled science; the evidence is unequivocal. Profound changes to the earth's thermal patterns are occurring (IPCC 2014) and appear to be accelerating (Herring et al. 2018). Furthermore, what were once worst-case and decades-distant consequences are now taking place (Hansen et al. 2017). There is hope that the Rio/Kyoto/Copenhagen/Cancun/Durban/Doha/Warsaw/Lima/Paris negotiating process has finally created a nascent global response. Nevertheless, few people are so optimistic as to believe this response will allow techno-industrial society to continue unchanged or for the planet to return to its preindustrial climate.

Even if the improbable happens (i.e. greenhouse gas emissions are immediately and entirely eliminated) there is enough warming baked into the system to disrupt the climate well into the next century. Apparently, the best to expect is eventually to stabilize the disruption that industrialisation caused. Scenarios that keep atmospheric CO_2 concentration levels below 450 ppm by 2100 (essential for keeping global temperature rise below a barely tolerable 2°C) all require quickly initiating and then indefinitely sustaining reductions in emissions (IPCC 2014). Achieving stabilisation at that level requires reductions that are frankly brutal: 40–70% lower global emission by 2050, with higher percentages required from techno-industrial countries and near zero global emission levels by 2100. Never before have we contemplated making such a massive reduction and then to maintain, if not deepen, that reduction forever.

The bleak nature of this new biophysical context is not easily contemplated. Thus, persuasively establishing its inevitability should only be done when serving a worthy purpose. The reason for stating this premise is the expectation that we will soon, one way or another, be consuming far fewer resources. The greater purpose in this chapter is to focus our efforts on discovering the conditions necessary to help citizens to pre-familiarise and pre-adapt themselves to this new reality before being forced to do so by biophysical circumstances.

13.3 New Behavioural Context

During a historically brief period of material affluence, it has been possible to ignore the biophysical foundation of civilisation. Behavioural scientists could focus on improving physical, mental and social well-being while remaining ignorant of resource constraints. During this time conservation psychology developed effective interventions for promoting environmental stewardship (Clayton 2012; Hamann et al. 2016) and responding to global climate change (Clayton et al. 2015). Recently, however, it has been questioned whether a consumer-focused, fossil-fueled techno-industrial society *can ever* be made sustainable (Bardi 2011; De Young 2014; Monbiot 2015; Princen 2014; Princen et al. 2002; Turner 2008, 2012).

13.3.1 A Predicament, Not a Problem

This new behavioural context cannot be framed as a problem, at least not in the common definition of that word. It is a predicament, an unsolvable situation that will play out over many decades, perhaps through this century and into the next. If it were a problem, we would seek a solution and by applying that solution we would return to normal (Greer 2008). In contrast, predicaments have no solution; instead, they must be endured. Society can respond, but even an effective response does not eliminate the predicament. A useful response does not alter but rather accommodates the new situation. This is adaptation in a classic sense: to change behaviour into new forms that better fit a new reality.

If we faced a problem (e.g. emergency, crisis) then we might be advised to weather the storm until we 'get back to normal'. However, even a functional response to a predicament is unlikely to get us back; accommodation is about 'getting to a new normal'. The new behavioural context is also different in another significant way. Responses will need to be broadly applied across one's entire behaviour pattern, then maintained and even expanded throughout a lifetime. Unfortunately, society has little familiarity with the long-drawn-out behavioural planning and management needed to respond in this way. For while we know behaviours adequate for addressing short-term challenges to health and well-being, there exists little guidance for behaviour change necessary for addressing a many decade- or century-long predicament.

13.3.2 Changing Multiple Behaviours

Early conservation research focused on promoting one or a small suite of behaviours (Hamilton et al. 2018). We designed interventions to promote household recycling, mass transit use and water conservation (see, for instance, Geller et al. 1982). Most early studies focused on either providing information (e.g. environmental education, enhancing procedural knowledge) or motivation (e.g. economic incentives, token rewards). More recently, the focus has shifted to using social norms (e.g. injunctive norms, declarative norms) and team-based interventions (e.g. eco-teams). However, seldom was the focus on promoting clusters of behaviours. Other research explored not how to promote a specific behaviour, but what we know about people who already practice conservation behaviours. Research on long-term participants in environmental stewardship programs report two consistent motivations: the opportunity to do something meaningful to benefit the environment and the chance to learn something new (Ryan and Grese 2005; Ryan et al. 2001).

Later, Stern and colleagues made sense out of the huge array of available behaviours by suggesting we concentrate on those with the greatest environmental significance (Gardner and Stern 2002; Stern 2000). This logic prioritised high-impact behaviours, those with the highest achievable reduction in carbon emissions or resource consumption. The choice is based not only on a behaviour's technical potential (i.e. degree of impact if adopted) but also upon the social scale of its adoption (i.e. realistic adoption rate across an extended time-scale; Stern 2011).

Unfortunately, this approach still easily defaults to the serial adoption of behaviours given the individual costs and efforts involved (e.g. upgrading heating systems, buying fuel-efficient vehicles). If circumstances allow us to be patient then we benefit from their joint effects over time being significant (see Stern and Wolske's (2017) perspective on Wynes and Nicholas (2017)). Implementation principles are being developed that attend to the differences between actions having immediate effects versus reductions that only occur over a decadal time-scale (Wolske and Stern 2018). We are also learning to design interventions that are durable (i.e. the behaviour is maintained long after the intervention has ended; Moore and Boldero 2017) and generalisable (i.e. the effect of an intervention spills over to other contexts and behaviours; Nilsson et al. 2017) both useful features for promoting and sustaining multiple behaviours.

13.3.3 Cannot Know the Behaviours Needed

Dietz et al. (2009) highlighted the importance of simultaneously changing multiple behaviours, each selected for their high short-term impact. However, they also predicted that "lifestyle changes may become necessary in the out-years under constrained energy supply or economic growth scenarios" (2009: 18455). This identifies an important concern. Embedded in our current approach is the assumption that we can know, well in advance, the appropriate environmental stewardship behaviours to promote. This prior-knowledge would be essential for the development of the policies, incentives or nudges (Thaler and Sunstein 2008) necessary to direct behaviour. Such knowledge might also be needed for a new behavioural change approach, that of developing boosts that enhance old, or create new, competencies (Hertwig and Grüne-Yanoff 2017). Yet, under the new context posited here, this assumption is not met. There exists only a general outline of required future behaviours, not their details. Indeed, it is nearly impossible to imagine what everyday life might involve after a drastic reduction in surplus energy coupled with accelerating climate disruption.

This behavioural predicament is twofold. We cannot prescribe the specific behaviours that will need adopting decades hence, other than to suggest that they may be very different from what is now familiar. Furthermore, there will be an urgency to respond, which will necessitate the adoption of whole clusters of behaviours; incremental and serial change will no longer suffice.

13.4 New Form of Intervention

There is a great difference between green consumerism and a newly emerging pattern of behaviours labeled green citizenship. This difference will become increasingly important as we confront the new behavioural context. Much of our current attention focuses on encouraging green consumerism. It is assumed that by modifying consumer choices it is possible to sustain a techno-industrial society. Green consumerism is fully compatible with efforts to make only incremental changes to techno-industrial society. Within this framework, consumers are treated as fully independent, self-determining and sovereign (Princen 2010; Princen et al. 2002).

Few, if any, constraints are to be placed on their decision-making, and their consumer choice, once made, is self-justifying and neither to be challenged nor judged. Furthermore, the behaviours promoted must be easily reversible thus preserving the individual's autonomy (Thaler and Sunstein 2008). Green consumerism is also a comfortable approach because it is not a complicated set of behaviours, does not require mentally draining decision-making and it contains the unspoken promise that after achieving an environmentally sustainable state, most of the benefits of modernity will remain. Unfortunately, green consumerism has proven ineffective in curbing collective rates of consumption. Despite greatly improved efficiencies and clever behavioural interventions, society's aggregate energy usage and emissions continue to climb (Dietz et al. 2007; Jackson 2009; Monbiot 2015; Rees 2010).

In contrast, green citizenship is an approach that promotes behaviours based on different motivations and a longer-term time horizon. Recent work suggests that green citizens identify alternate paths of engaging with environmental stewardship that are not limited to the consumptive, product-centric actions defined by green consumerism (Alexander 2011). By moving beyond a consumption focus, green citizens enjoy a broad set of benefits embedded within alternative life patterns. Empirical research reveals that individuals find the pursuit of competence (e.g. developing new skills), frugality (e.g. pursuing resourcefulness), community participation and opportunities for meaningful action to be intrinsically satisfying and durable motivators of long-term environmental stewardship (De Young 1996; Ryan and Grese 2005; Ryan et al. 2001). Furthermore, and most relevant to the issue at hand, green citizens are revealed to be explorers and problem-solvers (Hamilton et al. 2018). These citizens are engaged in anticipatory adaptation (Lyles 2015; Ryan 2016), a pro-active form of pre-familiarisation, planning and capacity-building (Wamsler et al. 2018). The emerging profile of green citizens suggests a need for interventions that dramatically differ from those aimed at promoting green consumerism (Guckian et al. 2017). However, green citizenship may involve more mentally taxing reflection and planning, an issue returned to shortly.

13.4.1 Small Experiments

The new behavioural context includes the stressful conditions of great and prolonged uncertainty, and grave stakes. These are circumstances where we would be advised to start with small steps. As Scott (1998: 345) advises, "Prefer wherever possible to take a small step, stand back, observe, and then plan the next small move". Scott's (1998) idea follows, in part, the 'small experiment' approach to environmental problem solving outlined by Kaplan (1996; see also Irvine and Kaplan 2001; Kaplan et al. 1998).

Small experiments are a framework for supporting problem-solving that is based on people's natural tendency to explore and understand (Kaplan and Kaplan 2003,

2009) and on their brain having evolved to prospect the future not just track the past (Seligman et al. 2013). The small experiment approach supports behavioural innovation, maintains local relevance and allows for the rapid dissemination of findings. It contrasts with the large-scale approach that dominates research these days, in that it helps non-scientists systematically discover what works in their community. Small experiments are going on all the time. They are often the basis of stories told by gardeners, teachers, do-it-yourself creators and community organisers. They are present when experts and citizens jointly apply their separate talents and knowledge to an issue of mutual concern. Small experiments are so common that they could be mistaken as inconsequential. In fact, they are a powerful means of behavioural experimentation.

13.4.2 Behavioural Entrepreneurship

Clearly, the needed interventions change when addressing the new behavioural context. No longer adequate are approaches focused on single and specific behaviours. If this were not challenging enough, even with our current expertise we are unable to know exactly which future behaviours will need promoting. Thus, what we must support is the capacity of future citizens to identify the needed behaviours without our being there. Furthermore, citizens also would need to innovatively execute and maintain those behaviours in that future. Taken together, such capacities constitute entrepreneurial thought, craft and action. In the present, this calls for a unique form of intervention. We need to support *behavioural entrepreneurs* by creating conditions today under which individuals develop the capacity to anticipate, envision and prospect a future context. Then, when later they are in that context, those individuals will be able to craft innovative responses and self-regulate their behaviour to carry out those responses. The shift here is subtle, and perhaps appears academic, but it is a move away from expert-driven, delivery-based interventions toward the facilitation of citizen-developed interventions occurring in a partially unknowable future context.

This is neither a radical nor an unfamiliar approach although it is rarely used in the current rush to promote behaviour change. It is derived from Lewin's (1952) pioneering work using citizen groups to affect fundamental change by first honestly presenting people with the situation being faced and then giving them the trust, time and support needed to craft their own responses. Programs based on Lewin's approach are being developed to promote environmental stewardship (Fisher and Irvine 2016; Matthies and Kromker 2000) including the community-based initiatives called Ecoteams (Davidson 2011; Nye and Burgess 2008; Staats and Harland 1995; Staats et al. 2004). There are also larger-scale examples including eco-housing and ecovillages (Litfin 2013; Nelson 2018) and transition towns (Hopkins 2008). It is significant that the larger-scale examples were neither initiated nor supported by corporations, governments or major environmental organisations, instead they self-initiated. Behavioural entrepreneurship is about self-initiating behaviour change. Yet, whether acting individually or in groups, these entrepreneurs will need the capacity to envision, craft and then initiate responses all while functioning within a radically changed context.

13.5 Capacities-First Approach

Given that today we cannot fully know the behaviour patterns needed later this century, we must instead ask *what are the conditions under which* future citizens can respond with competence and equipoise. There is an innovative means of extracting these conditions. It employs a method used within psychological discussions of intentionality (Baumeister et al. 2011; Mele 2001) and is referred to as a capacities-first approach (Seligman et al. 2013). This approach is a form of envisioning (Meadows 1996) and is wholly unlike our current tendency to construct interventions that are primarily past-driven.

A past-driven approach is a leveraging of traits, decision-making tendencies, knowledge, norms and motives from people's immediate and distant past. For instance, we assess whether an individual holds an eco-centric, ego-centric or social-centric value orientation and then create an intervention that leverages their dominant orientation. Another example starts with individuals who are inclined toward a specific environmental stewardship behaviour but lack the necessary procedural knowledge to carry out that behaviour. The intervention would then focus on providing the needed behavioural skills and strategies. A third example is making more salient an existing social norm using a public service announcement. In each instance, we, the experts, assume the role of creating interventions that manipulate existing factors to promote conservation behaviours among citizens.

In contrast, a *capacities-first* approach is future-centric. Citizens are imagined as actively coping with the challenges in that future context having successfully recast their behaviours into forms that fit that future ecological situation. Perhaps most significant, these future citizens are in no particular need of expert designed and managed interventions. However, perhaps we, the experts, could be of some help in the present. Although we cannot assume to know the specific future behaviours that citizens will be pursuing, we may assume that how they go about identifying and self-initiating those behaviours will be much the same as they do today. They will be using the same mental processes, cope with the same social challenges, be affected by the same emotions and need to develop skills well matched to the future context. Therefore, employing a reverse-engineering metaphor, we can imagine, in the present, what general capacities those future citizens must be in possession of, and the support they will come to rely upon while creating and initiating specific future behaviours. Providing for the development of those capacities now and supporting them in the future becomes a necessary, although perhaps not a sufficient, pre-condition for supporting future sustainability.

13.5.1 Needed Future Capacities

Applied here, this approach involves identifying the capacities that would be needed in order for citizens to plan, self-initiate and regulate their behaviour. A complete list of such capacities and their functional relationships would be long, drawing from the full range of social science research. For the purpose here, we can bound the list by considering only those features needed for conducting the mental work of envisioning, crafting and implementing behaviours in a future context.

Hertwig and Grüne-Yanoff (2017), in their explanation of the advantage of using boosting rather than nudging to change behaviour, mention creating competencies that are useful across a range of situations including, presumably, those for which we cannot in advance know the details. Their discussion of these capacities includes improving people's competencies to exercise their own agency. One example is the authors distinguishing between short- and long-term boosts with the latter focused on creating generic problem-solving capacities that would be useful in future situations (Sunstein 2016).

Wamsler et al. (2018) are more specific in their discussion of the relationship between mindfulness and sustainability. They highlight such individual capacities as being able to maintain an adaptive and flexible response to events, the minimising of impulsive and habitual reactions and similar self-regulation skills. Analogous capabilities were uncovered in the study of green citizenship (Hamilton et al. 2018) where participants identified the importance of a capacity for openness in approaching a situation so as to avoid habitual response. Green citizens also seek opportunities to learn new skills while simultaneously deriving intrinsic satisfaction from these same opportunities (Guckian et al. 2017; Hamilton et al. 2018).

These ideas suggest a preliminary set of three capacities necessary for effectively responding to the new biophysical and behavioural context.

Mental Clarity Clear-headedness would be necessary for envisioning desired future states. Conscious deliberation and reflection are needed to plan the intermediate and long-term goals, and relevant behaviours, needed for achieving those future states.

Building Competencies Given that future behaviours are unknowable in their details there is the need for a motivation to continuously develop new competencies rather than merely the training of specific skills. Particularly important is the ability to understand diverse and complex social and natural systems in order to be able to identify intended and unintended consequences of future actions.

Emotional Regulation The premise of this chapter cannot help but be unsettling. Nonetheless, given the likely need for social coordination, it will be necessary to maintain pro-social inclinations under the stress of difficult biophysical circumstances. Maintaining a positive emotional state will help to build and maintain social and behavioural resources.

13.5.2 Supporting Capacity Building

As disparate as the aforementioned capacities for clarity, competence building and emotional stability may seem at first, they share a common foundation: the ability to maintain attentional vitality (Basu 2015). Mental clear-headedness is a precondition for human effectiveness (Kaplan 1995) and thus vital to behavioural entrepreneurship. Envisioning future situations and, more importantly, imagining groups of behaviours that need to be adopted together for an effective response will need to be done while in the presence of the radically changing biophysical and behavioural contexts outlined above, the desperate needs of others and unmet personal needs.

It is here that the enormous adaptive significance of mental vitality becomes clear. It allows for pausing to insert our own intentions between the demands of the immediate environment and the future for which we are seeking to prepare a response (De Young 2010). With this ability, future citizens could envision multiple futures without undue confusion, contemplate alternate priorities and explore alternatives instead of jumping to first conclusions. In addition, and most relevant here, it allows imagining which combinations of behavioural responses will work well together. The importance of this ability cannot be overstated. Without this ability, future citizens could not override automatic functioning whether based on innate stimulus-driven patterns (e.g. inherited inclinations) or learned patterns (e.g. habitual responses). In short, the entrepreneurial thought, craft and action needed to respond well will depend on citizens maintaining their mental vitality.

Yet, preserving mental vitality is difficult even in the best of times since handling all the information we crave, as well as dealing with the onslaught of unbidden information, easily leads to our being overwhelmed and mentally exhausted. The challenge is all the more formidable under the premise of this chapter. Yet, while the cognitive demands placed on behavioural entrepreneurs will certainly tax their mental well-being, research has repeatedly highlighted the restorative effect of time spent in natural settings (see Marselle Chap. 7, this volume; Marselle et al. Chap. 9, this volume; Kaplan and Berman 2010; Kaplan and Kaplan 2009). This leads to a fascinating, if somewhat counterintuitive, aspect of the new biophysical context. It is possible that life will become less affluent, less easily mobile and less consumer-based. At the same time, everyday life may become more locally oriented with everyone more involved in their own provisioning. Thus, slowly over time, daily access to nearby nature may increase. Given that such access can improve mental, physical, social and spiritual well-being (see Cook et al. Chap. 11, this volume; Irvine et al. Chap. 10, this volume), the very restoration needed to effectively respond to the new context will be available within that same context.

Mental vitality is a state-of-mind essential to entrepreneurial behaviour but there is also a need for citizens to derive a motive from such engagement. Fortunately, the motives necessary to support behavioural entrepreneurship are embedded in the very challenges involved and are well-studied. It turns out that humans are intrinsically motivated to pursue capacity building (De Young 1996, 2000; Howell 2013; O'Brien and Wolf 2010; Sheldon et al. 2011; Van der Werff et al. 2013). Chawla

(1998) found that environmentally involved individuals credit intrinsic motivation when explaining the development of competence in both responding to difficulties and interacting effectively with others. There are also intrinsic satisfactions embedded in the pursuit of green citizenship (Guckian et al. 2017; Hamilton et al. 2018; Wolf 2011). It is indeed fortunate that people are able to derive a deep and direct intrinsic motivation from those behaviours that will need to be commonplace in the future.

There is a fascinating technique for focusing people's attention on the future by increasing their psychological connectedness to their future self (Schelling 1984). Zaval et al. (2015) were able to increase this connection by having participants write a brief essay about how they wished to be remembered. Envisioning their legacy had the effect of helping people to have a much longer time-horizon and be intrinsically motivated to pursue environmental stewardship behaviours.

Another means of helping people to develop future-oriented competencies is offered by Fredrickson's *Broaden and Build* model (1998). This model identifies the behavioural benefits of maintaining a positive emotional state. Fredrickson explored the paradox that while negative emotions are linked to specific action tendencies (e.g. anger promotes urge to attack, guilt leads to desire to make amends) there are no specific behaviours linked to positive emotions. Negative emotions also are known to greatly narrow the scope of attention, the information considered and the capacity for reflection. In contrast, positive emotional states expand cognition; inspire creativity, exploration and the development of future behavioural options. This has the effect of expanding our repertoire of behavioural responses. Fredrickson describes the broadening effect as widening the scope of thoughts that come to mind, and the building effect as increasing the resources available for responding (e.g. new plans, strategies, social relationships). Although positive emotional states are transitory, the physical, intellectual and social competencies, and resources built endure.

13.6 Conclusion

After having supported the capacity building of future behavioural entrepreneurs, we might imagine how their behaviour change strategies would develop. One vision has them analytically and rationally creating technically efficient responses to the new contexts and then adopting behaviours in well-organised packages having the highest environmental impact. A second vision imagines citizen-artists who have elegantly crafted lives functioning harmoniously within a diverse social community and vibrant natural environment with patterns of behaviour evolving and interacting beautifully. In the latter vision the slowly adapting structure of everyday life would comprise a behavioural aesthetic resulting in great contentment and sense of accomplishment.

These two visions of how behaviour change efforts may unfold are not mutually exclusive. Indeed, a mixture of the two seems plausible within a given community and across time. However, the second vision is much less common among experts who focus on changing people's conservation behaviour. Thus, providing support for this second vision seems a useful place to conclude. It turns out that the second vision, like behavioural entrepreneurship, is neither a radical nor an unfamiliar approach to environmental stewardship.

13.6.1 Conservation Aesthetic

Aldo Leopold (1933) is remembered for his promotion of a conservation and land ethic. However, near the end of his book, *A Sand County Almanac* (1949), he introduced the idea that the planet also could be restored using a conservation aesthetic. The distinction between these approaches to behaviour change is dramatic. A land ethic, whether voluntary or mandatory, involves "a limitation on freedom of action in the struggle for existence" (Leopold 1949: 202), an obligation to exercise restraint. In contrast, a conservation aesthetic would have us seek interactions with nature because we derive satisfaction from them. A conservation aesthetic is revitalising, unleashing pleasures derived from the hidden riches of interacting directly with the biodiversity of nature.

13.6.2 Behavioural Aesthetic

Modern industrial society rejoices in its many technical efficiencies and innovations. However, these accomplishments are challenged by new data (Bonaiuti 2017). What seems efficient from one perspective is brittle from another. Material production and consumption on a global scale turns out to require complex systems and demand massive energy inputs. This leads to increasing economic and social system vulnerabilities as the complexity reaches diminishing marginal returns (Tainter 1988) and as the production of natural resources both becomes less predictable and suffers from declining energy surpluses. Furthermore, focusing on the output from this vulnerable complex system reveals that consumer consumption, the end goal of the entire enterprise, is an astonishingly inefficient means of providing for social and spiritual well-being (De Young and Princen 2012; Kasser 2009; Kjell 2011; O'Brien 2008).

Critiques of modernity are not new. Nevertheless, there is a new claim that industrialisation destroys the aesthetic quality of everyday life. Berry (1987: 165–166) has made this observation about what one gains from daily work in non-industrial enterprises. He cites the work of Gill (1983: 65) on the higher calling that working manually fulfills, "…every [one] is called to give love to the work of [their] hands. Every [one] is called to be an artist". Berry makes this same claim throughout his poetry, fiction and non-fiction writing, frequently offering up small-scale agriculture as an instance of an artistic enterprise involving multiple and overlapping daily decisions centered on the concepts of beauty, resourcefulness and feeding of spiritual well-being as much as the body. Perhaps, as we endeavor to first repair and then maintain the planet, everyone will be called upon to be an artist, an idea consistent with Seligman's (1999) notion that authentic happiness comes from "living life as a work of art".

Thus, we have an idea, previously applied to agrarian pursuits but perhaps applicable to everyday enterprise, that would have us seek an aesthetic outcome to the behaviours we pursue. In addition to the environmental impact notion mentioned earlier, this current idea would involve selecting behaviours that, when they are considered in the whole, constitute something of beauty that enhances mental, social and spiritual well-being. This idea would have citizens weave together desired and valued outcomes matched to environmental stewardship goals, the use of old and the learning of new skills with all being adjusted through reflection and equipoise. The term *behavioural aesthetic* captures both the ongoing process and most certainly the outcome achieved across time; this is a form of performance art but at the everyday level and focused on sustainability.

References

Alexander S (2011) The voluntary simplicity movement: reimagining the good life beyond consumer culture. University of Melbourne, Melbourne Australia. https://doi.org/10.2139/ssrn.1970056. Accessed 21 June 2018

Bardi U (2011) The limits to growth revisited. Springer, London

Bardi U (2014) Extracted: how the quest for mineral wealth is plundering the planet. Chelsea Green Publishing, White River Junction

Basu A (2015) Bringing out the best in ourselves. In: Kaplan R, Basu A (eds) Fostering reasonableness. Maize Books, Ann Arbor, pp 87–104

Baumeister RF, Crescioni A, Alquist J (2011) Free will as advanced action control for human social life and culture. Neuroethics 4:1–11

Berry W (1987) Home economics. North Point Press, San Francisco

Bonaiuti M (2017) Are we entering the age of involuntary degrowth? promethean technologies and declining returns of innovation. J Clean Prod. https://doi.org/10.1016/j.jclepro.2017.02.196

Chawla L (1998) Significant life experiences revisited: a review of research on sources of environmental sensitivity. Environ Educ Res 4:369–382

Clayton S (ed) (2012) The Oxford handbook of environmental and conservation psychology. Oxford University Press, New York

Clayton S, Devine-Wright P, Stern PC, Whitmarsh L, Carrico A, Steg L, Swim J, Bonnes M (2015) Psychological research and global climate change. Nat Clim Chang 5:640–646

Cleveland CJ (2005) Net energy from the extraction of oil and gas in the United States. Energy 30:769–782

Cleveland CJ, Costanza R, Hall CAS, Kaufman R (1984) Energy and the US economy: a biophysical perspective. Science 225:890–897

Daly HE, Farley J (2010) Ecological economics: principles and applications. Island Press, Washington, DC

Davidson S (2011) Up-scaling social behaviour change programs: the case of EcoTeams. In: Whitmarsh L, O'Neill S, Lorenzoni I (eds) Engaging the public with climate change: behaviour change and communication. Earthscan, Washington, DC, pp 180–199

De Young R (1996) Some psychological aspects of reduced consumption behaviour: the role of intrinsic satisfaction and competence motivation. Environ Behav 28:358–409

De Young R (2000) Expanding and evaluating motives for environmentally responsible behaviour. J Soc Issues 56:509–526
De Young R (2010) Restoring mental vitality in an endangered world: reflections on the benefits of walking. Ecopsychology 2:13–22
De Young R (2014) Some behavioural aspects of energy descent: how a biophysical psychology might help people transition through the lean times ahead. Front Psychol 5:1255
De Young R, Princen T (2012) The localization reader: adapting to the coming downshift. The MIT Press, Cambridge, MA
Dietz T, Rosa EA, York R (2007) Driving the human ecological footprint. Front Ecol Environ 5:13–18
Dietz T, Gardner G, Gilligan J, Stern P, Vandenbergh M (2009) Household actions can provide a behavioural wedge to rapidly reduce US carbon emissions. Proc Natl Acad Sci 106:18452–18456
Fagnart JF, Germain M (2016) Net energy ratio, EROEI and the macroeconomy. Struct Chang Econ Dyn 37:121–126
Fisher J, Irvine KN (2016) Reducing energy use and carbon emissions: a critical assessment of small-group interventions. Energies 9:172
Fredrickson BL (1998) What good are positive emotions? Rev Gen Psychol 2:300–319
Gardner G, Stern P (2002) Environmental problems and human behaviour, 2nd edn. Pearson, Boston MA
Geller ES, Winett R, Everett P (1982) Preserving the environment: new strategies for behavioural change. Pergamon Press, New York
Gill E (1983) A holy tradition of working. Golgonooza Press, Suffolk
Greer JM (2008) The long descent: a user's guide to the end of the industrial age. New Society Publishers, Gabriola Island
Guckian ML, De Young R, Harbo S (2017) Beyond green consumerism: uncovering the motivations of green citizenship. Michigan J Sustain 5:73–94
Guilford MC, Hall CAS, O'Connor P, Cleveland CJ (2011) A new long term assessment of energy return on investment (EROI) for U.S. oil and gas discovery and production. Sustainability 3:1866–1877
Hall CAS (2011) Introduction to special issue on new studies in EROI. Sustainability 3:1773–1777
Hall CAS (2012) Energy return on investment. In: Butler T, Lerch D, Wuerthner G (eds) The energy reader: overdevelopment and the delusion of endless growth. The Foundation for Deep Ecology, Sausalito, pp 62–68
Hall CA (2017) The history, future, and implications of EROI for society. In: Energy return on investment: a unifying principle for biology, economics, and sustainability. Springer, Cham, pp 145–169
Hall CAS, Day JW (2009) Revisiting the limits to growth after peak oil. Am Sci 97:230–237
Hall CAS, Klitgaard KA (2011) Energy and the wealth of nations: understanding the biophysical economy. Springer, New York
Hall CAS, Balogh S, Murphy DJR (2009) What Is the minimum EROEI that a sustainable society must have? Energies 2:25–47
Hamann K, Baumann A, Loschinger D (2016) Psychology of environmental protection: handbook for encouraging sustainable action. http://www.wandel-werk.org/docs/20171007-Handbook_english.pdf. Accessed 21 June 2018
Hamilton EM, Guckian ML, De Young R (2018) Living well and living green: participant conceptualizations of green citizenship. In: Leal W, Callewaert J (eds) Handbook of sustainability and social science research, World sustainability series. Springer, Cham, pp 315–334
Hansen J et al (2017) Young people's burden: requirement of negative CO2 emissions. Earth Syst Dynam 8:577–616
Heinberg R, Fridley D (2016) Our renewable future. Post Carbon Institute, Island Press, Washington, DC
Herring SC, Christidis N, Hoell A, Kossin JP, Schreck CJ III, Stott PA (eds) (2018) Explaining extreme events of 2016 from a climate perspective. Bull Am Meteor Soc 99:S1–S157

Hertwig R, Grüne-Yanoff T (2017) Nudging and boosting: steering or empowering good decisions. Perspect Psychol Sci 12:973–986
Hopkins R (2008) The transition handbook: from oil dependency to local resilience. Chelsea Green Publishing, White River Junction
Howell RA (2013) It's not (just) "the environment, stupid!" values, motivations, and routes to engagement of people adopting lower-carbon lifestyles. Glob Environ Chang 23:281–290
IPCC (2014) Summary for policymakers. In: Climate change 2014: impacts, adaptation, and vulnerability. Part A: global and sectoral aspects. Contribution of working group II to the fifth assessment report of the Intergovernmental Panel on Climate Change. Cambridge University Press, Cambridge/New York
Irvine KN, Kaplan S (2001) Coping with change: the small experiment as a strategic approach to environmental sustainability. Environ Manag 28:713–725
Jackson T (2009) Prosperity without growth: the transition to a sustainable economy. Sustainable Development Commission, London
Jackson T, Webster R (2016) Limits revisited: a review of the limits to growth debate. (Report) London: All-Party Parliamentary Group on Limits to Growth. http://limits2growth.org.uk/revisited. Accessed 21 June 2018
Kaplan S (1995) The restorative benefits of nature: toward an integrative framework. J Environ Psychol 15:169–182
Kaplan R (1996) The small experiment: achieving more with less. In: Nasar JL, Brown BB (eds) Public and private places. Environmental Design Research Association, Edmond, pp 170–174
Kaplan S, Berman M (2010) Directed attention as a common resource for executive functioning and self-regulation. Perspect Psychol Sci 5:43–57
Kaplan S, Kaplan R (2003) Health, supportive environments, and the reasonable person model. Am J Public Health 93:1484–1489
Kaplan S, Kaplan R (2009) Creating a larger role for environmental psychology: the Reasonable Person Model as an integrative framework. J Environ Psychol 29:329–339
Kaplan R, Kaplan S, Ryan RL (1998) With people in mind: design and management of everyday nature. Island Press, Washington, DC
Kasser T (2009) Psychological need satisfaction, personal well-being, and ecological sustainability. Ecopsychology 1:175–180
Kjell ON (2011) Sustainable well-being: a potential synergy between sustainability and well-being research. Rev Gen Psychol 15:255
Leopold A (1933) The conservation ethic. J For 31:634–643
Leopold A (1949) A Sand County almanac. Oxford University Press, Cambridge
Lewin K (1952) Group decision and social change. In: Swanson E, Newcomb TM, Hartley EL (eds) Readings in social psychology. Holt, New York, pp 459–473
Litfin KT (2013) Ecovillages: lessons for sustainable community. Polity Press, Cambridge
Lyles W (2015) Compassion building practices to improve hazard mitigation and climate adaptation planning. Paper presented at the Association of collegiate schools of planning conference, Houston TX, USA
Matthies E, Kromker D (2000) Participatory planning: a heuristic for adjusting interventions to the context. J Environ Psychol 20:65–74
McKibben B (2010) Eaarth: Making a life on a tough new planet. Times Books, New York
Meadows DH (1996) Envisioning a sustainable world. In: Costanza R, Segura O, Martinez-Alier J (eds) Getting down to earth: practical applications of ecological economics. Island Press, Washington, DC
Meadows DH, Meadows DL, Randers J, Behrens WW (1972) Limits to growth. Potomac Associates, Washington, DC
Meadows DH, Randers J, Meadows DL (2004) Limits to growth: the 30-year update. Chelsea Green Publishing, White River Junction
Mele AR (2001) Autonomous agents: from self-control to autonomy. Oxford University Press, New York

Monbiot G (2015) Consume more, conserve more: sorry, but we just can't do both, The Guardian. http://www.theguardian.com/commentisfree/2015/nov/24/consume-conserve-economic-growth-sustainability. Accessed 21 June 2018

Moore HE, Boldero J (2017) Designing interventions that last: a classification of environmental behaviours in relation to the activities, costs, and effort involved for adoption and maintenance. Front Psychol 8:1874

Morgan T (2016) Life after growth. Harriman House, Hampshire

Murphy DJ (2014) The implications of the declining energy return on investment of oil production. Phil Trans R Soc A 372:20130126

Nelson A (2018) Small is necessary: shared living on a shared planet. Pluto Press, London

Nilsson A, Bergquist M, Schultz WP (2017) Spillover effects in environmental behaviours, across time and context: a review and research agenda. Environ Educ Res 23:573–589

Nye M, Burgess J (2008) Promoting durable change in household waste and energy use behaviour. University of East Anglia, Norwich

O'Brien C (2008) Sustainable happiness: how happiness studies can contribute to a more sustainable future. Can Psychol 49:289–295

O'Brien KL, Wolf J (2010) A values-based approach to vulnerability and adaptation to climate change. Wiley Interdiscip Rev Clim Chang 1:232–242

Odum HT (1973) Energy, ecology and economics. Ambio 2:220–227

Princen T (2010) Consumer sovereignty, heroic sacrifice: two insidious concepts in an endlessly expansionist economy. In: Maniates M, Myers J (eds) The environmental politics of sacrifice. The MIT Press, Cambridge, MA, pp 45–164

Princen T (2014) The politics of urgent transition. In: Wolinsky Y (ed) U.S. Climate change policy and civic society. CQ Press, Washington, DC, pp 218–238

Princen T, Maniates M, Conca K (eds) (2002) Confronting consumption. The MIT Press, Cambridge, MA

Rees WE (2010) The human nature of unsustainability. In: Heinberg R, Lerch D (eds) The Post carbon reader: managing the 21st century's sustainability crises. Watershed Media, Healdsburg, pp 194–203

Ryan K (2016) Incorporating emotional geography into climate change research: a case study in Londonderry, Vermont, USA. Emot Space Soc 19:5–12

Ryan RL, Grese RE (2005) Urban volunteers and the environment: forest and prairie restoration. In: Bartlett PF (ed) Urban place. The MIT Press, Cambridge, MA

Ryan RL, Kaplan R, Grese RE (2001) Predicting volunteer commitment in environmental stewardship programs. J Environ Plan Manag 44:629–648

Schelling TC (1984) Self-command in practice, in policy, and in a theory of rational choice. Am Econ Rev 74:1–11

Scott JC (1998) Seeing like a state: how certain schemes to improve the human condition have failed. Yale University Press, New Haven

Seligman MEP (1999) Teaching positive psychology. APA Monit 30:42

Seligman MEP, Railton P, Baumeister RF, Sripada C (2013) Navigating into the future or driven by the past. Perspect Psychol Sci 8:119–141

Sheldon K, Nichols C, Kasser T (2011) Americans recommend smaller ecological footprints when reminded of intrinsic American values of self-expression, family, and generosity. Ecopsychology 3:97–104

Staats H, Harland P (1995) The Ecoteam program in the Netherlands, study 4: a longitudinal study on the effects of the Ecoteam program on environmental behaviour and its psychological backgrounds. Centre for Environmental and Energy Research, Leiden University, Leiden

Staats H, Harland P, Wilke H (2004) Effecting durable change: a team approach to improve environmental behaviour in the household. Environ Behav 36:341–367

Stern PC (2000) Toward a coherent theory of environmentally significant behaviour. J Soc Issues 56:407–424

Stern PC (2011) Contributions of psychology to limiting climate change. Am Psychol 66:303–314

Stern PC, Wolske KS (2017) Limiting climate change: what's most worth doing? Environ Res Lett 12:091001

Sunstein CR (2016) The ethics of influence: government in the age of behavioural science. Cambridge University Press, Cambridge

Tainter JA (1988) The collapse of complex societies. Cambridge University Press, Cambridge

Thaler R, Sunstein CR (2008) Nudge: improving decisions about health, wealth and happiness. Simon and Schuster, New York

Turner G (2008) A comparison of the limits to growth with 30 years of reality. Glob Environ Chang 18:397–411

Turner G (2012) On the cusp of global collapse? updated comparison of the limits to growth with historical data. GAIA 21:116–124

Van der Werff E, Steg L, Keizer K (2013) It is a moral issue: the relationship between environmental self-identity, obligation-based intrinsic motivation and pro-environmental behaviour. Glob Environ Chang 23:1258–1265

Wamsler C, Brossmann J, Hendersson H, Kristjansdottir R, McDonald C, Scarampi P (2018) Mindfulness in sustainability science, practice, and teaching. Sustain Sci 13:143–162

Wolf J (2011) Ecological citizenship as public engagement with climate change. In: Whitmarsh L, O'Neill S, Lorenzoni I (eds) Engaging the public with climate change: behaviour change and communication. Earthscan, Washington, DC, pp 120–137

Wolske KS, Stern PC (2018) Contributions of psychology to limiting climate change: opportunities through consumer behaviour. In: Clayton S, Manning C (eds) Psychology and climate change: human perceptions, impacts, and responses. Elsevier, Amsterdam

Wynes S, Nicholas KA (2017) The climate mitigation gap: education and government recommendations miss the most effective individual actions. Environ Res Lett 12:074024

Zaval L, Markowitz EM, Weber EU (2015) How will I be remembered? conserving the environment for the sake of one's legacy. Psychol Sci 26:231–236

Chapter 14
Global Developments: Policy Support for Linking Biodiversity, Health and Climate Change

Horst Korn, Jutta Stadler, and Aletta Bonn

Abstract This chapter highlights key policy processes at the international level dealing with the alignment of policies for the biodiversity-climate-health nexus. Recent developments by UN Conventions and major international organisations, such as the Convention on Biological Diversity, the Ramsar Convention and the United Nations Framework Convention on Climate Change (UNFCCC), together with the World Health Organization (WHO) and the Intergovernmental Science-Policy Platform on Biodiversity and Ecosystem Services (IPBES), are discussed. Special attention is given to newly emerging integrative global policy processes and partnerships between the Convention on Biological Diversity and the WHO, also in the framework of the Agenda 2030 for Sustainable Development and avenues to translate them into local policy through the global partnership ICLEI – Local Governments for Sustainability. Conclusions are drawn to foster the joint implementation of policy goals.

Keywords Biodiversity-climate-health nexus · Science-policy interface · UN conventions · CBD partnership · IPBES · SDG goals

Highlights

- Policy agendas of health promotion, climate change adaptation and biodiversity conservation are starting to become aligned.

H. Korn (✉) · J. Stadler
Federal Agency for Nature Conservation (BfN), Isle of Vilm, Putbus, Germany
e-mail: horst.korn@bfn.de; jutta.stadler@bfn.de

A. Bonn
Department of Ecosystem Services, Helmholtz Centre for Environmental Research – UFZ, Leipzig, Germany

German Centre for Integrative Biodiversity Research (iDiv) Halle-Jena-Leipzig, Leipzig, Germany

Institute of Biodiversity, Friedrich Schiller University Jena, Jena, Germany
e-mail: aletta.bonn@ufz.de

M. R. Marselle et al. (eds.), *Biodiversity and Health in the Face of Climate Change*, https://doi.org/10.1007/978-3-030-02318-8_14

- Alignment of indicators, joint metrics and reporting for health, climate change adaptation and biodiversity is needed to work effectively across different sectors.
- Joint collaborative working and governance is needed to put policy agendas into practice and foster implementation across sectors.

14.1 Introduction

Biodiversity forms the foundation of life on Earth and human health, as it underpins the functioning of ecosystems and associated ecosystem services (Cardinale et al. 2012). We depend on the contributions from nature to people (Díaz et al. 2018) for providing our food and fresh water, regulating climate, preventing floods and disease, as well as providing recreational benefits and aesthetic and spiritual enrichment (see also Irvine et al. Chap. 10, this volume). Biodiversity contributes to both traditional and modern medicines and supports local livelihoods and economic development (Romanelli et al. 2015). Because of these fundamental linkages between biodiversity and human health, it is surprising that this important cross-cutting issue made it –only in the last few years – prominently onto the agendas of important international conventions and organisations such as the Convention on Biological Diversity (CBD), the Ramsar Convention on Wetlands and the World Health Organization (WHO). Given the fact that climate change increasingly has direct and indirect effects on both biodiversity and human health, it is even more important to stress the links between the topics in order to foster nature-based solutions for promoting health and adapting to climate change.

This chapter highlights some key policy processes to tackle the relationships between (1) biodiversity and climate change, (2) biodiversity and health, (3) climate change and health and (4) the biodiversity-climate-health nexus on the international level. The field is developing fast, and this chapter represents the status as of August 2018. The connection between biodiversity and health – sometimes also in relation to climate change – is also emerging in many practical regional and local initiatives, coming from both a nature conservation angle and a medical angle. (For an overview about European Nature and Health network initiatives see Keune et al. Chap. 15, this volume.)

14.2 Biodiversity and Climate Change

Much work has been done on the direct effects of climate change on biodiversity (e.g. changes in phenology and in species' distribution, composition and interactions; see Bellard et al. 2012; Parmesan 2006; Thomas et al. 2004) as well as indirect effects of these changes on human health (Pecl et al. 2017). But vice versa, biodiversity also affects the climate system and can also ameliorate climate change

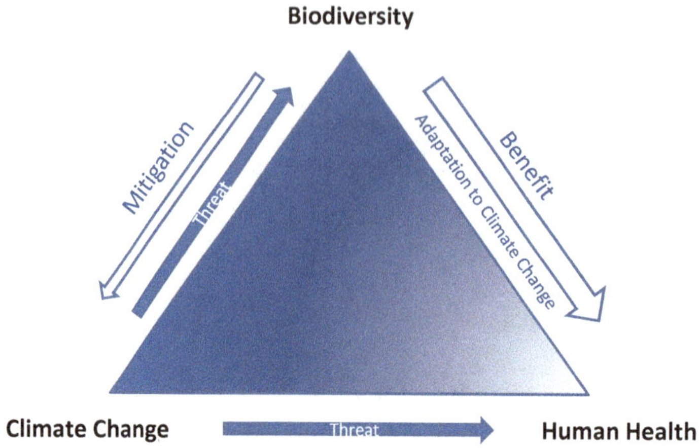

Fig. 14.1 Relationship between biodiversity, climate change and health. White arrows indicate a positive impact; dark arrows indicate a negative impact. The thickness of the lines corresponds to the strength of the impact

effects through nature-based mitigation (e.g. through carbon sequestration and carbon storage in vegetation or soils; see e.g. IPCC 2014) and adaptation measures (Lo 2016) (see Fig. 14.1). The latter – for example, reducing the urban heat island effect and disaster risk – have strong implications for human health and well-being. This was taken up and elaborated on by major international policy processes such as the Ramsar Convention on Wetlands in its resolutions (e.g. see Resolution XII.13: Wetlands and disaster risk reduction (Ramsar 2015)) and related activities reflected in the themes of the World Wetlands Days 2017 "Wetlands for Disaster Risk Reduction", and 2018 "Wetlands for a sustainable urban future". Ecosystem-based approaches to adapting to climate change and reducing disaster risk have also been an important topic in the processes of the CBD (Lo 2016).

14.3 Biodiversity and Health

The emergence of the ecosystem service concept led to the Millennium Ecosystem Assessment (MA 2005) with its synthesis report on health (Corvalan et al. 2005) followed by the Economics of Ecosystems and Biodiversity reports (TEEB 2010) and several national assessments (Schröter et al. 2016). These assessments mainly focused on economic benefits of nature and mention health benefits only little or less explicitly.

In the policy arena, the international treatment of the linkages of health and biodiversity began with the COHAB Initiative that was established in response to outputs of the First International "Conference on Health and Biodiversity – COHAB 2005", which took place in Galway, Ireland in August 2005 (see Box 14.1). The recommendations from that meeting addressed a number of key issues at the interface of biodiversity and human well-being, and raised issues of governance, equity

Box 14.1 Co-operation on Health and Biodiversity – COHAB Initiative
The COHAB Initiative operates through Partnership arrangements with a growing network of organisations worldwide, representing government and multi-lateral agencies, academic institutes, NGOs, indigenous communities and the private sector. These organisations share a common interest – to enhance co-operation between the health and biodiversity sectors, working together for a healthy planet with healthy people. Major areas of focus include:

- Poverty reduction and livelihood security
- Food security, nutrition and dietary health
- Emerging diseases
- Natural products and medicinal resources
- Disaster prevention, relief and recovery
- Traditional knowledge
- Indigenous community health
- Social and spiritual well-being and mental health.

COHAB Initiative Partnership arrangements provide a framework within which organisations may collaborate to increase the effectiveness of their efforts in addressing the issues linking the conservation and sustainable use of biodiversity with health, well-being and livelihood security. Partners range from Intergovernmental organisations (mainly from the UN-System), to international non-governmental organisations and a variety of country-based organisations.

(http://www.cohabnet.org, accessed 25.05.2018)

and participation. These were the core issues around which the COHAB Initiative was then established (COHAB 2005), and which provided the basis for further development of the topic. The COHAB Initiative, which is less active now, had a strong influence to put the topic on the agenda of the CBD and stimulated the joint work programme of the CBD and the WHO, which are now the main global actors in this field (see sect. 14.5.2).

14.4 Climate Change and Health

The direct link between climate change and health issues is well developed (e.g. WHO 2016; Wolf et al. 2015; see also Lindley et al. Chap. 1, Hunter et al. Chap. 17, both this volume). Already in 2008 the World Health Assembly developed a global Work Plan to support member states in climate change and health protection that was updated in 2014 (WHO 2015).[1] In 2015, the *Lancet* Commission on Health and Climate Change prominently recommended ten concise policy actions for the next 5 years on climate change adaptation to protect public health (Watts et al. 2015), which urged joint working across sectors and scaling up of investments to secure a climate-resilient public health system. Human health was also included as an important aspect in the European Environment Agency indicator report on climate change (Füssel et al. 2017). International policy commitments were documented in the Paris Agreement of the United Nations Framework Convention on Climate Change (UNFCCC), which recognised "the social, economic and environmental value of voluntary mitigation actions and their co-benefits for adaptation, health and sustainable development"(UN 2015a).

Unfortunately, the interlinkages between climate change, health and biodiversity only gained little attention within international climate policy, so far.

14.5 Biodiversity–Climate–Health Nexus

Despite the many activities in the individual fields of biodiversity conservation, climate change mitigation and adaptation as well as the improvement of human health, the benefits that intact ecosystems can provide to people's health in the face of climate change has only been recognised slowly during the last decade. There are many opportunities to bring the three topics of biodiversity, health and climate together in a constructive way and to tackle real issues. Biodiversity can help to prevent or minimise human-induced or natural disasters that are caused or accelerated by climate change.

For example:

1. Biodiversity can help human societies to adapt better to climate change induced heat waves in urban areas (see Lindley Chap. 1, this volume; overviews in Kabisch et al. 2017).
2. Biodiversity in the form of floodplain or mangrove ecosystems can help to protect human populations from the impact of severe floods partly caused by climate change (Temmerman et al. 2013).
3. Different species or varieties of plants and animals can help to adapt agricultural systems to climate change, so that they can provide sufficient nutrients and healthy diets (Lin 2011).

The emphasis of policy linkages was first on wetlands (see below) and nature-based solutions in urban areas (Kabisch et al. 2016, 2017; WHO Regional Office for Europe 2016), while the biodiversity-climate-health nexus has also been considered in much broader applications (see also Romanelli et al. 2015). In the following sec-

[1] For an overview of policy measures see http://www.who.int/globalchange/health_policy/en/ (accessed 8 August 2018).

tions we provide some examples of international policy processes that take an integrative approach.

14.5.1 RAMSAR-Convention

In 2012, the Ramsar Convention published a Technical Report "Healthy wetlands, healthy people" (Horwitz et al. 2012) that extensively reviewed the relationship between biodiversity (here in the form of wetland ecosystems), climate change and human health. The evidence of ecosystem services of wetlands and their benefits to human health and livelihoods was considered to be well established. Wetlands can provide food and shelter, flood control and mitigation of climate change through carbon storage as well as modes of transport and sources of beneficial drugs. As such the maintenance of 'healthy wetlands', including people as part of wetlands, was therefore considered to be very important. Nevertheless, it was also stated that the current understanding of climate change-induced increases in health and disease risks in wetlands should be taken into account when co-managing wetlands and human health. Decision-making should seek to maintain the capacity of wetlands to adapt to climate change, as functioning mangroves or floodplains and other wetlands can provide important buffers to climate-induced extreme events and associated risks of human health problems (Horwitz and Finlayson 2011), including risks of vector-borne diseases (see Müller et al. Chap. 4, this volume).

A draft version of the Ramsar report was already issued as a background document for the Ramsar COP 10 (Ramsar 2008) and led to Ramsar Resolution X.23, which recognised that the changing climate is expected to continue to increase the risk to human health of matters associated with wetland ecosystems. Importantly, the resolution emphasised tackling health risks, but also considered principles of equity and prevention in public health measures through wetlands. Contracting parties were urged to ensure that decision-making on co-managing wetlands and human health issues takes into account current understanding of climate change-induced increases in health and disease risk. The resolution text reflected the suggestions from the expert report (see above).

In Resolution XI.12 on Wetlands and Health (Ramsar 2012), the Conference of Parties to the Ramsar Convention raised the concern that threats to wetlands like climate change can act as drivers for disease emergence and re-emergence beyond natural cycles. Nevertheless, this link between wetlands, health and climate change is not directly addressed in the operative paragraphs of the resolution.

Three years later, as one of the outcomes of Ramsar COP 12 the Conference of Parties identified in Resolution XII.13 (Ramsar 2015) the link between wetlands and disaster risk reduction, and stated that healthy and well-managed wetlands can reduce disaster risk. Since many risks are expected to increase with climate change, joint work between technical and nature-based solutions to disaster risk reduction will be needed to secure human health.

Several resolutions of the Ramsar convention have led the way to link biodiversity with health issues and disaster risk reduction in a holistic way, also referring to climate change. This expertise now needs to support the aims of the 2030 Sustainable Development Goals (SDGs) and is an important contribution to the 2050-Vision of the CBD.

14.5.2 World Health Organization and Convention on Biological Diversity Partnership

Although health is already mentioned in the Preamble to the text of the Convention on Biological Diversity (CBD 1992)[2] and was included in the CBD Aichi Target 14, in 2010 (CBD 2010),[3] the first full CBD decision on biodiversity and human health, under the joint work programme with the World Health Organization, was only concluded at the 12th Conference of the Parties, held in November 2014 in Pyeongchang, South Korea (CBD 2014). "All human health ultimately depends on ecosystem services that are made possible by biodiversity and the products derived from them. While the inter-linkages between biodiversity, ecosystem services and human health are inherently complex, inter-disciplinary research is aiming to develop a more thorough understanding of these essential relationships".[4]

Important for preparation of the next COP was a joint report with the title "Connecting Global Priorities: Biodiversity and Human Health, a State of Knowledge Review" that was published in 2015 by the Secretariat of the Convention of Biodiversity together with the World Health Organization and numerous partners (Romanelli et al. 2015). It covers a wide range of topics concerning both terrestrial and aquatic ecosystems. A focus lies on the contribution of biodiversity to physical health through provision of food and nutrition as well as pharmaceuticals and traditional medicines. Further, the report deals with regulating services of water and air quality as well as the contribution of biodiversity to mental and cultural well-being. Health aspects include consideration of the microbial diversity as well as non-communicable and infectious diseases. Strategically, this report already considers links to global adaptation to climate change and associated disaster risk-reduction considerations, necessary tools, metrics and research avenues, and ultimately how

---

[2] CBD, Preamble: "Aware that conservation and sustainable use of biological diversity is of critical importance for meeting the food, health and other needs of the growing world population, for which purpose access to and sharing of both genetic resources and technologies are essential,…" (see: https://www.cbd.int/convention/articles/default.shtml?a=cbd-00, accessed 8 August 2018).

[3] Aichi target 14: "By 2020, ecosystems that provide essential services, including services related to water, and contribute to health, livelihoods and well-being, are restored and safeguarded, taking into account the needs of women, indigenous and local communities, and the poor and vulnerable." (see: https://www.cbd.int/decision/cop/default.shtml?id=12268, accessed 8 August 2018).

[4] For an overview of COP decisions and SBSTTA recommendations related to health see https://www.cbd.int/health/ accessed 8 August 2018).

strategies for health and biodiversity can contribute to achieving the SDGs and thereby align conservation, health and climate goals in a comprehensive way.

This report formed the basis for the further development of the topic on Biodiversity and Human Health at the CBD-COP13 in Mexico (CBD 2016b). In this decision, parties, other governments and relevant organisations are invited to carry out a wide range of comprehensive, integrative and far-reaching activities based on identified interlinkages at various levels and between different sectors. The Annex contains a comprehensive list of health-biodiversity linkages, which provides a good source of information when dealing with other sectors.

Following the COP13-Decision the field progressed rapidly, and already at the following meeting of the CBD-SBSTTA (Subsidiary Body on Scientific, Technical and Technological Advice) the subject on the scientific and technical side (CBD 2017) was further developed. SBSTTA draws on information *inter alia* from new reports issued by the Regional Office for Europe of the World Health Organization on the evidence of urban green spaces for health in 2016 (WHO Regional Office for Europe 2016), which was followed swiftly by a review of the impact of actual interventions in urban areas and their effectiveness (WHO Regional Office for Europe 2017). The SBSTTA-Recommendation stresses again the collaboration of different international organisations, and the national integration of biodiversity and health aspects into different sectors as vitally important, so that a holistic treatment of the topic is possible. The topic will therefore remain high on the international agenda.

A memorandum of understanding was signed between the CBD and the WHO in 2015, which provides a solid base for cooperation (WHO and CBD 2015), and also through an interagency liaison group on biodiversity and health that was established in 2017.[5] During its first meeting, important areas of further work were identified, such as the need for indicators for biodiversity and health and the development of simple messages around topics like: (1) ecosystem degradation, (2) diversity of diets/nutrition, (3) urban green spaces and (4) prevention. Climate change is treated here as a cross-cutting issue (CBD and WHO 2017).

In 2017, the WHO also co-sponsored the international conference "Biodiversity and Health in the face of climate change – Challenges, Opportunities and Evidence Gaps" (Marselle et al. 2018), which was organised by the German Federal Agency for Nature Conservation (BfN) and the European Network of Heads of Nature Conservation Agencies (ENCA), and which led to formal ENCA recommendations that are further elaborated on in the concluding chapter of this volume (Marselle et al. Chap. 20).

The CBD-COP-Decision XIII/3 to enhance implementation of the Aichi targets and to mainstream and integrate biodiversity within and across sectors (CBD 2016a) identified health as one of four key mainstreaming sectors for the 2050 Vision of Biodiversity, which should be taken up in post-2020 consideration of the CBD and is already an agenda topic of the 14th Conference of the Parties to take place in Egypt in November 2018.

[5] See: https://www.cbd.int/health/ilg-health/default.shtml

So far, the WHO European Health 2020 Framework mainly deals with the connection of health and the environment in relation to pollution and, for example, safe outdoor play for children (WHO 2017). However, the further collaboration between the CBD and the WHO may fuel the recognition of the importance of biodiversity for human health, in particular in the face of climate change within WHO policy more widely, both in Europe and globally.

14.5.3 Intergovernmental Science-Policy Platform on Biodiversity and Ecosystem Services (IPBES)

The Intergovernmental Science-Policy Platform on Biodiversity and Ecosystem Services (IPBES) is the intergovernmental body that assesses the state of biodiversity and of the ecosystem services it provides to society, in response to requests from decision-makers. As an outcome of its sixth meeting in Medellin/Columbia in March 2018 it decided on a procedure to determine the focal topics of its next assessments. The topic biodiversity and health is currently high on the international political agenda, but it is premature to speculate about a possible IPBES assessment on that topic. It is up to the CBD-COP to put this desire forward formally and the IPBES-Plenary as an independent body can decide to take it on board as a new subject or not (as of August 2018).

Due to this rapid development, with key events taking place towards the end of 2018 (CBD-COP14) and the beginning of 2019 (IPBES-7), we will know only by that time how the topic will have advanced on the agendas of these international treaties and organisations and if it will be considered as a priority for the Post-2020-system of the CBD. This would nicely link with the original Millennium Assessment report on health (Corvalan et al. 2005).

In the current IPBES thematic assessments, health is covered in the report on land degradation and restoration (IPBES 2018). It concludes that it is well established that land degradation adversely affects human well-being through the loss of biodiversity and ecosystem services, which has reached critical levels in many parts of the world. In many contexts, land degradation negatively impacts food and water security, as well as human health and safety. Land degradation generally harms psychological well-being by reducing benefits for mental balance, attention, inspiration and healing. Land degradation has particularly negative impacts on the mental health and spiritual well-being of indigenous peoples and local communities. Finally, land degradation, especially in coastal and riparian areas, increases the risk of storm damage, flooding and landslides, with high socio-economic costs and human losses (IPBES 2018). Therefore, there is a clear relationship between land degradation through the loss of biodiversity and ecosystem services on human well-being and health, and recognition that land degradation becomes more severe in the face of climate change.

14.5.4 Sustainable Development Goals

The establishment of IPBES coincided with the United Nation's 2030 Agenda on Sustainable Development (UN 2015b). Building on the Brundtland Commission (Brundtland Commission 1987), the Rio Declaration on Environment and Development (UN 1992) and the eight Millennium Development Goals established in 2000 (UN 2000), the SDGs were now developed as a holistic and integrated approach to global development. In 2016, the *2030 Agenda for Sustainable Development* comprising 17 SDGs with 169 targets was officially approved during a UN Summit (UN 2015b). The SDGs aim to foster action integrating economic, social and environmental issues (ICSU 2017). In particular, SDG 14 'Life below water' and SDG 15 'Life on land' directly deal with biodiversity, while SDG 13 'Climate change' considers actions for mitigation and adaptation to a changing climate. For health, most prominently the SDG 3 'Good health and well-being', seeks to ensure healthy lives by promoting well-being for all at all ages. Here, a close link with CBD and Ramsar will be beneficial, and the CBD already identified a good alignment of the 2030 Agenda and the Strategic Plan for Biodiversity with many synergies (CBD et al. 2017). Considering the many goals of the 2030 Agenda, it will require good joint sector working to overcome trade-offs and to focus on synergies. Implementation will also crucially depend on translation into policies and practical management at the national and local level to deliver on the targets. Having an overarching goal of 'One Health' (Zinsstag et al. 2015; see also Keune et al. Chap. 15, this volume) may strengthen the sustainable development and conservation agenda.

14.5.5 ICLEI – Local Governments for Sustainability

Since concerted efforts by main actors on the local level are pivotal to reach the integration of different policy goals in the fields of biodiversity, climate and public health on the ground, global networks are very important. As the majority of the world's population now lives in cities, and this trend will increase in the future, actions taken by local and regional governments in cities, towns and regions will have a high impact on future developments. ICLEI as a global network of local governments for sustainability with more than 1,500 members and regional offices announced at its World Congress in 2018 the "ICLEI Montréal Commitment and Strategic Vision" (ICLEI – Local Governments for Sustainability 2018), in which five interconnected pathways for change, highlighting the complex relationships among urban systems, are laid out. Climate change, health and biodiversity issues are addressed, with nature being mainstreamed throughout. In addition, one of the pathways to transformative action is through supporting nature-based development.

14.6 Conclusions

Within the last decade much emphasis has been placed on the individual linkages between (1) biodiversity and climate change, (2) biodiversity and health, and (3) health and climate. But so far addressing the three issues together is rare even though they are closely inter-related. Ultimately joint indicators and metrics need to be found to be slotted into sectoral policies.

Integrative research is urgently needed to better understand the triangular relationship between biodiversity in all its forms, levels and inter-relations, climate change effects (temperature and precipitation) and health, taking into account the 'One Health Approach' that goes beyond considering only human health by looking at the entire system.

As evidenced in this volume, there are many opportunities for synergies to tackle public health, biodiversity and climate change adaptation. International and regional conventions as well as international organisations and government programmes are increasingly addressing these issues jointly. They should be encouraged to go further in order to benefit from possible synergies and to avoid detrimental outcomes for society by either no action or by not taking into account aspects beyond a single sector. The World Health Organization already liaises with the global conventions – CBD, Ramsar as well as UNFCCC – and this cooperation could be strengthened. Synergies between the conventions on the issue of climate change, its possible impact on health and how well managed biodiversity could help human societies to better cope with the expected changes need to be further explored and developed. Alignment with the 2030 Agenda on Sustainable Development will further foster joint working.

A specific IPBES assessment on biodiversity and health, with associated scenario development under a changing climate, would be very helpful to provide a single up-to-date, policy-relevant document on the issue that could guide further policy development and the international research agenda.

Acknowledgements This work was supported by the German Federal Agency for Nature Conservation (BfN) with funds of the German Federal Ministry for the Environment, Nature Conservation, and Nuclear Safety (BMU) through the research project "Conferences on Climate Change and Biodiversity" (BIOCLIM, project duration from 2014 to 2017, funding code: 3514 80 020A).

References

Bellard C, Bertelsmeier C, Leadley P, Thuiller W, Courchamp F (2012) Impacts of climate change on the future of biodiversity. Ecol Lett 15(4):365–377

Brundtland Commission (1987) World commission on environment and development: our common future. Oxford University Press, New York

Cardinale BJ, Duffy JE, Gonzalez A, Hooper DU, Perrings C, Venail P, Narwani A, Mace GM, Tilman D, Wardle DA, Kinzig AP, Daily GC, Loreau M, Grace JB, Larigauderie A, Srivastava DS, Naeem S (2012) Biodiversity loss and its impact on humanity. Nature 486(7401):59–67

CBD (1992) Convention on biological diversity. United Nations, Montreal. https://www.cbd.int/convention/text/

CBD (2010) Decision CBD/COP/X/2. Strategic plan for biodiversity 2011–2020. Convention on Biological Diversity. https://www.cbd.int/sp/targets/default.shtml

CBD (2014) COP 12 Decision XII/21. Biodiversity and human health. https://www.cbd.int/decision/cop/default.shtml?id=13384

CBD (2016a) COP 13 Decision XIII/3. Strategic actions to enhance the implementation of the Strategic Plan for Biodiversity 2011–2020 and the achievement of the Aichi Biodiversity Targets, including with respect to mainstreaming and the integration of biodiversity within and across sectors. Cancun. https://www.cbd.int/decisions/cop/?m=cop-13

CBD (2016b) COP 13 Decision XIII/6. Biodiversity and human health. Cancun. https://www.cbd.int/health/cop-13-dec-06-en.pdf

CBD (2017) CBD/SBSTTA/REC/XXI/3. Health and biodiversity. Convention on Biological Diversity. https://www.cbd.int/recommendations/sbstta/?m=sbstta-21

CBD, WHO (2017) Report of the first meeting of the interagency liaison group on biodiversity and health. Geneva. https://www.cbd.int/doc/c/3ff0/ec82/94151f1a58f1d16ad21abe13/hb-lg-2017-01-01-en.pdf

CBD, FAO, WB, UNEP, UNDP (2017) Biodiversity and the 2030 Agenda for Sustainable Development, Technical Note. Convention on Biological Diversity; Food and Agriculture Organization of the United Nations; The World Bank; UN Environment; United Nations Development Programme. https://www.cbd.int/development/doc/biodiversity-2030-agenda-technical-note-en.pdf

COHAB (2005) COHAB's founding principles. http://www.cohabnet.org/COHAB2005ConferenceRecommendations.htm

Corvalan C, Hales S, McMichael AJ, Butler C, Campbell-Lendrum D, Confalonieri U, Leitner K, Lewis N, Patz J, Polson K, Scheraga J, Woodward A, Younes M (2005) Ecosystems and human well-being: health synthesis. A Report of the Millennium Ecosystem Assessment. Geneva, Switzerland. https://www.millenniumassessment.org/documents/document.357.aspx.pdf

Díaz S, Pascual U, Stenseke M, Martín-López B, Watson RT, Molnár Z, Hill R, Chan KMA, Baste IA, Brauman KA, Polasky S, Church A, Lonsdale M, Larigauderie A, Leadley PW, van Oudenhoven APE, van der Plaat F, Schröter M, Lavorel S, Aumeeruddy-Thomas Y, Bukvareva E, Davies K, Demissew S, Erpul G, Failler P, Guerra CA, Hewitt CL, Keune H, Lindley S, Shirayama Y (2018) Assessing nature's contributions to people. Science 359(6373):270–272

Füssel H-M, Jol A, Marx A, Hildén M, Aparicio A, Bastrup-Birk A, Bigano A, Castellari S, Erhard M, Georgi B (2017) Climate change, impacts and vulnerability in Europe 2016-An indicator-based report. Copenhagen. https://www.eea.europa.eu/publications/climate-change-impacts-and-vulnerability-2016

Horwitz P, Finlayson CM (2011) Wetlands as settings for human health: incorporating ecosystem services and health impact assessment into water resource management. Bioscience 61(9):678–688

Horwitz P, Finlayson M, Weinstein P (2012) Healthy wetlands, healthy people: a review of wetlands and human health interactions. Ramsar Technical Report No. 6. http://archive.ramsar.org/pdf/lib/rtr6-health.pdf

ICLEI – Local Governments for Sustainability (2018) The ICLEI Montréal Commitment and Strategic Vision 2018–2024. Bonn. https://worldcongress2018.iclei.org/wp-content/uploads/The%20ICLEI%20Montr%C3%A9al%20Commitment.pdf?utm_medium=email&utm_source=sharpspring&sslid=MzEzMzY3sDQzNzU1AwA&sseid=MzQzMDW2MDY0NwIA&jobid=a3e7a768-0ea3-4cf5-98c7-611b48026f2e

ICSU (2017) Guide to SDG interactions: from science to implementation. Paris. https://council.science/cms/2017/05/SDGs-Guide-to-Interactions.pdf

IPBES (2018) Thematic assessment report on land degradation and restoration of the Intergovernmental Science-Policy Platform on Biodiversity and Ecosystem Services. Bonn. https://www.ipbes.net/assessment-reports/ldr

IPCC (2014) Climate change 2014: mitigation of climate change. http://www.ipcc.ch/report/ar5/wg3/

Kabisch N, Frantzeskaki N, Pauleit S, Naumann S, Davis M, Artmann M, Haase D, Knapp S, Korn H, Stadler J, Zaunberger K, Bonn A (2016) Nature-based solutions to climate change mitigation and adaptation in urban areas: perspectives on indicators, knowledge gaps, barriers, and opportunities for action. Ecol Soc 21(2). https://doi.org/10.5751/ES-08373-210239

Kabisch N, Korn H, Stadler J, Bonn A (eds) (2017) Nature-based solutions to climate change adaptation in urban areas – linkages of science, policy and practice. Springer, Cham. https://doi.org/10.1007/978-3-319-56091-5

Lin BB (2011) Resilience in agriculture through crop diversification: adaptive management for environmental change. Bioscience 61(3):183–193

Lo V (2016) Synthesis report on experiences with ecosystem-based approaches to climate change adaptation and disaster risk reduction. CBD Technical Series No 85. Montreal. https://www.cbd.int/doc/publications/cbd-ts-85-en.pdf

MA (2005) Millenium ecosystem assessment. Island Press, Washington, DC. https://www.millenniumassessment.org/en/index.html

Marselle M, Stadler J, Korn H, Bonn A (eds) (2018) Proceedings of the European Conference "Biodiversity and Health in the Face of Climate Change – Challenges, Opportunities and Evidence Gaps". BfN-Skripten 509. Federal Agency for Nature Conservation, Germany, Bonn. https://doi.org/10.19217/skr509

Parmesan C (2006) Ecological and evolutionary responses to recent climate change. Annu Rev Ecol, Evolu Syst 37:637–669

Pecl GT, Araújo MB, Bell JD, Blanchard J, Bonebrake TC, Chen I-C, Clark TD, Colwell RK, Danielsen F, Evengård B, Falconi L, Ferrier S, Frusher S, Garcia RA, Griffis RB, Hobday AJ, Janion-Scheepers C, Jarzyna MA, Jennings S, Lenoir J, Linnetved HI, Martin VY, McCormack PC, McDonald J, Mitchell NJ, Mustonen T, Pandolfi JM, Pettorelli N, Popova E, Robinson SA, Scheffers BR, Shaw JD, Sorte CJB, Strugnell JM, Sunday JM, Tuanmu M-N, Vergés A, Villanueva C, Wernberg T, Wapstra E, Williams SE (2017) Biodiversity redistribution under climate change: impacts on ecosystems and human well-being. Science 355: eaai9214

Ramsar (2008) Ramsar COP10 DOC. 28 Healthy wetlands, healthy people – a review of wetlands and human health interactions. Draft Executive Summary and Key Messages Chnagwong. http://ramsar.rgis.ch/pdf/cop10/cop10_doc28_e.pdf

Ramsar (2012) Resolution XI.12. Wetlands and health: taking an ecosystem approach. Bucharest. https://www.ramsar.org/document/resolution-xi12-wetlands-and-health-taking-an-ecosystem-approach

Ramsar (2015) Resolution XII.13 Wetlands and disaster risk reduction. Punta del Este. https://www.ramsar.org/sites/default/files/documents/library/cop12_res13_drr_e_0.pdf

Romanelli C, Cooper D, Campbell-Lendrum D, Maiero M, Karesh W, Hunter D, Golden C (2015) Connecting global priorities: biodiversity and human health: a state of knowledge review. Geneva. https://www.cbd.int/health/stateofknowledge

Schröter M, Albert C, Marques A, Tobon W, Lavorel S, Maes J, Brown C, Klotz S, Bonn A (2016) National ecosystem assessments in Europe: a review. Bioscience 66(10):813–828

TEEB (2010) The economics of ecosystems and biodiversity: mainstreaming the economics of nature: a synthesis of the approach, conclusions and recommendations of TEEB. http://www.teebweb.org/

Temmerman S, Meire P, Bouma TJ, Herman PM, Ysebaert T, De Vriend HJ (2013) Ecosystem-based coastal defence in the face of global change. Nature 504(7478):79

Thomas CD, Cameron A, Green RE, Bakkenes M, Beaumont LJ, Collingham YC, Erasmus BFN, De Siqueira MF, Grainger A, Hannah L, Hughes L, Huntley B, Van Jaarsveld AS, Midgley GF,

Miles L, Ortega-Huerta MA, Peterson aT, Phillips OL, Williams SE (2004) Extinction risk from climate change. Nature 427(6970):145–148
UN (1992) Rio declaration on environment and development. United Nations, Rio de Janeiro. http://www.un.org/documents/ga/conf151/aconf15126-1annex1.htm
UN (2000) United Nations Millennium Declaration. United Nations, Department of Public Information, New York. http://www.un.org/millennium/declaration/ares552e.htm
UN (2015a) Adoption of the Paris Agreement. Paris. https://unfccc.int/sites/default/files/resource/docs/2015/cop21/eng/l09r01.pdf.
UN (2015b) Transforming our world: the 2030 agenda for sustainable development. A/RES/70/1. https://sustainabledevelopment.un.org/post2015/transformingourworld
Watts N, Adger WN, Agnolucci P, Blackstock J, Byass P, Cai W, Chaytor S, Colbourn T, Collins M, Cooper A, Cox PM, Depledge J, Drummond P, Ekins P, Galaz V, Grace D, Graham H, Grubb M, Haines A, Hamilton I, Hunter A, Jiang X, Li M, Kelman I, Liang L, Lott M, Lowe R, Luo Y, Mace G, Maslin M, Nilsson M, Oreszczyn T, Pye S, Quinn T, Svensdotter M, Venevsky S, Warner K, Xu B, Yang J, Yin Y, Yu C, Zhang Q, Gong P, Montgomery H, Costello A (2015) Health and climate change: policy responses to protect public health. The Lancet 386(10006):1861–1914
WHO (2015) WHO Workplan on climate change and health. Aims and objectives 2014–2019. Secretariat of the World Health Organisation, Geneva. http://www.who.int/globalchange/health_policy/climate-change-and-health-workplan-2014-2019.pdf?ua=1
WHO (2016) Fact sheet: climate change and health. Secretariat of the World Health Organisation, Geneva. http://www.who.int/en/news-room/fact-sheets/detail/climate-change-and-health
WHO (2017) Health 2020. A European policy framework and strategy for the 21st century. Copenhagen. http://www.euro.who.int/__data/assets/pdf_file/0011/199532/Health2020-Long.pdf?ua=1
WHO, CBD (2015) Memorandum of Understanding WHO and CBD. Secretariat of the World Health Organisation, Geneva. Secretariat of the Convention of Biological diversity, Montreal. https://www.cbd.int/doc/agreements/agmt-who-2015-07-23-mou-en.pdf
WHO Regional Office for Europe (2016) Urban green spaces and health: a review of evidence. Copenhagen. http://www.euro.who.int/__data/assets/pdf_file/0005/321971/Urban-green-spaces-and-health-review-evidence.pdf?ua=1
WHO Regional Office for Europe (2017) Urban green space interventions and health: a review of impacts and effectiveness. Copenhagen. http://www.euro.who.int/__data/assets/pdf_file/0010/337690/FULL-REPORT-for-LLP.pdf?ua=1
Wolf T, Lyne K, Martinez GS, Kendrovski V (2015) The health effects of climate change in the WHO European Region. Climate 3(4):901–936
Zinsstag J, Schelling E, Waltner-Toews D, Whittaker M, Tanner M (2015) One Health: the theory and practice of integrated health approaches. CABI, Wallingford/Boston

Chapter 15
European Nature and Health Network Initiatives

Hans Keune, Kerstin Friesenbichler, Barbara Häsler, Astrid Hilgers, Jukka-Pekka Jäppinen, Beate Job-Hoben, Barbara Livoreil, Bram Oosterbroek, Cristina Romanelli, Hélène Soubelet, Jutta Stadler, Helena Ströher, and Matti Tapaninen

Abstract Attention to the importance of nature and human health linkages has increased in the past years, both in science and in policy. While knowledge about and recognition of the importance of nature and human health linkages are increasing rapidly, challenges still remain. Among them are building bridges between relevant but often still somewhat disconnected sectors and topics. There is a need to bring together researchers in the fields of health sciences, ecology, social sciences, sustainability sciences and other interdisciplinary sciences, as well as for cooperation between governments, companies and citizens. In this chapter, we introduce European networking initiatives aimed at building such bridges.

Keywords European network · Nature health · Knowledge management · Community building · Transdisciplinarity · Integrative framework

---

H. Keune (✉)
Community of Practice Biodiversity & Health, Belgian Biodiversity Platform, Brussels, Belgium

Research Institute for Nature and Forest (INBO), Brussels, Belgium

Department for Interdisciplinary and Primary Care Antwerp (ELIZA), Faculty of Medicine and Health Sciences, The University of Antwerp, Antwerp, Belgium

Ecosystem Services Partnership (ESP) Thematic Working Group Ecosystem Services & Public Health, Brussels, Belgium

Network for Evaluation of One Health (NEOH), London, UK
e-mail: hans.keune@inbo.be; hans.keune@uantwerpen.be

K. Friesenbichler
Umweltdachverband, Vienna, Austria
e-mail: kerstin.friesenbichler@umweltdachverband.at

M. R. Marselle et al. (eds.), *Biodiversity and Health in the Face of Climate Change*, https://doi.org/10.1007/978-3-030-02318-8_15

Highlights

- Attention to the importance of nature and health linkages has increased.
- There is a need to build bridges between the nature and health sectors, and science, policy and practice.
- This chapter describes international/European and national nature and health network initiatives.
- Strengthened inter-network collaboration through capacity building, mainstreaming and integration is needed.
- More structural support is required to encourage better integration.

B. Häsler
Network for Evaluation of One Health (NEOH), London, UK

Department of Pathobiology and Population Sciences, Veterinary Epidemiology Economics and Public Health Group, Royal Veterinary College, University of London, London, UK
e-mail: bhaesler@rvc.ac.uk

A. Hilgers
Ministry of Agriculture, Nature and Food Quality, The Hague, The Netherlands
e-mail: a.k.hilgers@minez.nl

J.-P. Jäppinen
Biodiversity Centre, Finnish Environment Institute (SYKE), Helsinki, Finland
e-mail: Jukka-Pekka.Jappinen@ymparisto.fi

B. Job-Hoben · H. Ströher
German Federal Agency for Nature Conservation (BfN), Bonn, Germany
e-mail: beate.job-hoben@bfn.de; stroeher@arnold-janssen-stiftung.de

B. Livoreil · H. Soubelet
The French Foundation for Research on Biodiversity (FRB), Paris, France
e-mail: barbara.livoreil@fondationbiodiversite.fr; helene.soubelet@fondationbiodiversite.fr

B. Oosterbroek
Ecosystem Services Partnership (ESP) Thematic Working Group Ecosystem Services & Public Health, Brussels, Belgium

International Centre for Integrated Assessment and Sustainable Development, Maastricht University, Maastricht, The Netherlands
e-mail: bram.oosterbroek@maastrichtuniversity.nl

C. Romanelli
CBD-WHO Joint Work Programme on Biodiversity and Human Health, UN Secretariat of the Convention on Biological Diversity, Montreal, Canada
e-mail: cristina.romanelli@cbd.int

J. Stadler
Federal Agency for Nature Conservation (BfN), Isle of Vilm, Putbus, Germany
e-mail: jutta.stadler@bfn.de

M. Tapaninen
Metsähallitus Parks and Wildlife Finland, Kajaani, Finland
e-mail: matti.tapaninen@metsa.fi

15.1 Introduction

Attention to the importance of nature and human health linkages has increased in the past ten years, both in science and in policy. This relates to health benefits from nature-based health-care solutions, such as reducing stress, improving children's immune systems, and reducing the impact from environmental pollution or climate change. This also relates to health risks, such as pollen allergies or infectious diseases transmitted by ticks and mosquitoes. While knowledge about and recognition of the importance of nature and human health linkages are increasing rapidly, challenges still remain. Among them are building bridges between relevant, but often still rather disconnected, sectors and topics. There is a need to connect researchers in the fields of health sciences, ecology, social sciences, sustainability sciences and other interdisciplinary sciences, as well as for cooperation with governments, companies and citizens. This need is expressed by both health and nature sectors, and is considered crucial by many for facilitating integrated and practice-oriented approaches. In this chapter, we introduce European networking initiatives aimed at building such bridges.

The comprehensive State of Knowledge Review Report on Biodiversity and Human Health (WHO and CBD Secretariat 2015) opens with a double and mutually reinforcing message on cooperation: one from the Convention on Biological Diversity (CBD) Secretariat that "all sectors, policymakers, scientists, educators, communities and citizens alike can – and must – contribute to the development of common solutions to the common threats that we face". The other message is from the World Health Organization (WHO), acknowledging the WHO's awareness of the growing body of evidence that biodiversity loss is a risk to human health, stating "protecting public health from these risks lies outside of the traditional roles of the health sector" and that "it relies on working with partners engaged in conservation, and the sustainable use and management of natural resources".

In December 2017, the CBD's Subsidiary Body on Scientific, Technical and Technological Advice (SBSTTA) stated recommendations for health and biodiversity at its 21st meeting. It concluded with formally recommending promoting dialogue among ministries and agencies responsible for, among others, the sectors involved with health, environment, pollution, agriculture, urban planning, climate change adaptation and disaster risk reduction in order to foster integrated approaches. In 2018 this was accorded by the member states of CBD (CBD 2018).

In 2017, an expert consultation took place in the context of the Regional Assessment for Europe and Central Asia for the intergovernmental science-policy Platform on Biodiversity and Ecosystem Services (IPBES 2018). The expert panel included people with a wide range of expertise linked to biodiversity in Europe, such as food and nutrition, medicinal resources and infectious disease. The panel was, among other things, asked to assign importance to a number of possible key messages for policy makers regarding the nature-health theme. Survey results revealed that 97% of the expert panel considered 'integrated approaches to nature and health both in and between science, policy and practice' very important in such a key message. Moreover, 91% even considered this message regarding integrated approaches to be very important. Whilst the expert panel had to rate a number of other possible key messages for policy makers regarding the nature-health theme as well (such as the need for research on the human immune system), the need for integrated approaches ranked highest.

In this chapter, we introduce first several relevant international/European and then several national nature and health network initiatives that have the ambition to foster building bridges between nature and health both within and between science, policy and practice. The initiatives present themselves and their main activities, complemented with a self-assessment of what works well and what the challenges are. In this way this chapter provides an overview of initiatives that can offer inspiration to people and groups that have similar ambitions. Finally, we draw some conclusions, summarize challenges, and make suggestions for next steps involved in facilitating further networking, capacity building and integration. Although the purposes of these initiatives vary, all the described initiatives have in common that synthesising both nature- and health-related information, as well as facilitating discussion between experts and practitioners from both nature- and health-related sectors, forms a core part of their main activities.

15.2 International/European Initiatives

15.2.1 ESP Thematic Working Group Ecosystem Services and Public Health

15.2.1.1 Introduction

The Ecosystem Service Partnership (ESP) is an independent non-governmental worldwide network for enhancing the science, policy and practice of ecosystem services for conservation and sustainable development. Part of the work is organized in thematic working groups (TWGs). One of these TWGs is related to health. This TWG was set up in January 2013 to facilitate dialogue between scientists and stakeholders on the connections between ecosystems and human health. In its work, the Public Health TWG helps to build the evidence base on the linkages between ecosystems and human health, and to support communication of key messages to scientists, policy makers and stakeholders. It refers to several international initiatives and work programmes that embrace ecosystem approaches to health. The ESP TWG aims to support these by collating data and expertise, and contributing to the continuing development of conceptual frameworks for ecosystem approaches to health.

15.2.1.2 Main Activities

The main activities have been the organization of special sessions at ESP conferences (one in 2013 and one in 2016) and the organization of a survey.

Ecosystem Services and Human Health – Awareness and Attitudes Survey

The aim of this survey was to gain a clearer view of where and how human health perspectives are addressed by people working in the field of ecosystem services research, policy and practice (what we call the 'ecosystem services community'). We hoped to gauge the degree of awareness and interest in the topic, and to better understand the needs of those who aim to address links between ecosystems and human health within their fields of work. We also wanted to gain information on the main opportunities and barriers/needs and challenges. In Box 15.1, we present some highlights from the results. In light of nature-health collaboration initiatives, these findings suggest that the vast majority of the ecosystem services community would welcome collaboration with health experts, to inform politicians and through those collaborations maximize ecosystem benefits.

When asked about factors that act as barriers to interdisciplinary research on ecosystems and health, in particular collaboration barriers such as disciplinary differences and lack of mutual understanding were mentioned. Further, lack of awareness about ecosystem–health linkages, lack of scientific understanding of ecosystem–health linkages and lack of resources stand out. When asked about factors that act as opportunities for interdisciplinary research on ecosystems and health in their own area of work, a wide range of examples was mentioned, of which specifically ecosystem-relevant topics, concepts or practices as a sub-group stand out. Topical examples are the influence of urban green infrastructure on health, climate change mitigation and linking ecosystem services with food security; conceptual examples are ecological public health and valuation.

2016 European ESP Conference Session: Health as an Integrating Concept in Ecosystem Services and Nature-based Solutions

The main activity in 2016 concerned the organization of a session at the European ESP-conference. The session was very well attended and included both a diversity of presentations, mainly from on-going research projects, and group discussion. We highlight some issues from the group discussion.

Box 15.1: Some Respondent Highlights of the Ecosystem Services and Human Health – Awareness and Attitudes Survey

- 83% disagreed with the statement "human health is not relevant to my current work on ecosystem services" (including 36% strongly disagreeing).
- Over 50% indicated that "information about ecosystem–human health links is difficult to find", whereas human health seems to be relevant to most respondents.
- 96% agreed that "policy and practice on ecosystem services should account for human health aspects".
- 97% agreed that "the ecosystem services community should seek to develop/strengthen links to the health community".

Part of the discussion concerned the characteristics of ecosystem services related to health: quality of green spaces in relation to health and how people are exposed to different types of nature. Further, an overview of specific ecosystem services and disservices relevant to health were discussed. Apart from green space, the role of both food and perception were discussed.

Part of the discussion concerned issues important for research and mainstreaming. Dealing with complexity was at the core of the discussion about research challenges. In addition, the work could be well related to the health sector, both in terms of indicators and research methods, but also in terms of needs: what kind of information is needed for uptake in the health-care sector?

15.2.1.3 What Works Well

What works well is occasionally bringing together a diversity of experts interested in both ecosystem services and the links with human health. This helps to mainstream the health perspective in the field of ecosystem services and to discuss opportunities and challenges. Obviously, this seems to work best at ESP conferences. What also works quite well is collecting information about bridge-building challenges in the survey discussed here.

15.2.1.4 Main Challenges

The main challenges seem to be keeping momentum and activities alive in the TWG. This is based on voluntary work from the initiating experts, who often lack time and resources to work for the TWG and to participate in all international ESP conferences. Getting regular inputs from other experts interested in the theme and the TWG is not straightforward and needs more work.

Contact information: https://www.es-partnership.org/community/workings-groups/thematic-working-groups/twg-9-ecosystem-services-public-health/

15.2.2 Network for Evaluation of One Health

15.2.2.1 Introduction

One Health aims to bring together a collection of expertise, stemming mainly from the human and animal health fields, but over time broadening its perspective to the environment (Keune and Assmuth 2018). Zinsstag et al. (2011) propose One Health as an approach aimed at tackling complex patterns of global change, in which the inextricable interconnection of humans, pet animals, livestock and wildlife with their social and ecological environment is evident, and requires integrated approaches to human and animal health and their respective social and environmental contexts. The WHO – CBD State of Knowledge Review on Biodiversity and Health

(2015) proposes One Health as an overarching framework for integrated efforts, while also recognising and relating to other relevant approaches such as EcoHealth. Earlier a tripartite collaboration between FAO, OIE and WHO (2010) proposed a similar integrated effort also labeled 'One Health'. Wallace et al. (2015) extended the perspective of One Health to include the socio-economic perspective more clearly, in what they term 'Structural One Health'. They criticize the earlier One Health concept for omitting to address fundamental structural political and economic causes underlying collapsing health ecologies. Consequently, a One Health approach to address global health challenges such as malnutrition, disease emergence and biodiversity loss should accept that complex issues require a participatory and interdisciplinary process. The Network for Evaluation of One Health (NEOH) was an international network funded by the European Cooperation for Science and Technology (COST) from 2014 to 2018 with the aim to enable quantitative and qualitative evaluations of One Health activities and to further the evidence base by developing and applying a science-based evaluation protocol in a community of experts. While several One Health initiatives have been implemented across Europe, so far there has been no standardized methodology for the systematic evaluation of One Health activities and, more specifically, there have been only a few studies that measured the added value of One Health. The NEOH addressed this gap.

15.2.2.2 Main Activities

The Network's driving activity was the production of a handbook for evaluation of One Health and the validation of its content by applying it to a suite of international case studies. The full handbook is available as open access here: https://www.wageningenacademic.com/doi/book/10.3920/978-90-8686-875-9 and most case studies are published in a special issue in Frontiers journal entitle "Concepts and experiences in framing, integration and evaluation of One Health and EcoHealth": https://www.frontiersin.org/research-topics/5479/concepts-and-experiences-in-framing-integration-and-evaluation-of-one-health-and-ecohealth. The case studies conducted, and other published studies, are compared in a meta-study for the purpose of international comparison and reflection on the value of One Health. Finally, NEOH considered stakeholder engagement important to assess needs and to promote informed decision-making and resource allocation in One Health, and to facilitate training, learning and capacity building for evaluation of integrated approaches to health (e.g. training schools, workshops, short-term scientific missions and conference grants).

The Network was organized into four working groups who frequently exchanged information with a wider group of experts contributing to different tasks. WG1 was responsible for the development of the overall evaluation framework and the development of the handbook. WG2 applied the evaluation framework, protocol and index developed to different One Health initiatives. WG3 conducted a meta-study of the available case studies. WG4 was in charge of dissemination and stakeholder engagement.

15.2.2.3 What Worked Well

There was a focus on ensuring a friendly and integrative attitude in the Network, with adaptive leadership. By bringing together researchers, practitioners, decision-makers and other stakeholders from different fields with an interest in One Health and evaluation, and offering opportunities for knowledge, exchange and sharing with a clear task and purpose, NEOH managed to create a dynamic learning organization. By engaging a wide range of people with similar interests, but different (disciplinary) backgrounds, expertise, levels of seniority and professional roles, many different perspectives and skill-sets came together in an enabling environment. This contributed substantially to the innovation of methods and integration of existing knowledge, and resulted in enthusiastic participation and a good range of outputs and products.

15.2.2.4 Main Challenges

Given the large membership of the Network, which was spread across a number of countries, and the many opportunities to get involved, there was a risk that participants did not feel ownership of NEOH. Consequently, strong communication and pro-active engagement of participants was critical to ensure that the work was integrative and effective, and not just an assembly of individual tasks. Another major challenge was the risk of collaborating mainly with existing contacts who already buy into the One Health concept instead of recruiting people who have not yet engaged with One Health. Because of this, there was a dominance of animal health professionals in the Network. To mitigate this imbalance, NEOH interacted with other integrated health networks globally to promote wider engagement, conceptual and practical advances, and shaping of a joint agenda. As part of these activities, it formed closer ties with the EcoHealth community. 'EcoHealth' encompasses an "ecosystem approach to health": the biological, physical, social and economic environments and their relation to human health (Keune and Assmuth 2018). EcoHealth can be characterized by interdisciplinarity (e.g. health science, veterinary science, ecology, social science) and transdisciplinarity (collaboration with non-academic practice experts and stakeholders). Apart from the collaborative angle, the equity perspective was essential in EcoHealth (Lebel 2003). Later a more sophisticated set of EcoHealth principles was developed (Charron 2012). As a follow-up of the NEOH COST-Action, as well as an answer to the need for a European network, as was expressed during the 2016 European OneHealth/EcoHealth workshop in Brussels (see Sect. 15.2.3), NEOH has become the European Chapter of the Ecohealth International Trust and is now called Network for Ecohealth and One Health.

Contact information: http://neoh.onehealthglobal.net/ and http://www.cost.eu/COST_Actions/tdp/TD1404 and https://www.ecohealthinternational.org/regional-chapters/europe/

15.2.3 European One Health/Ecohealth Workshop

15.2.3.1 Introduction

The European OneHealth/EcoHealth (OH/EH) workshop took place in 2016 in Brussels (Keune et al. 2017). The organization was coordinated by the Belgian Community of Practice Biodiversity and Health (see also below), and involved a diversity of organizations, including NEOH, CBD and WHO. The workshop aimed at facilitating reflection and exchange, mapping future avenues and supporting collaboration of working on the linkages of biodiversity and human health, or linkages within an OH framework. The general objective of the workshop was to foster collaboration between OH/EH and related concepts and communities that endeavor to combine ecosystem, animal and human health, and to build bridges between science, policy and practice active in the domain of nature and health.

Given the similarities in their objectives to create synergies between health benefits for humans, animals and the environment, the OH and EH concepts appear to be supported by converging communities, working towards a shift from narrow and restricted frameworks towards systems approaches. The two approaches have different origins: EH stems more from a sustainable health action research perspective, and OH more from a human and animal health expert collaboration perspective. Still, the two approaches are united in emphasising "a holistic understanding of health beyond the purely biomedical" and championing "systems thinking as a way of achieving a greater understanding of health problems, and both espouse inter- and trans-disciplinary research and collaborative participation" (Keune et al. 2017).

15.2.3.2 Main Activities

Over 100 experts from different professional backgrounds (science, policy and practice) and different fields of expertise contributed to the workshop. They included natural scientists, animal and human health scientists, as well as social scientists, policy representatives from national governments and the EU, and experts working in Europe, but also in other regions in the world. The workshop programme featured a combination of specific topics and generic integrative sessions. In the topical sessions, participants exchanged experiences and views from their fields and projects, whilst exposing the arguments for and possible ways to apply the One Health perspective in their areas of expertise. Such a broad range of issues was selected in order to reflect the diversity of thematic areas presented in the CBD–WHO *State of Knowledge Review* as well as the cross-sectoral and interdisciplinary challenges faced by the OH community.

15.2.3.3 What Works Well

It was noted by participants that the wide array of cross-sectoral issues was not common in expert meetings. For example: biodiversity-related issues featured less in discussions of the OH community; and experts that tackle health benefits from nature contact or experience do not often engage with communities focusing on nature-related health risks such as infectious diseases. The more generic sessions on evaluation, social science and education were also appreciated and considered important. Lastly, the largely interactive character of the workshop was welcomed by participants. This facilitated networking, bridge building and joint reflection, as well as creative ‘out of the box’ thinking.

15.2.3.4 Main Challenges

During discussions at the European OH/EH workshop, the need for focused European networks was recognized. This will support implementation of OH/EH concepts, which can benefit from transdisciplinary and iterative processes between policy, science and practice. One should, however, be careful of creating big OH/EH institutions as this could result in building fences rather than creating openness to (new) collaborations. This may be avoided by focusing on open, collaborative networks like Communities of Practice, which are less (institutionally) bound and more flexible, and can be open to newcomers and new ideas and approaches. Such networks should not be limited to scientific experts, but also need to be open to policy experts, local knowledge, practitioners, grass-root organizations and all relevant stakeholders. Specific focused networks could concentrate on, for example, transdisciplinary One Health education, integration of social sciences in OH/EH actions and networks, and on translating research findings on the Environment-Microbiome-Health axis into policy-making. It was also suggested that a European Community of Practice could be initiated in order to support these several concrete networking initiatives, and to help to promote the building of other emerging initiatives. Currently, with NEOH (see Sect. 15.2.2 above), the establishment of such a European OH/EH network is under discussion. A follow-up European OH/EH meeting was organized in September 2018 in Bologna.

Contact information: http://www.biodiversity.be/health/58

15.2.4 Conference Biodiversity and Health in the Face of Climate Change

15.2.4.1 Introduction

Climate change poses significant challenges to biodiversity and human well-being in Europe. Biodiversity in urban as well as in adjacent rural areas can provide benefits for human health and well-being when nature-based climate change mitigation and adaptation activities are carried out. On the other hand, climate change can negatively influence human health via the spread of allergenic plants and vector-borne diseases. Both issues were tackled at the *European Conference on "Biodiversity and Health in the Face of Climate Change – Challenges, Opportunities and Evidence Gaps",* on 27–29 June 2017 in Bonn/Germany. The joint conference was held by the German Federal Agency for Nature Conservation (BfN) and the European Network of Heads of Nature Conservation Agencies (ENCA) in collaboration with the Helmholtz-Centre for Environmental Research (UFZ) / German Centre for Integrative Biodiversity Research (iDiv). The event was co-sponsored by the WHO Regional Office for Europe.

15.2.4.2 Main Activities

The European conference in Bonn brought together 220 experts from science, policy and practice to highlight and discuss the importance of biodiversity's positive contribution to human health in the face of climate change (Marselle et al. 2018). Indirect negative impacts of climate change on human health (e.g. the spread of allergenic plants or vector-borne diseases) were also discussed. The aim of the conference was to increase knowledge, share experiences and foster nature-based solutions to meet the challenges of climate change and health issues. In this context, health was considered in its physical, psychological and social dimension, including socio-environmental equity.

The latest scientific findings on the impacts of climate change on European biodiversity and links to human health were discussed. In addition, the implementation of nature-based solutions towards health and climate goals were outlined. Interactive sessions focused on case studies of successful demonstration projects and lessons learned. Resulting discussions led to recommendations for creating synergies between ongoing policy processes, scientific programmes and practical implementation. These recommendations were formally adopted by the ENCA network at its plenary session in October 2017.

At the conference, the WHO Regional Office for Europe (2016) launched a publication on "Urban green spaces – a brief for action", in which experiences from interventions to promote human health by fostering green spaces in urban areas are summarized.

15.2.4.3 What Works Well

The conference incorporated and stimulated close interaction between different scientific disciplines (interdisciplinarity) and between scientists and practitioners (transdisciplinarity) such as from policy institutions. It was attended by participants from more than 30 countries, with diverse professional backgrounds (e.g. biology, psychology, medicine, city planning, economy, law) and working on different levels ranging from local and community levels to the EU level. The conference results were distributed via various channels (e.g. the ENCA network) to reach several administrative and political spheres as well as different expert networks of scientists and practitioners.

15.2.4.4 Main Challenges

Despite the fact that there are many good examples of nature-based solutions for climate change adaptation and promotion of human health in place, there is still a need to increase both the evidence base as well as the awareness of decision makers and practitioners of biodiversity's contributions for human health and well-being. In addition, the co-benefits of nature-based solutions for climate change adaptation should be highlighted for policy-makers and regional planning authorities. In order to foster the wider application of nature-based solutions for climate change adaptation and promotion of human health, and to deliver positive results, the provision of guidance and the sharing of experiences on the effective design and management of green spaces are key factors.

Contact information: https://www.ecbcc2017jimdo.com/ and https://www.bfn.de/en/activities/climate-change-and-biodiversity/events/biodiversity-and-health-in-the-face-of-climate-change.html

15.2.5 Regional Capacity-Building Workshop on Biodiversity and Human Health for the WHO Europe Region

15.2.5.1 Introduction

The Regional capacity-building workshop on biodiversity and health for the WHO European region, held on 23–25 October 2017 in Helsinki, Finland, was jointly convened by the Secretariat of the CBD and the WHO. It was convened in collaboration with the Ministry of Environment, Housing and Energy and the Ministry of Health and Social Affairs, Finland. The WHO Regional Office for Europe also provided technical input and support through the European Centre for Environment and Health. The objective of the workshop was to build capacity among policy makers in the region and to strengthen collaboration, engagement and policy coherence between national agencies responsible for biodiversity and those responsible for health, its Aichi Biodiversity Targets, and to contribute to enhanced national implementation of the Strategic Plan for Biodiversity 2011–2020, and related Sustainable Development Goals.

It also aimed to assist in mainstreaming biodiversity-health linkages in national biodiversity strategies and action plans and national health strategies, and to contribute to the implementation of global commitments for sustainable development including decision XIII/6, concluded at the 13th Conference of the Parties (COP) to the Convention.[1] COP Decision XIII/6 considers the implications of the findings of *Connecting Global Priorities: Biodiversity and Human Health, a State of Knowledge Review*, led by CBD and WHO (WHO and CBD 2015), with contributions from over 100 multidisciplinary experts, and is the most comprehensive global policy commitment on biodiversity and health achieved to date.

15.2.5.2 Main Activities

The workshop, aimed at building capacity among policy makers in the region, brought together representatives from ministries responsible for biodiversity and those responsible for health from some 30 countries in the region, as well as a number of relevant organizations, and thematic regional experts. Participants discussed critical linkages at the biodiversity-health nexus and their relevance to the Strategic Plan for Biodiversity 2011–2020 and its Aichi Biodiversity Targets, discussing the need to further mainstream biodiversity and health linkages in public health strategies, and to incorporate public health considerations in biodiversity strategies and better align cross-sectoral policy action. The workshop format featured high-level keynote presentations from both sectors, and a vast array of expert presentations followed by question-and-answer sessions, presentations by country representatives, discussions in smaller working groups, interactive sessions, a guided health walk, as well as an optional field visit at the end of the workshop.

Presentations and group discussions focused on five thematic areas at the biodiversity and health nexus. These included: The human microbiome and the benefits of exposure to microbial diversity in the environment; supporting biodiversity and health for food security and nutrition; zoonotic and vector-borne diseases and One Health; biocultural diversity, mental health and community health; and promoting ecosystem and human health in urban landscapes.

15.2.5.3 What Works Well

The expert presentation provided an overview of the state of the evidence across each of the thematic areas in line with the findings of the State of Knowledge review on Biodiversity and Health, presented case studies and relevant regional and global initiatives that could be leveraged to support the mainstreaming of biodiversity and health linkages across national policies, plans and programmes in the region.

All nominated country representatives from both the environment and health sectors were then invited to make presentations based on their national experiences. This provided an opportunity for country representatives to highlight relevant national policy developments, best practices and related cooperation initiatives emphasising, where possible, main outcomes, experience gained and lessons learned.

[1] https://www.cbd.int/doc/decisions/cop-13/cop-13-dec-06-en.pdf

Smaller working groups and interactive sessions provided a unique opportunity for cross-sectoral exchange among policy makers at the national and regional levels. Participants identified opportunities and challenges associated with mainstreaming biodiversity and health linkages across sectors, highlighted data gaps and needs, and discussed how to strengthen policy coherence across sectors and global policy commitments in line with the 2030 agenda for sustainable development. Discussions also provided valuable input to supporting implementation on the ground and supporting policy developments. At the global level, for example, insights were discussed in view of the preparation of a biodiversity-inclusive One Health guidance prepared by the CBD-Secretariat in collaboration with the WHO, endorsed by CBD Parties and adopted as Recommendation XXI/3 of the Subsidiary Body on Scientific, Technical and Technological Advice (SBSTTA) that will inform the outcomes of the 14th meeting of the CBD Conference of the Parties.[2] Regional capacity-building workshops provide unique opportunities to bridge the frequent gaps between scientific findings and both their relevance and application to real-world policy settings, to foster cross-sectoral dialogue, to raise awareness and to strengthen policy engagement.

15.2.5.4 Main Challenges

A number of challenges in supporting biodiversity and health mainstreaming were identified by participants. Examples include:

- The need for additional forums and workshops to support implementation of regional and global policy commitments.
- The need to better integrate understanding of ecological and evolutionary processes that can help societies to manage the complex socio-ecological systems that encompass health systems, food systems and the way societies plan where and how to live.
- The need for more significant investment in preventive measures to reduce the inefficiencies associated with reactive response-driven approaches.
- The need to strengthen mainstreaming by integrating health-biodiversity linkages into national strategies and policies for health and for biodiversity, and in those for agriculture, fisheries and food production, planning, climate change and disaster risk reduction, as well as economy and finance.

Importantly, it was agreed that while more scientific research is always needed, enough is also known to move to action in many areas. There are a number of no-regret measures that could be better harnessed: investing in nature-based solutions such as the integration of biodiverse green spaces in urban development; better control and use of antimicrobials, pesticides and other biocides; addressing together the drivers of ill health and biodiversity loss; and better monitoring of environmental change. In particular, it is essential to raise further awareness among

[2] https://www.cbd.int/doc/c/72d6/b5bb/9244e977048688ec45735d2c/sbstta-21-04-en.pdf

different stakeholders, including policy-makers, and to build capacity on the ground to facilitate implementation and maximise synergies between actions taken across sectors.

Mechanisms and initiatives to support implementation at each the national, sub-national and global level were also identified as necessary both for strengthening the science policy-interface and for maximising policy coherence across sectors and levels of governance. Tools and mechanisms to support both the development and implementation of policies, plans and programmes based on biodiversity-inclusive holistic approaches such as One Health, EcoHealth and Planetary Health are also needed at each of the national, regional and global levels.

Contact information: https://www.cbd.int/health/european/default.shtml

The regional capacity-building workshop was made possible thanks to financial support from the European Commission and the Government of Finland (four ministries), and co-operational assistance from Finnish Environment Institute (SYKE). The full report of the regional workshop is available from https://www.cbd.int/doc/c/ab6d/0fed/3e795d2f62d288b6ee369c31/hbws-2017-01-02-en.pdf

15.2.6 Coalition of the Willing on Biodiversity and Health

15.2.6.1 Introduction

A potentially interesting collaborative but informal format for networking and capacity building among countries/member states of the CBD and WHO is a 'Coalition of the Willing on Biodiversity and Health'. Another voluntary and informal initiative is the International Coral Reef Initiative (ICRI) created in 1994 by eight states (Australia, France, Japan, Jamaica, Philippines, Sweden, the UK and the USA) and set up during the first CDB conference of the parties in December 1994. This coalition now brings together more than 60 members. No similar initiative exists at the moment regarding nature and health linkages, but informally a 'Coalition of the Willing on Biodiversity and Health' is already considered as a potentially relevant format to enhance the capacity among countries to implement the internationally agreed ambition of putting biodiversity and health recommendations into practice. The Coalition of the Willing on Pollinators, which was established in 2016, can function as a good reference and example, and will be briefly introduced here.

Promote Pollinators – Coalition of the Willing on Pollinators

One of the highlights of the 2016 Conference of the Parties of CBD was the set up and signing of the Declaration on the Coalition of the Willing on Pollinators. Thirteen countries signed the declaration in Cancun, Mexico (CBD COP-13) and many countries, organizations and businesses want to join. Pollinators play a key role in the conservation of biological diversity, ecosystems, food production and the global economy. The coalition believes that country-led politics can foster policy measures and innovative action on protecting pollinators.

The initiative to form a coalition was taken by the Ministry of Economic affairs of the Netherlands and was warmly welcomed by Anne Larigauderie, Executive Secretary for the Intergovernmental Platform on Biodiversity and Ecosystem Services (IPBES). The Coalition of the Willing on Pollinators believes that country-led politics can foster policy measures and innovative action on protecting pollinators. National pollinator strategies are an important tool for the conservation of pollinators. The coalition is reaching out to new partners with the aim of continuously expanding common efforts and sharing knowledge and innovations.

15.2.6.2 Main Activities

The main aim of the coalition is to share information among countries about how to take action to protect pollinators and their habitats by developing and implementing national pollinator strategies, consistent with the IPBES thematic assessment on pollinators, pollination and food production. The Coalition works by sharing experience and lessons learnt in developing and implementing national pollinator strategies, especially knowledge on new approaches, innovations and best practices. The Coalition also seek collaboration with a broad spectrum of stakeholders, in order to develop research on pollinator conservation and to enhance mutual support and collaboration.

15.2.6.3 What Works Well

The Coalition has a formal character in its aim and focus, and its procedural way of working. Still, it is not a consensus-oriented negotiation organization, as is CBD. In the Coalition, the focus is on mutual exchange, inspiration and learning among countries that share a positive interest in implementing internationally agreed upon recommendations (e.g. from CBD or IPBES).

15.2.6.4 Main Challenges

A crucial challenge is to keep the Coalition functional. Despite the informal practice of the Coalition, this demands some structural support function, secretariat, with sufficient resources.

Contact information: https://promotepollinators.org/

15.3 National Initiatives Within Europe

15.3.1 Austria

15.3.1.1 Introduction

The initiative "Biodiversity and health" led by Umweltdachverband (Austrian NGO and environmental umbrella organization) in cooperation with several partners started in 2012.[3] The aim of this Austrian project is to raise awareness for the benefits of biodiversity and nature for human health and well-being. By pointing out to the correlations and relationships between biodiversity and health aspects, the attention of decision-makers and the general public is drawn to the intrinsic value of unspoilt ecosystems, landscapes and services they provide for free. The aim is to promote acceptance and commitment for the conservation of biodiversity in order to facilitate achieving the national biodiversity goals along with the Biodiversity Strategy Austria 2020+. Another objective is to bring together the various stakeholders across all relevant sectors in order to enable mutual regard for their interests and to integrate biodiversity conservation in other sectoral policies and networks.

15.3.1.2 Main Activities

A 'Biodiversity and health' forum was established in 2015 as a cross-sector platform with the goal of mainstreaming issues of biodiversity conservation into other sectors, including the sense of health promotion. Stakeholders from various fields such as science, nature conservation, health, medicine, psychology, education as well as representatives from authorities participated. The forum meets annually and discusses priorities for cross-sector collaboration and possibilities on how to engage the general public. As an outcome, an action plan has been drafted with active support of the Austrian Federal Ministry for Sustainability and Tourism, and also in coordination with the Austrian Federal Ministry of Labour, Social Affairs, Health and Consumer Protection.

Another important part of the initiative consists of public relations work in order to encourage the general public to include actions for biodiversity conservation in their daily life. This was realized by producing an animated short video, which explains biodiversity and its benefits for health and well-being (www.youtube.com/watch?v=JWP4EEJ-l9k). The message of the short video was designed to be easy to understand. It is suitable for introducing people to the topic and for visualising the multiple associations of biodiversity and health. Furthermore, a book "Good for you and me. How Biodiversity promotes our health" (German) was published to enable a more detailed look at this complex relationship. The book draws attention to vari-

[3] This contribution has been drafted within the project "BIO.DIV.NOW II – Mainstreaming von Biodiversität erfolgreich umsetzen", funded by the Austrian Federal Ministry of Sustainability and Tourism and the European Union.

ous aspects, such as the value of species richness for the development of medicinal products, the importance of contact with nature for children and their development, the opportunities to recover and relax in natural areas, and the role of ecosystem services in providing clean air and water. In addition, the initiative participated in an international conference on Landscape and Human Health: Forests, Parks and Green Care (University of Natural Resources and Life Sciences 2017).

In summary, the initiative "Biodiversity and health" contributes in various ways to the facilitation of interdisciplinary communication as well as networking and to the integration of biodiversity protection and connected aspects of health and well-being into other sectoral policies.

15.3.1.3 What Works Well

The forum "Biodiversity and health" fulfills its purpose as a cross-sector platform in order to show and discuss the interlinkages of biodiversity and human health in consideration of all relevant aspects. The participants of the meetings are very eager to find out more about activities in other sectors. For this purpose, the presentation of best practice examples from different stakeholders works well, including in drawing attention to the synergies of biodiversity protection and health promotion.

Collecting measures and relevant requirements for the national action plan on biodiversity and health has also been part of the meetings of the forum. The action plan consists of six action fields and nine targets, and includes 48 recommendations for measures relating to the promotion of biodiversity conservation linked to its various benefits for the health sector as well as other parts of society. The plan has been drafted with input from this multi-sectoral platform and constitutes an important tool for promoting the topic and getting people engaged. It has been presented to Austria's national biodiversity commission, who is invited to recommend the broad implementation of the action plan. The plan is available online at the following link: www.umweltdachverband.at/inhalt/empfehlungen-fuer-einen-aktionsplan-2020-biodiversitaet-and-gesundheit?ref=137.

15.3.1.4 Main Challenges

Apart from gaining actual recognition for the interlinkages of biodiversity and human health among the various stakeholders, one of the main challenges is to get key players from other sectors to assume responsibility for the integration of biodiversity issues in their own agendas, strategies and fields of action. In order to make sure that biodiversity, ecosystems and the services they provide are protected, real actions need to take place. Biodiversity conservation needs to be acknowledged as a matter of high social importance in all relevant sectors, which is a challenging task.

Contact information: www.umweltdachverband.at/biodiversitaet-und-gesundheit/

15.3.2 *Belgium*

15.3.2.1 Introduction

Since 2011 the Belgian Community of Practice Biodiversity and Health (COPBH), facilitated by the Belgian Biodiversity Platform, has tried to enhance biodiversity and health-related science, policy and practice in Belgium. The Belgian Biodiversity Platform is a science policy practice interface related to biodiversity issues, and is funded by the Belgian Federal Science Policy Office (BELSPO).

15.3.2.2 Main Activities

Community Building and Networking Events

In 2011, the Belgian Biodiversity Platform organized a Belgian Biodiversity and Health conference (Keune et al. 2013). It was at this event that the COPBH was founded. The COPBH facilitates an online expert registry and newsletter, and some research project initiatives emerged from bigger and smaller meetings of the COPBH. Apart from scientific partners, there is also collaboration with practice organizations, both with policy institutions and NGOs. Recently, connections to the health sector have been strengthened through collaboration with the Faculty of Medicine and Health Sciences and the Province of Antwerp with the launch of the Chair Care and the Natural Living Environment at the University of Antwerp. An advisory expert committee working within the framework of the Belgian Superior Health Council was initiated at the end of 2017, with support from the COPBH. The aim is to better connect to health-care professionals and other relevant groups for collaboration. In 2016 the COPBH coordinated the organization of the European One Health/Ecohealth workshop in Brussels (see Sect. 15.2.3 above). This is another example of how the COPBH tries to enhance international contacts for Belgian experts and practitioners.

The COPBH also inspires research programmes related to health and biodiversity topics, both at a Belgian and an international level. An example is an overview of research needs and gaps, which was produced before the start of a BELSPO research funding programme called BRAIN, in order to inspire research calls regarding biodiversity and health; this overview was included as an addendum in the first BRAIN call where biodiversity and health issues were addressed. In addition, the COPBH works on mainstreaming and awareness raising by giving on-demand introductory presentations, such as in 2017 in the Flemish Parliament, and support with state-of-the-art overviews of scientific knowledge and practice projects. Finally, the COPBH also contributes to Belgian delegations to international processes such as Mapping and Assessment of Ecosystem Services (MAES), IPBES and CBD, focusing mainly on health-related issues.

15.3.2.3 What Works Well

In particular, the networking events and mainstreaming activities seem to work quite well. The presence in international processes seems fruitful in the sense of gaining attention for biodiversity and health at the international level and in other countries, and for support efforts in Belgium: the fact that biodiversity and health is more prominent on the international agenda also creates more interest and legitimacy for the work in Belgium.

15.3.2.4 Main Challenges

Several main challenges stand out. First, active involvement of experts and practitioners in community building is important. Even though there is an interest, clearly shown by the high attendance during events, in daily practice, often there is a lack of time and resources to further commit to such integrated and collaborative efforts. A second and related factor is that funding resources for more collaborative research and practices are still rather limited. There has been improvement over the years, but more interdisciplinary and transdisciplinary projects in particular, both in science and in practice, have a difficult time to find support. Thirdly, and again also related, a big challenge in bridge building is overcoming the divide between a focus on nature-related health benefits and risks. These issues are still treated by separate communities and departments, whilst a more integrated approach would be desirable. A more institutional challenge is the complex policy constellation of Belgium: several nature- and/or health-related policies are either a federal or a regional policy responsibility. To work in an integrated manner is more difficult in such an institutional constellation.

Contact information: http://www.biodiversity.be/health/

15.3.3 Finland

15.3.3.1 Introduction

General, professional and scientific discussion on the interlinkages of biodiversity and human health has been very active in Finland over the last years. The positive health effects of biodiversity and nature connection on human health especially have gained a lot of interest. Based on produced information, there is a good reason to believe that better contact with natural environments can enhance the cohesion of families and communities, citizens' health and well-being, prevent diseases and, as a consequence, also reduce national health costs.

Through the better knowledge of health effects from nature, there is also a very strong business case and job creation possibilities. Nature-connected innovations in health-care systems, well-being tourism and various approaches, such as Healthy Parks – Healthy People, health walks and Green Care, already support this business case.

15.3.3.2 Main Activities

Recently, Finnish scientists have produced results suggesting that biodiversity loss and rising trends of inflammatory diseases – two global megatrends – may be related (von Herzen et al. 2011). There is also scientific evidence supporting the differences in the presence of allergies between the people living in Finnish Karelia and Russian Karelia. According to the results, allergy is more common in Finnish Karelia than in Russian Karelia. People exposed to a greater number of nature contacts and diverse microbiota on the Russian side of the border seem to have more protection from allergic reactions (Hanski et al. 2012, see also the biodiversity hypothesis presented by Haahtela et al. 2013).

The project *Ecosystem Services and Human Health* (2013–2014), financed by the Finnish Cultural Foundation, stimulated national dialogue on biodiversity and human health between environmental and health researchers, experts and decision-makers (Jäppinen et al. 2014). Likewise, the project *Ability to read nature – creating business from green well-being* (Särkkä et al. 2013, available in Finnish only) and the Healthy Parks – Healthy People Finland (HPHPF) programme (Parks and Wildlife Finland 2016) have produced relevant and comprehensive knowledge for the needs of service design, national planning and wider discussion (see Box 15.2).

The Pan-European WHO-CBD Workshop on Biodiversity and Health for the European Region, held in Helsinki (23–25 October 2017) promoted international dialogue on the subthemes: Human microbiome and exposure to microbial diversity in the environment; Biodiversity, health, food security and nutrition; Zoonotic and vector-borne diseases and One Health; Biocultural diversity and mental health; Promoting ecosystem and human health in urban landscapes; and Biodiversity, health, food security and nutrition (see WHO-CBD Pan-European Workshop on Biodiversity and Health for the European Region, held in Helsinki (23–25 October 2017) https://www.cbd.int/health/european/default.shtml).

15.3.3.3 What Works Well

Finland has built a good basis for the future developments on biodiversity and health issues through the analyses, results, policies and practical delivery of policies of the recent activities described above. As a small country Finland also has the advantage that networks of national health and biodiversity experts and administrative sectors are already quite well established. Finland also strongly participates in international discussion, which has been an important part of positive developments in the field of biodiversity and human health. National challenges are often similar between countries, and learning from good practice is globally essential.

Box 15.2: Healthy Parks, Healthy People – Finland

Veikko Virkkunen, Metsähallitus, Parks and Wildlife Finland, veikko.virkkunen@metsa.fi

Parks and Wildlife Finland (PWF) manages all of Finland's national parks, other state-owned protected areas and cultural heritage sites, as well as their hiking services. As the global awareness and evidence on the benefits of diverse nature and outdoor recreation for human health and well-being have significantly increased over the last few years, PWF has been implementing the HPHPF programme since 2010. The programme is a policy example to deal with the spread of chronic illnesses, increasing welfare costs, and securing funding for biodiversity conservation. As such, the overall goal of HPHPF is that Finnish health and well-being is improved by diverse nature. HPHPF consists of three main themes, as well as prioritized measures, to attain these goals by 2025:

1. **From nearby nature to national parks**

   Major cities in Finland can contribute to health by offering well-functioning, continuous green space serving the outdoor recreation requirements of local people. PWF is working with partnership networks between managers of public greenspaces, for example in the cities of Oulu, Kajaani and Helsinki. The focus of the manager networks is to improve the quality, accessibility and awareness of the various sites and communicate them together effectively.
2. **Everyone outdoors**

   Everyone should have equal opportunities to enjoy the green environments. Bold initiatives lower the threshold for engaging in outdoor recreation, making it easy and fun throughout the year. PWF improves the service design of popular protected areas for new customers, e.g. disabled people (see Fig. 15.1a), and experts in the Finnish Adapted Physical Activity Federation.

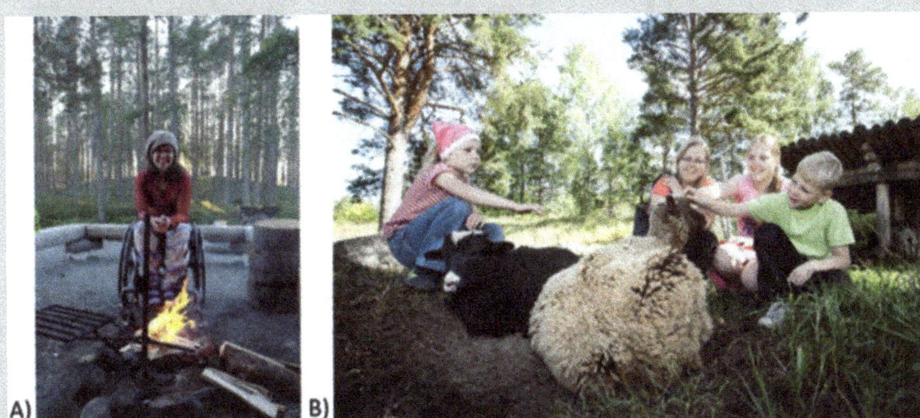

Fig. 15.1 Facilitating the use of the outdoors for all. (**a**) Accessible structures and trails for disabled people in Hossa National Park; (**b**) Family contributing during the Shepherd Weeks

(continued)

Box 15.2 (continued)

3. **Communications and cooperation**

   Increased knowledge of the connection between biodiversity and health needs to reach key actors and influence decision making. PWF has initiated cooperation with two regional hospital construction projects with the aim of enhancing customer experience and speeding up recovery by introducing strong green space imagery, natural soundscape and materials, as well as new operational models utilising the nearby nature.

   Enjoying the outdoors can also contribute to biodiversity. PWF runs national Shepherd Weeks attracting thousands of applicants each year, and so far over 1,500 volunteers (see Fig. 15.1b). During the Shepherd Weeks volunteers on 12 sites contribute to nature conservation and landscape management, taking care of grazing animals. The week in nature helps volunteers in recovery from stress, improving mood and enhancing family ties.

   The HPHPF programme continues to inspire PWF and partners in coming up with practical outcomes and new development projects.

In general, and perhaps more so than in most other European countries, the Finnish people are active, outdoor people, for whom nature is an essential part of everyday life and leisure time. This active relationship with nature has improved their social, physical and mental well-being, and the positive relationship towards nature provides a good basis for developing new positive synergies that are based on the natural environment. There is also a good number of private companies that have based their businesses on the positive interconnections between people and nature.

15.3.3.4 Main Challenges

At a national level there is still a need to promote cross-sectoral dialogue, especially between the Ministry of Social Affairs and Health, Ministry of the Environment and the Ministry of Agriculture and Forestry. These ministries and their research and development institutes can make progress through mainstreaming and enhancing national cooperation between governmental and other sectors, including private companies.

There is a need for more detailed scientific evidence on the interlinkages of nature and health, but at the same time, it is very clear that experts, practitioners and decision makers do know enough to act, which means integrating the known positive health effects of nature into national health-care strategies and policies. For instance, Finland could invest in nature-based solutions such as the integration of biodiverse green spaces in urban development, and better control the use of antimicrobials, pesticides and other biocides harmful for human health, and also for biodiversity.

In this regard, Finland could prepare a roadmap on biodiversity and human health, which would assist the preparation of national health and biodiversity policy and action plan. The identified policy and research needs could also be integrated in the updated version of the Finnish National Biodiversity Strategy and Action Plan (NBSAP), and if there is enough political will, it may be possible to develop a separate National Biodiversity and Human Health Strategy and Action Plan for the Post 2020 period.

Contact information: http://www.metsa.fi/web/en/healthbenefitsfromnationalparks and https://www.cbd.int/health/european/default.shtml

15.3.4 France

15.3.4.1 Introduction

Created in 2008, the Foundation for Research on Biodiversity is a national science-policy platform created by the main French public research establishments working on biodiversity. This platform was joined by Moët Hennessy Louis Vuitton (LVMH) in 2014. In 2018, more than 240 public and private entities (firms, non-governmental organizations, managers or publics authorities) have joined the FRB to face biodiversity challenges together.

The core mission of FRB is to generate innovation, promote good scientific projects in association with society and its stakeholders, develop studies, overviews and valuations, and communicate research results.

15.3.4.2 Main Activities

Supporting Research

The answer to a number of biodiversity and health questions requires assembling and combining multiple and heterogeneous data sets, allowing researchers to conduct new analyses that go beyond those related to data published in individual studies or research programmes. To tackle this challenge, FRB firstly promotes a new approach to biodiversity research, fostering better use of existing data from large data sets collected in different locations, on different scales, on different levels of biodiversity (from micro-organisms to ecosystems and landscapes) and through different scientific disciplines, time series, etc. This is made possible thanks to calls for synthesis launched at the synthesis centre *Centre de synthèse et d'analyse sur la biodiversité* (CESAB), which belongs to an international network of similar initiatives.

One project about the relationships between biodiversity and infectious diseases has been funded by FRB in this context, and it was led by Jean-François Guegan (France) working with 11 other scientists from France, the USA, Italy and Mexico.

Bringing together ecologists, public health scientists, veterinarians, modelers and parasitologists working in four different regions of the world, this project addressed three major issues: (1) which life-history characteristics may confer to hosts a better capacity to be 'good vessels', (2) how do we quantify the parasites' capacity to cross species boundaries; and (3) what is the role of biodiversity in transmission of infectious diseases on different spatial scales.

Deliverables were databases, disease modelling, reviews and exploratory articles, actionable public health policy information shared with health-protection agencies and the media; and training of young scientists in this new research.

Systematic Reviews on 'Resistance to Antibiotics', 'Biodiversity and Infectious Diseases'

FRB also promotes several other methods to highlight knowledge gaps or uncertainties on knowledge, the latter often related to the great disparity between experimental protocols. Systematic reviews are one of these approaches. This method aims to promote a more efficient use of knowledge as well as the assessment of scientific uncertainties in order to facilitate decision making, to validate the research results and to favour the development of targeted research programmes that effectively complement the knowledge already acquired.

FRB currently leads or contributes to several systematic reviews or evidence-synthesis works. Funded by the French Ministry of Environment, one addresses how antibiotic resistance in the environment is impacted by changes in practice concerning (1) the use of antibiotics, (2) the management of wastes and (3) the management of the natural environment. The protocol of this review is available on open-access and the review will deliver its final results in early 2019.

In 2003, the French government published its first national agenda for environment and health. The third one, launched in 2015, included for the first time several actions about biodiversity and health, two of which are managed by FRB. The first one was conducted within a group of European experts from the H2020 Eklipse programme of which the FRB is a partner. Experts will address one main issue: what is known about the effects of different types of habitats and certain components of green spaces on mental health and well-being? The results of this work are intended to guide more effectively the decisions to create new urban and peri-urban green spaces, to better inform landscape architects and environmental managers about the most reliable knowledge, and to highlight research gaps. The second one was financed by the French Agency for Biodiversity and will target the positive effects of biodiversity on the prevention and control of infectious diseases affecting humans. The aim of this systematic review is to analyse the scientific knowledge on the link between biodiversity and some infectious diseases in order to identify the research gaps and validated research results to support public policies and stakeholder actions on the biodiversity and infectious diseases interface.

Advocating Biodiversity Conservation and Its Sustainable Use Based on Scientific Results

The Foundation produces documents that synthesize research results for better ownership by public and private decision makers. The latest one was related to the epidemic of Lyme disease in Europe. FRB is also a member of several organizations such as IPBES, the European network Eklipse on science-based decision for biodiversity, the European research network on biodiversity (BiodivERsA) and CDB, all of which deal with Biodiversity and health. At the national level FRB is a member of the National group for Environment and Health and co-leader of the group 'Biodiversity and Health' with the French Ministry of Environment.

15.3.4.3 What Works Well

The networking, at national, European and international levels, is very efficient and several messages related to the preservation of biodiversity have been effectively passed to stakeholders (members of the Foundation's strategic orientation council), to the ministries, within the French delegation for the CBD and IPBES and to the European or international working groups. The first results (CESAB research project) have found a strong echo among stakeholders and are recognized within the scientific community. For more achievements of the project, see: Ezenwa et al. 2015; García-Peña et al. 2016; Suzán et al. 2015.

15.3.4.4 Main Challenges

The first challenge faced by the Foundation is to find money to support research to fill knowledge gaps and contribute to the building of sound evidence bases. The second challenge is to find more effective levers to transform knowledge into relevant action to preserve both biodiversity and the health of humans, animals and plants.

Contact information: http://www.fondationbiodiversite.fr/fr/ and http://www.cesab.org/index.php/fr/projets-passes/59-biodis

15.3.5 *Germany*

15.3.5.1 Introduction

The *German Federal Agency for Nature Conservation (BfN)* provides the German Federal Ministry for the Environment, Nature Conservation and Nuclear Safety (BMU) with professional and scientific assistance in all nature conservation and landscape management issues on the national, European and international levels. In these contexts, the BfN plays a central role as 'science-policy interface'. In this light, the BfN has been active in the field of biodiversity and health for almost 15 years, in an effort to cover the physical, mental and social dimensions of health (see Job-Hoben et al. 2010).

15.3.5.2 Main Activities

BfN Research and Development Project: 'Green-Natural-Healthy'

To support the inclusion of health promotion aspects in planning practice, the BfN-funded study 'Green, natural, healthy' (Rittel et al. 2014) included information on different user groups and their needs, criteria to determine health-promoting potentials of urban green spaces and a list of good arguments for planners concerning the positive effects of green spaces on human health. These scientific findings support municipalities with helpful arguments to safeguard and enhance the positive benefits of 'green spaces' on human health against the background of climate change, demographic change and environmental justice.

Transfer of Results

One prominent example of the transfer of scientific results to decision makers is the national follow-up of the international study 'The Economics of Ecosystems and Biodiversity' (TEEB). The 'Natural Capital Germany – TEEB DE' report on 'Ecosystem Services in the City – Protecting Health and Enhancing Quality of Life' contains comprehensive sections of the current knowledge of the nexus between urban green, human health, climate aspects and social cohesion (Naturkapital Deutschland – TEEB DE 2016).

Communication Related to the Topics of 'Biodiversity, Health and Climate Change'

One example of BfN's communication activities is the web portal 'NatGesIS' – short for 'nature conservation and health information system', a tool for communicating the interlinkages between nature conservation and health. The portal contains a comprehensive compilation of information about nature-related health courses and treatments, wellness and nature experience with children, as well as specific data on natural resources, health and climate change made available for the scientific community and the public. A second example of BfN's communication activities is a series of events concerning psychological aspects in the communication about nature conservation (regarding topics such as happiness, well-being, nature experience, climate change and mindfulness).

Another example of outreach activities to the general public are hiking events, organized by the BfN every year since 2010. Through this format it is possible to experience the linkages between nature and human well-being personally. In addition to a prominent opening event, local and regional organizers can join in and promote their hiking activities on a central web platform. In 2016, more than 1,600 hiking tours were offered.

15.3.5.3 What Works Well

The health-related activities of the German UN Decade on Biodiversity 2011–2020 contribute to an ongoing networking and communication process in Germany. Next to public relations, newsletters and social media, the UN Decade honors projects and contributions, which work in an exemplary manner to conserve biodiversity. For the years 2017/2018, the UN Decade placed the slogan 'Healthy – With the diversity of nature' at the centre of the competition. The objective is to highlight exemplary engagement shown in four key areas: (1) medicine from nature, (2) recreation areas and activities in nature and outdoors, (3) the healing power of nature, and (4) natural resources as a basis for health. Since the start of the main topic, around 20 projects in this thematic area have been awarded. The conferment of the title 'Official project of the UN Decade on Biodiversity' receives high public attention in the print media, social media and television. To further connect prospective partners from health-care and biodiversity, a special working group has been established. It also serves to present case studies and promotes the development of new ideas. Additionally, a conference on biodiversity and health was held in June 2018 which focused on the health prevention potential of nature.

15.3.5.4 Main Challenges

There is still a need to raise awareness among decision makers and practitioners in the health sector with regard to the contribution of biodiversity and nature to human health. Networks and intensive exchange have to be further established, and joint projects should be initiated.

Contact information: https://www.bfn.de/ or http://natgesis.bfn.de/ (in German only) or https://www.undekade-biologischevielfalt.de (in German and English).

15.4 Conclusions

The examples in this overview illustrate the variety of European nature–health network initiatives. This mirrors the emerging international interest in nature–health linkages across Europe; several initiatives are still quite recent. We should note that the contributions are based on self-assessment by key organizers or facilitators of the respective initiatives. We nevertheless hope that these self-reflections are inspiring and will encourage creation of sufficient critical mass in the European region for strengthening these kinds of networking activities, and collaboration and exchange among them, for the sake of further progress. In the rest of this final section, we summarize some of the key findings and describe lessons learned.

15.4.1 Aims of the Networking Initiatives

Important aims mentioned are capacity building (mainly knowledge capacity and expert capacity), mainstreaming (across disciplines and sectors between and beyond nature and/or health) and integration. Functional in this respect is strengthening of the evidence/knowledge base regarding nature – health linkages, but also linking existing insights to policy and practice, to the extent it is concluded that there is already sufficient understanding on particular items within the broader nature–health linkages. Regarding integration, this is mentioned in terms of both sectors (i.e. nature and health sectors and other relevant sectors, in science, policy and practice) and content (i.e. regarding both nature-related health risks and benefits), both within specific topical domains (e.g. infectious disease risks), as concerning generic angles, such as social science, evaluation or education. An example of reaping the fruits of a networking capacity is the expert consultation for the IPBES Regional Assessment Europe and Central Asia (IPBES 2018): experts can more easily be contacted and are already aware of ongoing work and important challenges.

15.4.2 Main Activities and Outputs

Knowledge generation or facilitation activities are part of the project, such as expert elicitation, knowledge synthesis, development of integrative and evaluative frameworks, and data support.

Network activities are aimed at stimulating dialogue, community building and several other forms of interdisciplinary and transdisciplinary interaction between experts and stakeholders. Other types of events or projects are mentioned, such as hiking events and communication activities through newsletters, books, video and the like. Other achievements include an expert registry, web portals, and guiding material – such as handbooks, policy briefs, best practices, action plans, case studies, innovations and practical solutions.

15.4.3 Conditions

An important condition for successful networking initiatives is the availability of structural resources including supporting infrastructure. Even when informal in character, structural, financial or other, support is important to keep momentum and activities going. Most networks seem to flourish best in an informal setting for exchange and collaboration, but some initiatives also require a more formal element such as development of joint action plans or other forms of recommendations. Another important element is the contribution of network members and experts: without commitment or a sense of ownership, and without a broad range of membership beyond the usual suspects, they may struggle to survive and to reach their goals.

Several network initiatives mention multi-scale activities, which may also be mutually supportive. For example, it may help local or national initiatives to link to or mention international developments supporting the direction of local propositions. Further, local cultural institutional conditions may promote or hinder the functioning of network initiatives. For example, the complex institutional constellation of Belgium is perceived to be a challenge, whereas the more intensive nature-connectedness of the Finnish lifestyle helps to trigger a positive response to nature–health activities.

15.4.4 Ways Forward

Several network contributions to this chapter mention future plans and needs. Clearly, they support significant capacity building and mainstreaming work, the importance of which is underlined at different occasions and steps. The existence of a diversity of nature–health network initiatives is mainly a strength, and even on an international scale, they all have their own history and context in which they are relevant. More structural support for these initiatives and strengthening inter-network collaboration offers a strong way forward.

Acknowledgements We thank all funding bodies supporting the different initiatives outlined in this chapter for their important contributions. We also thank the reviewers for their insightful comments and the editors of this book for making this publication possible.

References

CBD (2018) Decision adopted by the conference of the parties to the convention on biological diversity, 14/4. Health and biodiversity. CBD/COP/DEC/14/4

Charron DF (ed) (2012) Ecohealth research in practice: innovative applications of an ecosystem approach to health. Springer, Ottawa

Ezenwa VO, Prieur-Richard A-H, Roche B, Bailly X, Becquart P, García-Peña GE, Hosseini PR, Keesing F, Rizzoli A, Suzán G, Vignuzzi M, Vittecopq M, Mills JN, Guégan J-F (2015) Interdisciplinarity and infectious diseases: an Ebola case study. PLoS Pathog 11(8):e1004992. https://doi.org/10.1371/journal.ppat.1004992

García-Peña GE, Garchitorena A, Carolan K, Canard E, Prieur-Richard A-H, Suzán G, Mills JN, Roche B, Guégan J-F (2016) Niche-based host extinction increases prevalence of an environmentally acquired pathogen. Oikos. https://doi.org/10.1111/oik.02700

Haahtela T, Holgate S, Pawankar R, Akdis CA, Benjaponpitak S, Caraballo L, Demain J, Portnoy J, von Hertzen L, WAO Special Committee on Climate Change and Biodiversity (2013) The biodiversity hypothesis and allergic disease: world allergy organization position statement. World Allergy Organ J 6(1):3. https://www.ncbi.nlm.nih.gov/pmc/articles/PMC3646540/#

Hanski I, The Karelia Study Group (Leena von Herzen, Nanna Fyhrquist, Kaisa Koskinen, Kaisa Torppa, Tiina Laatikainen, Piia Karisola, Petri Auvinen, Lars Paulin, Mika J. Mäkelä, Erkki Vartiainen, Timo U. Kosunen, Harri Alenius & Tari Haahtela) (2012) Proceedings of the National Academy of Sciences of the United States of America PNAS May 2012. http://www.pnas.org/content/109/21/8334

IPBES (2018) Regional assessment Europe and Central Asia, Chapter 2. https://www.ipbes.net/assessment-reports/eca

Jäppinen J-P, Tyrväinen L, Reinikainen M, Ojala A (eds) (2014) Nature for health and well-being in Finland – results and recommendations from the Argumenta project ecosystem services and human health (2013–2014) (Abstract and Summary). Reports of the Finnish Environment Institute 35/2014. 104 pp. Helsinki. https://helda.helsinki.fi/handle/10138/153461

Job-Hoben B, Pütsch M, Erdmann K-H (2010) Human health protection – a 'new' issue area for nature conservation? Natur und Landschaft 85(4):137–141

Keune H, Assmuth T (2018) Framing complexity in environment and human health, In: Oxford research encyclopedia of environmental science. Oxford University Press, New York

Keune H, Kretsch C, De Blust G, Gilbert M, Flandroy L, Van den Berge K, Versteirt V, Hartig T, De Keersmaecker L, Eggermont H (2013) Science–policy challenges for biodiversity, public health and urbanization: examples from Belgium. Environ Res Lett 8(2):025015. https://doi.org/10.1088/1748-9326/8/2/025015

Keune H, Flandroy L, Thys S, De Regge N, Mori M, Antoine-Moussiaux N, Vanhove MP, Rebolledo J, Van Gucht S, Deblauwe I (2017) The need for European OneHealth/EcoHealth networks. Arch Public Health 75:64

Lebel J (2003) Health, an ecosystem approach. International Development Research Centre, Ottawa

Marselle M, Stadler J, Korn H, Bonn A (2018) Proceedings of the European conference "Biodiversity and health in the face of climate change - challenges, opportunities and evidence gaps". BfN-Skripten 509. Federal Agency for Nature Conservation, Germany, Bonn. https://doi.org/10.19217/skr509

Naturkapital Deutschland – TEEB DE (2016) In: Kowarik I, Bartz R, Brenck I (eds) Ecosystem services in the city – protecting health and enhancing quality of life. Technische Universität Berlin, Helmholtz-Zentrum für Umweltforschung – UFZ, Berlin/Leipzig. Accessed 6 Feb 2018 at: https://www.ufz.de/export/data/global/190507_TEEB_De_Broschuere_KF_Bericht3_Stadt_engl_web.pdf

Pan-European Workshop on Biodiversity and Health for the European Region, held in Helsinki (2017.) https://www.cbd.int/health/european/default.shtml

Parks and Wildlife Finland (2016) Healthy parks – healthy people Finland, Health and Wellbeing 2025 programme. http://www.metsa.fi/web/en

Rittel K, Bredow L, Wanka ER, Hokema D, Schuppe G, Wilke T, Nowak D, Heiland S (2014) Green, natural, healthy: The potential of multifunctional urban spaces. Accessed 6 Feb 2018 at: https://www.bfn.de/fileadmin/BfN/service/Dokumente/skripten/Skript371_EN.pdf

Särkkä S, Konttinen L, Sjöstedt T (eds) (2013) Ability to read nature – creating business from green well-being (in Finnish only). Sitra. 60 pp. Helsinki. https://www.sitra.fi/julkaisut/luonnonlukutaito-luo-liiketoimintaa-vihreasta-hyvinvoinnista/

Suzán G, García-Peña GE, Castro-Arellano I, Rico O, Rubio AV, Tolsá MJ, Rocher B, Hosseini PR, Rizzoli A, Murray KA, Zambrana-Torrelio C, Vittecoq M, Bailly X, Aguirre AA, Daszak P, Prieur-Richard A-H, Mills JN, Guegan JF (2015) Metacommunity and phylogenetic structure determine wildlife and zoonotic infections disease patterns in time and space. Ecol Evol 5(4):865–873. https://doi.org/10.1002/ece3.1404

University of Natural Resources and Life Sciences, Austrian Research and Training Centre for Forests, Natural Hazards and Landscape & Institute of Landscape Development, Recreation and Conservation Planning, Vienna (eds) (2017). Proceedings of the 3rd international conference on landscape and human health: forests, parks and green care. BFW, Vienna

von Herzen L, Hanski I, Haahtela T (2011) Natural immunity – biodiversity loss and inflammatory diseases are two global megatrends that might be related. EMBO Rep 12:1089–1093. http://embor.embopress.org/content/12/11/1089

Wallace RG, Bergmann L, Kock R, Gilbert M, Hogerwerf L, Wallace R, Holmberg M (2015) The dawn of structural one health: a new science tracking disease emergence along circuits of capital. Soc Sci Med 129:68–77

WHO Regional Office for Europe (2016) Urban green spaces and health: a review of evidence. WHO, Copenhagen. http://www.euro.who.int/__data/assets/pdf_file/0005/321971/Urban-green-spaces-and-health-review-evidence.pdf?ua=1

World Health Organization and Secretariat of the Convention on Biological Diversity (2015) Connecting global priorities: biodiversity and human health: a state of knowledge review. World Health Organization, Geneva. https://www.cbd.int/health/SOK-biodiversity-en.pdf

Zinsstag J, Schelling E, Waltner-Toews D, Tanner M (2011) From "one medicine" to "one health" and systemic approaches to health and well-being. Prev Vet Med 101(2011):148–156

Part IV
Planning and Managing Urban Green Spaces for Biodiversity and Health in a Changing Climate

Chapter 16
Nature-Based Solutions and Protected Areas to Improve Urban Biodiversity and Health

Kathy MacKinnon, Chantal van Ham, Kate Reilly, and Jo Hopkins

Abstract Biodiversity and healthy natural ecosystems, including protected areas in and around cities, provide ecosystem benefits and services that support human health, including reducing flood risk, filtering air pollutants, and providing a reliable supply of clean drinking water. These services help to reduce the incidence of infectious diseases and respiratory disorders, and assist with adaptation to climate change. Access to nature offers many other direct health benefits, including opportunities for physical activity, reduction of developmental disorders and improved mental health. Economic valuations of green spaces in several cities globally have found that nature provides billions of dollars in cost savings for health services. Protected areas are increasingly common in, and around, cities to protect biodiversity and ecosystem services, including these benefits for health. Many cities are also launching programmes to enhance the health and environmental benefits of parks, based on a model of Healthy Parks, Healthy People, by Parks Victoria in Australia. Partnerships between conservationists, city planners and health authorities are critical to maximise these benefits. In some places, medical professionals prescribe time in nature, and some cities specify standards for urban green spaces to enhance their health benefits. The United Nations Sustainable Development Goals provide an important global framework for such partnerships from global to local level.

Keywords Health · Protected areas · Nature · Urban · Climate change

---

K. MacKinnon (✉)
IUCN World Commission on Protected Areas, Gland, Switzerland
e-mail: kathy.s.mackinnon@gmail.com

C. van Ham · K. Reilly
IUCN European Regional Office, Brussels, Belgium
e-mail: chantal.vanham@iucn.org; kate.reilly@iucn.org

J. Hopkins
Parks Victoria, Melbourne, Australia
e-mail: jo.hopkins@parks.vic.gov.au

M. R. Marselle et al. (eds.), *Biodiversity and Health in the Face of Climate Change*, https://doi.org/10.1007/978-3-030-02318-8_16

Highlights

- Protected natural areas in, and adjacent to, cities provide ecosystem benefits and services that support human health and climate change adaptation.
- Urban green spaces provide billions of dollars in cost savings for health services.
- Partnerships between conservationists, city planners and health authorities are critical for the continued protection of protected nature areas in and around cities.

16.1 Introduction

Biodiversity and healthy natural ecosystems underpin and sustain human livelihoods and well-being by providing essential services such as food, clean air and water, and protection against floods, coastal storms and other natural disasters (Dudley et al. 2010). These functions will become ever more important in helping people to cope with, and adapt to, climate change and its impacts. Water scarcity, food security and biodiversity loss will be some of the greatest global challenges over the next few decades; all will be exacerbated by climate change and have consequences for human health and well-being. In Africa alone some 75 million–250 million people are expected to be experiencing water shortages by 2020, with a 50% reduction in yields from rain-fed agriculture, leading to more food shortages, poverty, insecurity and migration (World Bank 2010). In Asia, climate change is projected to lead to decreased freshwater availability and the increased prevalence of water-borne diseases, whereas coastal areas, especially the densely populated delta regions, will be exposed to a greater risk of flooding. These climate-induced changes will have a cost in terms of human health, with more endemic morbidity and mortality due to the rise of diarrhoea and other water-borne diseases and the spread of certain disease vectors (World Bank 2010; Müller et al. Chap. 4, this volume).

Land degradation and the continued erosion of the natural capital that underpins functioning ecosystems – including soil, water and biodiversity – are an increasing threat to human health and sustainable livelihoods. The World Health Organisation (WHO) suggests that up to a quarter of all deaths globally could be avoided simply by improved management of environmental issues such as air pollution, water contamination and dust from degraded drylands (WHO 2005).

Over half of the world's population now lives in cities, and it is predicted that nearly 70% of people will be living in urban environments by 2050 (United Nations 2014). In the coming decades, 95% of urban expansion is expected to occur in the developing world, including in some of the countries most likely to be impacted by climate change and more erratic weather patterns (United Nations 2014). Cities are not urban 'islands'; they depend on surrounding natural landscapes and seascapes, including protected areas, to provide critical ecosystem services, such as food, clean air, water supplies and protection against floods, coastal storms and other natural disasters (Dudley et al. 2010; Gómez-Baggethun et al. 2013). At the same time, rapid urbanisation is affecting the very ecosystems on which cities and urban citizens depend by exerting pressures on freshwater supplies and increasing pollution (Mcdonald et al. 2008). With the dual challenges of climate change and rapid urbanisation, improving the public health of urban residents will be of particular importance.

Increasing urbanisation brings its own challenges in terms of human health. Non-communicable diseases such as diabetes, cardiovascular disease, cancer and depression are now among the fastest growing health challenges around the world (WHO 2005, 2014). While many factors are involved in this increase, lifestyle factors such as physical activity, diet and stress are particularly important (WHO 2014). There is also increasing evidence that lack of access to nature in cities, and associated sedentary, indoor lifestyles, is linked with physical and mental health disorders including vitamin D deficiency, asthma, anxiety and depression (Gelsthorpe 2017). Better access to nature has been shown to have positive physical and mental health benefits and can even contribute to healing after surgery (Sandifer et al. 2015; Townsend et al. 2015, Cook et al. Chap. 11, this volume).

There is increasing evidence that biodiversity and healthy natural ecosystems, including protected areas, can help climate change adaptation by serving as a natural buffer against climate-related disasters, contributing to water and food security, and playing a critical role in maintaining human health and well-being (Dudley et al. 2010; IUCN 2016a, b; Gómez-Baggethun et al. 2013). A healthy ecosystem is one that is sustainable – that is, it has the ability to maintain its structure (organisation) and function (vigour) over time in the face of external stress (resilience) (Costanza et al. 1999). In this chapter, we argue that effective protection, management and restoration of protected areas and other natural ecosystems can be practical, cost-effective and help to meet the interlinked goals for biodiversity, health and climate change adaptation in a rapidly-urbanising world. Identifying and understanding the synergies between nature, health, urban development and national climate change policies and programmes will be critical for delivering many of the United Nations Sustainable Development Goals (SDGs), especially those relating to water, health and sustainable cities.

16.2 Protected Areas: Contributing to Healthy Societies

Protected areas and other natural ecosystems can contribute positively to human health in various ways, many of which are just beginning to be understood. These can be categorised as follows: (i) by providing ecosystem benefits and services that sustain life and regulate against detrimental health effects from climate, floods, infectious diseases, etc.; (ii) as botanical sources for both traditional and modern medicines; and (iii) by providing direct benefits to physical, spiritual and mental health through time spent in nature.

16.2.1 Ecosystem Benefits and Services

Protected areas and other natural ecosystems, such as wetlands and forested areas, including those within and adjacent to cities, can provide positive health benefits and services (Dudley et al. 2010; Townsend et al. 2015). Conserving or restoring forests can, for example, reduce the risk of malaria and certain other diseases. Watersheds retaining natural vegetation, particularly forests, provide cleaner water than more degraded watersheds. Protected areas can maintain dryland vegetation, stabilising soil, preventing desertification and dust storms, and reducing the suspended solids in air that create major respiratory problems (WCPA 2015). Marine protected areas and healthy wetlands boost fish stocks, contributing to food security and adequate protein for coastal and subsistence communities (Halpern 2003).

Access to clean water is an essential pre-requisite for public health, and especially important in densely populated cities. Poor planning, inefficient use, population growth and increasing demands for water all mean that the provision of adequate, safe supplies of water remains a major source of concern. One in five people in the developing world live without a reliable water supply and two billion city dwellers do not have adequate sanitation. Lack of clean water increases infant mortality and the prevalence of water-borne diseases, reducing productivity, straining health services, and causing millions of deaths every year (WHO 2005; Stolton and Dudley 2010; WCPA 2015). Furthermore, water shortages undermine agricultural productivity and food security, while excess water, as a result of storms and floods, creates not just immediate social and economic impacts but is often followed by disease and epidemics (Dudley et al. 2010). Protection of natural habitats helps regulate against flooding and other weather-related events and sustains the availability of high-quality water for health, social and economic development.

Functioning natural ecosystems within well-managed watersheds and protected areas provide efficient and cost-effective ways of supplying clean water (see Box 16.1). One-third of the world's largest 100 cities, including Jakarta, Dar es Salaam, New York, Melbourne and Sydney, rely on forest-protected areas for a substantial part of their domestic water supply (Dudley and Stolton 2003). High-altitude, tropical montane vegetation provides clean water supplies to major cities in Latin America. Protected areas in Colombia, for example, cover about 10% of the country and provide 50% of Colombians with water. In the capital, Bogotá, eight million people get 80% of their water from the *paramos vegetation* protected in the Chingaza National Park (WCPA 2012). Recognising the importance of this natural function, the mayors of the surrounding municipalities are supporting restoration of natural habitats within the Park.

Protected wetlands can also provide critically important water supplies and protection from flooding for many urban populations. The 89,000 hectare Lagoas de Cufada Natural Park in southern Guinea-Bissau was created to protect the largest freshwater reserve of the country. In a region where rainfall has been reducing, this Ramsar site plays a crucial role in supplying water for the city of Buba, as well as

Box 16.1: Protected Areas Providing Clean Water for Domestic Use

In many parts of the world adequate supplies of potable water depend on protected areas:

- Kerinci Seblat National Park in Indonesia protects the head waters of two of Sumatra's major rivers, the Musi and the Batanghari, which provide downstream water supplies for major cities such as Jambi, Padang and Palembang, as well as millions of hectares of irrigated farmlands.
- In Ecuador, about 80% of Quito's 1.5 million residents receive drinking water from two protected areas in the Andes.
- The 22,000 hectare Te Papanui Conservation Park, in New Zealand's Lammermoor Range, provides the Otago region with essential water flows valued at NZ$ 93 million for urban water supply.
- Protected areas are particularly valuable in water resource terms where they occur upstream of large population centres in dry environments. The Cholistan Wildlife Sanctuary upstream of Karachi, Pakistan (population 18 million), for example, provides water services estimated at US$ 100 million per year to the downstream population.
- Six reservoirs in the Catskills Mountains provide water to nine million people in the New York City area. Careful management of the landscape and protected areas provide good quality water through the largest unfiltered water supply in the USA, with a few million dollars spent on watershed protection saving billions of dollars in infrastructure costs for filtration.

Sources: Dudley et al. 2010; World Bank 2010.

contributing to local livelihoods and the survival of hundreds of plant and animal species (Dudley et al. 2010).

Elsewhere, natural ecosystems, including wetlands and grasslands, play a key role in reducing pollution levels and particulate matter in water, as well as absorbing storm-water run-off. Wetlands can reduce high levels of nutrients, and some water plants concentrate toxic materials in their tissues, thus purifying surrounding water. For example, Florida's cypress swamps remove 98% of all nitrogen and 97% of all phosphorus from wastewater entering the wetlands. Natural wetlands also help dilute contaminants derived from upstream agriculture, thus ameliorating water quality in agriculturally-dominated landscapes in the world's major river basins (Dudley and Stolton 2003).

However, maintaining healthy ecosystems to provide these environmental benefits, such as adequate water supplies for agriculture and domestic use, will become an increasingly challenging issue with climate change, habitat degradation and biodiversity loss, especially in the developing world (Dudley et al. 2010; WCPA 2011). In South Africa, for instance, invasive alien species are estimated to affect ten million hectares (more than 8% of the land area) with significant ecological and economic costs. With high evapotranspiration rates, invasive alien trees are an immense burden to already water-scarce regions and reduce the amount of water available to reservoirs, industry and downstream agriculture. Large-scale programmes to remove these species are being undertaken in many of South Africa's watersheds, providing benefits to biodiversity, water supplies and employment opportunities for poor and disenfranchised communities under the Working for Water Programme (World Bank 2010).

The multiple roles of protected areas will become more valuable as climatic events become more severe, helping to reduce the impact of natural hazards and disasters and buffering vulnerable communities against all but the most severe flood and tidal events, landslides and storms (Stolton et al. 2008). Intact mangroves provide protection and reduce the damage caused by tsunamis and hurricanes, while also harbouring vital fish nurseries. In Sri Lanka, the Muthurajawella marsh near Colombo affords flood protection valued at over US$5 million/year (Costanza et al. 2008). In some cases, investments in protecting and restoring natural habitats may be more cost-effective for reducing disaster risk than investing in hard infrastructure alone. In Vietnam, where local communities have been planting and protecting mangrove forests as a buffer against storms, an initial investment of $1.1 million has saved an estimated $7.3 million a year in sea dyke maintenance and significantly reduced the loss of life and property from Typhoon Wukong in 2000 in comparison with other areas (IFRC 2002).

Although the value of ecosystem services in terms of water regulation and supply of clean water alone has been estimated at US$2.3 trillion globally (Costanza et al. 1997), very little of this potential value is spent on ensuring that these ecosystem functions are sustained. Many protected area systems are inadequately funded (Watson et al. 2014). One promising trend is the implementation of payment for ecosystem services (PES) schemes to compensate protected areas, upstream communities, indigenous peoples and private landowners for maintaining forests and other water-regulating habitats, such as those being piloted in Colombia, Ecuador, Mexico and Nicaragua (WCPA 2012).

16.2.2 Local and Global Medicines

Natural ecosystems are an important source of local, traditional and global medicines. Indeed, more species of medicinal plants are harvested than of any other natural product, and many rural and urban communities, especially in the developing world, rely on medicinal plants for primary health-care (Stolton and Dudley 2010). The economic value of medicinal plants and their extracts and drug derivatives has been estimated in billions of dollars (Ahn 2017). Today many of these plants are conserved only in protected areas; indeed, some protected areas have been specifically established to protect plants used in traditional medicines. A good example is the Alto Orito Indi-Ande Medicinal Plants Sanctuary in Colombia proposed by the indigenous Kofán communities (Stolton and Dudley 2010).

The value of protected areas to provide primary and affordable health-care products is a global phenomenon. Medical drugs derived from natural products support a huge pharmaceutical industry; over half of today's synthetic medicines originate from natural species, including drugs like aspirin, digitalis and quinine. Bioprospecting in protected areas has already turned up compounds that are being used, or are in the process of development, for combatting high blood pressure, cancer, leukaemia, HIV, enlarged prostate and malaria, and for antibacterial and antifungal treatments. Protected areas are important sources of herbs and medicinal plants that provide important health-care, social, cultural and livelihood benefits to local people (Stolton and Dudley 2010).

16.2.3 Provision of Direct Health Benefits

There is growing evidence that access to protected areas, ecological reserves, wetlands and forest areas and other natural spaces sustains a variety of physical, psychological and social benefits and enhances the health and well-being of people across their lifespan (Sandifer et al. 2015; Townsend et al. 2015). In Australia, Parks Victoria's Healthy Parks Healthy People (HPHP) programme recognises that parks are fundamental to vibrant and healthy communities, fostering social connections that are vital to community cohesion and contribute to social well-being (Townsend et al. 2015). Recreation and time spent in protected areas can be linked to physical and mental health benefits among adults, including the elderly, while research has shown that parks foster active play in children and improve mental and social health of adolescents during what is often a challenging time of life (Townsend et al. 2015).

Several countries have now adopted HPHP programmes in their national parks and protected areas, including national parks in the USA, Colombia, Finland and New Zealand. Many studies find that access to protected areas and other green and blue spaces increases levels of physical activity and consequently physical and mental health, although the relationship varies between type of activity and population group, and is affected by other factors such as perceived safety and distance to amenities (Hartig et al. 2014). In India, for example, Keoladeo National Park provides free access to a designated 2-km stretch that up to a thousand 'morning walkers' enjoy every day between 5 a.m. and 7 a.m. Similarly, in the UK, many protected areas actively promote outdoor activity programmes, such as the 'Green Gym' scheme (Trust for Conservation Volunteers 2016) and the Walking for Health programme (Marselle et al. 2014), which use the natural environment as a health resource. In Japan, Shinrin-yoku is the traditional practice of taking in the atmosphere and energy of the forest to improve health and reduce stress (Dudley et al. 2010). Building on the therapeutic effects of nature, the Victoria HPHP programme has developed long-term cooperation with mental health facilities to bring patients into parks and protected areas. This increased physical activity and access to green space has clear benefits for physical health, while nature can reduce feelings of anger, sadness and anxiety (Hartig et al. 2014).

A growing body of evidence is also demonstrating that the sense of connectedness with nature that results from positive nature-based experiences, whether in a city, a national park, or another natural ecosystem, leads to the development of positive attitudes and behaviours towards nature and its protection (Wright and Matthews 2014; Teisl and O'Brien 2003). Policies and programmes that create opportunities for greater access to nature thus have the added benefit of building public support for biodiversity conservation and political will for the protection of intact natural ecosystems that underpin human health and well-being (for more information, see Davies et al. Chap. 12, this volume).

16.3 Nature and Health in an Urban Setting

Many of the benefits that derive from protected areas in the broader landscape also apply to natural spaces in urban settings. Urbanisation both intensifies biodiversity loss and presents its own unique health and lifestyle challenges and opportunities. Cities are dependent on surrounding natural landscapes and protected areas to provide critical ecosystem services, but parks, waterways and river corridors can provide links and 'stepping stones' from cities to the broader landscape. Maintaining natural habitats and green and blue spaces within cities can also provide ecosystem services that are important for climate change adaptation.

Urban parks, green spaces and wetlands absorb rainwater and stormwater run-off and alleviate air pollution. The roles and benefits of natural ecosystems as green infrastructure will become more important with climate change (Beatley 2014). Tree cover in urban settings has been shown to reduce rainwater run-off and reduce flood risk. A study of street trees in Manchester, UK, found that surface runoff was up to 62% lower in asphalt plots with a tree planted in the middle compared to asphalt plots with no trees. Grass plots almost completely prevented surface runoff, and therefore reduced flood risk (Armson et al. 2013; Lindley et al. Chap. 2, this volume). Similarly, urban green spaces can help reduce air pollution. More than three million people globally die each year from outdoor air pollution (WHO 2016). A study by the University of Exeter's medical school into the impact of urban greenery on asthma suggests that respiratory health can be improved by the expansion of tree cover in very polluted urban neighbourhoods (Alcock et al. 2017). In the UK, over 5.4 million people receive treatment for asthma, with an annual cost to the National Health Service of around £1 billion; asthma is estimated to lead to over 1,000 deaths a year. The findings of these studies provide strong evidence for promoting the role of trees in urban planning and public health policy.

Increasing urbanisation and changing lifestyles have resulted in more people spending less time in nature, doing less physical activity, and experiencing greater stress, and negative health outcomes such as greater obesity and physical and men-

Box 16.2: Addressing the Nature-Deficit Disorder

Richard Louv (2005) coined the term 'nature-deficit disorder' to describe the range of behavioural problems, such as diminished use of the senses, attention difficulties, and higher rates of physical and emotional illnesses, that result from less time spent outdoors. Protected areas, urban parks and other green spaces are crucial gateways for connecting people with nature (IUCN, Canadian Parks Council 2017; IUCN 2014). Although towns and cities may have considerably lower species densities than surrounding rural areas, urban settings can be important for biodiversity conservation and provide natural environments that can contribute to human health and well-being in many ways (IUCN 2014). For example, the Golden Gates National Recreational Area in San Francisco, California, USA, is important for both nature and health. It contains a range of marine, coastal and terrestrial habitats that support 1,300 animal and plant species, including 36 threatened species. It also includes an area of ancient redwood forest protected as a national monument. An institute of the non-profit cooperating association of the recreational area uses the park to pilot-test new ideas for using parks as solutions to wider social challenges. One of its projects aims to promote healthy and sustainable food choices in the park and to use the National Park Service's purchasing power to influence the food supply chain to address obesity, type 2 diabetes and other health issues (IUCN 2014).

tal health problems (see Box 16.2). Access to nature in urban environments can also provide benefits for physical and mental health and contribute to children's cognitive, physical and social development (Russell et al. 2013). Similarly, a recent study in New Zealand found that risk of cardiovascular disease was lower in neighbourhoods with more than 15% green space than those without (Richardson et al. 2013). Natural spaces present a cost-effective, high-return investment that provide direct benefits for public health and education, improve living conditions, and build resilience to climate and environmental change.

Several major cities now have protected and conserved areas and even national parks within or directly adjacent to the metropolitan areas (IUCN 2014). These range from small wetland areas managed by an NGO in central London and urban protected areas in central Sydney and Rio de Janeiro to the much larger Table Mountain National Park, which covers some 25,000 hectares in the centre of Cape Town, South Africa, which protects key habitats and Cape flora in the world's smallest floral kingdom. These parks come under a range of governance types from NGOs to park agencies and municipal authorities, including co-management arrangements (IUCN 2014). They provide a range of services including conservation, recreation, tourism, health benefits and water resource management, as well as providing opportunities for visitors to learn about biodiversity conservation and the impacts of climate change (see Box 16.3).

Box 16.3: ClimateWatch Trails for Schools and Communities (Australia)
ClimateWatch is a national citizen science programme designed to enable every Australian to be involved in collecting and recording data that helps shape the country's scientific response to climate change.

Parks and protected areas provide ideal locations in which to assess the impacts of climate change as they provide scientists with information on landscapes in contrast with developed and urban areas. ClimateWatch trails are a great opportunity for park visitors to engage in long-term climate change research by recording their observations of nature.

Parks Victoria is partnering with Earthwatch Australia to develop new ClimateWatch trails in parks. The programme is aimed at schools and community groups in areas of social disadvantage from regional Victoria, encouraging students and community members to get active in the outdoors by recording data that can be used by scientists to monitor the natural environment. School-based curriculum resources have been developed as part of this programme.

The programme connects education, inclusion and citizen science, along with the numerous health and well-being benefits of connecting people from all walks of life to parks.

Source: Parks Victoria.

Urban parks and other forms of natural infrastructure can conserve healthy ecosystems and improve human health and well-being, while addressing challenges related to climate change, such as heat stress, storm surges and flooding (IUCN 2014). Maintaining and expanding both terrestrial and aquatic natural spaces must therefore be a key consideration in urban planning if the health of residents is a priority. Since cities also depend on and affect their surroundings, planners should also consider connections between cities and the broader landscapes in order to ensure that impacts on natural ecosystems are minimised and positive contributions to biodiversity conservation are maximised (see also Heiland et al. Chap. 19, this volume). This is challenging to do effectively and equitably, given the conflicting demands for land, resources and development, particularly in developing and rapidly urbanising parts of the world. Therefore, it is important that biodiversity conservation is recognised as a valuable contribution to a range of policy objectives, such as job opportunities, youth and community development, public health, water, energy and adaptation to climate change.

Recommendations from the IUCN World Parks Congress in Sydney in 2014 (IUCN 2014) and the New Urban Agenda (United Nations 2016), agreed at Habitat III in Quito in 2016, recognise the relevance of protected areas and nature to sustainable cities. Other global policy processes have also explicitly made the connection between nature and health. The UNFCCC Paris Agreement recognised and promoted the valuable role of ecosystem-based adaptation, including protected areas, to address climate change impacts (United Nations 2015). The Convention on

Biological Diversity (CBD) COP13 Cancun Declaration on Mainstreaming the Conservation and Sustainable Use of Biodiversity for Well-being indicates that the Parties commit to "promote the conservation, sustainable use, and where necessary, restoration of ecosystems as a basis for achieving good health" (CBD COP13, 2016). At the IUCN World Conservation Congress in Hawai'i a resolution was adopted (IUCN WCC-2016-Res-064-EN) to strengthen cross-sector partnerships to recognise the contributions of nature to health, well-being and quality of life. See Korn et al. Chap. 14, this volume, for more detail on the policy support for biodiversity, health and climate change.

One way to increase health benefits is to incorporate nature-based solutions in urban policy through targets for the provision of parks and green spaces within a certain distance of people's homes (Shanahan et al. 2015). For example, East Dunbartonshire Council in Scotland sets out standards for the quantity, quality and accessibility of open space, including parks, gardens, play areas and nature reserves, for its population (East Dunbartonshire Council 2015). It is interesting to note that, along with other commitments to biodiversity conservation and environmental protection, the UK's new 25-Year Plan for the Environment includes the following commitment: "Making sure that there are high quality, accessible, natural spaces close to where people live and work, particularly in urban areas, and encouraging more people to spend time in them to benefit their health and well-being" (Her Majesty's Government 2018). Integrated policy and programmes that recognise the increasingly important contribution of nature and parks for our physical, mental, cultural and spiritual health and well-being are essential (see Box 16.4).

The close links between biodiversity conservation and health are also recognised in the *Victorian public health and well-being plan 2015–19* and Victoria's new biodiversity plan (State of Victoria Department of Environment, Land, Water and Planning 2017). The biodiversity plan was launched in 2017 at the 15th World Congress on Public Health in Melbourne accompanied by a joint ministerial statement, the Victorian Memorandum for Health and Nature (D'Ambrosio and Hennessy 2017). The memorandum provides direction for the Victorian Government's health and environment portfolios to collaborate in order to maximise the public health benefits that are associated with being in nature. Victorian Government departments and agencies are now developing a joint work programme that aligns with the Memorandum. This cross-government collaboration gives a mandate for strengthening partnerships across the health and environment sectors. It has also resulted in increased recognition of the contributions of nature to health, well-being and quality of life. This will ultimately lead to better public health outcomes and better environmental outcomes.

Protected areas, urban parks and other green and blue spaces not only benefit health and biodiversity but can often achieve significant cost savings in delivering health-care. For example, an evaluation of the largest 85 cities in the USA, covering a population of 57.2 million, identified an estimated $3.08 billion of cost savings in health-care due to the health benefits of parks (Healthy Parks Healthy People 2017). Similarly, Parks Victoria, Australia, has estimated that Victoria's parks may save up to $200 million annually in avoided health-care costs through physical activity in nature (Parks Victoria 2015). The cost savings for health-care also extend to mental

Box 16.4: Conservation and Health Benefits of Rouge National Urban Park, Canada

Protected areas in and near urban areas can have significant benefits for biodiversity conservation and human health and well-being. Canada's first national urban park – Rouge National Urban Park – was created in the Greater Toronto Area in 2015, thanks to the efforts of Parks Canada, and a diverse partnership of countless individuals, indigenous partners, other levels of government, the park's farming community, community organisations, conservation groups and volunteers.

Once fully established, Rouge National Urban Park will be one of the largest and best protected urban parks globally, spanning 79.1 km^2 in the heart of Canada's largest and most diverse metropolitan area and overlapping five municipalities. The location of this park, which is within easy access for 20% of the country's population, creates an excellent opportunity to engage current and future generations of Canadians with the natural, cultural and agricultural heritage of the area.

Parks Canada is collaborating with various community partners to develop and deliver initiatives for Rouge National Urban Park visitors and Greater Toronto Area residents. One programme is specifically focussed on the health benefits of the park. The Mood Walks programme, which is run by the Canadian Mental Health Association in partnership with Hike Ontario and Conservation Ontario builds on the fact that time in nature with others can improve symptoms of existing disorders by reducing anxiety or depression (e.g. Bratman et al. 2015). Guided walks are targeted at youth aged 13–24 years who are enrolled in the Child and Adolescent Mental Health Program at the Scarborough and Rouge Hospital. The walking activities aim to help these young people improve their physical and mental health as well as their social skills by developing outdoors and conservation interests, meeting fun and interesting people, and learning more about wildlife, forests, wetlands and farms.

Source: Rouge National Urban Park 2016.

health – a recent natural capital accounting for London found that the city's green spaces provide an estimated saving of £370 million annually for mental health-care and an additional £580 million from improved physical health (Vivid Economics Ltd 2017). More research is still needed, particularly on health benefits from nature for different demographic and social groups (Shanahan et al. 2015) to maximise understanding of the socio-economic benefits of protected areas, but there are now strong arguments that biodiversity conservation can be a key contributor to addressing both climate change adaptation and health-care (see Kabisch Chap. 5, this volume, and Cook et al. Chap. 11, this volume, for more detail).

16.4 Working Together to Promote Biodiversity Conservation and Health

The 2030 Agenda for Sustainable Development and the SDGs will be the driving force behind much of the global work on sustainable development and conservation for the next decade (WCPA 2017). Biodiversity conservation, protected areas and conservation of natural ecosystems are directly relevant to many of the goals of the 2030 Agenda: to ensure healthy lives and promote well-being for all at all ages (SDG 3), water (SDG6), sustainable cities (SDG11), climate change adaptation (SDG 13) and biodiversity (SDGs 14 and 15) (WCPA 2017).

It is becoming increasingly clear that it is essential to build new partnerships to accelerate transformational change that will contribute to the well-being of people and the planet. Initiatives such as #NatureForAll, which is led by the IUCN's World Commission on Protected Areas and Commission on Education and Communication and the Salzburg Global Seminar's Parks for the Planet Forum (Salzburg Global Seminar 2015), are efforts to do just that. #NatureForAll is engaging hundreds of partner organisations to scale up efforts to raise awareness of nature and its values and to facilitate opportunities for people from all walks of life to experience, connect with and benefit from nature. The aim of this initiative is not only to improve health and well-being outcomes but also to increase cross-sectoral support and action for nature conservation by promoting the relevance of biodiversity conservation to other sectors. The Parks for the Planet Forum is a collaborative platform for transformative leadership that brings thought leaders and change-makers from diverse disciplines together to find ways to put nature at the very heart of human health and well-being, security and prosperity across the planet. These processes are calling for greater collaboration among biodiversity and natural resource experts, medical scientists, health practitioners, urban and regional planners, educators, economists and others to recognise, quantify and maximise the many health and well-being benefits to society from parks and nature both inside and outside cities.

While the provision of nature-based solutions is traditionally in the realm of environmental organisations and planners, greater involvement of the health sector will be critical for maximising benefits for both health and nature. Integrating policy on biodiversity, health and urban planning to realise joint benefits requires data from all fields to be linked and communicated to policy makers, to be considered in impact assessments and economic valuation of decisions (WHO and UNEP 2008; WHO and CBD 2015). In Toronto, Canada, for example, the City Council increased investments in urban green space in the city, including an increase in tree canopy cover, after the Medical Officer of Health cited studies on the benefits this would provide for health and reduced pollution (Toronto Medical Officer of Health 2015). Elsewhere medical practitioners and parks agencies are promoting experiences of nature as part of overall health-care (see Box 16.5).

Box 16.5: Nature Is Good Medicine

- Dr. Robert Zarr, a paediatrician at Unity Health Care's Upper Cardozo Health Center in Washington DC, prescribes physical activity in parks to treat obesity, diabetes and mental health disorders (Washington Post 2015). His **park prescription programme** is based on the multiple medical benefits of spending time outdoors. Dr. Zarr is at the forefront of a movement among physicians who are making nature a fundamental part of their patients' health-care. They are now joined by the US National Park Service and the US Public Health Service.
- The British Trust for Conservation Volunteers has been promoting **Green Gyms**, which combine conservation volunteering with physical activity through planting trees. Doctors in the UK can refer people to Green Gyms to treat problems caused by mental health disorders, social isolation and physical inactivity (Trust for Conservation Volunteers 2016).
- **Elders back on Country** – The health and well-being benefits for Aboriginal people in Australia of being on 'Country' have been well documented. Two new projects were recently initiated in the State of Victoria to enable disabled Aboriginal Elders to get Back on Country by using Trail Rider wheelchairs. Parks Victoria was awarded both a Victorian Tourism Award and the Australian Tourism Award for its disability access programme.

16.5 Looking Forward

These examples highlight the need to work together and strengthen knowledge on the health benefits of parks and nature – across government, medical professions and the community to ensure a healthy environment to support a healthy society. This starts with dialogue, policy and action plans and the integration of biodiversity and natural ecosystems in urban and regional planning and development, addressing this at the level of neighbourhoods, cities and the wider landscape.

The SDGs present an important framework for collaborative action to respond to a range of global challenges and are premised on the notion that problems cannot be solved in isolation. To achieve the multiple goals of the SDGs, it will be important to protect, manage and restore key natural ecosystems, including protected and conserved areas, to improve natural resource management and to safeguard the ecosystem services and biodiversity that contribute to human well-being. The protection and effective management of natural ecosystems within and beyond city boundaries is critical to ensuring that urban environments are buffered from the effects of climate change and that vital services such as clean air, clean water and opportunities for outdoor recreation that are essential to human health and well-being can continue to be provided to an increasingly urban population. At the same time, rapid urbanisation will continue to put pressure on protected areas and other natural ecosystems. Conservation experts, municipal governments, city planners, health professionals and others will increasingly need to work together to ensure that urban planning and development proceeds in a way that ensures the ongoing protection of these critical natural systems and equitable access to natural spaces for all sectors of society.

There are many good arguments for extending and strengthening the management of protected areas and other natural areas (Stolton and Dudley 2010), but the clear links between healthy ecosystems and healthy people seem especially relevant at a time when societies are looking for new solutions to cope with climate change. The emphasis on biodiversity conservation, protected areas and natural landscapes as nature-based solutions for human health and climate change adaptation is now supported by a range of international policies and agreements. Investments in protected areas and other nature-based solutions offer cost-effective solutions that provide direct benefits for human welfare, public health and education, and build resilience to climate and environmental change. Achieving these multiple benefits will require new partnerships across different sectors but will become increasingly necessary in a world of changing climate and increasing urbanisation.

References

Ahn K (2017) The worldwide trend of using botanical drugs and strategies for developing global drugs. BMB Rep 50(3):111–116

Alcock I, White M, Cherrie M et al (2017) Land cover and air pollution are associated with asthma hospitalisations: a cross-sectional study. Environ Int 109:29–41

Armson D, Stringer P, Ennos AR (2013) The effect of street trees and amenity grass on urban surface water runoff in Manchester, UK. Urban For Urban Green 12(3):282–286

Beatley T (2014) Blue urbanism: exploring connections between cities and oceans. Island Press, Washington, DC

Bratman N, Hamilton JP, Hahn KS et al (2015) Nature experience reduces rumination and subgenual prefrontal cortex activation. PNAS 112(28):8567–8572

Convention on Biological Diversity (CBD) COP13 (2016) Cancun declaration on mainstreaming the conservation and sustainable use of biodiversity for well-being. https://www.cbd.int/cop/cop-13/hls/cancun%20declaration-en.pdf. Accessed 30 May 2018

Costanza R, d'Arge R, de Groot R et al (1997) The value of the world's ecosystem services and natural capital. Nature 387:253–260

Costanza R, Mageau M, Aquatic Ecology (1999) What is a healthy ecosystem. Aquat Ecol 33:105–115

Costanza R, Pérez-Maqueo O, Martinez ML et al (2008) The value of coastal wetlands to hurricane prevention. Ambio 37:241–248

D'Ambrosio L, Hennessy J (2017) Victorian Memorandum for health and nature. https://www.environment.vic.gov.au/biodiversity/victorian-memorandum-for-health-and-nature. Accessed 30 May 2018

Dudley N, Stolton S (2003) Running pure: the importance of forest protected areas to drinking water. WWF/Gland/World Bank, Washington, DC

Dudley N, Stolton S, Belokurov A et al (eds) (2010) Natural solutions: protected areas helping people cope with climate change. IUCN/World Bank/WWF, Gland

East Dunbartonshire Council (2015) East dunbartonshire open space strategy 2015–2020
Gelsthorpe J (2017) Disconnect from nature and its effect on health and Well-being: a public engagement literature review. Natural History Museum, London
Gómez-Baggethun E, Gren A, Barton DN (2013) Urban ecosystem services. In: Elmqvist T, Fragkias M, Goodness J et al (eds) Urbanization, biodiversity and ecosystem services: challenges and opportunities. A global assessment. Springer, Dordrecht
Halpern BS (2003) The impact of marine reserves: do reserves work and does reserve size matter? Ecol Appl 13:117–137
Hartig T, Mitchell R, de Vries S et al (2014) Nature and health. Annu Rev Public Health 35:207–228
Healthy Parks Healthy People (2017) Urban planning and the importance of green space in cities to human and environmental health. http://www.hphpcentral.com/article/urban-planning-and-the-importance-of-green-space-in-cities-to-human-and-environmental-health. Accessed 31 May 2018
HM Government (2018) A green future: Our 25-year plan to improve the environment. https://www.gov.uk/government/uploads/system/uploads/attachment_data/file/693158/25-year-environment-plan.pdf. Accessed 31 May 2018
International Federation of Red Cross and Red Crescent Societies (IFRC) (2002) Mangrove planting saves lives and money in Vietnam. World disasters report focus on reducing risk. IFRC, Geneva
International Union for the Conservation of Nature (2014) Urban protected areas: profiles and best practice guidelines. IUCN, Gland
International Union for the Conservation of Nature (2016a) World conservation congress resolution Res-064-EN, to strengthen cross-sector partnerships to recognise the contributions of nature to health, well-being and quality of life. https://www.iucn.org/sites/dev/files/content/documents/wcc_2016_res_064_en.pdf. Accessed 31 May 2018
International Union for the Conservation of Nature (2016b) Nature-based solutions to address global societal challenges. IUCN, Gland
International Union for the Conservation of Nature, Canadian Parks Council (2017) The #NatureForAll Playbook. An action guide for inspiring love of nature. https://natureforall.global/s/NatureForAll-Playbook-ENG.pdf. Accessed 31 May 2018
Louv R (2005) Last child in the woods: saving our children from nature-deficit disorder. Algonquin Books, Chapel Hill
Marselle MR, Irvine KN, Warber SL (2014) Examining group walks in nature and multiple aspects of well-being: a large scale study. Ecopsychology 6:134–147. https://doi.org/10.1089/eco.2014.0027
Mcdonald RI, Kareiva P, Forman RTT (2008) The implications of current and future urbanization for global protected areas and biodiversity conservation. Biol Conserv 141:1695–1703
Parks Victoria (2015) Valuing Victoria's Parks. http://parkweb.vic.gov.au/__data/assets/pdf_file/0008/666350/Valuing-Victorias-parks.pdf. Accessed 30 May 2018
Richardson EA, Pearce J, Mitchell R et al (2013) Role of physical activity in the relationship between urban green space and health. Public Health 127(4):318–324
Russell R, Guerry AD, Balvanera P et al (2013) Humans and nature: how knowing and experiencing nature affect well-being. Annu Rev Environ Resour 38:473–502
Salzburg Global Seminar (2015) Parks for the planet forum, nature, health and a new urban generation. http://www.salzburgglobal.org/topics/article/parks-for-the-planet-forum-nature-health-and-a-new-urban-generation-report-now-online.html. Accessed 31 May 2018
Sandifer PA, Sutton-Grier AE, Ward BP (2015) Exploring connections among nature, biodiversity, ecosystem services, and human health and Well-being: opportunities to enhance health and biodiversity conservation. Ecosyst Serv 12:1–15
Shanahan DF, Lin BB, Bush R et al (2015) Toward improved public health outcomes from urban nature. Am J Public Health 105(3):470–477
State of Victoria Department of Environment, Land, Water and Planning (2017) Protecting Victoria's environment – biodiversity 2037. https://www.environment.vic.gov.au/biodiversity/biodiversity-plan. Accessed 31 May 2018

Stolton S, Dudley N (2010) Arguments for protected areas: multiple benefits for conservation and use. Earthscan, London

Stolton S, Dudley N, Randall J (2008) Natural security: protected areas and hazard mitigation. WWF, Gland

Teisl MF, O'Brien K (2003) Who cares and who acts? Outdoor recreationists exhibit different levels of environmentalism. Environ Behav 35(4):506–522

Toronto Medical Officer of Health (2015) Green city: why nature matters to health, Report for Toronto Board of Health. Toronto Public Health, Toronto

Townsend M, Henderson-Wilson C, Warner E et al (2015) Healthy parks healthy people: the state of the evidence. Parks Victoria, Melbourne

Trust for Conservation Volunteers (TCV) (2016) Green gym evaluation report 2016. https://www.tcv.org.uk/sites/default/files/green-gym-evaluation-report-2016.pdf. Accessed 31 May 2018

United Nations (2014) World urbanisation prospects, 2014 revision. https://esa.un.org/unpd/wup. Accessed 31 May 2018

United Nations (2015) Paris agreement. https://unfccc.int/process-and-meetings/the-paris-agreement/the-paris-agreement. Accessed 31 May 2018

United Nations (2016) Draft outcome document of the United Nations conference on housing and sustainable urban development (Habitat III). New Urban Agenda. http://habitat3.org/the-new-urban-agenda. Accessed 31 May 2018

Vivid Economics Ltd (2017) Natural capital accounts for public green space in London. Report prepared for Greater London Authority, National Trust and Heritage Lottery Fund. https://www.london.gov.uk/what-we-do/environment/parks-green-spaces-and-biodiversity/green-infrastructure/natural-capital?source=vanityurl. Accessed 31 May 2018

Washington Post (2015) D.C. doctor's Rx: a stroll in the park instead of a trip to the pharmacy. https://www.washingtonpost.com/national/health-science/why-one-dc-doctor-is-prescribing-walks-in-the-park-instead-of-pills/2015/05/28/03a54004-fb45-11e4-9ef4-1bb7ce3b3fb7_story.html?utm_term=.41bc02788294. Accessed 31 May 2018

Watson J, Dudley N, Segan DB et al (2014) The performance and potential of protected areas. Nature 515:67–73

World Bank (2010) Convenient solutions to an inconvenient truth: ecosystem-based approaches to climate change. World Bank, Washington, DC

World Commission on Protected Areas (WCPA) (2011) Natural solutions: protected areas helping people to cope with climate change. https://portals.iucn.org/library/sites/library/files/documents/Rep-2011-021.pdf. Accessed 31 May 2018

World Commission on Protected Areas (WCPA) (2012) Natural solutions: protected areas maintaining essential water supplies. https://www.iucn.org/sites/dev/files/import/downloads/natsols_water_flyer_final.pdf. Accessed 31 May 2018

World Commission on Protected Areas (WCPA) (2015) Natural solutions: protected areas are vital for human health and well-being. https://www.iucn.org/sites/dev/files/import/downloads/natural_solutions_pas__health_and_well_being.pdf. Accessed 31 May 2018

World Commission on Protected Areas (WCPA) (2017) Natural solutions: protected areas helping to meet the sustainable development goals. https://www.iucn.org/sites/dev/files/natural_solutions_-_sdgs_final_2.pdf. Accessed 31 May 2018

World Health Organisation (2005) Preventing chronic diseases: a vital investment. World Health Organisation, Geneva

World Health Organisation (2014) Global status report on non-communicable diseases. World Health Organisation, Geneva

World Health Organisation and Secretariat of the Convention on Biological Diversity (2015) Connecting global priorities: biodiversity and human health. A state of knowledge review. World Health Organisation/Secretariat of the Convention on Biological Diversity, Geneva

World Health Organisation (WHO) 2016 Ambient air pollution: A global assessment of exposure and burden of disease. World Health Organisation, Geneva.

World Health Organisation and United Nations Environment Programme (2008) Health and environment: managing the linkages for sustainable development. A toolkit for decision makers. World Health Organisation, Geneva

Wright P, Matthews C (2014) Building a culture of conservation: state-of-knowledge report on connecting people to nature in parks. http://cpaws.org/uploads/buildingacultureofconservation-web.pdf. Accessed 31 May 2018

Chapter 17
Environmental, Health and Equity Effects of Urban Green Space Interventions

Ruth F. Hunter, Anne Cleary, and Matthias Braubach

Abstract As populations become increasingly urbanised, the preservation of urban green space becomes paramount. Despite the potential from cross-sectional evidence, we know little about how to design new, or improve or promote existing, urban green space for environmental, health and well-being benefits. This chapter highlights aspects to be considered when designing and evaluating urban green space interventions that aim to maximize environmental, social and health benefits, and address equity issues. Based on a review of international research evidence and a compilation of European case studies, the chapter addresses the variety of green space intervention approaches and their related impacts. There was strong evidence to support park-based and greenway/trail interventions employing a dual-approach (i.e. a physical change to the urban green space and promotion/marketing programmes particularly for park use and physical activity); strong evidence for the greening of vacant lots for health, well-being (e.g. reduction in stress) and social (e.g. reduction in crime) outcomes; strong evidence for the provision of urban street trees and green infrastructure for storm water management for environmental outcomes (e.g. increased biodiversity, reduced air pollution, climate change adaptation). Urban green space has an important role to play in creating a culture of health and well-being. Results show promising evidence to support the use of certain urban green space interventions for health, social and environmental benefits. The findings have important implications for policymakers, practitioners and researchers.

R. F. Hunter (✉)
UKCRC Centre of Excellence for Public Health/Centre for Public Health, Queen's University Belfast, Belfast, Northern Ireland, UK
e-mail: ruth.hunter@qub.ac.uk

A. Cleary
School of Medicine, Menzies Health Institute Queensland, Griffith University, Gold Coast, Queensland, Australia
e-mail: anne.cleary@griffithuni.edu.au

M. Braubach
European Centre for Environment and Health, WHO Regional Office for Europe, Bonn, Germany
e-mail: braubachm@who.int

M. R. Marselle et al. (eds.), *Biodiversity and Health in the Face of Climate Change*, https://doi.org/10.1007/978-3-030-02318-8_17

Keywords Urban green space · Interventions · Health · Well-being · Environment · Equity

Highlights We know little about how to design new, or improve or promote existing, urban green space for health and social outcomes.

- Interventions should employ a dual approach that incorporates promotion and marketing of urban green space as well as changing the physical environment.
- There is evidence to support a range of environmental, health and social benefits.
- Little is known about the equity impact of urban green space interventions.

17.1 Introduction

The links between green space and health are increasingly well understood and have been summarised in numerous publications (Frumkin et al. 2017; WHO 2016). More than half of the world's population lives in urban areas (i.e. towns and cities), and this number is projected to increase to two in three people by 2050. Providing adequate green space within urban areas is therefore paramount. We need to preserve, enhance and promote existing urban green spaces and create new ones. Of course, for green space to provide its intended benefits it must be maintained and well cared for. Certain types of green space, such as vacant lots, have well-reported negative impacts (Branas et al. 2011).

Various political frameworks underscore the need for suitable green spaces in our cities. For example, the New Urban Agenda calls for an increase in safe, inclusive, accessible, green and quality public spaces. Similarly, the 2030 Agenda for Sustainable Development pledges to "provide universal access to safe, inclusive and accessible, green and public spaces, in particular, for women and children, older persons and persons with disabilities" (see Heiland et al. Chap. 19, this volume, for more on landscape planning legislation).

However, despite this growing interest in and support for urban green space, current knowledge is reasonably limited regarding the effectiveness of interventions related to the environment, health, well-being and equity. The evidence of the impact of such interventions on biodiversity and climate change adaptation is particularly scarce. This may be because there is limited understanding of the mechanisms through which green space might impact climate change. A previous review by the WHO Regional Office for Europe investigated the various mechanisms through which urban green space impacts human health (WHO Regional Office for Europe 2016), including by improving mental health and reducing the risk of cardiovascular disease, obesity, type II diabetes and cancer. Purported mechanisms included increased physical activity, reduced exposure to air and noise pollution, and psychological relaxation. However, the mechanisms through which urban green space impacts climate change are much less understood.

To address the gaps in our understanding on the effectiveness of urban green space interventions, the WHO Regional Office for Europe gathered experts on green space and urban planning to discuss approaches to and experiences with urban green space interventions. Based on a review of international research evidence and a compilation of European case studies (WHO Regional Office for Europe 2017), the expert meeting addressed the variety of green space intervention approaches and their related impacts on environmental conditions, health status, social and mental well-being, and equity. This chapter outlines the findings from this research, highlighting aspects to be considered when designing and evaluating urban green space interventions that aim to maximize environmental, social and health benefits and to address equity issues.

17.2 Urban Green Space Interventions

17.2.1 What Are Urban Green Space Interventions?

Urban green spaces are considered to be urban spaces covered by vegetation of any kind. This includes smaller green space features (such as street trees and roadside vegetation), green spaces not available for public access or recreational use (such as green roofs and facades, or green space on private grounds), and larger green spaces that provide various social and recreational functions (such as parks, playgrounds or greenways).

Urban green space interventions are defined as urban green space changes that significantly modify green space availability and features by creating new green space, changing or improving existing green space, or removing or replacing green space. The use of the term ‘urban green spaces’ should not be considered to conflict with other commonly used terms and definitions, such as ‘green infrastructure’, ‘green corridors’ or ‘public open space’, which tend to be applied in urban and regional planning.

On the basis of the evidence review, four main categories of urban green space interventions were identified:

1. *Park-based*: Involve change to the physical environment only, or use a dual approach combining a change to the physical environment with programming or marketing events in order to promote use of parks.
2. *Greenways/trails*: Development of new greenways (typically continuous linear corridor of green space facilitating walking, cycling and other activities) and walking/cycling trails, or the modification of existing greenways or walking/cycling trails, for example, through the addition of signage, or using a dual approach (see above).

3. *Greening*: Generally aesthetic-based interventions including greening of vacant lots (typically involving removing rubbish, planting trees) and providing street trees.
4. *Green infrastructure*: For environmental purposes such as storm water management or cooling urban/suburban areas, representing benefits related to the ecosystem service approach (provisioning and regulation of environmental goods and services).

These four categories, while not considered to be exhaustive or absolute, broadly represent the majority of green space interventions currently being applied in urban settings.

The methodologies for undertaking the evidence and case-study reviews are detailed elsewhere (WHO Regional Office for Europe 2017). Briefly, the evidence review searched eight electronic databases (Medline, PsycINFO, Web of Science (Science and Social Science Citation Indices), PADDI (Planning Architecture Design Database Ireland), Zetoc, Scopus, Greenfiles, SIGLE (System for Information on Grey Literature in Europe)). Studies were included if they: (i) evaluated an urban green space intervention; and (ii) measured health, well-being, social or environmental outcome(s). Interventions involving any age group were included. Interventions must have involved: (i) physical change to green space in an urban-context including improvements to existing urban green space or development of new urban green space, or (ii) a combination of physical change to urban green space supplemented by a specific urban green space awareness, marketing or promotion programme to encourage use of urban green space. The case studies were submitted to the WHO in response to a call on urban green space interventions. An online survey questionnaire was used to gather data on characteristics of green space, type of intervention, project objectives and outcomes, impacts of the interventions, and lessons learned.

A summary of the evidence base for each intervention category and equity impacts, and case study examples illustrating intervention approaches are provided below.

17.2.2 Park-Based Interventions

There was strong evidence to support the use of park-based interventions that specifically combined a physical change to green space and promotion/marketing programmes, particularly for increasing park use and encouraging physical activity (7/7 studies showing a significant intervention effect) (see Table 17.1). A number of the studies in the review included control groups. Control groups allow researchers to assess whether the findings from the intervention tested are due solely to the intervention and help rule out alternate explanations. Typically control groups included green space sites that did not undergo any intervention (e.g. no change to the physical environment, and no new marketing events) during the study period,

Table 17.1 Summary of park-based interventions

Reference	Study design	Population	Intervention	Outcome
Cohen et al. (2009a) Los Angeles, CA, USA	Quasi-experiment: controlled, pre-post design	Predominantly Latino and African-American and low-income neighbourhood	5 parks (mean 8 acres) underwent major improvements including new/improved gyms, picnic areas, walking paths, playgrounds, watering and landscaping (cost: >$1 m each) Parks ranged from 3.4 to 16 acres (mean 8 acres) and served an average of 67,000 people within a 1-mile radius. Parks contained multi-purpose fields; playgrounds; gymnastics areas; and picnic and lawn areas.	−ve: Overall park use and PA declined in both intervention and control parks
Cohen et al. (2009b) Los Angeles, CA, USA	Quasi-experiment: controlled, pre-post design	Youths and seniors living within 2 mile radius of parks	2 parks (48–67 acres) underwent renovations: (1) improvements to skate park surfaces only (cost $3.5 m) (2) improvements to entrance, courtyard areas and gymnasium of senior centre (cost $3.3 m)	−ve: 510% increase in skate park use compared to 77% in comparison skate park Substantially fewer users of senior centre
Quigg et al. (2011) Dunedin, New Zealand	Quasi-experiment: controlled, pre-post design	Children aged 5–10 years from the local community	2 community playgrounds: (1) playground had 10 new components installed, including play equipment, seating, additional safety surfacing, and waste facilities; (2) playground had 2 new play equipment pieces installed	−ve: No statistically sig. difference in total daily PA compared with control.
Cohen et al. (2012) Los Angeles, CA, USA	Quasi-experiment: controlled, pre-post design	Residents within 1 mile radius of intervention parks	12 parks (mean 14 acres) involving installation of Family Fitness zones (outdoor gyms), 8 pieces of equipment at each park (average cost $45,000 for each park), mean park size 14.4 acres (range, 1–29 acres); served an average of 40,964 individuals within 1-mile radius	−ve: Park usage increased by 11% compared to control parks (not sig.)
Veitch et al. (2012) Victoria, Australia	Quasi-experiment: controlled, pre-post design	Most disadvantaged decile in state of Victoria	1 park (size 25,200 m^2): involving establishment of a fenced leash-free area for dogs (12,800 m^2); an all-abilities playground; a 365 m walking track; BBQ area; landscaping; fencing to prevent motor vehicle access to the park	+ve: Sig. increase from pre to post-improvement in number of park users for intervention park (T1 = 235, T3 = 985) and number of people walking (T1 = 155, T3 = 369) and being vigorously active (T1 = 38, T3 = 257)

(continued)

Table 17.1 (continued)

Reference	Study design	Population	Intervention	Outcome
Bohn-Goldhaum et al. (2013) Sydney, Australia	Quasi-experiment: controlled, pre-post design	2–12 year olds and their parents or care givers; low socioeconomic neighbourhood	1 park underwent renovations: new children's play equipment, upgrading paths, adding new greenery, lighting and facilities (e.g., park furniture), green space was created by opening the adjacent sports field to public use	−ve: No sig. difference between parks for usage or the number of children engaging in MVPA at follow-up. In the intervention park the number of girls engaging in MVPA significantly decreased ($p = 0.04$) between baseline and follow-up
Cohen et al. (2014) Los Angeles, CA, USA	Quasi-experiment: post data only	Residents living within 0.5 mile radius of parks; minority populations	Creation of 3 pocket parks (0.15–0.32 acres) from vacant lots and undesirable urban parcels; playground equipment and benches installed, walking path developed around the perimeter, all fenced and enclosed by lockable gates (average cost $1 m per park funded by local non-profit groups)	−ve: Pocket parks were used as frequently or more often than playground areas in neighborhood parks. However, they were vacant during the majority of observations
Peschardt and Stigsdotter (2014) Copenhagen, Denmark	Natural experiment: pre-post design	52% male; 88% Danish	A pocket park (932 m^2) in a dense urban area was redesigned to increase seating areas and walking trails	−ve: No sig. change in number of park users but demographics of park users changed slightly with more men, people aged 15–29 and more educated people using the park
Droomers et al. (2015), Gubbels et al. (2016), 24 most deprived neighbourhoods, Netherlands	Quasi-experiment: controlled, pre-post design	Adolescents (12–15 years) and adults in severely deprived neighbourhoods	Dutch District Approach (five million euros): new public parks replacing vacant land (n = 9), refurbishing existing parks (n = 9), n = 6 improving paths, drainage, landscaping, planting flower bulbs in front yards; constructing wall gardens; greening streets, developing a greenway	−ve: Intervention areas did not show more favourable changes in PA and general health compared to all the different groups of control areas for adults

NSW Health (2002) Sydney, Australia	Quasi-experiment: controlled, pre-post design	Residents aged 25–65 years	3 types of interventions in 3 parks: promoting PA and park use (via advertisements, walking maps), park modifications (signage, greening, improved paths, new playground) and the establishment of walking groups	+ve: Intervention group more likely to have walked in the 2 weeks prior to follow-up than control. Sig. group by gender interaction indicated, intervention males were 2.8 times more likely to walk than were males in the control ward
Tester and Baker (2009) San Francisco, CA, USA	Quasi-experiment: controlled, pre-post design	Resource poor neighbourhoods; primarily Latino community	Major renovations to two parks: lighting, fencing, artificial turf, landscaping, picnic benches, goal posts, walkways	+ve: Sig. increases of greater than fourfold magnitude among children and adults of both genders at the intervention park playfields, but not in the control park; sig. park use in non-play fields
Cohen et al. (2013) Los Angeles, CA, USA	RCT: parks randomized to 3 study arms (17 parks per study arm)	Parks users and residents living within 1 mile radius of park	2 intervention groups: (1) Park Director only; (2) Park Advisory Board-Park Director Involved in all aspects of research and in using baseline results to design park-specific interventions to increase park use and PA; Park Directors received five training sessions from a marketing consultant Each park received $4000 to spend on signage; promotional incentives; outreach and support for group activities	+ve: In both intervention parks, PA increased, generating an estimated average of 600 more visits/week/park, and 1830 more MET-hours of PA/week/park
Ward Thompson et al. (2013) Glasgow, Scotland, United Kingdom	Quasi-experiment: controlled, pre-post design	High socioeconomic deprivation areas with woods/green space within 500 m of the community	Regeneration of local community: construction of improved footpaths; clearing rubbish and signs of vandalism; signage and entrance gateways; silvicultural work to improve appearance and safety of trees and vegetation (improve views and visibility); publicity and group activities to encourage knowledge of woodlands and opportunities for use.	+ve: Quality of life sig. increased in both neighbourhoods (more in intervention) over time and a sig. difference in quality of the physical environment between sites in 2006 but not 2009. Sig. differences in perceptions of safety ($p < 0.05$) in the intervention site over time, compared with no sig. change in the control

(continued)

Table 17.1 (continued)

Reference	Study design	Population	Intervention	Outcome
King et al. (2015) Denver, CO, USA	Quasi-experiment: pre-post design	Residents of transitional housing (homeless and refugees)	Transformation of 2-acres of undeveloped green space into a recreational park and community garden The new park had clearly defined recreational spaces including a multi-purpose playing field; playground equipment; basketball court; benches, a large community garden; a walking path alongside a creek	+ve: Sig. increase in total number of people observed using the park post-intervention ($p = 0.004$); Increase in proportion of users engaging in moderate ($p = 0.007$) or vigorous PA ($p = 0.04$). Post-intervention average monthly visitors sig. increased ($p = 0.002$)
Cranney et al. (2016) Sydney, Australia	Quasi-experiment: pre-post time series design	Beachside suburb comprising relatively high socioeconomic status neighborhoods	Outdoor gym installed (60,000 Aus $), targeted marketing and promotional strategies to engage older adults and hosting exercise sessions by a professional Park is 16.08 ha, picnic shelters, barbecues, drinking fountains, toilets and change facilities, a skate park and children's playground	+ve: Small but sig. increase in senior park users engaging in MVPA at follow-up (1.6 to 5.1%; $p < 0.001$); sig. increases from baseline to follow-up in the outdoor gym area for MVPA (6–40%; $p < 0.001$); and seniors' use (1.4–6%; $p < 0.001$)
Slater et al. (2016) Chicago, IL, USA	Quasi-experimental: prospective, controlled, longitudinal design	Predominantly African American and Latino neighborhoods	Park renovations and community engagement (39 intervention parks) Renovations involved replacing old playground equipment and ground surfacing Mean park size 3.86 sq. acres (range 0.09–40.48)	+ve: Sig. increases between baseline and 12-month follow-up for park utilization and the number of people engaged in MVPA; increase in park utilization over time in intervention parks compared with control

MVPA Moderate-vigorous physical activity, *PA* physical activity, *RCT* Randomized Control Trial, *US* United States, *+ve* positive intervention effect, *−ve* no intervention effect but the green space was similar in size, with similar characteristics, and served a similar population to the intervention site.

Four studies that involved major park improvements coupled with promotion programmes showed a significantly positive post-intervention effect for: increasing usage (Tester and Baker 2009; Ward Thompson et al 2013; King et al 2015; Slater et al 2016); physical activity (Tester and Baker 2009; King et al 2015; Slater et al 2016); quality of life (Ward Thompson et al. 2013); and perception of safety (Ward Thompson et al. 2013). Tester and Baker (2009) evaluated the effects of major improvements to playing fields of two public parks as well as physical activity programmes, and training and skills development for park and recreation programme staff. Results showed that playing field improvements, with and without family and youth involvement initiatives, significantly increased visitation and overall physical activity (four- to ninefold increase) compared to the control group. Ward Thompson et al. (2013) investigated the impact of regeneration of deprived areas in Glasgow, UK. Green spaces were upgraded through clearing rubbish and signs of vandalism; construction of improved footpaths, installation of signage and entrance gateways; and publicity and organization of group activities to encourage opportunities for use. Quality of life ($p = 0.002$), perceptions of safety ($p < 0.05$) and usage ($p < 0.001$) significantly improved among local residents compared with the control site. King et al. (2015) demonstrated significant improvements in park usage ($p = 0.004$) and physical activity of users ($p = 0.007$) after the transformation of 2 acres of undeveloped green space into a recreational park (including footpaths, playing fields, benches and basketball courts) and a community garden in an area of transitional housing for the homeless and refugees.

Slater et al. (2016) showed significant improvements in park usage and physical activity levels of users over time (up to 12 months) in 39 intervention parks that undertook major improvements including replacement of old playground equipment and ground surfacing, coupled with extensive community engagement activities to encourage and promote park usage, compared with control sites.

Three studies showed significant intervention effects for minor park improvements including significant increases in walking (NSW Health 2002), park usage and physical activity of users (Cohen et al. 2013; Cranney et al. 2016). An intervention in Sydney (NSW Health 2002) involved park modifications (e.g. signage, greening, improved paths and a new playground), park promotion use via advertisements, walking maps and the establishment of walking groups. A large randomised controlled trial (RCT) by Cohen et al. (2013) involved 51 parks allocated to one of three management trials. Park Directors received training from marketing consultants regarding outreach, customer service and promotion events. Each park received $4000 to spend on park programmes, which included signage (e.g. banners, walking path signs), promotional incentives (e.g. water bottles, park-branded key chains, individually targeted e-mails), and outreach activities (e.g. hiring community engagement officers, buying activity materials). Cranney et al. (2016) investigated the effects of the provision of an outdoor gym in Sydney alongside hosting exercise sessions and targeted marketing and promotional strategies to engage older adults.

There was a small but significant increase in senior green space users engaging in moderate-vigorous physical activity at follow-up (1.6–5.1%; $p < 0.001$).

There was limited evidence regarding park-based interventions that only involved physical change to the green space (2/9 studies showed a significant intervention effect).

Two studies showed a positive outcome with increases in physical activity and park usage (Cohen et al. 2009b; Veitch et al. 2012). Cohen et al. (2009b) investigated the impact of two interventions that saw improvements made to a skate park and the green space surrounding a senior centre. Results showed a significant increase in skate park use but substantially fewer users of the green space surrounding the senior centre. There was also a significant increase in the perception of safety in both of the renovated green spaces ($p < 0.001$). An Australian study by Veitch et al. (2012) showed significant increases in the number of park users and number of people walking and being vigorously active after major park improvements (i.e. fenced leash-free area for dogs, playground, walking track, barbeque area and landscaping).

Seven studies showed no significant impact on physical activity, park usage or general health for urban green space interventions involving change to the built environment only (Cohen et al 2009a, 2012, 2014; Quigg et al 2011; Bohn-Goldhaum et al 2013; Peschardt and Stigsdotter 2014; Droomers et al 2015; Gubbels et al 2016). Cohen et al. (2009a) showed that park use and physical activity declined in parks that underwent major improvements including new/improved gyms, picnic areas, walking paths, playgrounds, watering and landscaping. A study by Quigg et al. (2011) investigated the impact of upgrading two community parks on children aged 5–10 years. Upgrades that involved installation of new play equipment, seating, additional safety surfacing, and waste facilities produced no change in physical activity levels among children.

Cohen et al. (2012) found that park usage increased by 11% compared to control parks (not statistically significant) following the installation of Family Fitness zones (i.e. outdoor gyms) in 12 parks.

The URBAN 40 study investigated the impact of changes in the quality or quantity of green space in different populations in 24 severely deprived neighbourhoods in the Netherlands. The intervention involved a suite of park-based and greening interventions (costing €5 million) to ameliorate problems with employment, education, housing, social cohesion and safety. The interventions involved: (i) provision of new public parks (from pocket parks up to 250 acres; n = 9), and (ii) renovating existing parks (n = 9). Renovations of existing parks involved: improving paths, drainage, landscaping and maintenance; planting flower bulbs in front yards; constructing wall gardens; greening streets, and/or developing a greenway. Investments were made in green space that could be utilised by residents for recreation ('green to be used') and improvements in the green appearance of the neighbourhood ('green character'). Eighteen neighbourhoods improved their parks, in half of the cases in combination with investments in the green character of the neighbourhood. Nine of these neighbourhoods invested in new public parks. The other nine neighbourhoods redeveloped and refurbished existing parks. Another six neighbourhoods improved only their green character (no parks). Repeated cross-sectional surveys from 2004 until 2011 yielded self-reported information on leisure-time walking, cycling and sports, perceived general health and mental health, of over 48,000 local residents. Results showed that the intervention sites did not show more favourable changes in physical activity and general health compared to all the different groups of control areas (Droomers et al. 2015). In a subset of these neighbourhoods, additional data were collected from the same individuals before and after the interventions (Gubbels et al. 2016). Also in this study, no significant health-related improvements were associated with the interventions, with two exceptions. Objective improvements in greenery were associated with a smaller decline in adolescents' leisure time cycling, and improvements in perceived greenery were related to a decrease in adults' depressive symptoms.

There was no evidence to support the provision of pocket parks (typically small green spaces with limited facilities or programming, if any) for increased usage and physical activity (Cohen et al. 2014; Peschardt and Stigsdotter 2014). Cohen et al. (2014) investigated the impact of the creation of three pocket parks on the number of park users and physical activity. This involved installation of playground equipment and benches and development of walking paths, and all areas were fenced and enclosed by lockable gates. Results showed that pocket parks were used as frequently or more often than playground areas in neighbourhood parks (control areas); however, they were vacant during the majority of observations. The authors concluded that pocket parks may act as catalysts for physical activity; however, additional marketing and programmes may be needed to encourage usage. Similarly, Peschardt and Stigsdotter (2014), in a dense urban area, found no significant change in number of park users following the redesign of a pocket park that increased seating areas and walking trails.

17.2.3 Greenways and Trail Interventions

There was inconclusive evidence (3/6 studies showed a significant intervention effect) to support the use of new or modified trails or greenways for promoting health benefits (see Table 17.2).

Fitzhugh et al. (2010) investigated the impact of an urban greenway trail designed to enhance connectivity of pedestrian infrastructure with nearby retail establishments and schools. The study showed significant changes between the intervention and control neighbourhoods for total physical activity ($p = 0.001$), walking ($p = 0.001$) and cycling ($p = 0.038$). A study in the USA (Clark et al. 2014) showed significantly positive effects for a marketing campaign and addition of signage for trail use. Usage of ten urban trails (six intervention and four control trails) were monitored following a marketing campaign promoting trail use and the addition of way-finding and incremental distance signage to selected trails.

Significant pre-post increases in trail usage were found for both comparison (31% increase) and intervention (35% increase) trails ($p < 0.01$). A large multisite natural experiment in the UK (n = 1796 participants) investigated the impact of new walking and cycling routes on physical activity (Sahlqvist et al. 2013; Brand et al. 2014; Goodman et al. 2014). Proximity to the intervention was strongly associated with greater use of the new infrastructure (32% of the study population reported using the new infrastructure at 1-year follow-up; 38% reported at 2-year

Case Study: Parque Ribeiro do Matadouro, Santo Tirso, Portugal

Led by the Santo Tirso municipality, the 'Parque Ribeiro do Matadouro' is a 1.54 ha park constructed on derelict land, near the Matadouro stream, close to the Santo Tirso city centre. Construction of the park was completed in 2013 costing approximately €1,400,000. This park-based intervention applied a dual approach. Open public forums engaged local community in the design of the park with feedback and suggestions from the community being included in the design (e.g. wi-fi access in the park). Guided tours occurred during the construction phase to keep the community updated on progress of the park's construction and the park's name was chosen via community voting in a naming contest. Signs, interactive art installations and organised community events within the park invite people to visit and use the park. Further work is planned to expand green space along the river to create green networks improving connectivity between Parque Ribeiro do Matadouro and other green spaces. This phase of works will also closely integrate social engagement, with community gardens and a youth house being established as part of the intervention (Fig. 17.1).

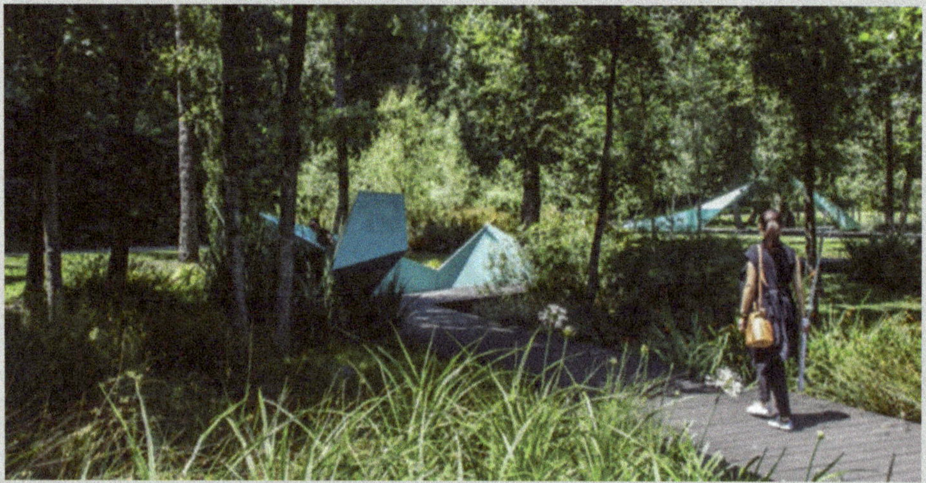

Fig. 17.1 Interactive art installations at Parque Ribeiro do Matadouro invite visitors to engage with the space. (Image: Victor Esteves, Oh!Land Studio)

Table 17.2 Summary characteristics of greenway and trail interventions

Reference	Study design	Population	Intervention	Outcome
Evenson et al. (2005) North Carolina, USA	Quasi-experimental: pre-post design	Adults aged >18 years living within 2 miles of the trail	A railway was converted to a multi-use trail Trail 2.8 miles/10 feet wide with 2 mile spur of 23 mile trail; trail passed by 2 schools, shopping areas, apartment buildings and neighbourhoods	−ve: Those who had never used the trail had sig. declines in median time spent in MVPA, vigorous PA and bicycling for transport. Those who had used the trail also had sig. declines in median time spent in vigorous PA.
Burbidge and Goulias (2009) Utah, USA	Quasi-experiment: longitudinal design	Individuals residing near the new trail	Construction of a trail (2-way multi-use trail separated from existing roads and sidewalks) for both transportation and recreation. The trail created a 2.5 mile loop connecting two currently existing sidewalks	−ve: Negative sig. effect on PA and walking between baseline and follow-up; 18–64 year olds sig. increased number of PA episodes between baseline and follow-up ($p = 0.024$)
Fitzhugh et al. (2010) Tennessee, USA	Quasi-experiment: controlled, pre-post design	Children, adolescents and adults in neighbourhood	Retrofit of an urban greenway (2.9 miles long; 8-foot wide) to enhance connectivity of pedestrian infrastructure with nearby retail establishments and schools (cost: $2.1 m)	+ve: Pre and post intervention changes between experimental and control neighbourhoods were sig. different for total PA ($p = 0.001$); walking ($p = 0.001$) and cycling ($p = 0.038$). There was no sig. change over time for active transport to school
West and Shores (2011) North Carolina, USA	Quasi-experiment: controlled, pre-post design	Residents living within 0.5 mile radius of greenway	5 miles of greenway developed and added to existing greenway along a river	−ve: No sig. difference between intervention and control group

(continued)

Table 17.2 (continued)

Reference	Study design	Population	Intervention	Outcome
Clark et al. (2014) Southern Nevada, USA	Quasi-experiment: controlled, pre-post design	Trails were in lower SES neighbourhoods	6 intervention trails: after a marketing campaign promoting PA and trail use (2012), signage was added/altered including: distance markings, way-finding signs, trail maps, trail names, and icons for acceptable uses	+ve: Sig. increases for both control and intervention, pre–post for trail usage per day; 31% increase for the control trails and 35% for the intervention trails ($p < 0.01$); non-sig. difference between the intervention and control group ($p = 0.32$)
Brand et al. (2014), Sahlqvist et al. (2013), Bird et al. (2014), Goodman et al. (2014) Cardiff, Kenilworth and Southampton, United Kingdom	Quasi-experimental, longitudinal design	Adults living within 5 km by road of the core Connect2 projects	Building or improvement of walking and cycling routes across the United Kingdom including a traffic-free bridge over Cardiff Bay; a traffic-free bridge over a busy trunk road; an informal riverside footpath turned into a boardwalk	+ve: Proximity to Connect2 associated with greater use of Connect2; 32% reported using Connect2 at 1 year and 38% at 2 years.; at 2 years, those nearer the intervention sig. increased walking and cycling (15.3 mins/week/km) and total PA (12.5 mins/week/km)

MVPA Moderate-vigorous physical activity, *PA* physical activity, *US* United States, *+ve* positive intervention effect, *−ve* no intervention effect

follow-up). At 2-year follow-up individuals living nearer the intervention versus those living further away did report significant increases in walking and cycling (effect of 15.3 min per week per km closer to the intervention after adjustments for baseline variables). Proximity was also associated with a comparable increase in total physical activity (effect of 12.5 min per week per km closer to the intervention). Further analyses showed that the intervention did not produce reductions in CO_2 emissions (Brand et al. 2014).

Three studies showed no significant impact for the provision of new trails/greenways on usage or physical activity. Evenson et al. (2005) found no significant effect for usage and physical activity on a new 2.8-mile (approx. 4.5-km) multiuse trail in the USA. Burbidge and Goulias (2009) found no significant effects for the construction of a multiuse trail designed for both active transport and recreational use. A study by West and Shores (2011) found no significant effect on physical activity behaviour for 5 miles (approx. 8 km) of greenway developed and added to an existing greenway along a river. None of these interventions included any promotion or marketing campaign of the new trails/greenways.

Case Study: Connswater Community Greenway, Belfast, Northern Ireland, UK

Developed by the East Belfast Partnership and led by Belfast City Council, the Connswater Community Greenway provides 9 km of linear park running along the course of the Connswater, Knock and Loop Rivers. The project, which cost approximately €47,000,000, was funded through the Big Lottery Fund, Belfast City Council and the Department for Social Development. The intervention delivers multiple social and environmental outcomes through the provision of foot and cycle paths for physical activity, tourism and heritage trails, hubs for education, and elements of the East Belfast Flood Alleviation Scheme. Social engagement occurred in parallel with physical changes to the intervention site. A so-called 'bottom-up' approach was applied, which involved the employment of a full-time community support officer. This project also recognizes that green space interventions are long-term investments as reflected by the 40-year management and maintenance plan for the greenway that was developed from the outset (Fig. 17.2).

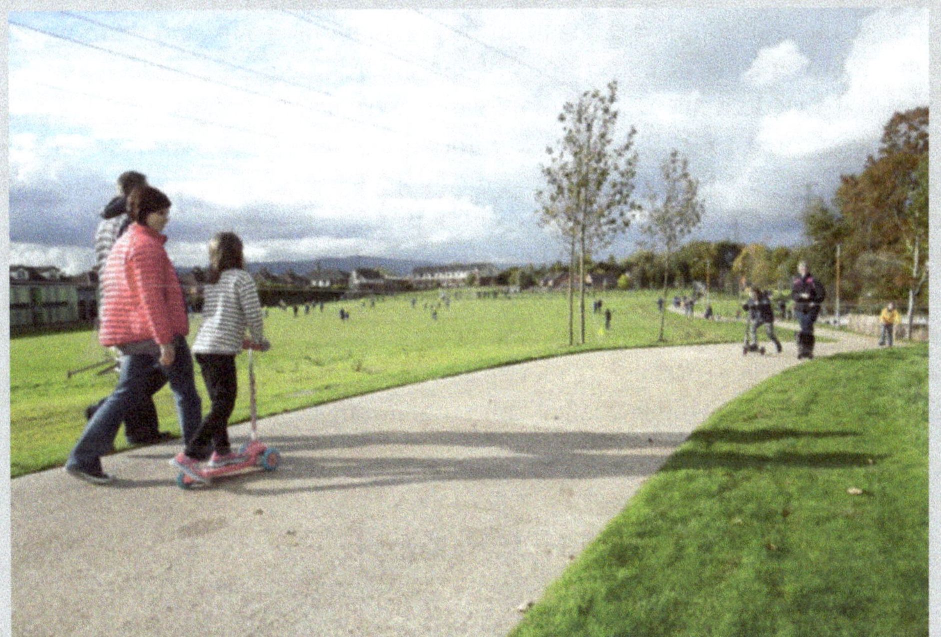

Fig. 17.2 Connswater Community Greenway delivers social and environmental outcomes. (Image: Connswater Community Greenway Trust)

17.2.4 Greening Interventions

There was strong evidence to support the greening of vacant lots (4/4 studies showed a significant intervention effect) and greening of urban streets (4/4 studies demonstrated a significant intervention effect), for environmental, physiological, psychological and improved social environment outcomes (see Table 17.3).

A decade-long study using a difference-in-difference design in the USA (Branas et al. 2011) showed that greening of vacant urban lots (>725,000 m^2) resulted in reductions in gun assaults ($p < 0.001$), vandalism ($p < 0.001$) and residents reporting less stress and more exercise ($p < 0.01$). In an RCT, Garvin et al. (2013) demonstrated a decrease in the number of total crimes and gun assaults, and increased safety around greened vacant lots compared with control lots ($p > 0.05$). Anderson et al. (2014) demonstrated significant biodiversity outcomes for a range of greening interventions in three deprived urban areas in South Africa. In a US-based study, South et al. (2015) found that heart rate lowered significantly in local residents living near greened compared to non-greened vacant lots (n = 2 clusters of vacant lots) ($p < 0.001$).

Four (out of four) studies showed significant impacts on health and environmental factors for interventions involving greening of urban streets. Ward Thompson et al. (2014) found evidence to support the provision of so-called 'DIY streets' in urban areas in the UK. Streets were made safer and more attractive (e.g. planting trees/plants), and traffic calming measures were added at nine different sites. Longitudinal data showed that participants perceived they were significantly more active post-intervention ($p = 0.04$) than the comparison group, and there were significant improvements in perceptions of the environment. Joo and Kwon (2015) found that illegal dumping of household garbage occurred at 55.4% of greened sites (n = 74) compared to 91.9% of sites without greenery (n = 74) in South Korea. Strohbach et al. (2013) showed a significant increase in bird species in a study investigating 12 community-driven greening projects involving tree plantings carried out in deprived areas compared to random urban sites without greening (p = 0.049). Adverse outcomes from greening interventions were also reported by Jin et al. (2014), who demonstrated that increased street tree canopy was positively associated with $PM_{2.5}$ (particulate matter with aerodynamic diameters of 2.5 mm or less) concentrations owing to reduced air circulation.

17.2.5 Green Infrastructure Interventions

There was promising evidence to support the provision of rain gardens (3/4 studies showed a significant positive effect) and strong evidence to support the provision of roof gardens (3/3 studies showed a significant positive effect) for managing the adverse impact of storm water. One study (1/1 study) demonstrated significant cooling effects for a roof garden in a suburban area (see Table 17.4).

Table 17.3 Summary characteristics of greening interventions

Reference	Study design	Population	Intervention	Outcome
Branas et al. (2011) Philadelphia, PA, USA	Quasi-experiment: difference-in-difference design	Cohort of 50,000 Philadelphians from household survey	Greening of vacant urban land (n = 4436); (> 725,000 m^2) from 1999 to 2008 involving removing trash and debris, grading the land, planting grass and trees, installing low wooden fences around perimeter	+ve: Greening associated with reductions in gun assaults ($p < 0.001$), vandalism ($p < 0.001$), residents reported less stress and more exercise ($p < 0.01$)
Garvin et al. (2013) Philadelphia, PA, USA	Pilot RCT: difference-in-difference analytical approach	People living approx. two blocks surrounding the randomly selected vacant lots; 97% African–American; median income $15,417–17,743	Greening of vacant lots (4500–5500 square feet); removing debris, grading the land and adding topsoil, planting grass and trees, building a wooden fence	+ve: Non-sig. decrease in the number of total crimes and gun assaults around greened vacant lots compared with control; people around the intervention lots reported feeling sig. safer after greening compared with control lots ($p < 0.01$)
Anderson et al. (2014) Cape Town, South Africa	Quasi-experimental, controlled (post data only)	Spectrum of socioeconomic neighbourhoods, ranging from middle to lower income areas	Civic-led greening interventions implemented via three sites	+ive: Biodiversity in the greening intervention sites was higher than the vacant lot and comparable to the conservation sites
South et al. (2015) Philadelphia, PA, USA	Quasi-experimental, controlled, pre and post	N = 12 participants completed pre- and post-intervention walks; all were African-American, eight male; majority had household income < S15, 000	Randomly selected cluster of vacant lots received standard greening treatment involving cleaning and removing debris, planting grass and trees, and installing a low wooden post-and-rail fence	+ve: Difference-in-difference estimates between greened and non-greened vacant lots was sig. lower for heart rate ($p < .001$) for the greened site; being in view of a greened vacant lot decreased heart rate sig. more than a non-greened vacant lot

(continued)

Table 17.3 (continued)

Reference	Study design	Population	Intervention	Outcome
Strohbach et al. (2013) Boston, MA, USA	Quasi-experimental, controlled (post data only)	Low SES areas; 617,594 inhabitants; population density of 4939 inhabitants per km^2; tree canopy covers 29% of the city area	12 community driven greening projects in low SES areas including creation of a small park (424 m^2),tree plantings in an existing park (4377 m^2) and tree plantings at residential houses (859 m^2)	+ve: Sig. difference between greening projects and random urban sites (p = .049); most greening projects had more species than the random urban sites in their vicinity
Jin et al. (2014) Shanghai, China	Quasi-experimental, controlled (post data only)	Area of 6340.5 km^2, 23.5 million population	Street trees on 6 streets (length 205–223 m; width 15.2–17.5 m) were treated with different pruning intensities (strong, weak and null) which would result in different canopy coverage across the four seasons	+ve: Increased street tree canopy was positively associated with $PM_{2.5}$ concentrations owing to reduced air circulation
Ward Thompson et al. (2014) England, Scotland and Wales, United Kingdom	Quasi-experiment: controlled, pre-post design	Mean age 75 years; 44% male; 22.5% non-white British	n = 56 residents pre and n = 29 post intervention 'DIY Streets': 9 intervention streets located in urban areas in United Kingdom. Streets were made safer, more attractive and traffic calming measures were added.	+ve: Sig. positive perceptions of intervention streets post-intervention (p = 0.04); longitudinal participants perceived they were sig. more active post-intervention (p = 0.04) than the control group
Joo and Kwon (2015) Suwon, South Korea	Quasi-experimental, controlled (post data only)	Population 1.2 m	74 sites with street greenery (e.g. planter boxes) installed by the city council, located in low-rise residential areas to reduce illegal dumping of household garbage	+ve: Illegal dumping of household garbage occurred at 55.4% of sites with installed greenery compared to 91.9% of sites without greenery installed

PM Particulate Matter, *SES* Socioeconomic status, *US* United States, *+ve* positive intervention effect, *−ve* no intervention effect

Mayer et al. (2012) explored whether voluntary incentives were effective at distributing storm water management throughout a small suburban catchment, and whether the number and placement of rain gardens and rain barrels were sufficient to alter the hydrology, water quality and aquatic biology of the catchment. In total, 83 rain gardens and 176 rain barrels were installed onto more than 30% of the 350 eligible residential properties in a 1.8 km^2 catchment area in Ohio, USA. The intervention had an overall small but statistically significant effect of decreasing storm water quantity at the sub-watershed scale. In a similar study in the same area (Shuster and Rhea 2013; Roy et al. 2014), the installation of 81 rain gardens and 165 rain barrels at four experimental areas was compared to two control areas. In contrast,

Case Study: Bristol Street Green Screens, Birmingham, England, UK

Bristol Street in Birmingham is a dual carriageway with a wide grassed central reservation along which runs, almost continuously, a metal highway pedestrian guardrail. This greening intervention involved fitting green vegetated screens to 141 m of existing guardrail. Installation of the green screens was completed in 2015 costing approximately €29,000. Follow-up analysis of particulate matter (PM_{10}, $PM_{2.5}$ and PM_1) 2 months post installation showed significant increases ($p < .001$) of particulates on green screen leaves in comparison to nursery stock of the same plants. In addition to the potential air quality improvement role of the green screens, they also improve the aesthetics of the street and may benefit local businesses through increased pedestrian traffic. The green screens require minimal maintenance and through utilizing existing infrastructure may provide a cost-efficient and practical solution to increasing green space within dense urban areas (Fig. 17.3).

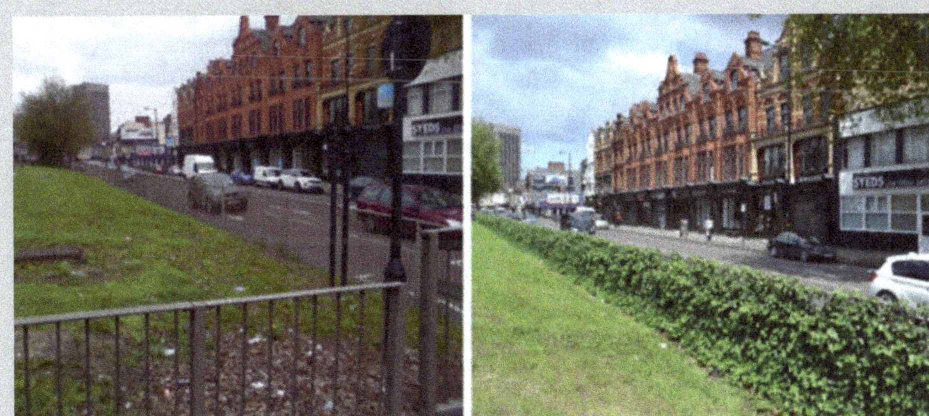

Fig. 17.3 The left panel shows Bristol Street, Birmingham in 2014 before green screen implementation and the right panel shows the street in 2016 after green screen implementation as part of the Bristol Street Green Screens Trial Project, Birmingham, UK. (Image: Chris Rance)

Table 17.4 Summary characteristics of green infrastructure interventions

Reference	Study design	Intervention	Outcome
Van Seters et al. (2009) Toronto, Canada	Quasi-experiment, controlled (post data only)	A 241 m^2 green roof vegetated with wildflowers installed on a multi-story, university building	+ve: The green roof retained 63% more rainfall than the conventional roof over the 18 month monitoring period
Carpenter and Kaluvakolanu (2011) Michigan, USA	Quasi-experiment, controlled (post data only)	Extensive green roof of 10.16 cm depth applied to the roof of a building on a university campus; a green roof section of 325.2 m^2 and 929 m^2 were monitored	+ve: Sig. higher total solids concentration ($p = 0.045$) for the green roof than the asphalt roof; lower total phosphate concentrations for the green roof (non-sig.); green roof retained 68% of rainfall volume and reduced peak discharge by an average of 89%
Mayer et al. (2012) Ohio, USA	Before-after-control-intervention (BACI) experimental design	Retro-fit storm water management: Installation of 83 rain gardens and 176 rain barrels onto more than 30% of the 350 eligible residential properties through an incentivised auction (2007–2008)	+ve: Intervention had an overall small but sig. effect of decreasing storm water quantity at the sub watershed scale
Fassman-Beck et al. (2013) Auckland, New Zealand	Quasi-experiment, controlled (post data only)	A 500 m^2 extensive green roof installed on a council civic centre	+ve: 57% retention of rain water in comparison to control
Shuster and Rhea (2013), Roy et al. (2014) Ohio, USA	Before–after–control–intervention (BACI) experimental design	Retro-fit storm water management: Installation of 81 rain gardens and 165 rain barrels onto 30% of properties through an incentivised auction (2007–2008) at 4 experimental subcatchments	−ve: No sig. difference between control and experimental sites with regards to stream water quality, periphyton, and macroinvertebrate metrics +ve: Small sig. decrease in runoff volume in treatment subcatchments
Kondo et al. (2015) Philadelphia, PA, USA	Quasi-experiment: difference-in-difference design	Installation of green storm water infrastructure at 52 sites: 152 tree trenches, 46 infiltration or storage trenches, 43 rain gardens, 29 pervious pavement installments, 20 bumpouts, 14 bio-swales, 5 storm water basins, 1 wetland, and 12 other	+ve: Sig. reductions in narcotics possession (18–27% less) ($p < .01$), ($p < .01$) at varying distances from treatment sites; sig. reductions in narcotics manufacture and burglaries; non-sig. reductions in homicides, assaults, thefts, public drunkenness, stress levels, blood pressure and cholesterol

(continued)

Table 17.4 (continued)

Reference	Study design	Intervention	Outcome
Jarden and Jefferson (2016) Ohio, USA	Before–after–control–intervention (BACI) experimental design	Installation of 91 rain gardens, street-connected bio-retention cells and rain barrels at 2 treatment streets. Rain gardens (< 25 m^2) were installed in front yards and backyards; bio-retention cells (~26–44 m^2) were installed between the sidewalk and street	+ve: Reduction in storm water flow at the treatment streets with reductions of up to 33% of peak discharge and 40% of total run-off volume
Peng and Jim (2015) Hong Kong, China	Quasi-experiment, controlled, pre and post design	A 484 m^2 extensive green roof was retrofitted on a 2-story railway station	+ve: Green roof displayed cooling effects in spring, summer, and fall, with slight warming effects in winter

BACI Before-after-control-intervention, *US* United States, *+ve* positive intervention effect, *−ve* no intervention effect

results showed no significant difference between control and intervention sites with regard to river water quality, periphyton and macroinvertebrate metrics. However, it did show a small significant decrease in runoff volume in intervention areas.

Kondo et al. (2015) investigated the effects of a range of green storm water infrastructures across 52 sites in Philadelphia on health and social outcomes using a difference-in-difference design. Installed infrastructure included 152 tree trenches, 46 infiltration/storage trenches, 43 rain gardens, 29 pervious pavements, five storm water basins, and one wetland. The comparator groups were matched control sites where no construction took place. Results showed significant reductions in narcotics possession (18–27% less; $p < 0.01$), narcotics manufacture and burglaries. There were non-significant reductions in homicides, assaults, thefts and public drunkenness. In addition, there were negative, non-significant effects on stress levels and increased reporting of high blood pressure and cholesterol.

Jarden and Jefferson (2016) found a significant reduction in storm water flow at the intervention sites with reductions of up to 33% of peak discharge and 40% of total run-off volume. The intervention involved provision of 91 rain gardens (< 25 m^2), street-connected bio-retention cells (~26–44 m^2) and rain barrels on two streets. Each intervention street had a matched control street (n = 4) of similar size, drainage area and characteristics.

Van Seters et al. (2009) found that the green roof on a building in Toronto, Canada (241 m^2) retained 63% more rainfall than the conventional (bitumen) roof over an 18-month monitoring period. In a similar study in Michigan, USA, Carpenter and Kaluvakolanu (2011) investigated the effects of an extensive green roof (325.2 m^2 and 929 m^2) on a university building compared to a stone-ballasted roof and an asphalt roof. Results showed that the green roof retained 68% of rainfall volume and reduced peak discharge by an average of 89%. Also, there were significantly higher total solids concentration ($p = 0.045$) for the green roof than for the asphalt roof. Finally, Fassman-Beck et al. (2013) found that a green roof (500 m^2 on a council civic centre) retained 57% of rain water in comparison to control (bitumen roof). All of these studies were quasi-experiments that collected post-implementation data only.

Peng and Jim (2015) found that a green roof displayed significant cooling effects in spring, summer and autumn, with slight warming effects in winter, in a suburban area in Hong Kong compared to a bare roof control site.

17.2.6 *Impact of Urban Green Space Interventions on Equity Factors*

There is currently too little evidence to enable us to draw firm conclusions regarding the impact of urban green space interventions on a range of equity indicators, for example those from disadvantaged backgrounds, migrants, the elderly, children, and those with disabilities. Twenty studies were based in disadvantaged neighbourhoods, with relatively mixed supporting evidence for urban green space interventions. For those studies that did show a positive intervention effect in disadvantaged neighbourhoods there is, however, insufficient reported information on whether the community used, or indeed, benefitted from, the urban green space interventions. Previous research demonstrating that urban green space may be 'equigenic' (Mitchell et al. 2015) (i.e. health benefits associated with access to green space are strongest among those in disadvantaged populations) suggests that this is an important area for future research.

17.3 Lessons Learned and Key Considerations

In summary, there was *promising evidence* to support the provision of urban green space interventions for environmental, health and well-being effects. In particular, there was *strong evidence* for park-based interventions employing a dual approach (i.e. a physical change to the urban green space and promotion/marketing programmes) particularly for increasing park use and physical activity; greening of vacant lots for health and well-being (e.g. reduction in stress) and social (e.g. reduction in crime, increased perceptions of safety) benefits; greening of urban streets particularly for environmental benefits (e.g. increased biodiversity, reduced air pollution, reduction in illegal dumping); and roof gardens for managing storm water impacts. There was *promising evidence* to support the provision of roof gardens for environmental benefits (temperature), which has an impact on climate change.

Case Study: Woods in and Around Towns, Multiple Locations, Scotland, UK

Led by Forestry Commission Scotland, this greening intervention targets deprived urban areas within Scotland. The intervention aims to enhance quality of life for local residents by restoring nearby wooded green spaces and improving access to these sites. The intervention sites undergo practical upgrades such as creating and maintaining paths and trails, providing seating and resting areas, installing signs and trail 'guideposts' and implementing initiatives to improve the safety of the sites through designing and maintaining paths with a clear line of sight. Social engagement is also a key component, with intervention sites hosting organised community events such as group walks, conservation events and family fun days. Analysis of cross-sectional data from residents living with 500 m of an intervention site has shown significant increases in visits to the green space, improved attitudes towards using the green space for physical activity, and greater perceptions of safety in comparison to a control site. Through implementing interventions in deprived urban areas this intervention helps to promote equity and provide health outcomes for those who are likely to benefit the most from green space access (Fig. 17.4).

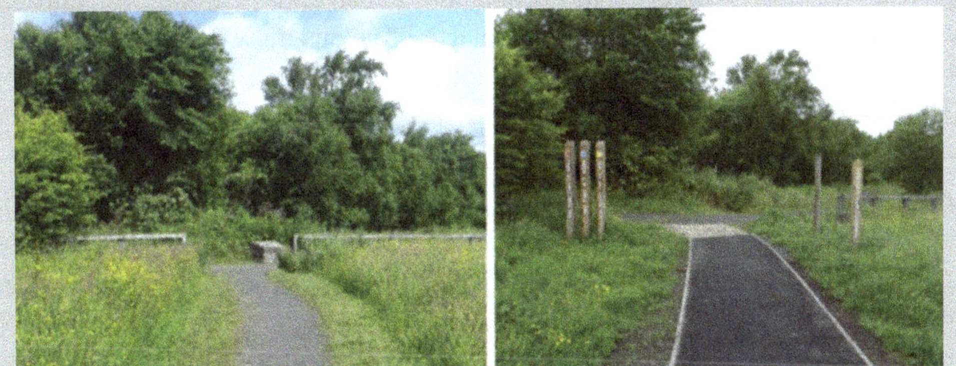

Fig. 17.4 The left panel shows the entrance to greenspace before intervention implementation and the right panel shows post intervention implementation as part of the Woods in and Around Towns programme, Scotland, UK. (Image: Left panel: Eva Silveirinha de Oliveira, Right Panel: Sara Tilley OPENspace Research Centre)

There was *inconclusive evidence* to support urban greenways or trails regardless of whether there were promotion and/or marketing activities to encourage use of the greenway/trails. There was *limited evidence* for park-based interventions that only involved physical change to the urban green space (i.e. they did not include programmes to promote the use of the green space), including pocket parks for health and well-being benefits, and *no evidence* (i.e. an absence of studies) for green walls, allotments/community gardens and urban agriculture-based interventions. There was a *lack of evidence* regarding adverse or unintended consequences, the long-term impact, economic benefits or the differential impacts of urban green space interventions on various equity indicators. There was also a lack of studies from low income countries. None of the studies directly assessed their impact on climate change. This could be due to inadequate observation time to detect such changes.

The next section outlines recommendations for practitioners (including urban planners, urban designers, landscape architects, civil engineers, transport engineers, property developers and public health professionals), policy-makers and researchers regarding intervening in urban green space. These recommendations were informed by the evidence review, case studies and discussions at a WHO expert working group on urban green space interventions.

17.3.1 Practice Recommendations

The following section builds on the previous recommendations by the WHO (2006) and NICE (2018), Public Health England (2014) and Institute for European Environmental Policy (IEEP) (2016), and also broadens these recommendations to incorporate other health, social and environmental outcomes.

The following factors should be considered when designing urban green space interventions:

1. Given the complex social and economic dynamics that occur at scale, implementation of green infrastructure requires both a multi-disciplinary (urban planning, landscape architecture, civil engineering, ecology, environmental science, urban design, public health, health economics, environmental science) and multi-sector (academic, government, nongovernmental organizations, private sector) approach.
2. Urban green space interventions should be designed with foreseen long-term impacts from the outset. Those responsible for planning and delivering interventions should 'design-in' components that specifically focus on long-term health, social and environmental effects, ensuring to take direction from the large and conclusive cross-sectional evidence base in their intervention design.
3. Local communities, and indeed different subgroups within these communities, use urban green space in a variety of ways. Future interventions need to consider how the green space may be used and what the needs of the local community are.
4. Engage the local community throughout the design process and across the life course (i.e. children to older adults) to ensure that their needs are incorporated into the intervention. This will also encourage community to take ownership for the urban green space and its future management and maintenance at a commu-

nity level. Examples of community engagement processes include group workshops, roundtable discussions and charrettes.
5. Need to design urban green space interventions that incorporate and maximize health, environmental and social benefits.
6. Need to use a dual approach that incorporates promotion and marketing of urban green space as well as changing the physical environment (i.e. more complex than 'build it and they will come'), particularly for health and social benefits.
7. Local practitioners need to actively engage with the evaluation process, for example by engaging with local universities, organisations and the local community.

17.3.2 Policy Recommendations

Providing and protecting urban green space presents a significant policy opportunity to improve multiple facets of quality of life and the environment with well-developed and sensitive urban green space interventions. Whilst the evidence summarised here and in other reviews is sometimes mixed, there is a preponderance generally supporting the association between urban green space and health, well-being, and social and environmental outcomes. Policy-makers must also ensure that any provision or improvement of urban green space is done so through an 'equity lens'. The few published economic evaluations of urban green space interventions are positive. Bird et al. (2014) suggest significant financial savings could be made as a result of increased numbers of people walking and cycling. Similarly, a modelling study suggested that effectiveness estimates as low as a 2% gain in population physical activity levels would be cost-effective (£18, 411/disability-adjusted life-year) (Dallat et al. 2014). Although the direct health gains are predicted to be small for any individual, summed over an entire population they are substantial (e.g. health value of physical activity in natural environments in England has been estimated at £2.2bn/year) (White et al. 2016).

17.3.3 Research Recommendations

Findings from the recent WHO Regional Office for Europe report (2016) demonstrate substantial evidence to support the association between urban green space for environmental, health and well-being impacts, alongside suggested mechanisms of action. We must now move towards intervention-based research that will help policy-makers and practitioners. Findings from the evidence review suggest that areas in need of specific attention include research investigating the impact of urban green space interventions on equity indicators and economic factors (for more information, see Kabisch, Chap. 5 this volume). Research should also move beyond assessing the effects of such interventions on physical activity and usage, towards mental and social measures. This type of research has direct policy implications. Research is needed on the impact of interventions in a variety of green space settings, including low- and middle-income countries. Due to the scarcity of the evidence base, research on the effects of urban green space interventions on climate change and biodiversity are required. It is imperative that research is provided in a timely and accessible manner, which has implications for current publication and funding models. It is important to note the significant cost in undertaking this type of research. Researchers, practitioners and policy-makers should work together to devise novel strategies to ensure cost-effective and timely research processes, for example, exploring the use of 'virtual' research experiments. Researchers should develop relationships with key stakeholders who are responsible for urban green space provision and maintenance, for example, local authorities and housing associations, thus enabling opportunities for rigorous evaluations of urban green space interventions.

There is a considerable gap in the theoretical basis to guide intervention approaches, and further, the current intervention approaches largely negate the large and conclusive cross-sectional evidence base. Future studies should include a more complete description of their intervention strategies and logic models that describe the assumed causal pathways by which they affect the outcomes in order to better understand the underpinning theoretical mechanisms and improve future intervention design. The intervention processes logic model should also be used to inform and design the evaluation approach.

17.4 Conclusions

Urban green space cannot be seen in isolation from other local government priorities such as transport and housing. It must be framed holistically and viewed as a complex system in which the interplay between physical, economic, social and natural ecosystems affects health, behaviours and communities. The growing diversity of our towns and cities is transforming how green space is required and negotiated for health, well-being, and social and environmental benefits. Preserving and enhancing existing green spaces, and creating new green spaces, is critical. Significant urban green space investment is made worldwide, and many researchers and policy-makers alike have gradually shown increased support to implement cost-efficient and effective urban green space interventions to improve population-level health, well-being, social and environmental factors. Urban green space interventions can deliver health, social and environmental benefits for all population groups – and particularly among lower socioeconomic status groups. There are very few – if any – other public health interventions that can achieve all of this.

Acknowledgements Funding for this work was provided by the WHO Regional Office for Europe, based on a project grant from the German Federal Ministry for the Environment, Nature Conservation, Building and Nuclear Safety. The work draws on discussion at a WHO expert panel meeting in September 2016 on urban green space interventions.

References

Anderson PML, Avlonitis G, Ernstson H (2014) Ecological outcomes of civic and expert-led urban greening projects using indigenous plant species in Cape Town, South Africa. Landsc Urban Plan 127:104–113

Bird E, Powell J, Ogilvie D et al (2014) Health economic assessment of walking and cycling interventions in the physical environment: Interim findings from the iConnect study. Paper presented at the South West Public Health Scientific conference, Weston-Super-Mare, UK, 5 Feb 2014

Bohn-Goldhaum E, Phongsavan P, Merom D et al (2013) Does playground improvement increase physical activity among children? A quasi-experimental study of a natural experiment. J Environ Public Health 2013:109841

Branas CC, Cheney RA, MacDonald JM et al (2011) A difference-in-differences analysis of health, safety, and greening vacant urban space. Am J Epidemiol 174:1296–1306

Brand C, Goodman A, Ogilvie D (2014) Evaluating the impacts of new walking and cycling infrastructure on carbon dioxide emissions from motorized travel: a controlled longitudinal study. Appl Energy 128:284–295

Burbidge SK, Goulias KG (2009) Evaluating the impact of neighborhood trail development on active travel behavior and overall physical activity of suburban residents. Transp Res Rec J Transp Res Board 2135:78–86

Carpenter DD, Kaluvakolanu P (2011) Effect of roof surface type on storm-water runoff from full-scale roofs in a temperate climate. J Irrig Drain Eng 137:161–169

Clark S, Bungum T, Shan G et al (2014) The effect of a trail use intervention on urban trail use in southern Nevada. Prev Med 67:S17–S20

Cohen DA, Golinelli D, Williamson S et al (2009a) Effects of park improvements on park use and physical activity: policy and programming implications. Am J Prev Med 37:475–480

Cohen DA, Sehgal A, Williamson S et al (2009b) New recreational facilities for the young and the old in Los Angeles: policy and programming implications. J Public Health Policy 30:S248–S263

Cohen DA, Marsh T, Williamson S et al (2012) Impact and cost-effectiveness of family fitness zones: a natural experiment in urban public parks. Health Place 18:39–45

Cohen DA, Han B, Derose KP et al (2013) Physical activity in parks: a randomized controlled trial using community engagement. Am J Prev Med 45:590–597

Cohen DA, Marsh T, Williamson S et al (2014) The potential for pocket parks to increase physical activity. Am J Health Promot 28:S19–S26

Cranney L, Phongsavan P, Kariuki M et al (2016) Impact of an outdoor gym on park users' physical activity: a natural experiment. Health Place 37:26–34

Dallat MA, Soerjomataram I, Hunter RF et al (2014) Urban greenways have the potential to increase physical activity levels cost-effectively. Eur J Pub Health 24:190–195

Droomers M, Jongeneel-Grimen B, Kramer D et al (2015) The impact of intervening in green space in Dutch deprived neighbourhoods on physical activity and general health: results from the quasi-experimental URBAN40 study. J Epidemiol Community Health 70:147–154

Evenson KR, Herring AH, Huston SL (2005) Evaluating change in physical activity with the building of a multi-use trail. Am J Prev Med 28:177–185

Fassman-Beck E, Voyde E, Simcock R, et al (2013) 4 Living roofs in 3 locations: does configuration affect runoff mitigation? Journal of Hydrology 490:11–20

Fitzhugh EC, Bassett DR, Evans MF (2010) Urban trails and physical activity: a natural experiment. Am J Prev Med 39:259–262

Frumkin H, Bratman GN, Breslow SJ et al (2017) Nature contact and human health: a research agenda. Environ Health Perspect 125:075001–075001

Garvin EC, Cannuscio CC, Branas CC (2013) Greening vacant lots to reduce violent crime: a randomised controlled trial. Inj Prev 19:198–203

Goodman A, Sahlqvist S, Ogilvie D et al (2014) New walking and cycling routes and increased physical activity: one- and 2-year findings from the UK iConnect study. Am J Public Health 104:e38–e46

Gubbels JS, Kremers SP, Droomers M et al (2016) The impact of greenery on physical activity and mental health of adolescent and adult residents of deprived neighborhoods: a longitudinal study. Health Place 40:153–160

Institute for European Environmental Policy (IEEP) (2016) The health and social benefits of nature and biodiversity protection stakeholder workshop, 27–28 January 2016

Jarden KM, Jefferson AJ, Grieser JM (2016) Assessing the effects of catchment-scale urban green infrastructure retrofits on hydrograph characteristics. Hydrol Process 30:1536–1550

Jin S, Guo J, Wheeler S et al (2014) Evaluation of impacts of trees on PM2.5 dispersion in urban streets. Atmos Environ 99:277–287

Joo Y, Kwon Y (2015) Urban street greenery as a prevention against illegal dumping of household garbage-a case in Suwon, South Korea. Urban For Urban Green 14:1088–1094

King DK, Litt J, Halec J et al (2015) 'The park a tree built': evaluating how a park development project impacted where people play. Urban For Urban Green 14:293–299

Kondo MC, Low SC, Henning J et al (2015) The impact of green stormwater infrastructure installation on surrounding health and safety. Am J Public Health 105:e114–e121

Mayer A, Shuster WD, Beaulieu J et al (2012) Building green infrastructure via citizen participation: a six-year study in the Shepherd Creek (Ohio). Environ Pract 14:57–67

Mitchell RJ, Richardson EA, Shortt NK et al (2015) Neighborhood environments and socioeconomic inequalities in mental Well-being. Am J Prev Med 49:80–84

National Institute for Health and Care Excellence (NICE) (2018) Physical activity and the environment. https://www.nice.org.uk/guidance/ng90. Accessed 22 May 2018

New South Wales Department of Health (2002) The effect of park modifications and promotion on physical activity participation. Summary report

Peng LLH, Jim CY (2015) Seasonal and diurnal thermal performance of a subtropical extensive green roof: the impacts of background weather parameters. Sustainability 7:11098–11113

Peschardt KK, Stigsdotter UK (2014) Evidence for designing health promoting pocket parks. Archnet-IJAR 8:149–164

Public Health England (2014) Local action on health inequalities: Improving access to green spaces. Health Equity Evid Rev 8. https://www.gov.uk/government/uploads/system/uploads/attachment_data/file/357411/Review8_Green_spaces_health_inequalities.pdf. Accessed 22 May 2018

Quigg R, Reeder AI, Gray A et al (2011) The effectiveness of a community playground intervention. J Urban Health 89:171–184

Roy AH, Rhea LK, Mayer AL et al (2014) How much is enough? Minimal responses of water quality and stream biota to partial retrofit stormwater management in a suburban neighborhood. PLoS One 17:e85011

Sahlqvist S, Goodman A, Cooper AR et al (2013) Change in active travel and changes in recreational and total physical activity in adults: longitudinal findings from the iConnect study. Int J Behav Nutr Phys Act 10:28

Shuster WD, Rhea LK (2013) Catchment-scale hydrologic implications of parcel-level stormwater management (Ohio USA). J Hydrol 485:177–187

Slater S, Pugach O, Lin W et al (2016) If you build it will they come? Does involving community groups in playground renovations affect park utilization and physical activity? Environ Behav 48:246–265

South EC, Kondo MC, Cheney RA et al (2015) Neighborhood blight, stress, and health: a walking trial of urban greening and ambulatory heart rate. Am J Public Health 105:909–913

Strohbach MW, Lermana SB, Warren PS (2013) Are small greening areas enhancing bird diversity? Insights from community-driven greening projects in Boston. Landsc Urban Plan 114:69–79

Tester J, Baker R (2009) Making the playfields even: evaluating the impact of an environmental intervention on park use and physical activity. Prev Med 48:316–320

Van Seters T, Rocha L, Smith D et al (2009) Evaluation of green roofs for runoff retention, runoff quality, and leachability. Water Qual Res J Can 44:33–47

Veitch J, Ball K, Crawford D et al (2012) Park improvements and park activity: a natural experiment. Am J Prev Med 42:616–619

Ward Thompson C, Roeb J, Aspinall P (2013) Woodland improvements in deprived urban communities: what impact do they have on people's activities and quality of life? Landsc Urban Plan 118:79–89

Ward Thompson C, Curl A, Aspinall P et al (2014) Do changes to the local street environment alter behaviour and quality of life of older adults? The 'DIY streets' intervention. Br J Sports Med 48:1059–1065

West ST, Shores KA (2011) The impacts of building a greenway on proximate residents' physical activity. J Phys Act Health 8:1092–1097

White MP, Elliott LR, Taylor T et al (2016) Recreational physical activity in natural environments and implications for health: a population based cross-sectional study in England. Prev Med 91:383–388

WHO Regional Office for Europe (2016) Urban green spaces and health. WHO Regional Office for Europe, Copenhagen, Denmark

WHO Regional Office for Europe (2017) Urban green space interventions and health. WHO Regional Office for Europe, Copenhagen, Denmark

World Health Organisation (WHO) (2006) Promoting physical activity and active living in urban environments. The role of local governments. The solid facts. World Health Organization Europe, WHO Regional Office for Europe, Copenhagen

Chapter 18
Resilience Management for Healthy Cities in a Changing Climate

Thomas Elmqvist, Franz Gatzweiler, Elisabet Lindgren, and Jieling Liu

Abstract Cities are experiencing multiple impacts from global environmental change, and the degree to which they will need to cope with and adapt to these challenges will continue to increase. We argue that a 'complex systems and resilience management' view may significantly help guide future urban development through innovative integration of, for example, grey, blue and green infrastructure embedded in flexible institutions (both formal and informal) for multi-functionality and improved health. For instance, the urban heat island effect will further increase city-centre temperatures during projected more frequent and intense heat waves. The elderly and people with chronic cardiovascular and respiratory diseases are particularly vulnerable to heat. Integrating vegetation and especially trees in the urban infrastructure helps reduce temperatures by shading and evapotranspiration. Great complexity and uncertainty of urban social-ecological systems are behind this heatwave-health nexus, and they need to be addressed in a more comprehensive manner. We argue that a systems perspective can lead to innovative designs of new urban infrastructure and the redesign of existing structures. Particularly to promoting the integration of grey, green and blue infrastructure in urban planning through institutional innovation and structural reorganization of knowledge-action systems may significantly enhance prospects for improved urban health and greater resilience under various scenarios of climate change.

Keywords Resilience management · Nature-based solutions · Urban health · Climate change · Urban complexity · Knowledge-action systems

---

T. Elmqvist (✉) · E. Lindgren
Stockholm Resilience Center, Stockholm University, Stockholm, Sweden
e-mail: thomas.elmqvist@su.se; elisabet.lindgren@su.se

F. Gatzweiler
Institute of Urban Environment (IUE), Chinese Academy of Sciences (CAS), Xiamen, China
e-mail: franz@iue.ac.cn

J. Liu
Institute of Social Sciences (ICS), University of Lisbon, Lisbon, Portugal
e-mail: jielingliu@campus.ul.pt

M. R. Marselle et al. (eds.), *Biodiversity and Health in the Face of Climate Change*, https://doi.org/10.1007/978-3-030-02318-8_18

Highlights

- Cities are experiencing multiple impacts from global environmental change.
- A systems perspective can lead to innovative designs of new urban infrastructure and the redesign of existing structures to address complex urban health challenges.
- The integration of grey, green and blue infrastructure in urban planning through institutional innovation and structural reorganization of knowledge-action systems may result in large health improvements and increase urban resilience.

18.1 Introduction

Urban health and well-being is an outcome of urban complexity. In this chapter we argue that cities are complex adaptive social-ecological-technological systems, a perspective needed in order to untangle this complexity and define the types of problems we are confronted with (Alberti et al. 2018). By framing complexity conceptually we suggest pathways for urban governance for urban health and well-being, pathways that address problems of great scientific and economic complexity and radical uncertainty, of which climate change is a prime example. One example of such a pathway is using multiple ecosystem services as a means to create resilience to climate change in cities and thus reduce negative impacts on health and well-being, or so-called 'nature-based solutions' (NBSs) (Secretariat of the Convention on Biological Diversity 2009), such as the 'Sponge City' initiative for flood water treatment currently taking place in China and the green roof design thriving across many European cities. Whereas technology can be helpful for solving complicated engineering problems by seeking solutions for optima and equilibria, complex or inexact problems require the recognition of deep uncertainty and non-linearity.

18.1.1 Urban Systems as Complex Adaptive Systems

A social-technological approach has, up until now, been the traditional way of analyzing urban complexity (e.g. Geels 2011; Hodson and Marvin 2010), and in this context, many have struggled to define exactly what is meant by a city. Here we expand on an emerging framework of cities as complex *social-ecological-technological* systems, as cities include much more than a particular density of people or area covered by human-made structures (Bai et al. 2016; Alberti et al. 2018).

Cities are places where social, ecological and technological systems connect and integrate; where various types of capital and infrastructures intersect in multi-dimensional spaces; and where connectivity, interaction, exchange and communication accelerate in time. Urban socio-ecological-technological systems are complex and dynamic because multiple agents from various types of networks interact with each other and their environments, and on multiple scales (Table 18.1). The health and well-being outcomes that emerge from these complex adaptive systems are not entirely plannable (Alberti et al. 2018).

Urban systems (which include social, technological and ecological dimensions) provide functions (Table 18.1) that are similar but not identical to those provided by ecosystems (Gatzweiler et al. 2016, 2018).

A key difference between urban and natural ecosystems is that most goods and services in urban systems are produced by people and are a result of secondary production, while natural ecosystems consist of primary (autotroph) and secondary producers. Nevertheless, recognizing cities as complex adaptive systems that provide numerous categories of functions (Table 18.1) is the basis for resilience management for healthy cities in the context of climate change.

Table 18.1 Functions of urban systems

Function	Description
Supporting	Benefits provided by physical space (habitat) and infrastructure for basic life support functions such as waste management, water treatment and sanitation, and energy provision (electricity). Enables the flow of energy (captured in the form of low-entropy goods) and information. They are necessary for all other functions to be produced. Markets sometimes require physical space for exchange, but market exchange can also take place in virtual spaces
Provisioning	Benefits derived from providing manufactured goods and knowledge, and providing infrastructure for access to water, energy, food, transportation, social interaction and market exchange to maintain the population's health, internal structure, procedures and processes; e.g. (processed) food, (purified) drinking water, construction materials, machines, artifacts (e.g. furniture, bicycles), education and knowledge infrastructure (universities)[a]
Regulating	Benefits derived from providing rules and regulation mechanisms to keep the infrastructure running; e.g. regulating access to social space, legal systems and markets (although not exclusive to urban areas, their significance may often be higher here because of higher institutional density and economic activity in urban areas). The means are laws, norms, cooperatives, law enforcement, disease and disaster management and emergency response systems, hospitals and health service systems, and environmental protection agencies
Cultural	Benefits provided for humans in cities that are created in socio-cultural spaces (again not exclusive to cities). Social space and liberties for economic and political exchange, exchange of ideas, social exchange, recreation and leisure, space for spiritual enrichment, art and cognitive development; e.g. cultural events, "Heimat" (sense of belonging), exhibitions, libraries, cultural heritage values (e.g. historical places), cultural diversity

[a]*Note:* The raw materials and natural resources, like oil, gas and wood, are also used directly in cities; however, that is rather a provisioning function of natural ecosystems

18.1.2 Urban Complexity, Sustainability and Governance

The complexity of urban systems poses enormous challenges for sustainability in identifying causal mechanisms because of the many confounding variables that exist. At the same time, scientific findings from empirical studies are difficult to generalize due to variations in socio-economic and biophysical contexts, and the great heterogeneity that characterizes urban regions (Grimm et al. 2008). Key challenges are scale mismatches, cross-scale interactions and limited transferability across scales (Cumming et al. 2012). Furthermore, the limited predictability of system behaviour over the long term requires a new consideration of uncertainty (Polasky et al. 2011).

The research and application of urban sustainability principles have until now rarely been applied beyond city boundaries and are often constrained to either single or narrowly defined issues (e.g. population, climate, energy, water) (Marcotullio and McGranahan 2007; Seitzinger et al. 2012). Although local governments often aim to optimize resource use in cities, increase efficiency and minimize waste, cities can never become fully self-sufficient. Therefore, individual cities cannot be considered 'sustainable' without acknowledging and accounting for their dependence on the natural ecosystems, resources and populations from other regions around the world (Folke et al. 1997; Seitzinger et al. 2012). Consequently, there is a need to revisit the concept of sustainability, as its narrow definition and application may not only be insufficient but can also result in unintended consequences, such as the 'lock-in' of undesirable urban development trajectories (Ernstson et al. 2010).

Governance failures and their negative outcomes can at least partly be understood as the result of a constrained ability and willingness to understand the dynamics of urban complexity. Governing dynamic complex urban systems for improving urban health and well-being, therefore, requires a better understanding of urban system complexity and the institutions that inhibit or enable solution-oriented actions (cf. Duit and Galaz 2008).

The dynamics and temporality of changes of a system determine adaptive governance styles. Under short-term shocks or longer-term stresses the styles of action can be control-oriented or adaptive (Fig. 18.1). Control-oriented styles of governance

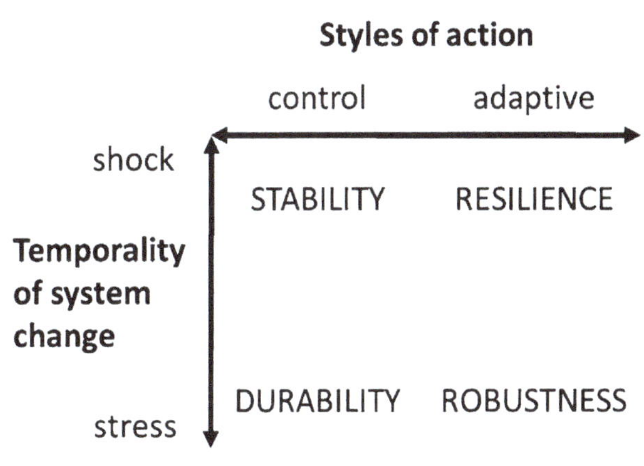

Fig. 18.1 Governance styles are determined by control and adaptive styles of action and how the temporality of system changes is perceived. (Modified from Leach et al. 2010)

assume less uncertainty and more calculable risks. Under such governance, stability (against shocks) or endurance (against stresses) of a system are believed to be maintained or restored by actions of control and order. Recognizing the inherent uncertainty of complexity also acknowledges limits to a control-style of governance.

Managing the resilience of an urban system for health depends on how system changes are perceived and on whether controlled or adaptive, flexible actions are performed (Fig. 18.1). The co-production of knowledge for urban health resilience management and integrated systems of flexible governance for urban health are responses to urban complexity and an attempt to harness it for sustainability.

The World Health Organization's Global Outbreak Alert and Response Network[1] is an example of governance strategies for resilience. It is set up to respond to unpredictable external shocks (outbreaks) with a flexible response network that can be mobilised when needed. Another example of resilience management for health is the Epidemic Intelligence and outbreak responses provided by the European Centre for Disease Prevention and Control (ECDC) to the EU Member States. ECDC continuously monitors and assesses epidemic outbreaks in the EU region. In case of emergencies and response needs, ECDC provides both assessment missions and different levels of epidemic response actions. An example of integrated, flexible systems governance for urban health in the context of climate change are the urban Knowledge-Action Systems (KAS) analysed by Muñoz-Erickson et al. (2017). KAS are social networks of actors involved in the production, sharing and use of knowledge for action and all other types of infrastructure, facilitating the flow of resources, including data and knowledge, and thereby enabling feedback, response and learning for action. Such KAS, once institutionalised as an organisational entity, could be referred to as the collective mind of a city, or the 'urban brain'. An example is the Southeast Florida Regional Climate Compact,[2] which came together to upgrade their resilience knowledge systems for climate adaptation.

18.1.3 Urban Complexity and Resilience

When people think of urban resilience, it is generally in the context of response to sudden impacts, such as a hazard or disaster recovery (see Alberti et al. 2003; Alberti and Marzluff 2004; Vale and Campanella 2005; Cutter et al. 2008; Wallace and Wallace 2008). However, the resilience concept goes far beyond recovery from single disturbances, as demonstrated by the above example of knowledge-action systems. Resilience is a multi-disciplinary concept that explores persistence, recovery, and adaptive and transformative capacities of interlinked social and ecological systems and subsystems (Holling 2001; Folke et al. 2002; Walker et al. 2004; Biggs et al. 2012).

---

[1] https://extranet.who.int/goarn/

[2] http://www.southeastfloridaclimatecompact.org/about-us/what-is-the-compact/

Resilience thinking is part of systems thinking in complexity science, and has two central foci: one is to strengthen the current social-ecological-technological system to live with change by enhancing the ability to adapt to potential external pressures, in order to retain its essential functions and identity; the other is the ability to shift development pathways from those that are less desirable or unsustainable to ones that are more desirable or sustainable –also referred to as transformability (Walker et al. 2004; Folke et al. 2010).

A distinction is often made between general resilience and specified resilience (Walker and Salt 2006). General resilience refers to the resilience of a system to all kinds of shocks, including novel ones, whereas specified resilience refers to the resilience 'of what, to what' – in other words, resilience of some particular part of a system (related to a particular control variable) to one or more identified kinds of shocks (Walker and Salt 2006; Folke et al. 2010). While sustainable development is inherently normative and positive, this is not necessarily true for the resilience concept (Pickett et al. 2013). For example, development may lead to traps that are very resilient and difficult to break out of. The desirability of specified resilience, in particular, depends on careful analysis of resilience 'of what, to what' (Carpenter et al. 2001) since many examples can be found of highly resilient systems (e.g. oppressive political systems) locked into an undesirable system configuration or state. It also may refer 'to whom' as a recognition of environmental inequity (e.g. Pickett et al. 2011).

In general, both the sustainability and the resilience concepts (particularly general resilience) are not easily applicable to the city scale (Elmqvist et al. 2013a). Cities are centres of production and consumption, and urban inhabitants are reliant on resources and ecosystem services – including everything from food, water and construction materials to waste assimilation – secured from locations outside of cities. Although cities can optimize their resource use, increase their efficiency and minimize waste, they can never become fully self-sufficient (Grove 2009). For that reason, it is not sufficient to de-couple cities from resource use (UNEP 2013), rather, cities need to be re-coupled with the regional and global ecosystems in which they are contained (Zhu et al. 2017). Therefore, individual cities cannot be considered "sustainable" without acknowledging and accounting for their teleconnections (Seto et al. 2012) – in other words, the long-distance dependence and impact on ecosystems, resources and populations in other regions around the world (Folke et al. 1997).

Virtually all living systems from the local to the global scale are open and interconnected networks. To achieve resilience for urban health, there is a need to better understand the health and well-being effects of interventions at multiple scales of complex urban systems (Brelsford et al. 2017). Further, as Markelova and Mwangi (2012) point out, referring to Cash and Moser (2000), it is necessary to ascertain the appropriate scale for evaluating benefits from complex systems, and choosing the appropriate scale depends on numerous factors such as the specific objectives of a study, the level of accuracy, and the value system chosen by the evaluator. In addition, interventions will not be effective "when a particular problem issue is managed at an institutional scale whose authoritative reach does not correspond with the geographical scale or particular spatial dynamics of a (…) problem".

However, despite the complex nature of urban systems, there exist relatively simple universal laws that are useful to be aware of when designing systems of governance for urban health resilience. One refers to the urban scaling effect and similarly counts for living organisms. It says that the bigger the organisation becomes, the less energy per capita is needed. For cities, this means that with a doubling of population size, energy supply, for example, increases sublinearly by 85% (one petrol station can serve more people), implying an economy of scale savings effect of 15% for energy and infrastructure. With regard to average wages, the amount of crime and incidence of infectious diseases, the number of patents produced, or the number of restaurants, there is a superlinear scaling effect of 1.15, manifesting systematic increasing returns to scale (West 2017, Bettencourt et al. 2010).

18.2 Climate Change Aggravating Existing Urban Complexity

Demographic and technological changes have resulted in anthropogenic forces on the climate system, greatly exacerbating the flow of energy and materials within urban systems, increasing the complexity levels of urban systems and their functions. In addition, climate change aggravates the complexity of urban systems by imposing direct and indirect impacts on the urban system variables and their functions. Climate change effects include increased intensities and frequency of rainfall, droughts, storms and heat waves, due to warmer sea and land surface temperatures, rising sea levels and reduction of albedo, which further exacerbates the warming, and a range of climate uncertainty. These effects challenge the sensitivity of each variable of the urban social-ecological systems and subsystems (da Silva et al. 2012). The geo-demographical change shows an overall trend of increasing population in increasingly multi- and intercultural urban areas, which challenges the already precarious concept of sustainability of urban systems. The different magnitudes of climate change, therefore, accelerate and complicate both the general and specified resilience of urban systems of multiple scales.

Resilience as a concept has been argued frequently for the case of climate change for the reasons presented above. It is also primarily referred to as the adaptation of climate change impacts. As urban systems are composed of complex environments in which ecological, social, cultural and economic factors interact on multiple scales and across different subsystems, climate change imposes not only direct impacts on the grey, green and blue infrastructure in urban systems, basic life support functions and manufactured goods, such as food, water, energy, transportation and their management and provision, but also indirect impacts on the health and well-being of urban dwellers. Therefore, we argue that health should be an end goal of climate change adaptation and a proxy to examine the level of resilience of complex urban social-ecological-technological systems. Comprehensively acknowledging the value of ecosystem services, incorporating them into urban planning practices for climate change impacts, and institutionalizing this process can help us achieve this end goal.

18.3 Climate Change, Urban Ecosystems and Health

Despite the fact that "…human health is better now than at any time in history…" (Haines 2018), this progress has come at social and environmental costs such as increasing inequality, increasing energy use and related greenhouse gas emissions, soil degradation, biodiversity loss and severe water stress. Together with increasing urban population pressures, this mixture can become a backlash to what we may perceive as progress in human development. In 2012 approximately 7 million people died prematurely as a result of exposure to air pollution, making air pollution the world's largest single environmental health risk. Despite improved availability of health systems and other public services, urban health risks remain: exposure to noise, water and air pollution, diseases related to urban lifestyle, contagious diseases connected with crowding (e.g. tuberculosis, sexually transmitted diseases, influenza, and certain rodent- and vector-borne diseases such as dengue fever, etc.), and risks associated with homelessness, violence and inequality. Understanding the complex interactions of climate change, urban system functions and health has been identified as a research priority for cities in the future (Bai et al. 2018).

Climate change will have numerous impacts on human health and well-being in urban environments depending on local conditions and vulnerabilities. The risk of deaths, injuries and epidemics (especially water-, food-, rodent- and vector-borne diseases) from storms, coastal storm surges and floods will increase in disaster-prone areas, exacerbated by damages to important infrastructure and societal services. Cities are particularly vulnerable to heatwaves since temperatures in certain parts of a city can reach several degrees higher than in surrounding peri-urban and rural areas, due to the so-called urban heat island effect (Zhang et al. 2017). It has been shown that the risk both of death and of acute episodes of chronic diseases, such as acute respiratory illness, heart attacks and stroke, increases markedly in relation to heat wave events (Michelozzi et al. 2009). The elderly, persons with chronic cardio-vascular and respiratory diseases, and individuals who have difficulties implementing heat-reducing actions during a heat wave are particularly vulnerable, and so are outdoor workers in cities where temperatures may soar during working hours (IPCC 2014; Kovats and Hajat 2008). It is well known that air pollution increases the risks associated with heat, and vice versa, which further increases health risks from heat waves in cities.

The urban ecosystem service and urban social-ecological-technological approach have recently developed into several programs exploring the scope and potential of nature-based solutions (Kabisch et al. 2016). Nature-based solutions are actions that are inspired by, supported by or copied from nature, and often with the potential to address a variety of societal challenges in sustainable ways, and contribute to green growth (EU DG Research and Innovation 2015). Nature-based solutions for sustainable urbanization rely in large part on natural areas and features in and around cities to perform essential ecosystem services. This concept may also be used in climate change adaptation to reduce climate change-related impacts on health (Gill et al. 2007), or to gain health co-benefits from climate change adaptation within other sectors of society.

Urban green areas and vegetation can reduce some of the environmental health risks within the urban systems (Elmqvist et al. 2013b). Urban green and water areas, such as city gardens and ponds, and nearby forests, lakes and sea, have a strong potential to locally buffer heat extremes (Hardin and Jensen 2007). In summertime, high temperatures are absorbed by water areas. Greenery, in particular trees, reflects solar radiation and lower temperatures locally through evapotranspiration and shading (Bowler et al. 2010). By increasing urban vegetation through the planting of trees, creating parklands, green rooftops, green walls, and so on, local temperatures in cities can be better regulated and maintained. Urban greenery has also been shown to be effective in reducing air pollutants such as particles and nitrogen and sulphur oxides (Hartig et al. 2014).

Not only do urban green and blue areas reduce health risks associated with high temperatures and air pollutants, but urban vegetation also contributes to reduce flood-related health risks. Vegetation stabilizes the soil and reduces surface runoff following precipitation events. Keeping or adding vegetation will decrease the risk of landslides, as well as the pressure on drainage systems around human settlements. By increasing the vegetation cover and reducing the impermeable surface area in built environments, the volumes of surface storm-water runoff can decrease, thus increasing the resilience to flooding. Increased urban green space will thus increase permeability and water runoff mitigation, as well as decrease flood risk by intercepting rainwater (Pataki et al. 2011).

In addition, urban vegetation has other beneficial health effects. Several studies have shown that vegetation contributes to reducing noise pollution and creating tranquil environments for conducive to mental health (González-Oreja et al. 2010). Urban green areas and vegetation support and facilitate human health and well-being by alleviating stress and allowing space for physical activity and community interaction, which sustain mental health, physical fitness and cognitive and immune functions (WHO 2017).

As the fundamental ecological base of urban social-ecological systems, biodiversity and ecosystem services play a significant role in reducing the negative impacts of climate change on health, both at present and in the future, therefore reducing vulnerability and strengthening resilience of the urban systems and subsystems.

18.4 Organizing Resilience Management for Urban Health

Lessons from the knowledge of complexity science for urban health and well-being (Gatzweiler et al. 2018) have taught us that "a system for governing knowledge and action would need to have as much variety in the actions it can take as exists in the system it is regulating". That means organizing resilience management for urban health needs to respond to some inherent features of complex urban systems. Complex urban systems are not only multi-dimensional, they are multi-sectoral, and the functions they provide (Table 18.1) provide goods and services that have private, public and common pool features.

Nature-based solutions to urban health under climate change are capable of addressing the required variety of such complex urban systems. Resilience management for urban health must combine and link the components addressed above:

1. Knowledge of urban system functions, climate change and health
2. Nature-based solutions (action)
3. Monitoring and impact evaluation
4. Learning and adaptation.

Setting up and governing knowledge-action systems (Fig. 18.2) is a response to the need for solving urban health risks by resilience management. This can be and is being done by scientific analysis of complex urban systems, involving stakeholders in the co-production of knowledge, and implementing that knowledge in decision-making processes. Setting up and governing knowledge-action systems requires: (1) recognition of all urban inhabitants as the stakeholders of urban health, and (2) collective learning. For all urban inhabitants – policymakers, business managers, scientists, citizens and communities – not only are their health and well-

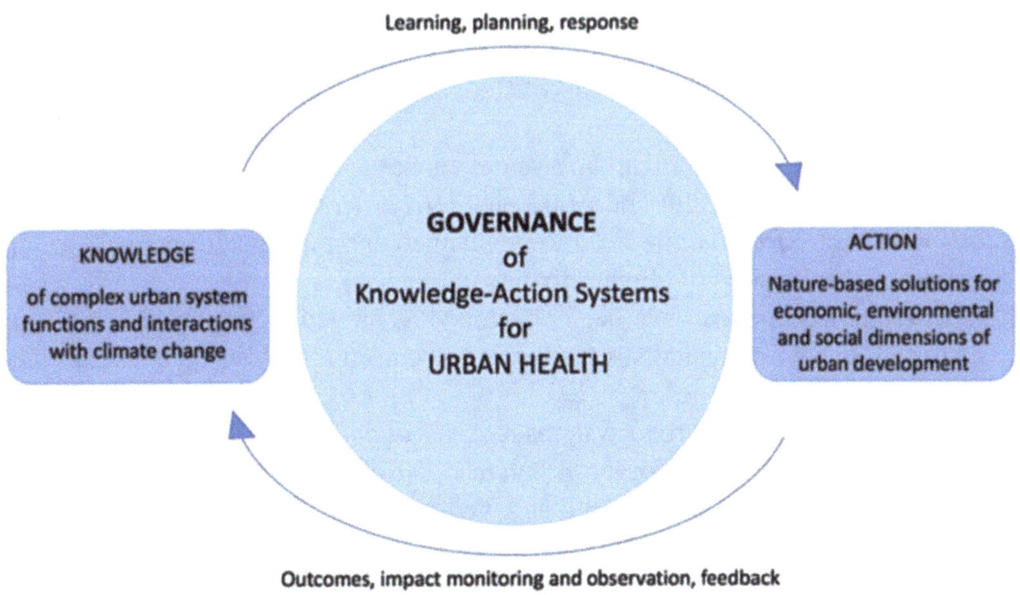

Fig. 18.2 Managing resilience for urban health by implementing and governing of knowledge-action systems

being compromised under climate change, they themselves are also (partially) accountable for the climate-health problems, and, therefore, should be included in resolving them. In addition to knowledge co-creation, policy co-design and implementation and actions to respond to urban climate-health challenges based on the three-dimensional principles of nature-based solutions, governing knowledge-action systems, also requires collective learning. The outcomes of nature-based interventions need to be monitored and observed by stakeholders as feedback to the knowledge pool of climate change, urban ecosystems and health, thereby enabling knowledge-action systems governance, also known as resilience management for urban health, to co-evolve with the changing complexity of urban systems resulting from further impacts of climate change.

18.5 Conclusions

Urban health and well-being outcomes are the product of systems that function to produce services of value to humans. The degree to which urban system functions deliver services for human health and well-being depends on the human capability to manage complexity and create healthy urban environments. Institutions, understood as being made up of rules enabling and constraining interactions, provide the space and freedom for action as well as the organisational constraints.

As human dominance of ecosystems spreads across the globe, humankind must become more proactive not only in trying to preserve components of earlier ecosystems and services that they displace, but also in imagining and building new kinds of ecosystems and nature-based hybrid solutions that allow for a reconciliation between human development, functioning ecosystems and biodiversity. To address this, we offer the following five approaches:

1. *Resilience management for healthy cities* in the context of climate change must be based on a deep understanding of the *complexity of urban systems* and the functions they provide.
2. Climate change affects all urban system functions directly or indirectly, and thereby also human health and well-being. *Urban green areas and greening of other types of infrastructure* need to be planned and managed to respond to the increasing health risks of climate change in cities.
3. *Nature-based solutions* have been developed as an action response to increase resilience to environmental stresses and can be used to *help reduce health risks* of climate change in cities.
4. Managing resilience in urban systems requires *adaptive and flexible governance* styles on several scales in order to enhance multi-functionality of systems and functions that support urban health and well-being.
5. Our knowledge of urban system complexity and urban system functions needs to be translated into actions that are not only nature-based, but also governed by *knowledge-action systems* that recognize all urban inhabitants as stakeholders and enable collective learning for urban health under climate change.

References

Alberti M, Marzluff J (2004) Ecological resilience in urban ecosystems: linking urban patterns to human and ecological functions. Urban Ecosyst 7:241–265

Alberti M, Marzluff J, Shulenberger E, Bradley G, Ryan C, Zumbrunnen C (2003) Integrating humans into ecology: opportunities and challenges for studying urban ecosystems. Bioscience 53:1169–1179

Alberti M, McPhearson T, Gonzales A (2018) Embracing urban complexity. In: Elmqvist et al (eds) Urban planet. Cambridge University Press, Cambridge. https://doi.org/10.1017/9781316647554

Bai X, Surveyer A, Elmqvist T, Gatzweiler FW et al (2016) Defining and advancing a systems approach for sustainable cities. Curr Opin Environ Sustain 23:69–78. https://doi.org/10.1016/j.cosust.2016.11.010

Bai X, Dawson RJ, Urge-Vorsatz D, Delgado GC et al (2018) Six research priorities for cities and climate change. Nature 555:23–25

Bettencourt LMA, Lobo J, Strumsky D, West GB (2010) Urban scaling and its deviations: revealing the structure of wealth, innovation and crime across cities. PLoS One 5(11):e13541. https://doi.org/10.1371/journal.pone.0013541

Biggs R, Schlüter M, Biggs D et al (2012) Towards principles for enhancing the resilience of ecosystem services. Annu Rev Environ Resour 37:421–448

Bowler DE, Buyung-Ali L, Knight TM, Pullin AS (2010) Urban greening to cool towns and cities: a systematic review of the empirical evidence. Landsc Urban Plan 97:147–155

Brelsford C, Lobo J, Hand J, Bettencourt LMA (2017) Heterogeneity and scale of sustainable development in cities. PNAS 114(34):8963–8968

Carpenter S, Walker B, Anderies JM, Abel N (2001) From metaphor to measurement: resilience of what to what? Ecosystems 4(8):765–781

Cash D, Moser SC (2000) Linking global and local scales: designing dynamic assessment and management processes. Glob Environ Chang 10:109–120

Cumming GS, Olsson P, Chapin FS III, Holling CS (2012) Resilience, experimentation, and scale mismatches in social-ecological landscapes. Landsc Ecol 28(6):1139–1150. https://doi.org/10.1007/s10980-012-9725-4

Cutter SL, Barnes L, Berry M et al (2008) A place-based model for understanding community resilience to natural disasters. Glob Environ Chang 18(4):598–606

da Silva J, Kernaghen S, Luque A (2012) A systems approach to meeting the challenges of urban climate change. Int J Urban Sustain Dev 4(2):125–145

Duit A, Galaz V (2008) Governance and complexity—emerging issues for governance theory. Gov: Int J Policy Adm Inst 21(3):311–335

Elmqvist T, Barnett G, Wilkinson C (2013a) Exploring urban sustainability and resilience. In: Pearson L, Newton P, Rpberts P (eds) Resilient sustainable cities. Routledge, New York

Elmqvist T et al (eds) (2013b) Urbanization, biodiversity and ecosystem services: challenges and opportunities: a global assessment. Springer, Dordrecht. https://doi.org/10.1007/978-94-007-7088-1_1

Ernstson H, van der Leeuw SE, Redman CL et al (2010) Urban transitions: on urban resilience and human dominated ecosystems. AMBIO J Hum Environ 39(8):531–545

EU DG Research & Innovation (2015) Nature-based solutions & re-naturing cities. Towards an EU Research and Innovation policy agenda. https://doi.org/10.2777/765301

Folke C, Jansson Å, Larsson J, Costanza R (1997) Ecosystem appropriation by cities. Ambio 26:167–172

Folke C, Carpenter S, Elmqvist T et al (2002) Resilience and sustainable development: building adaptive capacity in a world of transformations. AMBIO J Hum Environ 31(5):437–440

Folke C, Carpenter SR, Walker B et al (2010) Resilience thinking: integrating resilience, adaptability and transformability. Ecol Soc 15(4):20

Gatzweiler FW et al (2016) Advancing health and wellbeing in the changing urban environment. Implementing a systems approach. Zhejiang University Press and Springer, Hangzhou

Gatzweiler FW, Boufford JI, Pomykala A (2018) Harness urban complexity for health and well-being. In: Elmqvist et al (eds) Urban planet. Cambridge University Press, Cambridge. https://doi.org/10.1017/9781316647554

Geels F (2011) Role of cities in technological transitions. In: Bulkeley et al (eds) Cities and low carbon transitions. Routledge Taylor and Francis Group, London/New York, p 13e28

Gill SE et al (2007) Adapting cities for climate change: the role of the green infrastructure. Built Environ 33:115–133

González-Oreja J, Bonache-Regidor C, Fuente-Díaz-Ordaz A (2010) Far from the noisy world? Modelling the relationships between park size, tree cover and noise levels in urban green spaces of the city of Puebla, Mexico. Interciencia 35:486–492

Grimm NB, Faeth SH, Golubiewski NE et al (2008) Global change and the ecology of cities. Science 319:756–760

Grove JM (2009) Cities: managing densely settled social-ecological systems. In: Chapin FS III, Kofinas GP, Folke C (eds) Principles of ecosystem stewardship: resilience-based natural resource management in a changing world. Springer, New York, pp 281–294

Haines A (2018) Planetary health: is human health at risk in the Anthropocene? Lecture, March 8, Lecture Theatre at the Oxford Martin School. https://www.oxfordmartin.ox.ac.uk/event/2526

Hardin PJ, Jensen RR (2007) The effect of urban leaf area on summertime urban surface kinetic temperatures: a Terre Haute case study. Urban For Urban Green 6:63–72

Hartig T, Mitchell R, de Vries S, Frumkin H (2014) Nature and health. Annu Rev Public Health 35:207–228

Hodson M, Marvin S (2010) Can cities shape socio-technical transitions and how would we know if they were? Res Policy 39:477–485

Holling CS (2001) Understanding the complexity of economic, ecological, and social systems. Ecosystems 4(5):390–405

Intergovernmental Panel on Climate Change (IPCC) (2014) Smith KR, Woodward A, Campbell-Lendrum D et al. Human health: Impacts, adaptation, and co-benefits. In: Field CB, Barros VR, Dokken DJ et al (eds) Climate Change 2014: impacts, adaptation, and vulnerability. Part A: Global and sectoral aspects Working Group II contribution of to the fifth assessment report of the Intergovernmental Panel on Climate Change. Cambridge University Press, Cambridge/New York, pp 709–754

Kabisch N, Frantzeskaki N, Pauleit S et al (2016) Nature-based solutions to climate change mitigation and adaptation in urban areas: perspectives on indicators, knowledge gaps, barriers, and opportunities for action. Ecol Soc 21. art39

Kovats RS, Hajat S (2008) Heat stress and public health: a critical review. Annu Rev Public Health 29:41–55

Leach M, Scoones I, Stirling A (2010) Governing epidemics in an age of complexity: narratives, politics and pathways to sustainability. Glob Environ Chang 20:369–377

Marcotullio P, McGranahan G (2007) Scaling the urban environmental transition, from local to global and Back. Earthscan, London

Markelova H, Mwangi E (2012) Multilevel governance and cross-scale coordination for natural resource management: lessons from current research. In: Bollier D, Helfrich S (eds) The wealth of the commons: a world beyond market and state. Levellers Press, Amherst

Michelozzi P, Accetta G, De Sario M et al (2009) High temperature and hospitalizations for cardiovascular and respiratory causes in 12 European cities. Am J Respir Crit Care Med 179(5):383–389

Muñoz-Erickson T, Miller C, Miller T (2017) How cities think: knowledge co-production for urban sustainability and resilience. Forests 8(12):203. https://doi.org/10.3390/f8060203

Pataki DE, Carreiro MM, Cherrier J et al (2011) Coupling biogeochemical cycles in urban environments: ecosystem services, green solutions, and misconceptions. Front Ecol Environ 9:27–36

Pickett STA, Cadenasso ML, Grove JM et al (2011) Urban ecological systems: scientific foundations and a decade of progress. J Environ Manag 92:331–362

Pickett STA, Boone CG, McGrath BP et al (2013) Ecological science and transformation to the sustainable city. Cities 32:S10–S20

Polasky S, Carpenter SR, Folke C, Keeler B (2011) Decision-making under great uncertainty: environmental management in an era of global change. Trends Ecol Evol 26:398–404. https://doi.org/10.1016/j.tree.2011.04.007

Secretariat of the Convention on Biological Diversity (2009) Connecting biodiversity and climate change mitigation and adaptation: report of the second ad hoc technical expert group on biodiversity and climate change. Montreal

Seitzinger S et al (2012) Planetary stewardship in an urbanizing world: beyond city limits. Ambio 41:787–794. https://doi.org/10.1007/s13280-012-0353-7

Seto KC, Reenberg A, Boone CG et al (2012) Urban land teleconnections and sustainability. Proc Natl Acad Sci U S A 109:7687–7692. https://doi.org/10.1073/pnas.1117622109

UNEP (2013) City-level decoupling: urban resource flows and the governance of infrastructure transitions. A Report of the Working Group on Cities of the International Resource Panel

Vale LJ, Campanella TJ (2005) The resilient city: how modern cities recover from disaster. Oxford University Press, Oxford

Walker B, Salt D (2006) Resilience thinking: sustaining ecosystems and people in a changing world. Island Press, Washington, DC

Walker B, Holling CS, Carpenter SR, Kinzig A (2004) Resilience, adaptability and transformability in social-ecological systems. Ecol Soc 9(2):5

Wallace D, Wallace R (2008) Urban systems during disasters: factors for resilience. Ecol Soc 13(1):18

West G (2017) Scale. The universal laws of growth, innovation, sustainability, and the pace of life in organisms, cities, economies, and companies. Penguin Press, New York

WHO (2017) Urban green spaces: a brief for action. WHO Regional Office for Europe, Copenhagen

Zhang Y, Murray AT, Turner BL (2017) Optimizing green space locations to reduce daytime and nighttime urban heat island effects in Phoenix, Arizona. Landsc Urban Plan 165:162–171. https://doi.org/10.1016/j.landurbplan.2017.04.009

Zhu YG, Reid BJ, Meharg AA, Banwart SA, Fu BJ (2017) Optimizing Peri-URban ecosystems (PURE) to re-couple urban-rural symbiosis. Sci Total Environ 15(586):1085–1090

Chapter 19
Linking Landscape Planning and Health

Stefan Heiland, Julia Weidenweber, and Catharine Ward Thompson

Abstract Aims and measures in landscape planning often align with aims for positive health outcomes, even if these are not explicitly mentioned in the planning documents. This chapter examines whether, and if so how, health issues are already being tackled in formal and informal landscape planning instruments in Germany and the UK at present and how this could be enhanced in the future. Thus, the focus is on planning issues, practice and methods. In addition, health-promoting features of green spaces, regarding both single green spaces and entire green space systems, are considered, as well as a method for planning greenway systems for daily physical mobility. Addressing health issues in landscape planning is a necessary part of sustainable planning in order to be able to cope with future developments, such as increasing climate change impacts and accelerating societal changes. For this reason, interdisciplinary corporation between landscape planning and the health sector should be strengthened.

Keywords Landscape planning · Open space planning · Local plans · Health promotion · Greenways for mobility · Green infrastructure

Highlights Integrating health issues into landscape planning holds manifold benefits for both sides.

- Potentials to include health issues in landscape planning are not yet fully used.
- Considering human health in landscape planning can be done in different ways and with different intensities.

S. Heiland (✉) · J. Weidenweber
Department of Landscape Planning and Development, Technische Universität Berlin, Berlin, Germany
e-mail: stefan.heiland@tu-berlin.de; julia.weidenweber@googlemail.com

C. Ward Thompson
OPENspace Research Centre, University of Edinburgh, Edinburgh, Scotland, UK
e-mail: c.ward-thompson@ed.ac.uk

M. R. Marselle et al. (eds.), *Biodiversity and Health in the Face of Climate Change*, https://doi.org/10.1007/978-3-030-02318-8_19

- Planning 'greenways for mobility' is an appropriate way to include health issues.
- Landscape planning must tackle key societal problems to be socially acknowledged.

19.1 Introduction

Multiple studies now suggest that access to green or natural environments may play an important role in supporting public health, including mitigating air and water pollution, offering opportunities for healthy activities and contributing to better mental health (WHO 2016). This has been triggered in part by the challenges of climate change, especially increases in the urban heat-island effect, and the effects of urban densification in an increasingly urbanised society, which may have both positive and negative consequences for the health of urban residents. To tackle these challenges, health issues must be integrated into spatial and urban as well as landscape planning, taking into account the potential for multiple positive health effects from urban green spaces and elements. However, there are many difficulties in determining how to guide and regulate such plans in the context of other demands for sustainable and cost-effective urban development (Wolch et al. 2014).

While green spaces exert many positive effects on human health, or at least have the potential to do so, they can at the same time be of great importance for protecting developing biodiversity. However, it should be noted that 'green' space, especially in urban areas, does not necessarily contribute to biodiversity (especially its in situ protection) as it comprises, for example, sport grounds, intensively used grassland, private gardens and monoculture cropland or forests. Nonetheless, even sites like these, despite certain adverse environmental effects (e.g. groundwater pollution), can also have positive environmental and human health benefits that should not be overlooked, even if they often could be enhanced, especially in terms of biodiversity.

In this chapter, health is understood according to the definition of the World Health Organization (WHO) as a state of complete physical, mental and social well-being (WHO 2017a). Consequently, for the purpose of our interest in environment-health links, health can be divided into social, mental, physical and aesthetic-symbolic components (the last category meaning that urban green could, for example, symbolise good human-nature relationships to a person, which might support their well-being), which need to be considered equally (Rittel et al. 2014, 2016).[1] Moreover, health promotion should be distinguished from health protection: health protection refers to preventing potential health risks and diseases, whereas health promotion focuses on maintaining health, strengthening health resources and establishing health-promoting environments (ibid.).

[1] The publications by Rittel et al. (2014, 2016) are identical, the version from 2016 is the English translation of the original publication in German (2014). From here on we quote only Rittel et al. (2016).

By the term 'landscape planning' we refer to all formal and informal planning instruments and procedures aimed at protecting, managing, designing, redesigning and maintaining green spaces and green elements, especially in an urban environment, including elements such as street trees and façade greening. Thus, the term covers a broad range of instruments in the realm of nature conservation, landscape architecture and urban or land use planning. Referring to the planning systems and instruments of Germany and the UK, respectively, we focus on the official instruments of landscape planning in Germany and on Local Plans or Core Strategies of Local Development Frameworks (official) as well as Green Infrastructure strategies (informal) in England as a part of the UK. This concentration on two countries is due, first, to the authors' main areas of expertise, and second, to the heterogeneity of planning systems in different countries across Europe, to which we cannot do justice in one book chapter. Nonetheless, we think that many recommendations might also be applicable to or adaptable by other countries.

This chapter does not concentrate on the health effects of urban green space and biodiversity, as these have been covered comprehensively in previous chapters (see Part I; Marselle et al. Chap. 9; Cook et al. Chap. 11, all this volume). Instead, our aim is to show whether and how health issues are already being tackled in formal and informal landscape planning instruments in Germany and the UK, and how this could be enhanced in the future. As research and practical gaps can be found in the incorporation of health aspects into landscape and spatial planning, our chapter focuses on planning issues, practice and methods. Furthermore, we present health-promoting features of green spaces, including single green spaces as well as entire green space systems, and present a method for planning a greenway system for daily physical mobility.

19.2 Benefits of Considering Health Issues in Landscape Planning

Aims and measures in landscape planning often align with positive health effects, even if those are not explicitly mentioned. To give some examples: the conservation of biodiversity and species-rich habitats often also safeguards aesthetically pleasing recreational areas; clean lakes and rivers can serve as important habitats as well as bathing waters or for the supply of drinking water; soil conservation contributes to food security and to groundwater recharge and rainwater retention during heavy rains, and thus reduces the risk of flooding, including associated health risks. Furthermore, climate change, demographic changes, changes in lifestyle, and – not least – increased urbanization demanding new residential areas can have effects on urban, but also rural, green spaces. Consequently, these factors have implications for landscape planning and for human health and health protection and promotion. Recreation is strongly related to health and is a topic that has been thoroughly considered for some time in landscape planning. Even here, however, it must be acknowledged that conflicts in landscape planning might also appear, for example, regarding the use of allergenic plants or the promotion of vector-borne diseases as an unintended side effect of promoting urban green (Damialis et al. Chap. 3, this volume; WHO 2016).

Consequently, there is considerable evidence that addressing health issues in landscape planning is helpful, indeed necessary, in order for planning authorities to be able to cope with future developments, and in order to make use of potential synergies and to mitigate conflicts and unintended negative side effects of planning. Furthermore, under conditions of increasing climate change impacts and accelerating societal changes, landscape planning, landscape architecture and nature conservation will only play a significant role for politicians and decision-makers if such disciplines are able to contribute to the solution of urgent societal challenges – such as health protection and promotion (see Heiland 2017, 183ff.). As Prüss-Ustün et al. (2017, p. 474) have said, "Investing in environmental interventions pays off for governments; it reduces the transfer of hidden costs from other sectors to the health sector". Conversely, there will be no future for landscape planning if it concentrates only on biodiversity, as it will always take a backseat against other interests – however important from an expert's perspective – such as health, social issues, drinking water supply and economic questions for the broader public and in politics.

It is important, therefore, to underline the need for interdisciplinary cooperation between landscape planning and the health sector (see Cook et al. Chap. 11, this volume). A mere consideration of health in landscape planning is not sufficient; there are greater opportunities for both sides from fuller collaborative working, and these should therefore be a priority: "While a new environmental conceptualisation of health [Ecological Public Health] might seem a difficult and complex task, that is the 21st century's unavoidable task" (Rayner and Lang 2012, p. 52). Nonetheless: It is a challenging task as it requires cooperation across disciplines and administrations with different approaches, aims, values and languages. For example, whereas landscape planners' thinking is primarily spatially based, the approach of health promotion is oriented towards the individual (Rittel et al. 2016, p. 20). As shown by Rittel et al. (2016) in the example of four case-study municipalities in Germany, an intensified cooperation between authorities responsible for nature conservation, landscape and green space planning on the one hand and health authorities on the other is hampered by factors that differ according to the size of municipality: in smaller municipalities, health authorities do not exist (as they are located at a county level), whereas in bigger cities they exist in a very differentiated, non-standardised way, which makes it difficult to identify the appropriate contact person for every planning issue. Furthermore, public health planning and longer term visions for supporting health may be beyond the usual concern of the relevant tier of health authority, e.g. of local clinical commissioning groups in the UK, which manage delivery of local health services. In the UK, landscape planning issues may be better understood at a national level, e.g. by Public Health England. Limited resources and competence are additional reasons that make cooperation difficult, factors that may well apply to other countries as well as the UK and Germany. Nonetheless: "The 'healthy city' (…) can only be understood as an interdisciplinary task and as the product of a concerted effort of many actors" (Klages 2012, p. 323, translation by the authors). This statement also applies to the 'climate-resilient, green and biodiverse city'.

19.3 Health as an Issue in Local Landscape Planning in Germany and the UK – The Status Quo

In order to understand how health issues are considered in landscape planning in Germany and the UK, it is necessary to know some basics about their planning systems, which are briefly introduced. This serves to clarify why we have chosen certain instruments for a deeper investigation. Finally, at the end of this section, we note our findings regarding the recent considerations of health in landscape planning.

19.3.1 The (Landscape) Planning System in Germany

Landscape Planning in Germany is an independent official planning instrument regulated by §§ 8–12 of the German Federal Nature Conservation Act (Bundesnaturschutzgesetz – BNatSchG) and the respective sections of the nature conservation acts of the 16 German federal states.[2] Landscape Planning generally exists on four different spatial-administrative levels or tiers: federal state, region (or similar administrative units, e.g. counties), municipalities, and partial areas of municipalities. On each of these levels, landscape plans cover the entire planning area, which means they comprise settlements as well as non-settlement areas (the only exception being North Rhine-Westphalia). Landscape planning aims to achieve the objectives of nature conservation as laid down in § 1 of the Federal Nature Conservation Act (BNatSchG) through protection, management, development and restoration of nature and landscapes. These objectives are the long-term safeguarding of: (1) biological diversity; (2) the performance and functioning of ecosystems, including their ability to regenerate, and the sustainable provisioning of natural resource functions; and (3) the diversity, uniqueness and beauty as well as the recreation value of nature and landscapes. Thus, landscape planning serves as a spatially oriented sectoral planning instrument for nature conservation, and delivers an 'ecological contribution' to comprehensive land use and spatial planning and other sectoral plans, such as traffic, agricultural and forestry planning. Requirements formulated by the landscape plans have to be integrated into the respective spatial or land-use plans at the same spatial level in order to become legally binding. Nonetheless, spatial or land use plans and sectoral plans have to consider the

[2] In detail, legal regulations for Landscape Planning differ between the German federal states, e.g. in terms of planning levels and the integration of landscape planning issues into spatial planning. These differences can be neglected for the purposes of this chapter.

requirements of landscape plans, but can deviate from them if appropriate reasons are given in the planning process. Thus, there is a strong link between landscape and spatial planning (at the regional and federal state level) and land use planning (at the local level), even if landscape planning remains independent. Furthermore, all spatial and land use plans (and in some federal states, also landscape plans), are usually subject to a Strategic Environmental Assessment (SEA) according to the EU SEA Directive, by which potential impacts of plans on the environment and on human health are assessed. In the following text we concentrate on landscape plans at municipal level (aka 'The local landscape plan'), as this is a sufficiently concrete level (scale usually 1:10.000), appropriate for considering health issues related to distinct areas; although health topics could also be an issue at other levels in the planning system.

19.3.2 The (Landscape) Planning System in the UK

In the UK, planning is devolved to the four countries of England, Wales, Scotland and Northern Ireland, whose enabling legislation and guidance tools are largely country-specific (Winter et al. 2016). The English planning system, on which we put a certain focus here, differs strongly from the German one; with the 'Localism Act' of 2011 the regional planning tier was abolished and almost all planning responsibility was conferred to the local level. The only guidance for local planning is given by the 'National Planning Policy Framework' (NPPF, Department for Communities and Local Government 2012), which has to be "taken into account in the preparation of local and neighbourhood plans, and is a material consideration in planning decisions" (ibid., p. 1), the legislative basis of which are the 'Planning & Compulsory Purchase Act' (2004) and the 'Town and Country Planning Regulations' (2012). Local Plans have taken over the function of the former 'Local Development Frameworks,' which were a portfolio of different planning documents, with a 'Core Strategy' as their central element. Both kinds of local planning documents still coexist and have to consider environmental and landscape issues, according to sections 9 ('Protecting Green Belt land') and 11 ('Conserving and Enhancing the Natural Environment') of the NPPF. Under the Town and Country Planning (Environmental Impact Assessment) Regulations 2017, local planning authorities have a general responsibility to consider the environmental implications of developments that are subject to planning control. The 2017 Regulations integrate Environmental Impact Assessment (EIA) procedures into this framework but apply only to those projects that are likely to have significant effects on the environment, e.g. airports, major road developments; power generation installations; mining, etc.

Despite environmental issues only playing a subordinate role in the formal UK planning systems, no separate or independent landscape planning system exists. One could argue that this obvious neglect of environmental and landscape issues in UK land-use planning has led to attempts to fill that gap, for example, by a considerable amount of local and (sub-)regional level, informal planning instruments such as

'Green Infrastructure Frameworks' and 'Green Infrastructure Strategies' (for a comprehensive overview on the political and neo-liberal background of this development see Hehn 2016). Green Infrastructure (GI) is "a network of multi-functional green space, urban and rural, which is capable of delivering a wide range of environmental and quality of life benefits for local communities" (Department for Communities and Local Government 2012, p. 52). The respective definitions of GI can differ and include different types of 'green' (e.g. even light railway lines) or aquatic features such as rivers, canals and ponds (ibid.). GI strategies are prepared at a local level to establish, maintain and enhance a municipality's GI, often not only to achieve ecological aims but also economic and social benefits (e.g. economic growth, property values, labor productivity, social cohesion, or quality of place) (Manchester City Council 2015). Many GI-strategies are explicitly aimed – amongst other things – at improving the health and well-being of residents. To some extent, aims or measures stated in GI strategies are incorporated into the Local Plans and/or Core Strategies and thereby influence official, legally binding plans. In the following sections we concentrate on Local Plans/Core Strategies and GI strategies, particularly regarding possible differences in how they tackle health issues.

19.3.3 Landscape Planning and Health in Germany

As there is a certain 'traditional' (even if criticised and contested) emphasis on biodiversity in landscape plans in Germany, human health has never been an important topic there. Although human health is mentioned in §1 BNatSchG as one reason for protecting nature, it doesn't have the status of a 'natural asset,' which landscape planning is obliged to deal with. Consequently, considering health issues is a voluntary task, unless landscape plans are subject to a SEA, as is the case in some federal states. In such a case, potential health impacts of the landscape plan have to be assessed and valued, but still no kind of 'pro-active planning for health,' especially regarding health promotion, is required. Furthermore, differentiated knowledge about health effects of biodiversity, landscape and green spaces is often lacking amongst conservationists and landscape planners, at least if it reaches beyond the general notion that 'a good environmental condition is the basis of human life.' At the same time, health authorities are seldom involved in planning decisions. Consequently, very few landscape plans explicitly and pro-actively refer to human health (Rittel et al. 2016). Where this is done, it happens in the context of experiencing nature, urban green spaces and recreation, as in the local landscape plan of the city of Hohen Neuendorf (Stadt Hohen Neuendorf 2014) as an example.

Nonetheless there are many links to health issues in landscape planning in general, but also in the respective single planning documents. Human health is often addressed implicitly, e.g. when dealing with 'recreation,' but also when dealing with other issues, such as air purification, groundwater protection, soil conservation, climate change, etc. (see examples in Sect. 19.2 and more comprehensively in Sect. 19.4). But these connections – and therefore the relevance of conserving and enhancing landscape and green spaces for human health – are not explicitly set out. As such, it has to be assumed that landscape-health relationships are largely irrelevant as a basis for political and administrative decisions, even if health impacts of intended land use changes have to be assessed by the SEA for local land-use plans, which, again, are mainly restricted to the avoidance or minimization of potential negative impacts of the plan, e.g. by noise and air pollution or the release of hazardous waste. More attention is paid to health in some informal planning concepts on urban development (Claßen and Mekel 2017; Rittel et al. 2016), but there is no strong link to landscape plans.

During the last few years, health has received increasing consideration in different documents (and sometimes additional funding) related to issues of landscape and urban green space planning, published by the German Ministry for Environment and Building (German Federal Ministry for the Environment, Nature Conservation, Building and Nuclear Safety, BMUB)[3] and the Federal Agency for Nature Conservation (BfN). In some cases, this is linked to the concepts of Green Infrastructure and Ecosystem Services, which, despite many possible points of critique (e.g. Heiland et al. 2016; Silvertown 2015), suggest an intention to raise awareness for a stronger consideration of health (and other human needs and interests) in nature conservation, landscape planning and landscape architecture. Examples include the 'Federal Green Infrastructure Concept' (BfN 2017a) and its underlying research report (Heiland et al. 2017), the reports of TEEB Germany for urban and rural areas (Naturkapital Deutschland – TEEB DE 2016a, b), the 'Urban Green Infrastructure' brochure with recommendations for municipalities (BfN 2017b) and the 'White Paper on Urban Green' (BMUB 2017). Rittel et al. (2016), being a result of a research project funded by the BfN, directly addresses municipalities in order to use synergies between landscape planning and health. It remains to be seen how these efforts and documents affect planning practice in the mid- to long-term perspective.

19.3.4 Landscape Planning and Health in the UK

As in Germany, public health has only become a formal consideration within the UK planning system relatively recently, although it should be noted that the promotion of public parks in urban areas in 19th century UK was premised on the need to protect the health of industrial workers. The current planning system is based conceptually on post-WW2 Town and Country Planning legislation, which made implicit (but not explicit) assumptions about the desirability of separating industrial zones from residential and recreational areas, in order to protect health.

Currently, Health Impact Assessment (HIA) across the UK is promoted by the government's Department of Health (DH) as a means to assess the health impact of

[3] Since 2018: Federal Ministry for the Environment, Nature Conservation and Nuclear Safety (BMU).

new government policy and its implementation (DH 2010a, b). Government guidance on the planning system states that local planning authorities should ensure that health and well-being and health infrastructure are considered in local and neighbourhood plans and in planning decision making. However, the use of HIA in the UK is only recommended as one way of considering the issues: "A health impact assessment may be a useful tool to use where there are expected to be significant impacts" (Ministry for Housing, Communities and Local Government 2014). Nonetheless, this guidance regards GI as a tool to link health and planning. It names safe and green open spaces as places for active play and food growing, and identifies green space accessibility by walking, cycling and public transport as attributes of a healthy community.

To gain insight into the current trend of incorporating health issues into the UK's spatial plans, an analysis of ten English planning documents has been carried out: six Core Strategies/Local Plans and four GI Strategies, all published or adopted in 2010 or later.[4] The planning documents were chosen to cover municipalities differing from one another in terms of inhabitants, size and geographical location as well as legal liability (Local Plans and Core Strategies being statutory, GI Strategies being informal and voluntary).[5]

The findings show that all planning documents deal with human health, but in different ways. All six Core Strategies/Local Plans mention health issues only implicitly, mainly in the context of climate change adaptation and mitigation as well as flood defense, thereby strongly targeting health protection. In contrast, all four GI Strategies explicitly name the improvement of health, due to the establishment or improvement of GI, as an objective, aim, or vision, and clearly refer to health promotion (e.g. encouraging active exercise in green spaces), while health protection plays a subordinated role in most cases. Nonetheless, both kinds of planning documents address physical activity by identifying the need for high-quality walking and cycling routes. However, differing reasons are given: Core Strategies/Local Plans mainly justify this on the basis of reduced vehicle emissions, improved safety of pedestrians and cyclists, as well as less congestion; whereas GI Strategies strongly promote access to the outdoors to encourage physical activity, leading to reduced obesity and respiratory diseases. Again, GI Strategies connect green structures and health more directly and explicitly.

---

[4]Core Strategies/Local Plans: Aylesbury Vale; South Kesteven; Bath & North East Somerset; Manchester; Lewisham; and Oxford. GI Strategies: Aylesbury Vale; South Kesteven; Bath & North East Somerset; and Manchester.

When investigating the chosen planning documents, implicit as well as explicit references to health aspects have been documented to ensure a thorough analysis. A keyword-search was conducted. To find explicit references to health issues, search terms like 'health,' 'physical activity,' etc. were used. Implicit references were documented when statements revealed links to health issues without explicitly naming them (e.g. recreation, air pollution control, groundwater purification, climate change adaptation, and mitigation, etc.). Finally, the documented statements were assigned to either health protection or health promotion.

[5]Note that ten planning documents only depict a small extract of the recent situation in the UK's planning system where legislative requirements differ between the countries of England, Wales, Scotland and Northern Ireland. Therefore, a generalization on the entire UK situation is not possible. However, this analysis can be seen as a starting point for further investigation.

Two important requirements of health are recreation and food supply. Recreation is frequently mentioned in the two kinds of planning documents: Green spaces are recognised as recreational opportunities and thus their maintenance or improvement is generally seen as an important goal of planning in all of the ten analyzed documents, even though they are more often and more intensively mentioned in GI strategies. Most of the investigated GI documents draw an explicit connection between healthier lifestyles and the improvement of areas for recreation. The investigated Local Plans/Core Strategies (with a few exceptions) do not draw this connection but rather look at recreational areas from a planning point of view (e.g. maintenance and development of a network of recreational routes that provide easy access to countryside areas ensuring that the need for recreational areas of all residents is met).

Regarding food supply, half of the investigated documents – three Core Strategies/Local Plans and two GI Strategies – promote 'grow your own' schemes. These include community food groups as well as individual growing plots and allotments. It should be noted that the health benefits of growing one's own food are not only from healthy nutrition but also arise from the physical outdoor activity (and potential social cohesion benefits) related to it. Van den Berg et al.'s (2010) study of 120 allotment holders and 60 non-gardeners in the Netherlands found that allotment gardeners are more physically active; 84% of allotment gardeners met the national recommendations for physical activity, compared to 62% of non-gardeners.

To sum up, as far as our selection of ten case studies allows, it can be said that the contribution of green spaces and elements to human health is already integrated into England's planning approaches, but it is more explicit in the informal and voluntary GI documents. Core Strategies/Local Plans refer to health issues in an implicit way by dealing with topics such as climate change adaptation and mitigation, walking and cycling routes, recreation, or 'grow your own' schemes, without clearly mentioning the health effects of the respective aims and actions. Therefore, it can be assumed that the *status quo* in official planning documents is similar to Germany. Recently, Public Health England has issued guidance (2017) to try to link HIA to EIA, and to encourage public health teams to engage with the planning system in this regard. It recognises that, for major developments at least, the consideration of impacts needs to be multi-dimensional and consider health as well as the landscape and other environmental issues.

19.4 Ways to Include Health Issues in Planning Processes and Documents

Three options to promote human health in landscape planning have been identified by Rittel et al. (2016). Whilst mainly referring to urban landscape planning in Germany, they could also be transferred and applied to other planning instruments or systems. The three options differ in methodological intensity and breadth of scope:

1. Health as a factor to be assessed by Strategic Environmental Assessment
2. Health as an argument to further support 'traditional' landscape planning goals
3. Health as an independent topic in landscape planning.

1. Health as a factor to be assessed by Strategic Environmental Assessment

Integration of human health in a SEA (being a part of Sustainability Appraisal in England) is already legally required by the EU SEA Directive 2001/42/EC. The positive and negative health impacts of the proposed objectives and measures in a plan need to be thoroughly addressed. As a result, adverse health effects will be avoided and positive effects of (landscape) planning can be identified. These positive health effects of goals and measures, which are primarily aimed at landscape and biodiversity conservation, could be more explicitly named as they justify those goals and measures from a different, more antropocentric, perspective. This could lead to a higher societal and political acceptance than pure 'environmental conservation arguments' might get. Nonetheless, this approach does not allow for proactively taking means to directly enhance the health benefits of green spaces.

2. Health as an argument to further support 'traditional' landscape planning goals

'Traditional' landscape planning in Germany aims at improving the state of the environment mainly in terms of biodiversity, but also in terms of landscape, soil, water, air and climate. Very often goals and measures identified for these purposes have positive side effects for human health, which are usually not explicitly mentioned in the plans. Hence, this option seeks to draw more attention to health effects by identifying and exposing them, and is therefore similar to the first option, but can also be used where no SEA is required. It is still the case, however, that no predominantly health-related objectives, goals, or measures are pursued with this option. Table 19.1 gives an overview of objectives often included in German landscape plans, and their potential health-related side effects. By naming these health effects, they could become effects pursued in landscape planning more consciously and proactive, rather than simply remaining unintended 'side effects' as at present. Methodologically, this option requires a survey and evaluation of health-related characteristics of specific green spaces as well as the likely health outcomes of implementing landscape planning objectives and measures. While the potential health benefits may be straightforward to identify based on current knowledge and evidence (e.g. WHO 2016), the scale and reach of the benefits may require more sophisticated tools than are conventionally available to planning officers.

Many planning documents encourage walking, cycling and the use of public transport. Here too, links to human health and well-being could be drawn, which not only result from minimised negative impacts of traffic (noise and air pollution), but also from enhanced physical fitness and mental health. As access to green spaces and their use is associated with a decrease in health risks such as high blood pressure and cholesterol, path and cycleways could be equipped with green structures or set up in green areas of the municipality.

Table 19.1 Examples of possible health-related effects of landscape planning objectives

Objectives of landscape planning	Health-related effects
Biological diversity	
Conservation of biological diversity	Species diversity (if not regarded as 'wild' or 'unmanaged') is often considered beautiful and can thereby contribute to relaxation and stress reduction, consequently enhancing well-being (e.g. via such mechanism as soft fascination, attention restoration, connecting self with nature, place identity)
	Depending on the type of urban green and its management, species diversity can reduce or increase vector-borne diseases (e.g. lyme disease)
Water	
Protection of groundwater and surface waters from pollutants	Health protection by preventing the contamination of drinking water or natural bathing/swimming areas
Protection and development of water areas	Health protection and promotion by positive bioclimatic effects during the day (cooling)
	Health promotion and enhancement of well-being due to the attractiveness of water bodies and their suitability for recreational uses
	Promotion of mental well-being by positive effects on mental relaxation and stress reduction
Protection of groundwater resources	Health protection by ensuring an adequate drinking water supply
Climate/Air	
Protection of functions of green spaces regarding bioclimatic conditions and air quality	Health protection by the preservation and development of bioclimatic comfort islands and areas for production and transport of cool and fresh (cleaned) air
	Filtration of air-borne pollutants
	Health protection by implementing appropriate measures to reduce bioclimatic stress due to climate change
Soil	
Protection of the retention and water storing function of soils	Health protection by storing and evaporation of precipitation and flood water, reducing flood damage to homes and livelihoods
Protection of the filtering and buffering functions of soils	Health protection by avoiding contamination of soil and groundwater
	Health protection by remediation of contaminated sites and improved groundwater protection
Protection of the natural yield function	Health protection by ensuring the natural preconditions for food production
Protection of the archive function of geotopes	Health promotion by securing historically important geotopes which could contribute to recreation, a sense of place and regional identity

(continued)

Table 19.1 (continued)

Objectives of landscape planning	Health-related effects
Diversity, uniqueness and beauty of nature and landscape, open space recreation	
Protection of landscape and recreational functions	Health promotion and protection by preservation and development of natural, semi-natural and cultural characteristic landscape elements and green spaces, which contribute to the aesthetic attractiveness of a landscape and to local or regional identity
	Health promotion by prevention, reduction or elimination of factors impairing recreation
	Health promotion by preservation and development of various types of green spaces with potential for a diversity of different uses (physical exercise, social interaction, relaxation and restoration, nature experience, growing food, etc.)

Based upon Rittel et al. (2016, 77ff)

3. Health as an independent topic in landscape planning

Here, health related aspects are not just used to provide further support for 'traditional' landscape planning objectives. Instead, specific goals and measures are developed for the purposes of health protection, and health promotion. From a health promotion perspective, this is the preferred option, as it is the only one which allows for explicit pro-active measures promoting health, regardless of other landscape planning issues, such as biodiversity, water protection etc. This means, however, that landscape planning enters previously uncharted territory. Consequently, landscape planners require new knowledge, as they are usually not trained in health planning, and cooperation with health authorities. This is the most comprehensive and complex of the three options for including health concerns in landscape and green space planning, and requires the following working steps (Rittel et al. 2016, p. 41):

- Survey and assessment of the potential or actual health-promoting effects of green spaces
- Identifying and resolving conflicts between health-related requirements or aspirations and other landscape planning objectives
- Development of health-promoting measures in green spaces and the entire system of green spaces in a city
- Redesign of green spaces to improve their health-promoting potential and effects, if necessary
- Analysis of existing and potential user groups and others whose health might benefit: As health-related potentials and effects of green spaces heavily depend on user-specific requirements, an analysis of user groups is recommended. In every step of the planning process, it is useful to consider their needs and interests, as many health potentials of green spaces can only be realised if the spaces are actually used and/or considered as community places. Therefore, green

spaces must be adapted to the users' demands and stakeholder participation should play an important role in the planning processes (as, of course, should generally be the case, also regarding other planning issues besides health).

As the investigation of the ten English planning documents revealed, even explicit references to health issues are generally quite vague, e.g. 'GI promotes healthier lifestyles'. *How* this happens is often not explained, nor the means to plan green space to achieve this goal. To strengthen such kinds of statements it would be helpful to refer to scientific studies which give evidence of positive effects of urban green space on human health, and the likely magnitude of that effect. Examples of such studies include: Abraham et al. (2007), Bedimo-Rung et al. (2005), Bell et al. (2008), Fuller et al. (2007), Francis et al. (2012), Grahn and Stigsdotter (2010), Kaczynski et al. (2008), Lee and Maheswaran (2011), Mitchell and Popham (2007), Newton (2007), Pretty et al. (2010), Roe et al. (2013, 2016), Stigsdotter et al. (2010), Ward Thompson et al. (2012, 2016) and the Germany TEEB-study on urban areas (Naturkapital Deutschland – TEEB-DE 2016b) which gives an overview of the German context. A recent review of evidence on the many ways in which urban green space is linked to health can be seen in WHO 2016 and evidence on environmental interventions in green space to enhance health is summarised in Hunter et al. Chap. 17, this volume, and WHO (2017b). These and other similar publications can be helpful for landscape planners (in private offices as well as in public administration) as they offer sound evidence when it comes to decisions on conflicts or competition between different land uses, e.g. traffic, settlement and green space.

19.5 Health-Promoting Features of Green Spaces

The potential of green spaces to benefit human health, and their actual effects on health, depend on a variety of features and elements. These features and elements are presented in this section. For landscape planners, especially if pursuing the third option described in the last section, such features must be taken into consideration when assessing the health relevance of existing green spaces as well as designing new and redesigning existing ones. Unfortunately, to date it has not proved possible to attribute distinct health potentials and effects to certain, more generally defined, green space types, such as park, pocket-park, cemetery, garden, forest and so on, because in practice, these types are too heterogeneous in terms of size, location, vegetation, design, surrounding (infra-)structures or potential user groups, to allow for a similarly simplistic categorization of effect (Rittel et al. 2016, p. 50). Consequently, the consideration of each individual green space is required. However, it is not only the individual green space which should be considered, but also the entire open space system, or green infrastructure in a given area (municipality, city), as one green space rarely includes all desirable features and elements, but the entire system could or should do so. Sugiyama et al. (2010) make a good case for this in relation to physical activity, where size of park and the opportunities it offers for walking may be more important than simple proximity. Ward Thompson (2013) considers ways that open space planning and design can support physical activity and Ward Thompson (2015) discusses links between landscape planning and design and human health more generally.

Features and elements of green spaces and the green space system should do justice to all of the four components (aesthetic-symbolic, social, mental and physical) relevant for human health. The following Sects. 20.5.1 and 20.5.2 show how this could be achieved. The sections mainly refer to Rittel et al. (2016), where a more comprehensive overview can be found.

19.5.1 Individual Green Spaces

Before considering specific health benefits that green spaces can offer, general quality criteria must almost always be fulfilled in order to ensure, at least in principle, that people may be willing and able to use a green space and therefore take advantage of its health potential. The criteria that support inclusive use include: safety issues (e.g. ensuring good visibility), cleanliness (e.g. provision and emptying of waste bins, lack of vandalism), appropriate equipment for different types of uses (e.g. benches, playgrounds, providing shade), sufficient pathways, accessibility and approachability (e.g. enough entrances, including step-free ones, consideration of potential obstacles such as busy roads).

Aesthetic-symbolic health potentials can be promoted by designing green spaces in a way which enables people to perceive a green space as attractive, 'unique' and to identify with it. This is closely related to its perceived beauty (evoked, e.g. by the play of light and shadow, water in various forms, sightlines, trees and different types of vegetation, attractive leaves and flowers) and to the emphasis or creation of features that reflect typical local characteristics. Of course, 'beauty' and 'place identity' are based on different individual and community values and experience, a fact reinforcing the importance of user analysis and/or stakeholder participation.

Social health can be promoted by allowing for interaction and integration, e.g. by areas usable for picnics, playing, growing food or organising community gatherings and events, etc., by separating areas for different, conflicting uses, and by use of barrier-free design, e.g. allowing access for wheelchairs and pushchairs and for people with mobility and sensory impairments. Enabling and fostering nature experience (e.g. by a variety of plant species also providing food for insects and birds, areas managed to promote wildlife and maintained less intensively; see Davies et al. Chap. 12, this volume), opportunities for gardening and self-harvesting, but also retreats which offer the possibility for quiet relaxation and restoration are important for mental health and stress-reduction (see Marselle et al. Chap. 9, this volume).

With regard to physical health, a range of options for play and sports should be provided, as well as for walking (by far the most common form of physical activity), although possible conflicts between nature conservation and health must be taken into account. This applies to allergenic plants (see Damialis et al. Chap 3, this volume), plants with thorns and toxic parts (especially near playgrounds for children), or meadows managed for wildlife, rather than closely mown lawns, which could increase the risk of tick infestation (WHO 2016; Müller et al. Chap. 4, this volume).

In conclusion, two points must be emphasised: Firstly, one single green space will not usually include all recommended features and elements, as this is unlikely to be possible in a limited space and as individual elements and uses can be in conflict with each other. Secondly, all points described in this section exclusively refer to health aspects, not to other requirements green spaces should fulfill, e.g. in terms of biodiversity and nature conservation or climate adaptation. Of course, in landscape planning these other demands have to be considered as well, and sound decisions have to be made in favour of one of them if conflicts cannot be avoided or minimised.

19.5.2 Green Space Systems

Especially in urban areas, it is not individual green spaces which determine the 'green quality' of a city, but the entire system of green spaces, which is unique to every city. Relevant questions for human health regarding this are as follows: How are different green spaces distributed within a city (and its surrounding regions)? Is there a spatial concentration of green spaces or are they evenly distributed across the city? How many inhabitants have easy access to these spaces and are they close to their homes? Do different green spaces offer possibilities for different uses and requirements, so that the whole green space system enables a good variety of uses and offers possibilities for many different user preferences? Are the green spaces interlinked (for example by smaller 'greenways') that allow for walking, hiking or cycling in a green environment for a longer distance? Only after these questions are answered, can the potential health effects of 'local green' be assessed for an entire municipality or city.

To ensure a minimum supply of public green spaces to their inhabitants, different cities have come up with standard values on recommended accessibility standards for green space per inhabitant. Some consider a minimum size of green space that should be available within a maximum distance from every inhabitant's home, e.g. Natural England's 2010 recommendation (by no means always met) of a minimum of 2 ha of green space within 300 m (5 minutes' walk) of home. Others consider a minimum of green space per inhabitant. In Berlin, for example, 6 m^2 per inhabitant are considered necessary, even if this standard is not fulfilled in all parts of the city (Umweltatlas Berlin 2017). Beyond this, distinctions are made between different types of green spaces regarding their proximity to housing areas (Rittel et al. 2016, 56f; WHO 2016). Furthermore, the spatial network of all green spaces and greenways of a city is crucial. Beyond supporting walking or hiking during leisure time (e.g. '20 green main routes' in Berlin, the Highline Park in New York), this should encourage daily physical activity as an integral part of people's life, which is, according to health scientists, one of the most important aspects of health promotion in settlement areas (Rittel et al. 2016, p. 59; Ward Thompson 2013). The journey to work, to school, going shopping, etc. should be covered as much as possible - not by car - but on foot or by bike. Special attention to this issue is paid in the next section.

19.6 Greenways for Sustainable and Healthy Mobility in Daily Life

To allow for daily active travel by people, attractive, safe and largely noise-free connectivity of routes in green spaces are an important precondition (Greenspace Scotland 2008). Accordingly 'green connections' for cyclists and pedestrians should be created between residential areas and highly frequented places such as community and shopping centres, schools, kindergartens and areas with a high density of work places. To implement such a network of greenways for everyday physical activity and mobility, pre-existing green spaces could build the backbone, supplemented by newly planned routes, but especially by linear green structures, such as clearly demarcated pedestrian and cycle paths safe from motorised traffic and accompanied by tree avenues, hedgerows and other appropriate linear green elements. An overlap with parts of a habitat network or land within a green belt is possible, but conflicts should be avoided or at least minimised. Seen from a landscape planning perspective, this would ideally result in a city-wide network of green infrastructure, consisting of multi-functional green spaces with high amenity values and linear, but 'green', path connections. Such a network could contribute to the reduction of car traffic, thereby reducing noise, accidents and air pollution, and in this way would also improve healthy environmental conditions.

How such an approach could be pursued in (landscape) planning has been shown by Bloß (2016) in the example of the city of Oranienburg, a medium-sized municipality with about 42.000 inhabitants, located ca. 20 km north of Berlin. In order to identify suitable routes in an area of limited available space, Bloß made use of the GIS-based least-cost path (LCP) model (see Conine et al. 2004; Teng et al. 2011) for greenway alignment purposes. The LCP combines a land suitability assessment with an algorithm in order to identify the most suitable routes. Simplifying the working procedure somewhat, the following main steps were taken:

1. Identification of demand areas. Residential areas and highly frequented urban centres were identified as areas with a high demand for interconnection by greenways. These 'demand areas' were used to determine start and destination points for greenways (see Fig. 19.1).
2. Suitability assessment. The suitability of different areas for being a part of the greenway network was assessed using five criteria: land availability, road types, attractiveness, demand for connectivity and protection status (nature conservation). For each of these, all spatial features were categorised into levels of suit-

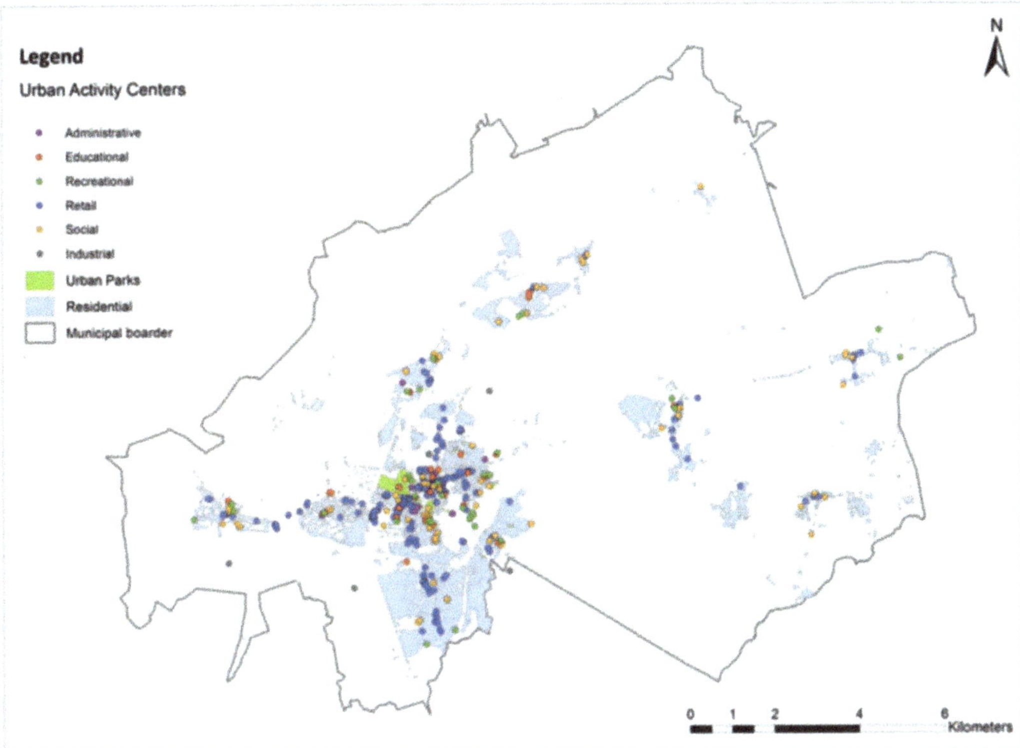

Fig. 19.1 Demand areas: residential areas and urban activity centres in Oranienburg that are to be connected by greenways (Bloß 2016, p. 33)

ability in single maps (see Fig. 19.2, example 'protection status'). After that, the criteria were weighted by their relative importance for greenway implementation and an overall suitability map was created.

3. Delineating the most suitable routes. The suitability assessment was the basis upon which the LCP algorithm was used to delineate the most suitable routes between the demand areas. The results of a first run of the model was discussed with local planning officials to evaluate its validity within the Oranienburg context. The discussion showed some deficits in the results and led to a modified second model run, leading to an adjusted greenway network (see Figs. 19.3 and 19.4 for the results of both model runs).

The resulting greenway network fulfilled the intended functions of alternative travel provision and nature protection to a large extent. However, although some constraints of the first network (e.g. physical barriers not considered by the model) could be eliminated by the second one, this still includes some undesirable tradeoffs, such as route alignment along main roads. Besides reflecting some imperfect weight allocations within the model, this is mainly a consequence of the scarcity of suitable sites which limited routing options – certainly not only a problem in Oranienburg, but found in most cities. This can be regarded as a major challenge and a problem to be overcome by landscape planners on the one hand, and as a fact which should lead to realistic expectations and compromises on the other hand.

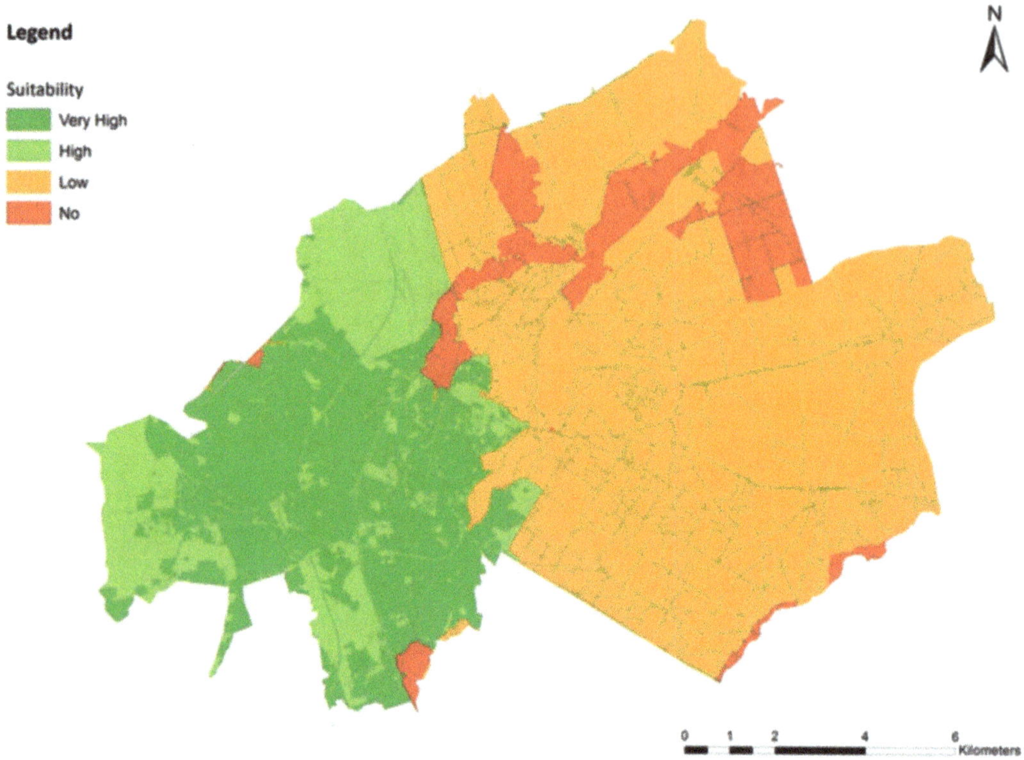

Fig. 19.2 Suitability of areas for the greenway network according to their nature conservation protection status (Bloß 2016, p. 37)

Even if no 'ideal' green network can be achieved, the example shows that good results are possible. Therefore, an approach as pursued by Bloß (2016) could be integrated into landscape planning, by adapting the method as well as the criteria for the suitability assessment to the respective local conditions and requirements.

19.7 Conclusions and Outlook

This chapter has shown that health issues are already implicitly touched upon or, in rare cases, explicitly named in landscape planning in England and Germany. In general, the potentials for including health issues into landscape planning are used neither frequently nor extensively, even if mutual benefits for health protection and promotion on the one hand and nature conservation and green space development on the other can be expected. One likely reason for this deficit is that to overcome it would require additional efforts by landscape planners and the respective planning and development authorities as well as by health authorities. There are some examples of recent attempts to overcome these disciplinary and professional silos, such as the 2015 development of the Place Standard Tool (NHS Health Scotland 2017), jointly promoted by the Scottish Government, the National Health Service, Scotland, and Architecture and Design Scotland – the Government body responsible for

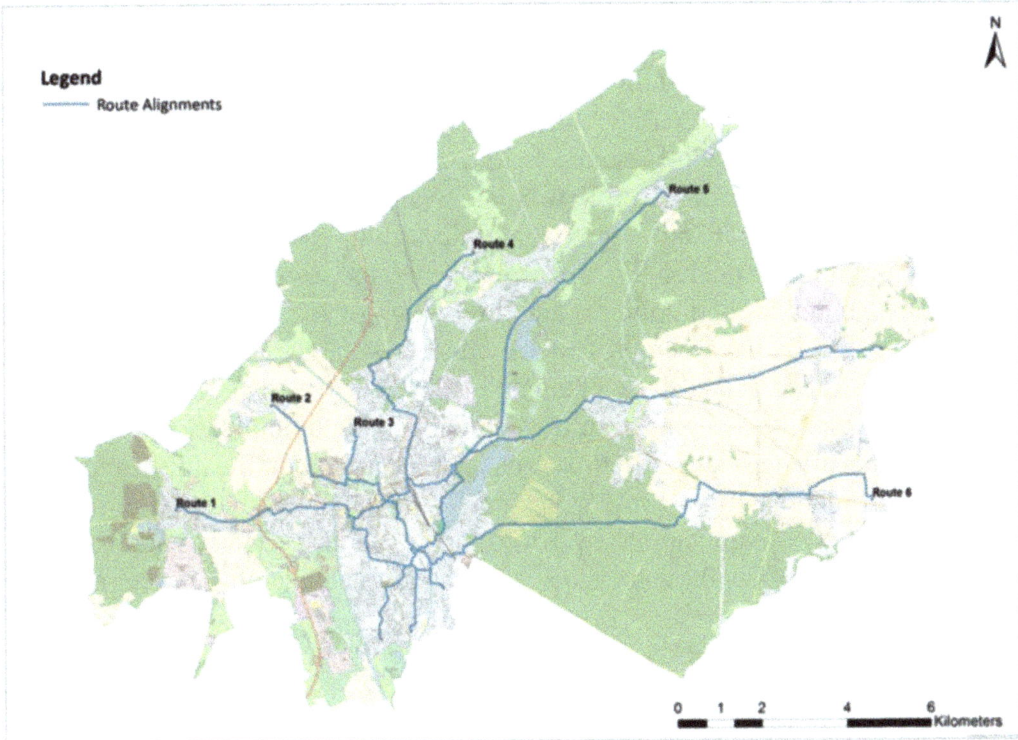

Fig. 19.3 Results for the first run of the Least-Cost Path model for the greenway network (Bloß 2016, p. 39)

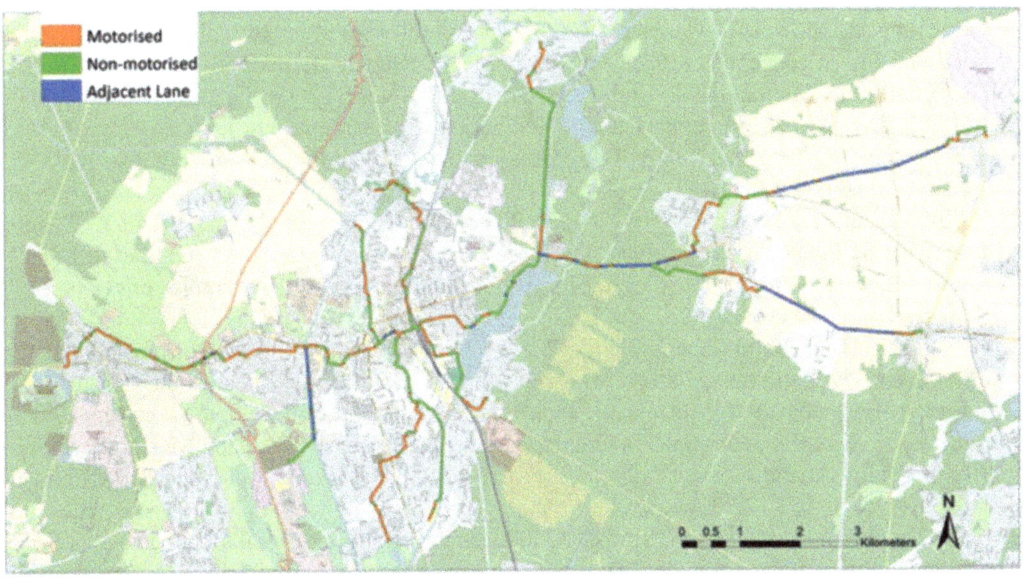

Fig. 19.4 Results for the second run of the Least-Cost Path model for the greenway network (adjusted model) showing sections of the network which are currently motorised, non-motorised or adjacent lanes to motorised roads (Bloß 2016, p. 48)

promoting policy on architecture and 'place'. The intersectoral public health action plan (Fachplan Gesundheit), promoted by the North Rhine-Westphalia Centre for Health since 2009, is intended for use by the public health sector in optimizing participation in the municipal policy and planning cycle (Claßen and Mekel 2017). Additionally, the 'Leitfaden Gesunde Stadt', an adopted version of the Healthy Urban Development Checklist of New South Wales (NSW 2009), has been published for use by local and regional public health and planning authorities (Landeszentrum Gesundheit NRW 2016). However, the results of the implementation of such guidelines and policies, and the linking of EIA and HIA in England, remain to be seen. In the absence of such evidence, we argue for the importance of these efforts because, if landscape planning is to have a socially acknowledged role in the face of rapidly changing natural, technological and political conditions and global grand challenges such as climate change, urbanization, health inequity and an ageing population, it must tackle key societal problems. This position is supported by a variety of publications by governmental bodies, scientists and NGOs. It remains to be seen if and how they will affect landscape planning in the mid- and long-term perspective.

References

Abraham A, Sommerhalder K, Bolliger-Salzmann H, Abel T (2007) Landschaft und Gesundheit. Das Potential einer Verbindung zweier Konzepte. Universität Bern, Institut für Sozial- und Präventivmedizin, Abteilung Gesundheitsforschung. Bern. Online at http://www.sl-fp.ch/getdatei.php?datei_id=817. Accessed on 14.01.2013

Bedimo-Rung AL, Mowen AJ, Cohen DA (2005) The significance of parks to physical activity and public health – a conceptual model. Am J Prev Med 28(Suppl. 2):159–168

Bell S, Hamilton V, Montarzino A, Rothnie H, Travlou P, Alves S (2008) Greenspace and quality of life: a critical literature review. greenspace Scotland research report. Online at http://www.greenspacescotland.org.uk/SharedFiles/Download.aspx?pageid=133&mid=129&fileid=95. Accessed on 09.08.2012

BfN (Bundesamt für Naturschutz) (2017a) Federal concept green infrastructure. Nature Conservation Foundations for plans adopted by the German Federation.). Online at: https://www.bfn.de/fileadmin/BfN/planung/bkgi/Dokumente/BKGI_Broschuere_englisch.pdf. Accessed on 15.12.2017

BfN (Bundesamt für Naturschutz) (Hrsg) (2017b) Urbane Grüne Infrastruktur. Grundlage für attraktive und zukunftsfähige Städte. Hinweise für die kommunale Praxis, Bonn

Bloß L (2016) A greenway for sustainable mobility. The potential of developing a greenway network for cyclists and pedestrians in Oranienburg using the Least-Cost Path. Master thesis. TU Berlin. Online at: http://www.landschaft.tu-berlin.de/menue/studium_und_lehre/abschlussarbeiten/. Accessed 03.12.2017

BMUB (Bundesministerium für Umwelt, Naturschutz, Bau und Reaktorsicherheit) (2017) Weißbuch Stadtgrün. Grün in der Stadt – Für eine lebenswerte Zukunft, Berlin

Claßen T, Mekel O (2017) Empowering local public health authorities as key drivers of an intersectoral municipal public health action plan: the experience of North Rhine-Westphalia, Germany. In: WHO Regional Office for Europe (ed) Sustainable development in Wales and other regions in Europe – achieving health and equity for present and future generations. World Health Organization, Copenhagen, pp 38–42

Conine A et al (2004) Planning for multi-purpose greenways in Concord, North Carolina. Landsc Urban Plan 68(2–3):271–287. Available at: http://www.sciencedirect.com/science/article/pii/S0169204603001592

Department for Communities and Local Government (2012) National Planning Policy Framework. Available from: https://www.gov.uk/government/publications/national-planning-policy-framework%2D%2D2. Accessed 05 Dec 2017

Department of Health (2010a) Health impact assessment tools. Available from: https://www.gov.uk/government/uploads/system/uploads/attachment_data/file/216008/dh_120106.pdf. Accessed 23 Jan 2018

Department of Health (2010b) Health impact assessment: evidence on health. Available from: https://www.gov.uk/government/uploads/system/uploads/attachment_data/file/216006/dh_120109.pdf. Accessed 23 Jan 2018

Francis J, Wood LJ, Knuiman M, Giles-Corti B (2012) Quality or quantity? Exploring the relationship between public open space attributes and mental health in Perth. W Aust Soc Sci Med 74(10):1570–1577

Fuller RA, Irvine KN, Devine-Wright P, Warren PH, Gaston KJ (2007) Psychological benefits of greenspace increase with biodiversity. Biol Lett 3(4):390–394

Grahn P, Stigsdotter U (2010) The relation between perceived sensory dimensions of urban green space and stress restoration. Landsc Urban Plan 94(3–4):264–275

Greenspace Scotland (2008) Health impact assessment of greenspace. A guide. Stirling (UK). Online at http://www.greenspacescotland.org.uk/SharedFiles/Download.aspx?pageid=133&mid=129&fileid=41. Accessed 12.01.2018

Hehn C (2016) The emergence and evolution of Green Infrastructure planning in North West England. A policy arrangement approach. Master thesis, TU Berlin. Online at: http://www.landschaft.tu-berlin.de/menue/studium_und_lehre/abschlussarbeiten/. Accessed 03.12.2017

Heiland S (2017) Perspektiven der Landschaftsplanung. In: Wende W, Walz U (Hrsg) Die räumliche Wirkung der Landschaftsplanung. Wiesbaden. S. 170–192

Heiland S, Kahl R, Sander H, Schliep R (2016) Integration von Ökosystemleistungen in die kommunale Landschaftsplanung. Naturschutz und Landschaftsplanung 48(10):313–320

Heiland S, Mengel A, Hänel K, Geiger B, Arndt P, Reppin N, Werle V, Hokema D, Hehn C, Mertelmeyer L, Burghardt R, Opitz S (2017) Bundeskonzept Grüne Infrastruktur – Fachgutachten. Bundesamt für Naturschutz (Hrsg.), BfN Skripten 457, Bonn-Bad Godesberg

Kaczynski AT, Potwarka LR, Saelens BE (2008) Association of Park Size, distance, and features with physical activity in neighborhood parks. Am J Public Health 98(8):1451–1456

Klages A (2012) Starke Sportvereine – starke Kommunen: Neue Perspektiven für die Stadtentwicklung. Stadt und Raum 6/2012, 320–324

Landeszentrum Gesundheit Nordrhein-Westfalen (2016) Leitfaden Gesunde Stadt. Hinweise für Stellungnahmen zur zur Stadtentwicklung aus dem Öffentlichen Gesundheitsdienst. Bielefeld

Lee AC, Maheswaran R (2011) The health benefits of urban green spaces: a review of the evidence. J Public Health (Oxf) 33(2):212–222

Manchester City Council (2015) Manchester's great outdoors. A Green and Blue infrastructure strategy. Online at: http://www.manchester.gov.uk/downloads/download/6314/manchester_green_and_blue_strategy. Last access 12.01.2018

Ministry of Housing, Communities and Local Government (2014) Guidance – Health and Wellbeing: the role of health and wellbeing in planning. Available from: https://www.gov.uk/guidance/health-and-wellbeing. Accessed 23 Jan 2018

Mitchell R, Popham F (2007) Greenspace, urbanity and health: relationships in England. J Epidemiol Community Health 61(8):681–683

Natural England (2010) 'Nature Nearby'. Accessible natural greenspace guidance. Online at http://webarchive.nationalarchives.gov.uk/20150902180000/http://publications.naturalengland.org.uk/publication/40004. Accessed 12.01.2018

Naturkapital Deutschland – TEEB DE (2016a) Ökosystemleistungen in ländlichen Räumen – Grundlage für menschliches Wohlergehen und nachhaltige wirtschaftliche Entwicklung. Hrsg.

von C. von Haaren, C.Albert. Hannover, Leipzig. Online at http://www.naturkapitalteeb.de/publikationen/projekteigene-publikationen/bericht-2.html. Accessed 17 Jan 2018

Naturkapital Deutschland – TEEB DE (2016b) Ökosystemleistungen in der Stadt – Gesundheit schützen und Lebensqualität erhöhen. Hrsg. von I. Kowarik, R. Bartz, M. Brenck. Berlin, Leipzig. Online at http://www.naturkapitalteeb.de/publikationen/projekteigene-publikationen/bericht-3.html. Accessed 17 Jan 2018

Newton J (2007) Wellbeing and the natural environment: a brief overview of the evidence. Online at http://archive.defra.gov.uk/sustainable/government/documents/Wellbeing_and_the_Natural_Environment_Report.doc. Accessed on 17 Jan 2018

NHS Health Scotkland (2017) The place standard tool. Available from: http://www.healthscotland.scot/tools-and-resources/the-place-standard-tool. Accessed 27 Jan 2018

NSW (New South Wales) Health (2009) Healthy urban development checklist. A guide for health services when commenting on development policies, plans and proposals. NSW Department of Health, Sydney

Pretty JN, Barton J, Colbeck I, Hine R, Mourato S, MacKerron G, Wood C (2010) Health values from ecosystems. UK National Ecosystem Assessment: technical report. Understanding nature's value to society, Cambridge. Online at http://uknea.unep-wcmc.org/LinkClick.aspx?fileticket=S901pJcQm%2fQ%3d&tabid=82. Accessed 27.02.2013

Prüss-Ustün A, Wolf J, Corvalán C, Neville R, Bos R, Neira M (2017) Diseases due to unhealthy environments: an updated estimate of the global burden of disease attributable to environmental determinants of health. J Public Health 39(3):464–475. https://doi.org/10.1093/pubmed/fdw085

Public Health England (2017) Health and Environmental Impact Assessment: a briefing for public health teams in England. Available from: https://www.gov.uk/government/uploads/system/uploads/attachment_data/file/629207/Health_and_environmental_impact_assessment.pdf. Accessed 15 Jan 2018

Rayner G, Lang T (2012) Ecological public health: reshaping the conditions for good health. Routledge/Earthscan, Abingdon

Rittel K, Bredow L, Wanka E, Hokema D, Schuppe G, Wilke T, Nowak D, Heiland S (2014) Grün, natürlich, gesund: Die Potenziale multifunktionaler städtischer Räume. Ergebnisse des gleichnamigen F+E-Vorhabens (FKZ 3511 82 0800). BfN-Skripten 371. Bonn-Bad-Godesberg. Online at: https://www.bfn.de/fileadmin/BfN/service/Dokumente/skripten/Skript371.pdf. Accessed 17 Jan 2018

Rittel K, Bredow L, Wanka E, Hokema D, Schuppe G, Wilke T, Nowak D, Heiland S (2016) Green, natural, healthy: the potential of multifunctional urban spaces. R&D Project FKZ 3511 82 800. BfN-Skripten 371. Bonn-Bad-Godesberg. Online at: https://www.bfn.de/fileadmin/BfN/service/Dokumente/skripten/Skript371_EN_barrierefrei.pdf. Accessed 17 Jan 2018

Roe JJ, Ward Thompson C, Aspinall PA, Brewer MJ, Duff EI, Miller D, Mitchell R, Clow A (2013) Green space and stress: evidence from cortisol measures in deprived urban communities. Int J Environ Res Public Health 10:4086–4103

Roe J, Aspinall P, Ward Thompson C (2016) Understanding relationships between health, ethnicity, place and the role of urban green space in deprived urban communities. Int J Environ Res Public Health 13(7):681. https://doi.org/10.3390/ijerph13070681

Silvertown J (2015) Have ecosystem services been oversold? Trends Ecol Evol 30(11):641–648

Stadt Hohen Neuendorf (2014) Landschaftsplan. Stadt Hohen Neuendorf. Online: https://hohen-neuendorf.de/de/bauen-wirtschaft/stadtplanung/landschaftsplan/landschaftsplan. Accessed17 Jan 2018

Stigsdotter UK, Ekholm O, Schipperijn J, Toftager M, Kamper-Jorgensen F, Randrup TB (2010) Health promoting outdoor environments – associations between green space, and health, health-related quality of life and stress based on a Danish national representative survey. Scand J Public Health 38(4):411–417

Sugiyama T, Francis J, Middleton NJ, Owen N, Giles-Corti B (2010) Associations between recreational walking and attractiveness, size, and proximity of neighbourhood open space. Am J Public Health 100:1752–1757

Teng M et al (2011) Multipurpose greenway planning for changing cities: a framework integrating priorities and a least-cost path model. Landsc Urban Plan 103(1):1–14. Available at: http://www.sciencedirect.com/science/article/pii/S0169204611002088

Town and Country Planning (2017) The Town and Country Planning (Environmental Impact Assessment) regulations 2017. Available from: http://www.legislation.gov.uk/uksi/2017/571/pdfs/uksi_20170571_en.pdf. Accessed 15. Jan 2018

Town and Country Planning, England (2012) The Town and Country Planning (Local Planning) (England) regulations 2012. Available from http://www.legislation.gov.uk/uksi/2012/767/pdfs/uksi_20120767_en.pdf. Accessed 15 Jan 2018

Umweltatlas Berlin (2017) 06.05 Versorgung mit öffentlichen, wohnungsnahen Grünanlagen (Ausgabe 2017). Online at http://www.stadtentwicklung.berlin.de/umwelt/umweltatlas/ib605.htm. Accessed 17 Jan 2018

van den Berg AE, van Winsum-Westra M, van Dillen SME (2010) Allotment gardening and health: a comparative survey among allotment gardeners and their neighbours without an allotment. Environ Health 9:74

Ward Thompson C (2013) Activity, exercise and the planning and design of outdoor spaces. J Environ Psychol 34:79–96. https://doi.org/10.1016/j.jenvp.2013.01.003

Ward Thompson C (2015) Is landscape life. In: Doherty G, Waldheim C (eds) Is landscape…? Essays on the identity of landscape. Routledge, Abingdon

Ward Thompson C, Roe J, Aspinall P, Mitchell R, Clow A, Miller D (2012) More green space is linked to less stress in deprived communities: evidence from salivary cortisol patterns. Landsc Urban Plan 105:221–229. https://doi.org/10.1016/j.landurbplan.2011.12.015

Ward Thompson C, Aspinall P, Roe J, Robertson L, Miller D (2016) Mitigating stress and supporting health in deprived urban communities: the importance of green space and the social environment. Int J Environ Res Public Health 13(4):440. https://doi.org/10.3390/ijerph13040440

WHO (World Health Organization) (2016) Urban green spaces and health – a review of evidence. WHO Regional Office for Europe, Copenhagen

WHO (World Health Organization) (2017a) Constitution of WHO: principles. Available from: http://www.who.int/about/mission/en/. Accessed 04. Dec 2017

WHO (World Health Organization) (2017b) Urban green space interventions and health – a review of impacts and effectiveness. WHO Regional Office for Europe, Copenhagen

Winter G, Smith L, Cave S, Rehfisch F (2016) Comparison of the planning systems in the four UK countries. Research paper 713–2015. Available from: http://www.niassembly.gov.uk/globalassets/documents/raise/publications/2016/joint-publication/joint-briefing-paper-ni-interactive.pdf. Accessed Feb 2018

Wolch JR, Byrne J, Newell JP (2014) Urban green space, public health, and environmental justice: the challenge of making cities 'just green enough'. Landsc Urban Plan 125:234–244

Part V
Conclusions

Chapter 20
Biodiversity and Health in the Face of Climate Change: Perspectives for Science, Policy and Practice

Melissa R. Marselle, Jutta Stadler, Horst Korn, Katherine N. Irvine, and Aletta Bonn

Abstract Increases in non-communicable diseases, biodiversity loss and climate change are among the greatest global challenges society is facing today. At the same time, biodiverse natural environments can buffer the negative effects of climate change to society and support human health. Contributions in this volume demonstrate the growing interest in the impact of biodiversity on human health and well-being in the face of climate change. The chapters in this volume present and critically review the growing body of literature on the associations of biodiversity and human health, with mounting evidence of positive effects for physical health and well-being. In this concluding chapter, we summarise the key outcomes of the chapters in this book. Synthesising the main results with a link to current policy, we develop

M. R. Marselle (✉)
Department of Ecosystem Services, Helmholtz Centre for Environmental Research – UFZ, Leipzig, Germany

German Centre for Integrative Biodiversity Research (iDiv) Halle-Jena-Leipzig, Leipzig, Germany
e-mail: melissa.marselle@ufz.de

J. Stadler · H. Korn
Federal Agency for Nature Conservation (BfN), Isle of Vilm, Putbus, Germany
e-mail: jutta.stadler@bfn.de; horst.korn@bfn.de

K. N. Irvine
Social, Economic and Geographical Sciences Research Group, The James Hutton Institute, Aberdeen, Scotland, UK
e-mail: katherine.irvine@hutton.ac.uk

A. Bonn
Department of Ecosystem Services, Helmholtz Centre for Environmental Research – UFZ, Leipzig, Germany

German Centre for Integrative Biodiversity Research (iDiv) Halle-Jena-Leipzig, Leipzig, Germany

Institute of Biodiversity, Friedrich Schiller University Jena, Jena, Germany
e-mail: aletta.bonn@ufz.de

M. R. Marselle et al. (eds.), *Biodiversity and Health in the Face of Climate Change*, https://doi.org/10.1007/978-3-030-02318-8_20

recommendations to address the urgent health and sustainability challenges in science, policy and practice.

Keywords Synthesis · Biodiversity · Climate change adaptation · Non-communicable disease · Policy recommendations · Science-policy interface

Highlights

- Contributions in this volume present growing evidence of the linkages between biodiversity and physical, mental and spiritual aspects of health and well-being.
- Evidence seems to suggest strong links between biodiversity and physical health and well-being, which points to important avenues for health treatments and natural resource management.
- Currently disjointed policy sectors of biodiversity conservation and management, public health and climate change need to work together to foster the foundation of our society – considering the ecosystem and human health in a One Health agenda.
- Arguing for health as a central benefit to society that results from nature conservation and good biodiversity management should improve the public and political interest in the subject.
- Evidence is sufficient to implement 'no regret' actions now that are mainly based on nature-based solutions.
- Key steps to integrate considerations of biodiversity, public health and climate change into research, policy and management agendas are provided.

20.1 Introduction

The rise in non-communicable diseases (World Health Organization [WHO] 2017a, b) combined with biodiversity loss and climate change (Bellard et al. 2012; Steffen et al. 2015) are among the greatest global challenges society is facing today. While biodiversity provides the foundation for human well-being, human societies also provide the greatest drivers for biodiversity loss and climate change. Central to addressing these critical challenges are the questions '*How* does biodiversity matter for human health and well-being?' and '*What* implications does this have for efforts to address our current predicament?' (WHO and CBD 2015). Increasingly, science is starting to unravel relationships of how biodiversity impacts human health and well-being, and we are at the beginning of an exponential rise in research activity, as shown by the contents of this book. The chapters critically review the growing body of literature that examines biodiversity's contribution to physical health as well as mental and spiritual well-being in the face of climate change. In their totality, these chapters encompass the mounting evidence of positive effects on physical health and well-being (see Lindley et al. Chap. 2, Dadvand et al. Chap. 6, Cook et al. Chap. 11, Hunter et al. Chap. 17, this volume). Some effects on physical health related to physical activity and obesity remain inconclusive, possibly because of study design and confounding variables such as socio-economic factors, which need to be considered carefully when designing studies (Kabisch Chap. 5, this volume). Some specific biodiversity-health associations are negative, especially with regard to allergies and vector-borne diseases (Damialis et al. Chap. 3, Müller et al. Chap. 4, this volume), whereas effective spatial planning and management actions can mitigate these effects (Elmqvist et al. Chap. 18, Heiland et al. Chap. 19, this volume). There is also some evidence of the positive effects of biodiversity on mental health and well-being (Marselle et al. Chap. 9, this volume). Importantly, this volume also considers spiritual well-being (Irvine et al. Chap. 10, this volume), which to date has been subject to little attention. Management of biodiversity could therefore form a globally important natural health service.

By reviewing and synthesising the available literature and recent findings, the authors in this volume develop an evidence base for how biodiversity can contribute to physical, mental and spiritual aspects of health and well-being. Importantly, the volume starts to further develop the theory of biodiversity-health relationships (Marselle Chap. 7, this volume), a necessary component for future studies. The authors identify the different mechanisms for biodiversity-health pathways by building on existing work (e.g. Hartig et al. 2014; Markevych et al. 2017; Potschin and Haines-Young 2011; van den Bosch and Ode Sang 2017). As this is an emerging research area, it was at times challenging for some chapters to relate to primary data and analyses where all three topics – biodiversity, health and climate change – were assessed together. Similarly, while the contributions draw on expertise from different disciplines, an additional challenge encountered was moving beyond analyses of green space in general to focus on the specific contribution of biodiversity in particular, for which few studies exist to date, although research has grown in the past decade (e.g. Aerts et al. 2018; Fuller et al. 2007; Dallimer et al. 2012; Lovell et al. 2014). To foster further research, the chapters identify knowledge gaps and areas for new research avenues as well as improvement through enhanced or better aligned indicators and metrics (de Vries & Snep, Chap. 8, this volume). These metrics should also link to existing policy targets in public health and nature conservation (Davies et al. Chap. 12, Korn et al. Chap.14, MacKinnon et al. Chap. 16, this volume). We need to move further in our research efforts to quantify the benefits and risks that biodiversity provides for human health, and how interaction with plants and animals shapes our physical, mental and spiritual health and well-being as well as societal and cultural practices. Studies have started to explore dose-response relationships of nature and health (e.g. Cox et al. 2017; Shananhan et al. 2015), which need to be further expanded in order to foster our understanding of the impact of duration and exposure of contact with biodiversity on health. This knowledge is required to aid development of 'health treatments', both through natural resource management interventions via configuration of green and blue spaces and through active social interventions, such as health walks (Marselle et al. 2014; Cook et al. Chap. 11, MacKinnon et al. Chap. 16, Hunter et al. Chap. 17, all this volume). Importantly, unravelling the different mechanisms requires a targeted and innovative study design and consideration of confounding factors to account for different configurations of green spaces as well as socioeconomic contexts in different cultural and ethnic settings.

By evaluating a broad range of case studies, the authors also demonstrate how managing green spaces for biodiversity and health can additionally contribute to adapting to the effects of a changing climate (Keune et al. Chap. 15, MacKinnon et al. Chap. 16, this volume), both as communities and as individuals (De Young Chap. 13, this volume). The chapters lay out practical recommendations for policy and practice as well as how to integrate existing knowledge into urban planning and management (Hunter et al. Chap. 17, Elmqvist et al. Chap. 18, Heiland et al. Chap. 19, this volume). Importantly, proactive planning can contribute actively to the public health agenda (Cook et al. Chap. 11, this volume) and help to increase a city's resilience in the face of climate change (Elmqvist et al. Chap. 18, this volume). Managing green spaces may also alleviate health equity issues (Kabisch Chap. 5, Cook et al. Chap. 11, this volume). In many areas we already know enough to act and to implement 'no regret' actions. It becomes obvious that the global challenges and goals related to biodiversity and health in a changing climate cannot be tackled by one discipline or one sector alone. Informed transdisciplinary dialogue and collaboration is clearly required to address the pressing research questions and to implement actions. The linkages between biodiversity and health are increasingly becoming recognized in both local and regional conservation management and in international policy development (Korn et al. Chap. 14, this volume). Fundamentally, the 2050 Vision of Biodiversity of the Convention of Biological Diversity (CBD) and the United Nations 2030 Agenda for Sustainable Development depend on joint action from many sectors and the alignment of environmental and societal goals. Implementation on the ground will need to be monitored and evaluated for effectiveness (see Hunter et al. Chap. 17, this volume), both for health outcomes and for synergies and trade-offs with conservation and climate policy goals.

Overall, quantifying the health benefits of interventions should also be supported by economic cost-benefit analysis to assess the value and cost-effectiveness of nature-based solution (NBS) measures for health and related co-benefits. These analyses should also support scenario development to assess different future trajectories at regional and global levels to inform decision making in policy and practice. Here, ongoing work with the scenarios and modelling expert group of the Intergovernmental Science-Policy Platform on Biodiversity and Ecosystem Services (IPBES) should pay special attention to the effects of biodiversity scenarios for public health. Finally, coordinated governance systems need to be developed and established to foster the sustainable use and enhancement of biodiversity to promote human health for all people in a changing climate.

In this concluding chapter, we synthesize the main results from the chapters and link them to current policy developments on a European and a global scale. Based on the evidence provided in this volume and drawing from the recommendations of the European Network of Heads of Nature Conservation Agencies (ENCA) derived from the European conference 'Biodiversity and Health in the face of climate change – Challenges, Opportunities and Evidence Gaps' (Marselle et al. 2018), we develop recommendations to address the urgent health and sustainability challenges in science, policy and practice.

20.2 Evidence of Effects of Biodiversity on Physical Health

Biodiverse natural environments and climate change interact to influence human physical health and well-being in positive and negative ways. Case study examples illustrate these interrelationships for extreme heat, allergenic plants and vector-borne diseases. The effects of nature and health relationships on specific populations groups – children and different socio-economic groups – are highlighted.

There are important links between biodiversity and physical health as demonstrated by the review of *Sarah Lindley and co-authors*. They argue that both biodiversity and climate change set important boundary conditions for human health, as they influence many elements that impact on health and well-being of individuals, for example through altered ecosystem functions and services. The authors point out that, especially in the face of a changing climate, NBS are needed to adapt to or mitigate negative climate-induced stressors, such as heat waves, reduced air quality, flooding or water quality regulation, that have serious impacts on human health. Many of the available studies are drawn from urban environments where climate effects may be experienced most dramatically due to the urban heat-island effect, and evidenced by the presented case study from Greater Manchester, England. The authors point to the need to consider socio-economic confounding factors to fully address the challenges of understanding the links between biodiversity and physical health, and for research to develop robust metrics and indicators to measure not only the state but also trends of linkages. Overall, it will be important to identify what configurations of green spaces in cities are most beneficial to promote health in order to provide input to urban planning and management.

Athanasios Damialis and co-authors discuss the negative effects of biodiversity and physical health by highlighting the specific issue of pollen allergies. As allergy prevalence has increased worldwide, partly due to a warming climate, their review provides a greater understanding of the emerging challenges. In particular, the authors call for better spatial and temporal risk mapping and forecasting of potential pollen exposure to advise allergy-sensitive individuals as well as to inform urban planning measures to develop green spaces that can minimise allergenic pollen exposure. Importantly, pollen can be a carrier of biochemical complex particles that can additionally affect health, and only recently has an understanding of the pollen microbiome begun to emerge. With the spread of invasive and alien allergenic species in a changing climate, such as ragweed (*Ambrosia artemisiifolia*), we need to better understand how these distributions can be assessed, predicted and proactively managed. Here, the development of automated, near-real-time pollen measurements is exciting and needs operationalisation on a greater scale to provide exposure risk alerts, environmental health-service infrastructure and personalised forecasts.

Another health issue derived from biodiversity-human contacts as discussed by *Ruth Müller and co-authors* is vector-borne diseases (VBDs), i.e. illnesses caused by parasites, viruses and bacteria transmitted by a vector, often insects, like blood sucking mosquitos. These are estimated to account for 17% of the global burden of non-communicable diseases, often affecting poorer populations living in degraded ecosystems in the Global South. In Europe, on average 77,000 people are affected by VBDs, and this figure is expected to rise, as abundance and regional distribution of these vectors are shaped by a changing climate as well as human transport. A warming climate may facilitate the spread of alien invasive species such as the Asian tiger mosquito (*Aedes albopictus*) and disease-transmitting ticks to Northern Europe as well as alter vector and host behaviour. Understanding and forecasting these changes is needed to inform pro-active natural resource management to prevent and halt establishment of vector populations. Notably, the diversity of pathogens as well as the diversity of vectors and hosts are as yet largely unknown and requires further research. Since biodiverse environments can contribute to discovering natural and novel insecticides as well as medially active compounds, global conservation efforts for biodiversity hotspots are needed to maintain options for vector control and pharmaceutical development. In addition, genetic tools in vector control need to be understood and further developed whilst, possibly more importantly, the socio-ecological systems need to be considered and traditional knowledge within local communities incorporated to manage VBDs. As the authors argue, most VBDs can be prevented through vector control if managed effectively, and a transdisciplinary approach across sectors is needed for successful implementation. It is not mainly the lack of scientific expertise but a lack of capacity and capabilities for implementation of good practice that hinder effective management. Comprehensive national strategies, community engagement and the application of varied intervention toolboxes are needed. At a policy level the WHO Global Vector Control Response 2017–2030 provides strategic guidance to deal with VBDs, and should be incorporated in climate adaptation and conservation policies.

Nadia Kabisch highlights in her review that socio-economic and socio-demographic effects are strong co-determinants of health, and confound the association of the impact of green space on health in many studies. Whilst these confounding effects will always be strong predictors, associations between green space and health vary in strength across different case studies and evidence appears strongest with respect to cardiovascular diseases and mental health. As several studies reported a moderating effect of urban green spaces on health inequalities between different socio-economic groups, this points to important avenues for green space urban planning especially in deprived neighbourhoods. The perceived quality and safety of green spaces seems to play a particularly important role in determining actual use of those spaces. Appreciation of different green space qualities varies between age groups, and therefore management should focus on providing safe and high-quality green spaces for all members of the community. For future research, the author suggests mixed methods approaches that employ both quantitative and qualitative investigations based on both empirical observations and experimental designs in order to disentangle the determining factors for urban green space and health relationships.

For children, considered as an especially vulnerable group of health beneficiaries, *Payam Dadvand and co-authors* show that even before birth, prenatal exposure of mothers to green space can improve pregnancy outcomes. Contact with green space may further aid cognitive and behavioural development in children, and has been reported to have some effects on reducing attention-deficit hyperactivity disorder (ADHD) symptoms. The authors identify potential mechanisms including: stress reduction; a higher level of social contacts and increased physical activity; reduction of urban environmental stressors, including noise, heat and air pollution; and increased contact with environmental microbiota. The latter has been shown to increase immunoregulation in several studies. The evidence of the impact of green space contact on respiratory and allergic conditions is inconsistent, as green spaces can provide positive effects whilst they are also a source of fungal spores and pollens. Proactive green space management can help to reduce asthma through careful plant species selection, increasing species diversity and mitigating exposure to air pollution. Despite the opportunity for greater physical activity in green spaces, there was inconsistent evidence of a reduction in obesity and overall increase in physical activity, possibly as studies did not sufficiently account for the quality of green spaces. The authors recommend that investigations should be carefully designed in order to account for confounding factors, such as quality of green space. Overall, in their synthesis, the authors advocate that biodiverse natural areas, especially in urban settings, are important factors for child health and development.

20.3 Mental Health and Spiritual Well-Being Benefits of Biodiversity

Biodiverse natural environments not only have physical health effects and climate change adaptation potential, they also offer mental health and spiritual well-being benefits.

As an introduction to the second part of the book, *Melissa Marselle* provides an overview of the conceptual frameworks that provide a perspective into the ways that biodiversity can influence mental health and well-being. Coming mostly from the field of environmental psychology, the frameworks discussed are environmental preference (Biophilia Hypothesis, Preference Matrix and Fractal dimensions of nature), theories of restorative environments (Stress Reduction Theory and Attention Restoration Theory) and the Ecosystem Service Cascade Model. Each framework is described and its conceptualisation of biodiversity and mental well-being are detailed. Analysis of these frameworks found that no single framework details both biodiversity and mental well-being. As such, the author recommends that future researchers empirically test these frameworks using biodiversity indicators in order to further delineate which of these frameworks are 'fit for purpose' for describing the inter-relationships between biodiversity and mental well-being.

Sjerp de Vries and Robbert Snep discuss methodological issues for consideration in future biodiversity–mental health research studies. The authors point out that within studies assessing relationships between biodiversity and mental health and well-being, the concept of biodiversity is frequently adapted from its original, ecological definition. To public health and psychology researchers, a focus on species richness may imply that having more species in a habitat is always better. However, to ecologists, this interpretation has little value as they are interested in the distinct assemblages of species, including functional characteristics, or if any key species are missing. Such adaptations to the ecological definition of biodiversity, the authors argue, could result in biodiversity and mental health studies having relevance for public health and psychology, but not for nature conservation. Given that mental health promotion and nature conservation are two separate goals, the authors suggest that a more relevant research question is: can the same environment constitute a healthy, biodiverse ecosystem and enhance mental health at the same time? Suggestions are presented for future biodiversity and mental health research, with guidance for epidemiological studies assessing biodiversity in and around the residential environment on mental health and well-being. The authors recommend that future research studies should focus not on biodiversity per se, but on healthy biodiverse ecosystems that help keep people mentally healthy.

Melissa Marselle and co-authors provide a comprehensive review of the scientific literature investigating the influence of biodiversity on mental health and well-being. The authors present a synthesis of 24 biodiversity and mental health and well-being studies. There is some evidence to suggest that biodiversity promotes better mental health and well-being, although more studies show a non-significant effect. Due to the heterogeneity in the studies, the authors examine the pattern of results in the 24 studies by level of biodiversity (from ecosystems/habitats to single species levels), which taxonomic groups are assessed (e.g. birds, trees) and mental health or well-being outcome variables. In this way, the authors identify at which level of biodiversity, group and outcome variable non-significant effects are found. Consistent non-significant relationships were only found at the ecosystem/habitat level with mental health outcomes, as most of the other results were mixed. Clear gaps in the research were also found, as none of the 24 studies investigated the effect of perceived species richness on mental health. The researchers make several recommendations for future biodiversity and mental health and well-being studies with regard to improved, theoretically-grounded research designs, measurements of biodiversity and mental health and well-being, and investigation of mediators and dose-response relationships.

As spiritual well-being is increasingly considered an important dimension of human health, *Katherine Irvine and colleagues* examine the inter-relationship between biodiversity and this aspect of human health and well-being. In their review, the authors develop an expanded understanding of spiritual well-being as encompassing one's relationships with the self, the community, the environment and transcendent Other(s), and consider this in relation to four themes from the literature. The first theme focuses on the influence of spiritual traditions on biodiversity, in which religious world views regarding nature and biodiversity can foster meaning, connection with nature, and feelings of transcendence. These experiences may result in nature conservation behaviours. The second theme, sacred places as repositories of biodiversity, highlights how spiritual values and taboos associated with specific natural sites can help to preserve biodiversity. The third theme considers the spiritual domain within ecosystems services through an examination of the measurement of spiritual well-being as a cultural ecosystem service. For the final theme, the effects of biodiversity on spiritual well-being, the authors found few empirical research studies that specifically investigated how biodiversity and biodiverse settings contribute to spiritual well-being. The authors thus examine the biodiversity–spiritual well-being relationship through an interpretation of several strands of research, for example wilderness recreation, urban green space usage, place attachment, and Attention Restoration Theory. The chapter ends with a detailed conceptual model to inform future research.

20.4 Importance of Biodiversity, Health and Climate Change Relationships for Professionals, Practitioners and Policy-Makers

Evidence of the health effects of biodiverse natural environments has implications for both policy and practice. This part of the book deals with the implications of the inter-relationships of biodiversity and health in the face of climate change for professionals and managers concerned with public health, nature conservation and pro-environmental behaviour, as well as how these inter-relationships are being supported by policy. Good practice examples using nature and biodiversity for human health and climate change adaptation in European countries are highlighted.

Penny Cook and co-authors discuss the implications and inter-relationships between public health, climate change and biodiversity, with specific consideration for disadvantaged groups and health inequalities. The authors provide a comprehensive overview of the numerous connections between public health and biodiversity in the face of climate change, such as: food, nutrition and water supply; environmental stress; aesthetic appreciation and spiritual well-being; socio-cultural well-being; physical and mental health; promotion of physical activity; and infectious diseases. From these interconnections, the authors consider the reasons why public health professionals should care about biodiversity loss and climate change, and support nature conservation and climate change legislation. At a local level, public health professionals could better link with local policies and practitioners to encourage greater access to and use of biodiverse urban green spaces through 'nature-based activities' like walking groups and gardening. The authors demonstrate how access to and use of natural environments can reduce social inequalities in health, a key goal of modern public health policies and programmes. However, individuals from socio-economically deprived areas are often less likely to be exposed to, and experience the benefits of, green spaces. As such, the authors highlight 'nature-based social prescriptions' as a public health intervention to facilitate contact with biodiverse natural environments for those who are less well-off in society. Specific recommendations by the authors that help implement biodiversity and climate change impacts into public health practice include linking nature conservation, public health and climate change priorities in existing local, national and international policies. In addition, working with planners and managers to ensure that green spaces are evenly distributed in urban areas is needed to avoid social inequalities in health, and robust evaluations of 'nature-based' interventions are vital in order to demonstrate causality.

Zoe Davies and co-authors discuss the impact that different nature conservation management options can have for both biodiversity and human health. The first management option, managing green spaces for people, involves no or little explicit consideration of the biodiversity quality of those spaces. These green spaces are typically in cities and designed for people rather than nature, which often results in small, isolated islands of green space that contain paved paths, recreation equipment, easy-to-maintain plants, and frequent pruning and mowing. The second management option, green spaces managed for biodiversity, involves explicit consideration of biodiversity conservation. These spaces tend to be protected areas that can be geographically distant from cities. Recreational activities of humans in protected areas are mainly managed to protect biodiversity. The authors highlight that the third management option, nature for people and nature, is rare, and discuss opportunities to manage green spaces in cities for both biodiversity and human health. For example, nature conservation professionals could work with city planners and landscape architects to add biodiversity into urban green spaces. Recommendations for managing nature for people and biodiversity from the authors include: maximizing the size of urban green spaces to sustain more species and contribute to greater health outcomes; maximizing the health benefits of nature by creating smaller urban green spaces that can be accessed and used by people; and a more international scope to understand how biodiversity and health relationships differ by cultural context.

As the consequences of climate change and biodiversity loss will require humans to change their behaviour to consume far fewer resources, *Raymond De Young* discusses how to initiate long-term behaviour change. This new behavioural context – characterised by the necessity for fundamental change across multiple behaviours and a lack of clarity about what future behaviours will be needed – requires a different approach to behaviour change. The author argues for a 'capacities-first approach' to support future citizens to become 'behavioural entrepreneurs' who can identify, execute and maintain the needed behaviours themselves. Supporting behavioural entrepreneurs requires ensuring they have mental clear-headedness in order to identify, plan, self-initiate and regulate behaviour. As mental clear-headedness is a limited cognitive resource, behavioural entrepreneurs will need to spend time in nature to help restore their depleted cognitive resources and cope with the stress of living in their new world.

To embed health agendas in conservation management and vice versa, national and global policy agendas need to be aligned across the biodiversity, health and climate sectors. *Horst Korn and co-authors* detail these first steps and highlight the developments in the Convention on Biological Diversity (CBD) and the collaboration of CBD with the WHO on the issue of health and biodiversity. In parallel, the 2020 Health Policy Framework of the WHO European region considers environmental conditions; such considerations need to be strengthened to include specific biodiversity linkages in the next review. The UN 2030 Agenda on Sustainable Development already links various Sustainable Development Goals (SDGs) relating to health, biodiversity and climate change, and it will now depend on regional, national and local implementation to achieve its ambitious goals.

As attention on the importance of nature and health linkages increases, *Hans Keune and co-authors* argue that there is a need to build bridges between the nature conservation and public health sectors. Giving case-study examples of nature and health network initiatives from several European countries, the authors demonstrate how professionals from science, policy and practice can work together to address both nature and health goals. To facilitate future linkages between these sectors, the authors recommend strengthening inter-network collaboration through capacity building and integration. They additionally emphasize the need for structural support to encourage capacity-building activities. The authors stress the importance of linking existing priorities in local, national and international policies to mainstream the importance of natural environments for human health; in this regard, the One Health approach may be one way to mainstream biodiversity and health issues.

20.5 Implications for Planning and Managing Urban Green Spaces for Biodiversity and Health in a Changing Climate

The inter-relationships between biodiversity, human health and climate change have implications for both urban planning and management. This fourth part of the book deals with the implications of the inter-relationships of biodiversity and health in the face of climate change for protected area managers, city authorities, urban planners and landscape architects. Evaluations of urban green space interventions to improve human health and the environment and weaken the impact of climate change are also presented.

Kathy MacKinnon and colleagues review the ecosystem services that protected areas and NBS provide for biodiversity conservation, human health and climate change adaptation. Examining different case studies across the world, the authors illustrate how protected areas can become 'health hubs' by facilitating physical activity and stress reduction through health walks and other organized activities. As such, protected areas provide an opportunity for people to get away and experience nature and wilderness. The economic value of protected areas in cost-savings for human health, as well as climate change adaptation is examined. In order to foster the use of protected areas and NBS for both biodiversity conservation and human health, the authors recommend increased and improved collaboration between sectors and stakeholders, and propose the UN 2030 Agenda for Sustainable Development and its 20 SDGs as a mechanism for collaborative action.

Ruth Hunter and co-authors examine the environmental and human health and equity benefits of urban green space interventions. In a review of the evidence, the authors find strong support for park-based and greenway or trail interventions for encouraging physical activity and park use – but only if those interventions involved both physical changes and promotion and marketing events. There was also strong evidence that greening of vacant lots in order to improve human health and well-being also led to a reduction in crime. Strong evidence was also found for the environmental benefits from urban greening and roof gardens – specifically, increased biodiversity, reduced air pollution, climate change adaptation and storm water management. The authors found a lack of evidence for the impact of urban green space interventions on equity indicators. Specific recommendations for future urban green space interventions for research, policy and practice are made, such as the importance of robust evaluation research designs, economic evaluations of green space, involvement of the local community in the design of urban green spaces and using a dual approach consisting of both promotion/marketing and physical design. The authors underscore that few other public health interventions can achieve the multiple health, social and environmental benefits for all population groups that can be achieved with urban green space interventions.

As climate change imposes direct impacts on the grey, green and blue infrastructure in cities, as well as indirect impacts on the health and well-being of urban dwellers, *Thomas Elmqvist and co-authors* propose the concept of systems thinking to foster sustainable urban development and resilience for urban health. As a starting point, the authors argue that health should be an end goal of climate change adaptation and a proxy to examine the level of resilience of cities. The authors point out that cities are complex systems because agents from different social, ecological and technological networks connect and interact with one another at multiple scales. This complexity of different actors and networks poses enormous challenges for urban sustainability. As such, considering cities from a systems perspective – in which all actors involved in the production, sharing and use of knowledge for action are connected in a social network – can be helpful for resilience management. The authors maintain that such a systems perspective can lead to innovative designs of new urban infrastructure and the redesign of existing structures, such as the use of NBS to create resilience to climate change in cities in order to reduce negative health impacts and well-being.

Reflecting on the policy opportunities and challenges for considering human health in landscape planning projects, *Stefan Heiland and co-authors* highlight the need for increased and improved collaboration between landscape architecture, urban planning and the health sector. Examining landscape planning instruments in both Germany and the UK, the authors show how human health and biodiversity are currently considered in the design of urban green spaces through green infrastructure and ecosystem services, recreation planning, and climate change legislation. The authors conclude that health issues are implicitly touched upon or, in rare cases, explicitly named in landscape planning legislation in the UK and Germany. Consequently, the authors argue, opportunities for including health issues into landscape planning are not frequently used, and suggest this could be because health authorities are seldom involved in planning decisions. They strongly argue that including environmental interventions for health in pro-active planning may reduce other hidden costs for a range of sectors, while greenspace and conservation planning cannot really go without health considerations anymore. The authors recommend legislation to overcome these disciplinary silos by requiring public health professionals to participate in urban landscape planning decisions.

20.6 Recommendations for Research, Policy and Practice

A number of important conclusions can be drawn from the chapters presented in this book. In this next section we identify 30 specific recommendations for research, policy and practice. These suggestions arise from those presented by the authors of this book, and incorporate recommendations debated by the European Network of Heads of Nature Conservation Agencies (ENCA) interest group on climate change at the European conference on 'Biodiversity and Health in the Face of Climate Change' held on 27–29 June 2017 in Bonn, Germany (Marselle et al. 2018).

20.6.1 Recommendations and Challenges to Integrate Biodiversity, Health and Climate Change in Research

Whilst there is increasing research activity to assess the linkages between biodiversity and health (Lindley et al. Chap. 2, Marselle et al. Chap. 9, Irvine et al. Chap. 10, Cook et al. Chap. 11, this volume), the chapters in this book highlight the need to expand the evidence base for the contributions of biodiversity to human health and well-being. In order to further this transdisciplinary field of biodiversity and health as an effective instrument for climate change adaptation, we identify key research challenges to integration:

1. *Investigating biodiversity-health linkages in a changing climate*: Future research should consider the potential positive and negative effects of biodiversity on human health and well-being in a changing climate. How biodiversity can help to adapt to climate pressures, e.g. through greenspace planning in urban areas or restoration of climate resilient wetlands, but also how vector-borne diseases and allergenic plants may shift in distribution with climate change, in order to identify appropriate management measures to foster positive and reduce negative health impacts.
2. *Broadening research to assess the effects of biodiversity on physical, mental, spiritual and social health and well-being*: Whilst there is considerable evidence of the physical health effects of biodiversity through shelter, food and medicines, there is, to date, limited evidence of the influence that biodiversity has on mental, spiritual and social well-being. This is especially relevant given that these latter health effects drove forward early conservation policy and link to intrinsic values of nature. Research should identify the influence of biodiversity on these under-investigated health and well-being outcomes.
3. *Further developing theory for biodiversity-health effects*: Evaluations of the impact of biodiversity on human health, or the effectiveness of nature-based interventions, require a solid theoretical basis to guide selection of health and well-being outcomes and identify causal mediators. Tending to such conceptual considerations is a necessary component for further research and integration across disciplines and sectors.
4. *Identifying mechanisms*: Different models have been developed to understand the various mediating pathways through which green spaces influence human health and well-being. Future research should investigate the specific mechanistic pathways through which biodiversity benefits health and well-being, for example ecosystem services, psychological restoration and perceived biodiversity. These mechanisms should be assessed through synthesis and meta-analysis of the existing literature in addition to well-designed empirical research.
5. *Identifying moderators*: Health effects may not be equally distributed in society and certain groups of people may experience greater health benefits from exposure to, or use of, green space and biodiverse environments. The impact of biodiversity on the health and well-being of specific socio-demographic (e.g. age and gender) and socio-economic (e.g. most disadvantaged) groups needs further scientific attention.
6. *Considering 'dose-response' relationships*: At present, there is a lack of knowledge on the quality and intensity of biodiversity that is required for an effect

(how much?), the length of exposure needed before effects take place (how long?), or the duration of lasting effects for mental health and well-being. As such, future research should usefully investigate the effects of species richness, diversity and distinctiveness, the quantity of time spent in biodiverse environments, and/or the frequency of visiting a biodiverse environment that might be required for a significant change in mental health or well-being.

7. *Evaluating effectiveness of interventions*: Nature-based interventions need to be evaluated for their effectiveness for health and well-being, biodiversity conservation and climate change adaptation. Socio-economic factors should also be included to ensure evaluations consider potential disproportional effects across different beneficiaries. Proof of causality is important to establish when assessing the effectiveness of an intervention. Whilst randomised controlled trials may not be feasible or appropriate, nature-based interventions are complex interventions and researchers should use more robust research designs such as natural experiments, quasi-experimental before-and-after repeated-measures designs, or longitudinal studies (e.g. gain/loss in biodiversity or access to green space). Complex analyses such as stepped wedge, interrupted time series or structural equation modelling analyses warrant more scientific attention.
8. *Analysing cost-benefits*: Economic evaluations of biodiversity and interventions for human health are a significant driver for decision makers. As such, cost-benefit evaluations of the anticipated reduction in health-care costs of biodiverse green spaces are recommended. Overall, the cost-benefit analyses should be holistic, addressing all multiple benefits provided, with the specific cost reduction potential to health-care seen as just one aspect.
9. *Developing models and scenarios*: Scenarios and models need to be developed to investigate and forecast the human health and well-being effects of current biodiversity loss and reduced access to natural environments in a changing climate.
10. *Integrating better across disciplines*: By its nature, the questions considered within the field of biodiversity and health in the face of climate change are transdisciplinary and thus require integration of the natural, social and health sciences. Research should therefore be transdisciplinary in order to fully understand and measure biodiversity as well as human health impacts.
11. *Increasing international scope*: Current literature is geographically biased. Whilst many findings will be applicable across the Global North, we acknowledge that cultural settings matter for the appreciation of green space and more research also needs to include the Global South. As such, there is a research need to broaden understanding to include different conditions around the globe, as biodiversity-health relationships will be influenced by climate, cultural contexts and social norms.

20.6.2 Recommendations to Foster Wider Application of Nature-Based Solutions for Health Promotion and Climate Change Adaptation in Policy

The chapters in this volume provide challenges and recommendations for policy. These recommendations concern two main challenge areas in increasing awareness and advancing integration across sectors and policies:

20.6.2.1 Increasing Awareness recommendations of the Human Health and Well-Being Effects of Natural Environments and Biodiversity

12. *Raising awareness of multiple co-benefits*: Nature-based solutions for climate change adaptation provide multiple co-benefits for human health and biodiversity. Yet policy-advisors, politicians and the public may not always be aware of these interconnections. It is thus important not only to highlight the interlinkages between climate change, human health and biodiversity but also to understand current levels of and gaps in knowledge among practitioners and policy-makers. There is an additional need to identify the type of information that would be useful to help these individuals implement actions that are based on evidence from biodiversity and health research.
13. *Enhancing communication and dissemination*: In order to raise awareness, communication of the health benefits of nature and biodiversity needs to be tailored to the interests of different stakeholders, practitioners and policy-makers. Social media with strategic messages, brief video clips on Twitter, YouTube and other platforms as well as TV and radio are good ways to communicate and disseminate simple messages about the health benefits of biodiversity. Working with environmental charities can help disseminate these messages to larger audiences.
14. *Developing manuals, guidance and tools*: Manuals and guidelines for policy-makers and practitioners need to be developed based on scientific evidence and good practice in applied management and policy development. Evidence and experience-based guidelines describing the key features of biodiversity required for increased health and well-being should be developed for park managers, landscape architects, urban planners and designers. Public health professionals require concrete guidance on how to use natural environments for health promotion as a complement to other already established measures. Demonstrating successful interventions or case studies where cross-sector working led to cost-effective and efficient delivery of ecosystem services that provided multiple benefits will foster learning and encourage further uptake. Integrated tools of analysis and metrics from different disciplines, sectors and areas of expertise could help raise awareness and application. Building on and enhancing established decision-making process tools may be useful starting points, for example Environmental Impact Assessment and Health Impact Assessment.

20.6.2.2 Greater Integration recommendations of Biodiversity, Health and Climate Change Issues

15. *Highlighting the mutual, multiple co-benefits*: Improving health and well-being and reducing harm and social inequalities are key policy priorities of governments at all levels of governance. As such, communications with decision-makers should focus on human health and well-being as a *central benefit* of nature-based solutions for climate change adaptation. The *co-benefits* of nature-based solutions for climate change adaptation are nature conservation and enhancement of biodiversity and ecosystem services. Importantly, framing and justifying the need to protect natural environments by highlighting the enormous impact on the health of the human population, as well as delivering additional co-benefits, is more likely to be persuasive to decision-makers than a rationale based solely on conservation.
16. *Building capacity*: Network activities aimed at stimulating dialogue, community building and several other forms of transdisciplinary interaction between experts and stakeholders should be encouraged, as they have been shown to be successful at helping to establish cooperative working for the enhancement of biodiversity, health promotion and climate change adaptation.
17. *Providing structural support*: An important condition for successful networking initiatives is the availability of structural resources including supporting infrastructure. Structural support – such as financial support for cooperative networks with leadership and the support of network members and experts – is essential for cross-sectoral and cross-disciplinary working.
18. *Supporting international and national policy development*: To successfully introduce biodiversity and health linkages at a strategic international level, it is important to consider biodiversity, health and climate change relationships in post-2020 CBD decision-making, the implementation of the 2030 Sustainable Development Agenda, and further development of the Health 2020 policy framework of the WHO European Region. Future national, regional and global ecosystem service assessments, for example the strategic framework of a rolling work programme of the Intergovernmental Science-Policy Platform on Biodiversity and Ecosystem Services (IPBES) up to 2030 or future activities of the Mapping and Assessment of Ecosystem Services (MAES) programme, should give special attention to the health values of biodiversity and to tackling the interlinked challenges and fostering action.
19. *Adopting a One Health approach to integrate biodiversity and health issues*: One Health is an integrative approach, advocated by the WHO and the CBD, to address biodiversity and human health by investigating the interconnection between humans, animals, plants, agriculture, wildlife and the environment in general. The One Health approach aims to design and implement programmes, policies, legislation and research in which multiple sectors communicate and work together to achieve better public health outcomes. Policy approaches need to adopt a One Health approach, to facilitate the interlinkages of biodiversity and health in the face of climate change.

20. *Linking priorities in existing local, national and international policies*: Existing policies, strategies and guidelines may, individually, address the issues of public health promotion, climate change adaptation and nature conservation. For example, health is often implicitly named in landscape and urban planning legislation when discussing climate change adaptation actions, and this provides an opportunity for linking climate change, human health and natural environment issues. Linking these existing documents and policy goals fosters a win-win, low-cost scenario in which the multiple co-benefits for human health and biodiversity conservation can be achieved. Public health leaders should work with governments, planners and ecologists to ensure that health considerations are incorporated into national and local planning and development regulations as well as environment and sustainability strategies and action plans.
21. *Linking to United Nations Sustainable Development Goal (SDG) indicators*: The 2030 Agenda for Sustainable Development and its 20 SDGs present a framework for collaborative action to respond to a range of global challenges that cannot be solved in isolation. SDGs relating to biodiversity and health in the face of climate change are SDG 3 'good health and well-being', SDG 11 'sustainable cities and communities', SDG 13 'climate action', SDG 14 'life below water' and SDG 15 'life on land'. To achieve the multiple aims of the SDGs, it will be important to work across sectors to protect, manage and restore the biodiversity and ecosystem services that contribute to human well-being, and reduce the impacts of climate change. SDGs provide a focus on a specific challenge to monitor progress, success and sustainability. They can also guide regional, national and local policies and practices.
22. *Fostering continued dedication to climate change agreements*: In order to combat the impact that climate change will have on human health and biodiversity, it is important to ensure continued commitment to existing international policy accords. As such, it is paramount that nations adhere to the climate change mitigation policies under the 2015 Paris Agreement. Linking these climate change-focused policies to the health agenda will help to create alliances and innovative implementation and funding schemes.

20.6.3 Recommendations to Implement Existing Knowledge into Practice

We know enough to act now. The chapters in this volume provide good practice case studies that demonstrate how research informs implementation of nature-based solutions to foster human health in the face of climate change. We identify two key challenges with regards to design and planning as well as management for integrating biodiversity and health issues when addressing climate change adaptation in practice:

20.6.3.1 Design and Planning recommendations to Enhance Contact with and Experience of Nature and Biodiversity

23. *Designing in biodiversity*: Landscape architects should be encouraged to 'design in biodiversity' by fostering native plants and wildlife in public parks or conservation areas as well as in the urban matrix. This increases the opportunities for people to interact with biodiversity and obtain its health benefits, whilst enhancing biodiversity conservation and also contributing to climate change adaptation.
24. *Creating a mixture of 'everyday' green spaces*: It is important for people to have contact with natural environments in their daily life (e.g. on their way to school or work, around the home). Various urban green spaces (ranging from street trees, 'pocket parks' and green school yards to larger urban parks) should be created to increase the opportunities for people to be exposed to biodiversity for their own health and well-being. To use green spaces for health promotion, city planners should create publicly accessible green spaces that are evenly distributed across the spatial extent of towns and cities; this may be mandated in urban planning guidelines. In addition, urban green spaces can contribute significantly to adaptation to climate change.
25. *Creating 'green' corridor connections*: Cities should be planned to include 'green corridors' through which citizens can travel from smaller urban green spaces to larger green spaces or protected areas. These 'green corridors' create additional opportunities for recreation and restoration, which have health, well-being and social benefits. Further, 'green corridors' can contribute to biodiversity conservation by increasing the amount of green space and providing links between different habitats for migration and sustaining metapopulations of species. In addition, green corridors can serve as important avenues for fresh air.
26. *Promoting and managing protected areas as 'health hubs'*: Protected areas provide opportunities for nature conservation as well as human health benefits. Thus, protected areas have the potential to be 'health hubs' for both nature and people. To encourage use, social interventions, such as guided health walks, can be used to highlight the value that a protected area delivers for human health and well-being. Such positive nature experiences can deepen people's commitment to conserve natural spaces and support protected areas. Dedicated management is needed in order to offer *natural* health services to humans in protected areas whilst protecting biodiversity.
27. *Co-designing with stakeholders*: The needs of the local community and other stakeholders must be taken into consideration in order to build ownership, cooperation and collaboration on biodiversity, health and climate change issues. A co-designed framework plan for biodiversity, health and climate change strategies and management is likely to be the most successful.

20.6.3.2 Management Recommendations to Improve the Use of Urban Green Spaces

28. *Utilising physical interventions*: Access to a green space does not necessarily result in its use. Physical design and management can improve the biodiversity quality and aid the use of green spaces. Physical interventions to facilitate use involves considering the needs of different users in the local community as well as long-term health, social and environmental effects. Management plans for green spaces should ensure these spaces are maintained in order to avoid perceptions of neglect, as overgrowth and/or broken benches/play structures/rubbish can increase fear of crime and reduce use.
29. *Employing social interventions*: To further encourage use, promotion and marketing events should be used in combination with physical interventions. It is especially important to target interventions to individuals in socially-deprived neighbourhoods. Practitioners should use nature-based social-prescribing interventions, such as health walks in forests, conservation volunteering or therapeutic gardens, to encourage use of and contact with biodiverse green spaces.
30. *Monitoring impact*: In order to develop evidence of impact and economic value, it is important to implement robust monitoring and evaluation of the effect of nature-based solutions on climate change adaptation, human health and well-being, and biodiversity. This will help to advance both management and policy in the interconnected field of biodiversity, health and climate change.

20.7 Outlook

Facing global challenges, we need concerted action to foster human health and biodiversity, the foundation of life. It is time to act now and to urgently address increasing health issues and to harness NBS to health promotion. In a changing climate the importance for nature-based solutions for human health will increase. In the long run modern combinations of nature-based solutions with technical solutions will be the cheaper alternative in comparison with choosing technical solutions on their own. Nature-based solutions have additional advantages in that they can pose win-win-win solutions for biodiversity, human health and adaptation to climate change, and their management actions are more easily reversible and adaptable.

In international policy, practice and research, the issue of biodiversity and human health, with a link to climate change as a major stressor for both, is high on the agenda. Research is focusing attention on this topic with new transdisciplinary research programmes. Since climate change will exacerbate societal problems with respect to health, policy needs to act now to put scientific evidence into real action. We hope this volume provides a critical overview and evaluation of the interlinkages of climate, health and biodiversity, and will inform and trigger further policy development and practical implementation, as well as stimulate ongoing scientific debate and open innovative research avenues.

Acknowledgements We are grateful to the ENCA interest group on climate change for initial discussions in June 2017. This work was supported by the German Federal Agency for Nature Conservation (BfN) with funds from the German Federal Ministry for the Environment, Nature Conservation, and Nuclear Safety (BMU) through the research project 'Conferences on Climate Change and Biodiversity' (BIOCLIM, project duration from 2014 to 2017, funding code: 3514 80 020A). Dr. Irvine's involvement was funded by the Rural and Environment Science and Analytical Services Division of the Scottish Government.

References

Aerts R, Honnay O, Van Nieuwenhuyse A (2018) Biodiversity and human health: mechanisms and evidence of the positive health effects of diversity in nature and green spaces. Br Med Bull 127(1):5–22

Bellard C, Bertelsmeier C, Leadley P, Thuiller W, Courchamp F (2012) Impacts of climate change on the future of biodiversity. Ecol Lett 15:365–377

Cox DT, Shanahan DF, Hudson HL et al (2017) Doses of neighborhood nature: the benefits for mental health of living with nature. Bioscience 67:147–155

Dallimer M, Irvine KN, Skinner AMJ et al (2012) Biodiversity and the feel-good factor: understand associations between self-reports human well-being and species richness. Bioscience 62(1):47–55

Fuller RA, Irvine KN, Devine-Wright P et al (2007) Psychological benefits of greenspace increase with biodiversity. Biol Lett 3:390–394

Hartig T, Mitchell R, de Vries S, Frumkin H (2014) Nature and health. Annu Rev Public Health 35:207–228

Lovell R, Wheeler BW, Higgins SL et al (2014) A systematic review of the health and wellbeing benefits of biodiverse environments. J Toxicol Environ Health B Crit Rev 17(1):1–20

Markevych I, Schoierer J, Hartig T et al (2017) Exploring pathways linking greenspace to health: theoretical and methodological guidance. Environ Res 158:301–317

Marselle MR, Irvine KN, Warber SL (2014) Examining group walks in nature and multiple aspects of well-being: a large-scale study. Ecopsychology 6:134–147

Marselle M, Stadler J, Korn H, Bonn A (eds) (2018) Proceedings of the European conference "Biodiversity and Health in the Face of Climate Change – Challenges, Opportunities and Evidence Gaps". BfN-Skripten 509. Federal Agency for Nature Conservation, Germany, Bonn. https://www.bfn.de/fileadmin/BfN/service/Dokumente/skripten/Skript509.pdf

Potschin MB, Haines-Young RH (2011) Ecosystem services: exploring a geographical perspective. Prog Phys Geogr 35:575–594

Shanahan DF, Fuller RA, Bush R et al (2015) The health benefits of urban nature: how much do we need? Bioscience 65:476–485

Steffen W, Richardson K, Rockström J et al (2015) Planetary boundaries: guiding human development on a changing planet. Science 347:736–747

van den Bosch M, Ode Sang Å (2017) Urban natural environments as nature-based solutions for improved public health – a systematic review of reviews. Environ Res 158:373–384

WHO (2017a) Fact sheets on sustainable development goals: health targets for noncommunicable diseases. World Health Organization Regional Office for Europe, Copenhagen, Denmark. http://www.euro.who.int/__data/assets/pdf_file/0007/350278/Fact-sheet-SDG-NCD-FINAL-25-10-17.pdf?ua=1. Accessed 30 July 2018

WHO (2017b) Noncommunicable diseases. World Health Organization Regional Office for Europe, Copenhagen, Denmark. http://www.euro.who.int/en/health-topics/noncommunicable-diseases. Accessed 13 July 2018

WHO & CBD (2015) Connecting global priorities: biodiversity and human health. A state of the knowledge review. World Health Organization & Secretariat of the Convention on Biological Diversity. http://www.who.int/globalchange/publications/biodiversity-human-health/en/. Accessed 30 July 2018

Correction to: Biodiversity and Health in the Face of Climate Change

Melissa R. Marselle, Jutta Stadler, Horst Korn,
Katherine N. Irvine, and Aletta Bonn

Correction to:
M. R. Marselle et al. (eds.), *Biodiversity and Health in the Face of Climate Change*, https://doi.org/10.1007/978-3-030-02318-8

This book was inadvertently published with the incorrect copyright holder "Springer Nature Switzerland AG". This has now been amended in the copyright page to the correct copyright holder "The Editor(s) (if applicable) and The Author(s)".

The updated online version of this book can be found at
https://doi.org/10.1007/978-3-030-02318-8

M. R. Marselle et al. (eds.), *Biodiversity and Health in the Face of Climate Change*, https://doi.org/10.1007/978-3-030-02318-8_21

Glossary

Adverse effects of climate change Changes in the physical environment or biota resulting from climate change that have significant deleterious effects on the composition, resilience or productivity of natural and managed ecosystems; on the operation of socio-economic systems; or on human health and welfare (United Nations Framework Convention on Climate Change 1992, p. 7).

Arboviruses Viruses transmitted by arthropods (such as phlebotomine sand flies, mosquitoes or ticks) that cause arboviral diseases, e.g., West Nile fever, Chikungunya fever, tick-borne encephalitis, borreliosis or leishmaniasis (Müller et al. Chap. 4, this volume).

Arthropod-borne diseases Diseases caused by infectious agents (pathogens) such as parasites, viruses or bacteria that are transmitted by an arthropod vector (such as a mosquito, fly or tick) (Müller et al. Chap. 4, this volume).

Biodiversity Biological diversity (biodiversity) is the variability among living organisms from all sources including, inter alia, terrestrial, marine and other aquatic ecosystems and the ecological complexes of which they are part; this includes diversity within species, between species and of ecosystems (United Nations Convention on Biological Diversity 1992, p.3).

Climate change Any change in the state of the climate that can be identified by changes in the mean and/or variability of its properties, and that persists for an extended period, typically decades or longer. Climate change may be due to natural internal processes, or to persistent anthropogenic changes in the composition of the atmosphere or in land use (IPCC 2007, p. 943).

Ecosystem services The direct and indirect contributions of ecosystems to human well-being (TEEB n.d.,a). There are four types of ecosystem services: provisioning, regulating, supporting and cultural (TEEB n.d.,b).

Green infrastructure A strategically planned network of high-quality natural and semi-natural areas with other environmental features, which is designed and managed to deliver a wide range of ecosystem services and protect biodiversity in both rural and urban settings (European Commission 2013, p.7).

M. R. Marselle et al. (eds.), *Biodiversity and Health in the Face of Climate Change*, https://doi.org/10.1007/978-3-030-02318-8

Health A state of complete physical, mental and social well-being and not merely the absence of disease or infirmity (World Health Organization 1948, p.1).

Introduced species Species that have been intentionally or unintentionally introduced outside their native distribution range. The introduction can be human-mediated (Müller et al. Chap. 4, this volume).

Invasive species Introduced species that affect the abiotic or biotic environment, the economy or human health in their exotic range (Müller et al. Chap. 4, this volume).

Integrated vector management Management approach aiming at the optimal use of available vector control tools in terms of efficacy, cost-effectiveness, ecological soundness and sustainability (Müller et al. Chap. 4, this volume).

Mental health A state of well-being in which an individual realizes his or her own abilities, can cope with the normal stresses of life, can work productively and is able to make a contribution to his or her community (World Health Organization 2016).

Mental well-being The psychological, cognitive and emotional quality of a person's life. This includes the thoughts and feelings that individuals have about the state of their life, and a person's experience of happiness (Linton et al. 2016, p.12).

Nature-based climate change adaptation Nature-based actions that preserve ecosystem services, which are necessary for human life in the face of climate change and reduce the impact of anticipated negative effects of climate change (e.g. more intense rainfall, more frequent floods, as well as heat waves and droughts) (Naumann et al. 2014).

Physical health The body's ability to function. It has many components, such as exercise, nutrition, sleep, weight management and intake of alcohol and drugs (Owen 2013).

Physical well-being The quality and performance of bodily functioning. This includes having the energy to live well, the capacity to sense the external environment, and our experiences of pain and comfort (Linton et al. 2016, p.12).

(Re-) emerging infectious diseases Newly emerged or associated pathogens that have gained renewed virulence due to other emerging or chronic diseases or the spread of antibiotic, antiviral and antifungal medication resistance (Müller et al. Chap. 4, this volume).

Reservoir host A human or animal that is infected by the pathogen and does not experience disease. From the reservoir host, the maintained pathogen is transmitted to the definite host population (Müller et al. Chap. 4, this volume).

Social well-being How well an individual is connected to others in their local and wider social community. This includes social interactions, the depth of key relationships and the availability of social support (Linton et al. 2016, p.12).

Spiritual well-being A connection to something greater than oneself, and in some cases faith in a higher power (Linton et al. 2016, p.12).

Species richness The number of different species (Marselle et al. Chap. 9; Cook et al. Chap. 11, this volume).

Urban green space Urban space covered by vegetation of any kind, including smaller green space features (such as street trees and roadside vegetation), green spaces not available for public access or recreational use (such as green roofs and facades, or green space on private grounds) and larger green spaces that provide various social and recreational functions (such as parks, playgrounds or greenways) (Hunter et al. Chap. 18, this volume).

Urban heat island Phenomenon in which cities and towns are much warmer than surrounding rural areas, particularly at night. It is primarily generated as a result of the physical properties of urban materials, their structure and – to a lesser extent – their use, e.g. through anthropogenic heat emissions (Lindley et al. Chap. 2, this volume).

Vectors Organisms that transport a pathogen from an infected host to an uninfected individual. The infectious agent may or may not pass through a developmental cycle within the vector. Climate change supposedly does not alter mechanical transmission but has a profound impact on biological vector competence and capacity (Müller et al. Chap. 4, this volume).

Vector-borne diseases Diseases caused by parasites, viruses or bacteria that are transmitted by a vector such as arthropods (Müller et al. Chap. 4, this volume).

Vector competence The ability of an animal to transmit a pathogen; this animal thus serves as a disease vector (Müller et al. Chap. 4, this volume).

Zoonosis An infectious disease in an animal that can be transmitted to humans (Müller et al. Chap. 4, this volume).

References

European Commission (2013) Building a green infrastructure for Europe. Luxembourg. https://doi.org/10.2779/54125

IPCC (2007) Climate change 2007: The physical science basis. In: Solomon S, Qin D, Manning M et al (eds) Contribution of working group I to the fourth assessment report of the intergovernmental panel on climate change. Cambridge University Press, Cambridge. http://www.ipcc.ch/publications_and_data/ar4/wg1/en/contents.html

Linton M, Dieppe P, Medina-Lara A (2016) Review of 99 self-report measures for assessing well-being in adults: exploring dimensions of well-being and developments over time. BMJ Open 6(7). https://doi.org/10.1136/bmjopen-2015-010641

Naumann S, Kaphengst T, McFarland K, Stadler J (2014) Nature-based approaches for climate change mitigation and adaptation. Federal Agency for Nature Conservation (BfN), Bonn

Owen S (2013) Health Triangle. http://www2.gsu.edu/~wwwche/. Accessed 12 July 2018

TEEB (n.d.-a) Glossary of terms. http://www.teebweb.org/resources/glossary-of-terms/. Accessed 12 July 2018

TEEB. (n.d.-b) Ecosystem services. http://www.teebweb.org/resources/ecosystem-services/. Accessed 12 July 2018

United Nations Convention on Biological Diversity (1992) Convention on biological diversity. https://www.cbd.int/doc/legal/cbd-en.pdf. Accessed 12 July 2018

United Nations Framework Convention on Climate Change (1992) United nations framework convention on climate change https://unfccc.int/files/essential_background/background_publications_htmlpdf/application/pdf/conveng.pdf. Accessed 2 Aug 2018

World Health Organization (1948) Constitution of WHO. http://apps.who.int/gb/bd/PDF/bd47/EN/constitution-en.pdf?ua=1. Accessed 2 Aug 2018

World Health Organization (2016) Mental health: strengthening our response. Fact Sheet. Available via http://www.who.int/mediacentre/factsheets/fs220/en/. Accessed 17 May 2018

Index

M. R. Marselle et al. (eds.), *Biodiversity and Health in the Face of Climate Change*, https://doi.org/10.1007/978-3-030-02318-8